Lasers in Aesthetic Surgery

Lasers in Aesthetic Surgery

Edited by

Gregory S. Keller, M.D.
Assistant Clinical Professor of Surgery
University of California Los Angeles
Los Angeles, California
Private Practice
Santa Barbara, California

Victor G. Lacombe, M.D.
Clinical Instructor of Facial Plastic Surgery
Division of Head and Neck Surgery
University of California Los Angeles
Los Angeles, California
Private Practice
Santa Rosa, California

Patrick K. Lee, M.D.
Assistant Clinical Professor
Departments of Medicine and Dermatology
University of California Los Angeles
Los Angeles, California

James P. Watson, M.D.
Assistant Professor of Plastic Surgery
Department of Surgery
University of California Los Angeles
Los Angeles, California

Associate Editor:
Kenneth M. Toft, M.D.
Clinical Instructor of Facial Plastic Surgery
Division of Head and Neck Surgery
University of California Los Angeles
Los Angeles, California
Private Practice
Carmichael, California

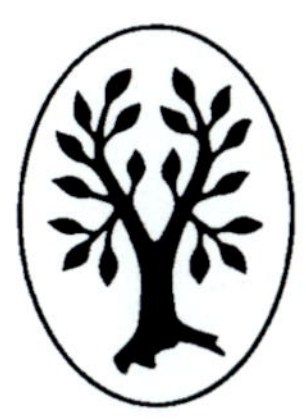

2001
Thieme
New York • Stuttgart

Thieme New York
333 Seventh Avenue
New York, NY 10001

Lasers in Aesthetic Surgery
Gregory S. Keller, M.D.
Victor G. Lacombe, M.D.
Patrick K. Lee, M.D.
James P. Watson, M.D.

Editor: Kathleen Lyons
Assistant Editor: Michelle Schmitt
Director, Production and Manufacturing: Anne Vinnicombe
Senior Production Editor: Eric L. Gladstone
Marketing Director: Phyllis Gold
Sales Manager: Ross Lumpkin
Chief Financial Officer: Peter van Woerden
President: Brian D. Scanlan
Development: Textbook Writers Associates, Inc.
Cover Designer: Michael Mendelsohn
Compositor: Prepare
Printer: Grafiche Fover

Library of Congress Cataloging-in-Publication Data is available from the publisher.

Important note: Medical knowledge is ever-changing. As new research and clinical experience broaden our knowledge, changes in treatment and drug therapy may be required. The authors and editors of the material herein have consulted sources believed to be reliable in their efforts to provide information that is complete and in accord with the standards accepted at the time of publication. However, in view of the possibility of human error by the authors, editors, or publisher of the work herein, or changes in medical knowledge, neither the authors, editors, publisher, nor any other party who has been involved in the preparation of this work, warrants that the information contained herein is in every respect accurate or complete, and they are not responsible for any errors or omissions or for the results obtained from use of such information. Readers are encouraged to confirm the information contained herein with other sources. For example, readers are advised to check the product information sheet included in the package of each drug they plan to administer to be certain that the information contained in this publication is accurate and that changes have not been made in the recommended dose or in the contraindications for administration. This recommendation is of particular importance in connection with new or infrequently used drugs.

Some of the product names, patents, and registered designs referred to in this book are in fact registered trademarks or proprietary names even though specific reference to this fact is not always made in the text. Therefore, the appearance of a name without designation as proprietary is not to be construed as a representation by the publisher that it is in the public domain.

Printed in Italy

5 4 3 2 1

TNY ISBN 0-86577-850-7
GTV ISBN 3-13-116381-X

To my family and the many patients and colleagues who made this book possible.

GSK

Contents

PART I Basic Laser Science

PART II Lasers for Skin Resurfacing and Treatment

PART III   Lasers for the Treatment of Vascular Lesions

PART IV   Laser Hair Removal

PART V   Laser Treatment of Pigmented Lesions and Tattoos

PART VI   Other Laser Treatments

PART VII   Aesthetic Surgical Uses of Lasers

Preface

Laser textbooks are never "up-to-date." The field of laser surgery moves so quickly that it is impossible to stay current. New machines and technologies evolve so quickly that book publishing, with a two-year lead time, cannot keep up with the onslaught.

This book was conceived as a cutting edge comprehensive textbook. To a great extent, we have succeeded. The newer technologies of non-invasive resurfacing are covered. The rapid expansion of laser systems and laser manufacturers, however, surpassed our ability to cover them all and still deliver the text on time to the publisher.

There is, however, a wide range of topics that are presented. Many of these are useful, but have not yet achieved great notoriety. The authors of this text should be commended for presenting "treasures" for those willing to probe more deeply into laser science.

A trend in laser technology is a movement away from the use of lasers for "cutting" surgery. While this is not universal, newer applications of laser science use selective photothermolysis and non-ablative methods to achieve their goals. Hair removal, non-ablative resurfacing, and photofacial technology are examples of the trend toward the selective use of lasers. Photodynamic therapy, perhaps the ultimate expression of the trend toward selective laser usage, may yet emerge as the therapy of the future.

Gregory S. Keller, M.D.

Acknowledgments

The most important group of people to acknowledge is the editorial and production staff of any textbook. The conversion of raw text and slides into a beautiful book is one of the miracles that occur in textbook publishing. Avé McCracken, Kathleen Lyons, Michelle Schmitt, and Eric Gladstone have badgered, cajoled, and worked this book into a respectable tome.

Another group deserving thanks is all of the authors and editors who labored on this textbook, especially Ken Toft and Victor Lacombe, who performed last minute rewrites, and were responsible for an incredible amount of work.

Another group that should be acknowledged is all of the laser scientists who have contributed to my understanding of the effects of this machinery on tissue. Dan Doiron, Ted Maiman, Cliff Morrow, David Harris, Nick Razum, Michael Slatkine, Tom Dougherty and many others have helped me understand the interaction of light with its target issue and how to quantify these reactions.

Finally, my office staff helped to turn this book into a reality, in particular Gretchen Ostergren and Isabel Thompson, who worked on all the details of our laser project.

Gregory S. Keller, M.D.

Contributors

Tina S. Alster, M.D.
Director
Washington Institute of Dermatologic Laser Surgery
Clinical Assistant Professor of Dermatology
Georgetown University School of Medicine
Washington, D.C.

David B. Apfelberg, M.D.
Assistant Clinical Professor
Department of Plastic Surgery
Stanford University Medical Center
Stanford, California
Director
Atherton Plastic Surgery Center
Atherton, California

William H. Beeson, M.D.
Director
Beeson Aesthetic Surgery Institute
Carmel, Indiana
Assistant Clinical Professor
Indiana University School of Medicine
Indianapolis, Indiana

Patrick H. Bitter, Sr., M.D.
Medical Director
Institute for Dermatology and Cosmetic Surgery
Los Gatos, California

Keith E. Blackwell, M.D.
Assistant Professor
Division of Head and Neck Surgery
Department of Surgery
University of California Los Angeles
Los Angeles, California

William K. Boss, Jr., M.D., F.A.C.S.
Vice Chairman
Department of Plastic Surgery
Hackensack University Medical Center
Hackensack, New Jersey

Brian D. Bucalo, M.D.
Private Practice
Boca Raton, Florida

W. Gregory Chernoff, M.D.
Clinical Assistant Professor
Division of Facial Plastic Surgery
Indiana University
Indianapolis, Indiana

Julene E. Cray, B.S.N.
Private Practice
Windsor, California

Thomas J. Dougherty, M.D.
Photodynamic Therapy Center
Roswell Park Cancer Institute
Buffalo, New York

Shimon Eckhouse, Ph.D.
ESC/Sharplan
Tel Aviv, Israel

Michael A. Fiorillo, M.D., F.A.C.S.
Assistant Professor
Department of Plastic Surgery
University of Medicine and Dentistry of New Jersey
Newark, New Jersey

Gregory S. Keller, M.D.
Assistant Clinical Professor of Surgery
University of California Los Angeles
Los Angeles, California
Private Practice
Santa Barbara, California

Maurice M. Khosh, M.D.
Assistant Professor
Department of Otolaryngology—Head and Neck Surgery
Columbia University
New York, New York

R. James Koch, M.D.
Assistant Professor of Surgery
Department of Facial Plastic and Reconstructive Surgery
Division of Otolaryngology—Head and Neck Surgery
Stanford University Medical Center
Stanford, California

Michael Kreindel, Ph.D.
ESC/Sharplan
Tel Aviv, Israel

Victor G. Lacombe, M.D.
Clinical Instructor of Facial Plastic Surgery
Division of Head and Neck Surgery
University of California Los Angeles
Los Angeles, California
Private Practice
Santa Rosa, California

Wayne F. Larrabee, M.D.
Clinical Professor of Otolaryngology
University of Washington
Seattle, Washington

Gary Lask, M.D.
Director
Dermatology Laser Center
Clinical Professor
Department of Dermatology
University of California Los Angeles
Los Angeles, California

Patrick K. Lee, M.D.
Assistant Clinical Professor
Departments of Medicine and Dermatology
University of California Los Angeles
Los Angeles, California

Paul C. Levins, M.D.
Department of Dermatology
Massachusetts General Hospital
Boston, Massachusetts

Timothy Lian, M.D.
Fellow
Department of Otolaryngology—Head and Neck Surgery
Louisiana State University Medical Center
Shreveport, Louisiana

Nicholas J. Lowe, M.D.
Clinical Professor
Department of Dermatology
University of California Los Angeles School of Medicine
Clinical Research Specialists
Santa Monica, California

Phillipa L. Lowe, M.B., Ch.B.
Clinical Research Fellow
Cranley Clinic for Dermatology
London, United Kingdom

Sue E. McCoy, M.B.B.S.
Laser Skin and Vein Clinic
North Adelaide, Australia

Clifford E. Morrow, B.S.S.E.
Morrow Photonics
North Kingstown, Rhode Island

Ronald L. Moy, M.D.
Assistant Clinical Professor
Department of Dermatology
University of California Los Angeles
Los Angeles, California

Christopher A. Nanni, M.D.
Washington Institute of Dermatologic Laser Surgery
Washington, D.C.

Geoffery Paul Nase, Ph.D.
Department of Physiology and Biophysics
Indiana University School of Medicine
Indianapolis, Indiana

Allen J. Oseroff, M.D.
Photodynamic Therapy Center
Roswell Park Cancer Institute
Buffalo, New York

Louie L. Patseavouras, M.D.
Private Practice
Greensboro, North Carolina

Nicholas J. Razum
Head, Education and Training
Miravant Medical Technologies
Santa Barbara, California

William Russell Ries, M.D., F.A.C.S.
Director
Division of Facial Plastic Surgery
Associate Professor
Department of Otolaryngology
Vanderbilt University Medical Center
Nashville, Tennessee

David Sawyer, M.S., M.B., Ch.B.
Past Clinical Research Fellow
Clinical Research Specialists
Santa Monica, California

Michael Slatkine, Ph.D.
ESC/Sharplan
Tel Aviv, Israel

Bruce Smoller, M.D.
Department of Pathology
University of Arkansas
Little Rock, Arkansas

Fred J. Stucker, M.D., F.A.C.S.
Professor and Chairman
Department of Otolaryngology—Head and Neck Surgery
Louisiana State University Medical Center
Shreveport, Louisiana

Emil A. Tanghetti, M.D.
Clinical Professor
Department of Dermatology
University of California Davis
Sacramento, California

Isabel M.Thompson, PA-C
Certified Physician Assistant
Laser Specialist
Gregory S. Keller Facial Plastic Surgery and Laser Center
Santa Barbara, California

Kenneth M. Toft, M.D.
Clinical Instructor of Facial Plastic Surgery
Division of Head and Neck Surgery
University of California Los Angeles
Los Angeles, California
Private Practice
Carmichael, California

Hakan Usal, M.D.
Clinical Instructor
Department of Plastic Surgery
University of Medicine and Dentistry of New Jersey
Newark, New Jersey

Amir Waldman, Ph.D.
ESC/Sharplan
Tel Aviv, Israel

Milton Waner, M.D.
Director
The University Hospital Laser Center
Associate Professor
Department of Otolaryngology—Head and Neck Surgery
University of Arkansas for Medical Sciences
Little Rock, Arkansas

James P. Watson, M.D.
Assistant Professor of Plastic Surgery
Department of Surgery
University of California Los Angeles
Los Angeles, California

Margaret A. Weiss, M.D.
Assistant Professor
Department of Dermatology
Johns Hopkins University School of Medicine
Hunt Valley, Maryland

Robert A. Weiss, M.D.
Assistant Professor
Department of Dermatology
Johns Hopkins University School of Medicine
Hunt Valley, Maryland

Brummette Dale Wilson, M.D.
Photodynamic Therapy Center
Roswell Park Cancer Institute
Buffalo, New York

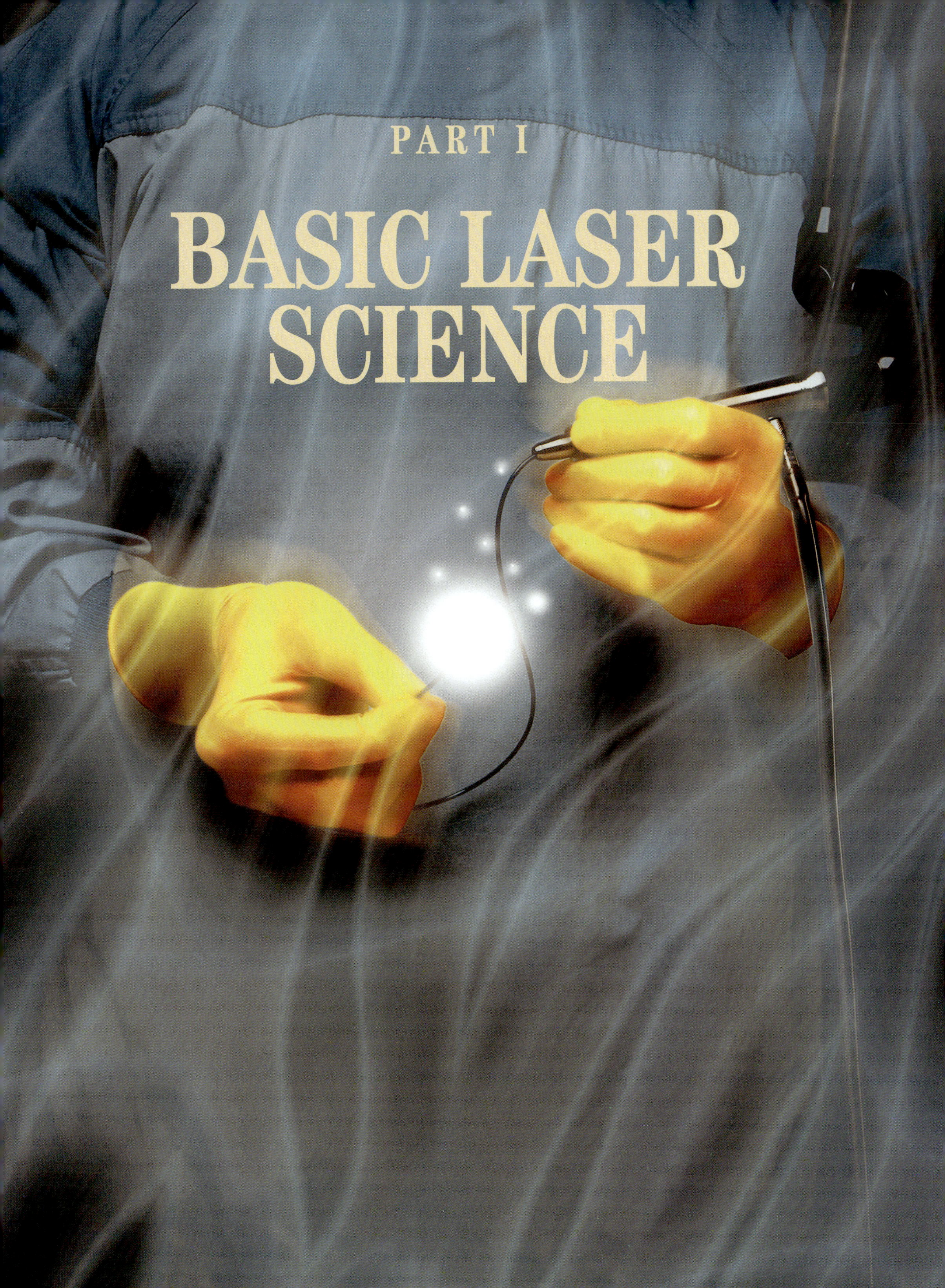
PART I
BASIC LASER
SCIENCE

CHAPTER 1

Laser Physics for Surgical Applications

NICHOLAS J. RAZUM

Einstein theorized about the possibility of lasers early in the twentieth century, but it was not until 1960 that T.H. Maiman demonstrated the first production of laser energy and made lasers a reality. In the 40 years since their invention, lasers have revolutionized many areas of medicine, science, and industry, and each year new applications of lasers are identified.

The basic physics of lasers has not changed since Einstein's hypothesis in 1917. The term *laser* is an acronym for *l*ight *a*mplification by the *s*timulated *e*mission of *r*adiation. The amplification of light that occurs in a laser produces an intense beam, and the radiation emitted is light energy, not harmful ionizing radiation. In this chapter basic information about the light energy produced by lasers, the role of atomic structure in the creation of laser light, the basic setup of a laser, and how certain substances can be stimulated to produce laser beams is presented. How laser light interacts with various living tissues in the body and how that light is delivered to spe-

cific areas of the body are also covered. Finally, the types of lasers employed in medicine and the concept of photodynamic therapy are examined.

LIGHT ENERGY

Lasers emit a beam of light, which is a form of energy that falls within what is called the *electromagnetic spectrum* (Fig. 1–1). Electromagnetic energy consists of an electric wave and a magnetic wave traveling together. Similar to the manner in which ocean waves travel, electromagnetic waves have speed, length, and frequency (or period). Electromagnetic waves travel at the speed of light, that is, 186,000 miles/second. Although this speed is not significant in medicine, it is interesting to note that a slight slowing of laser light occurs in dense materials such as water and tissue. The length of an electromagnetic wave is the distance from one peak to the next (Fig. 1–2). This

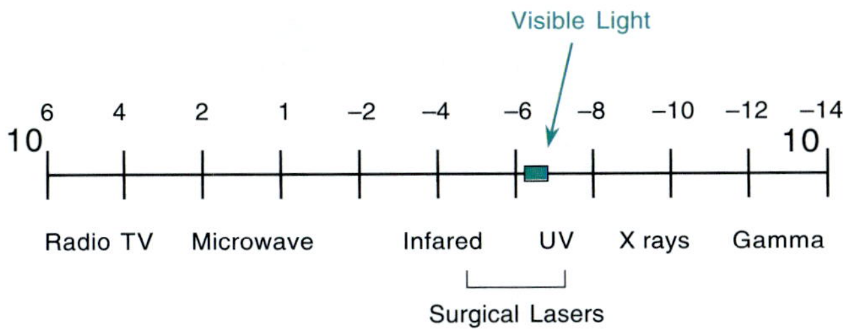

Figure 1–1. Electromagnetic spectrum.

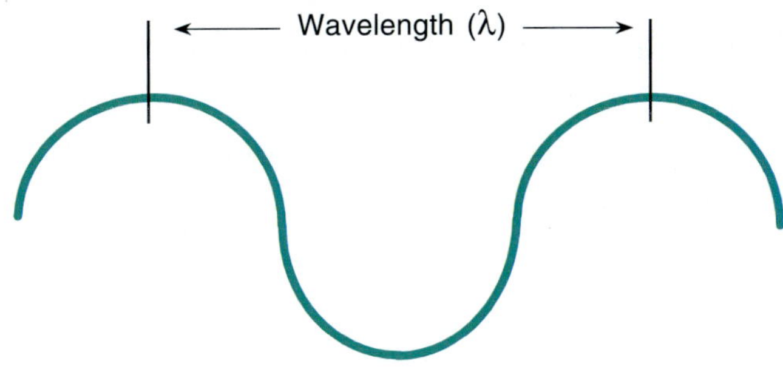

Figure 1–2. Measuring wavelength.

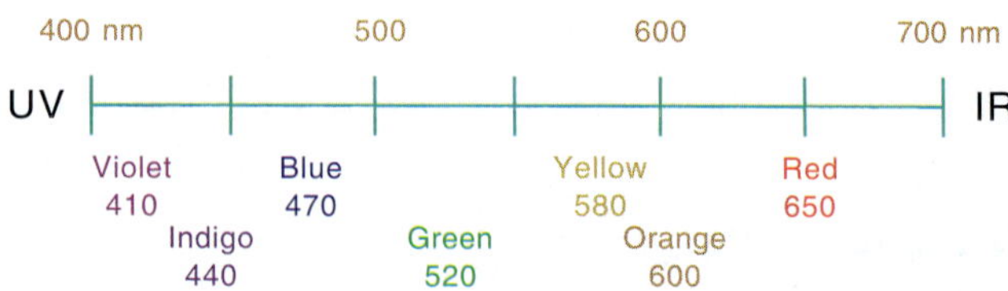

Wavelength (1x10⁻⁹ Meters)
1nm = 1 billionth of a meter

Figure 1–3. Visible light.

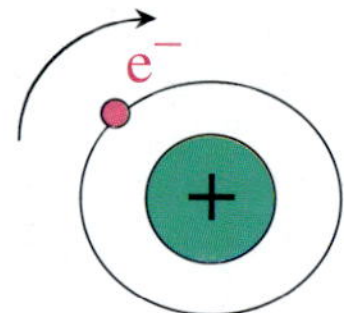

Electrons at their lowest energy
state orbiting the nucleus

Figure 1–4. Atom in ground state.

distance constitutes one *wavelength*, designated by the Greek letter lambda (λ). The frequency, or period, of an electromagnetic wave is the number of oscillations or cycles that occur during a specific period of time. Frequency can be visualized as the number of wave crests that pass a specific point in a known period of time, for example, 1 second. In fact, frequency is measured in *hertz* (Hz), and 1 hertz is equal to one cycle, or period, per second. The frequency of laser light varies with the type of laser, which is discussed in more detail later.

Electromagnetic energy ranges in wavelength from $\frac{1}{2}$ mile (AM radio waves) to 400 billionths of an inch (gamma waves). However, when referring to *visible light*, which is a very small part of the electromagnetic spectrum (see Fig. 1–1), wavelength is synonymous with color. The human eye is sensitive to an extremely narrow range of electromagnetic energy and can detect wavelengths from 400 to 700 nm, that is, violet to red (Fig. 1–3). One nanometer $= 1 \times 10^{-9}$ m, or 1 billionth of a meter. The human eye detects 650 billionths of a meter when looking at something deep red. Surgical lasers operate in the visible spectrum as well as just below it (in the *ultraviolet*, or UV, region) and just above it (in the *infrared*, or IR, region). Each wavelength, or color, has a different effect on tissue.

ATOMIC STRUCTURE

An atom consists of a nucleus and one or more electrons traveling around it in defined orbits (Fig. 1–4). Just as the planets revolve around the sun, electrons revolve at

various distances from their atomic nucleus. When an atom's electron travels in its normal orbit, the atom is said to be in the resting or *ground state*. However, an electron's normal orbit can be changed. An atom can act like a storage battery and absorb energy. When this occurs, the atom uses the absorbed energy to send its electrons into orbits that are farther away from the nucleus. This is called the *excited state* (Fig. 1–5). An atom remains in the excited state, with its electrons in a higher orbit, for only a brief period of time and must give off energy to move an electron closer to the nucleus and back to the ground state. This release of energy is often in the form of a single unit of light, called a *photon*.

Right now in the room around you, atoms are absorbing energy, holding it for a brief moment, and then releasing that stored energy as photons of light. This serendipitous release of photons is called *spontaneous emission*

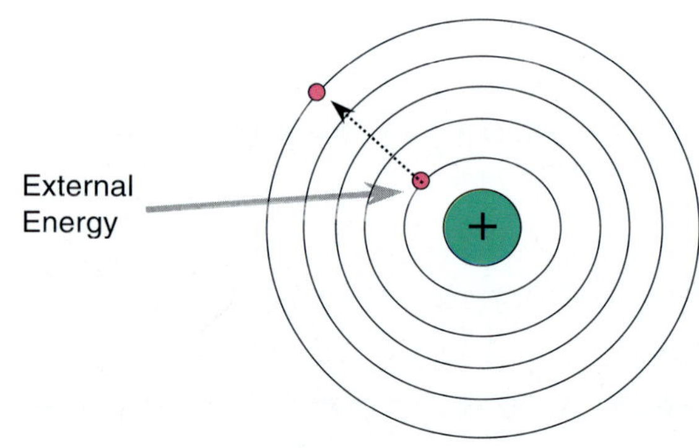

Energy absorbed by electron, moves
to orbit further away from nucleus

Figure 1–5. Excited state.

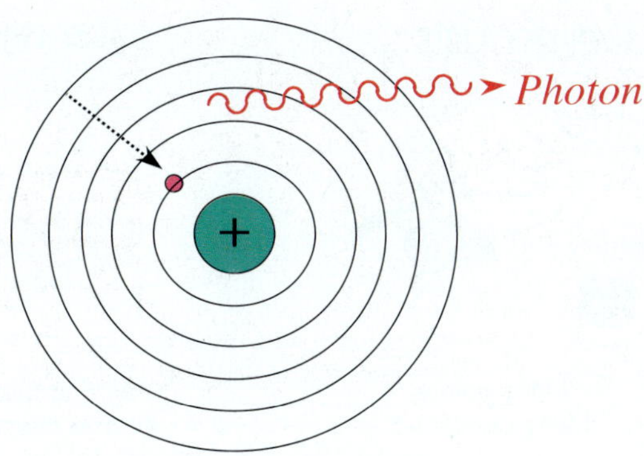

Electron gives off energy
and returns to lower energy state

Figure 1–6. Spontaneous emission.

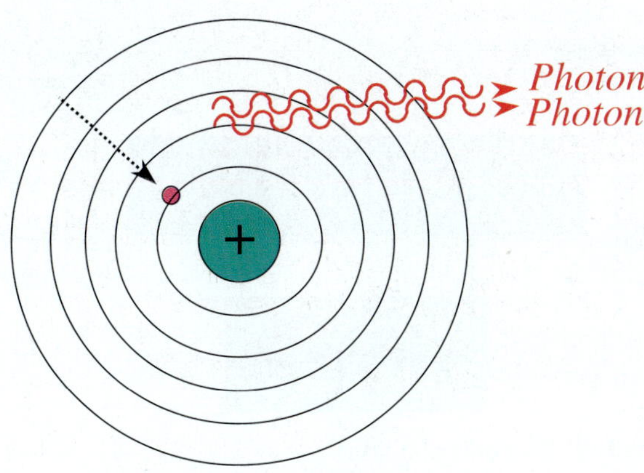

Creates identical photon

Figure 1–7. Stimulated emission.

(Fig. 1–6). You can actually see these spontaneous emissions in a darkened room with the aid of a military night scope or image intensifier that amplifies light 40,000 to 80,000 times.

Certain substances known as *gain mediums*, which we examine more closely later, can achieve *metastable* excited states, which means that some of their electrons can move into an excited state and stay there for a while. When many atoms or molecules of such a substance have been excited to a metastable state by the addition of energy, the result is a *population inversion*. Einstein theorized that in such a condition, you could force, or stimulate, an excited atom into giving off an additional photon. In this *stimulated emission*, an excited electron is struck by a photon that has energy equal to that which caused the electron to jump to the higher energy state (or orbit). When the stimulating photon strikes the excited electron and forces it down, an identical photon is created (Fig. 1–7). The result is two identical photons. These two photons now can go on to stimulate other excited electrons to create four photons, those four can create sixteen, and so on. Within the blink of an eye, billions of identical photons can be created if the excited electrons are available. Establishing a gain medium capable of allowing stimulated emission for many atoms or molecules is the basis for building a laser.

The new photon released when an excited electron is struck by a stimulating photon travels in the exact same path and is said to be in *phase* with the stimulating photon. This means that the peaks and valleys of the two photons' waves are perfectly aligned with one another. The resulting light therefore is coherent and monochromatic, as opposed to light from, for example, an incandescent light bulb, which is incoherent and consists of light of all wavelengths, or colors. Coherence is a fundamental property of lasers that distinguishes laser light from any other form of light energy (Fig. 1–8).

LASER PRINCIPLES

More than one atomic element can be stimulated by a power source to produce laser light. Various elements (e.g., argon) and even certain molecules (e.g., carbon dioxide, or CO_2) can be stimulated to metastable states, and each releases photons of a different wavelength, which, as explained earlier, means that each produces light of a different color.

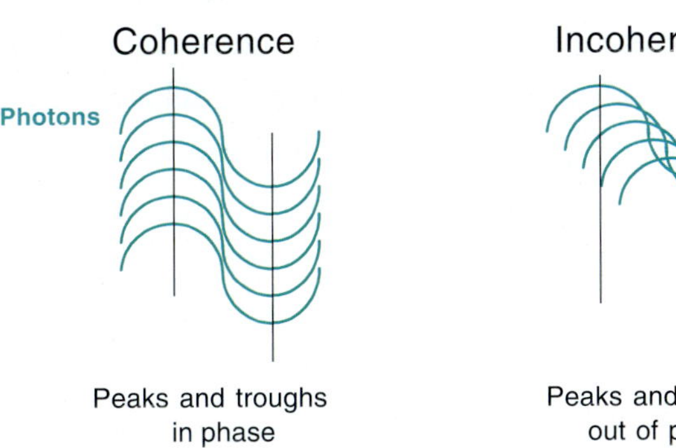

Figure 1–8. Coherence.

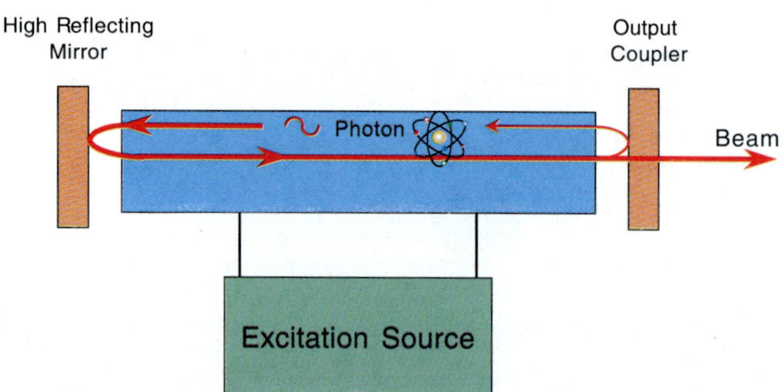

Figure 1–9. Elements of a laser.

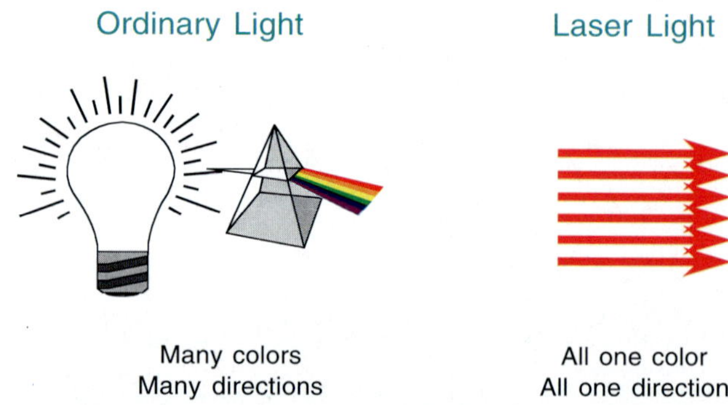

Figure 1–10. Monochromatic/collimated.

Gases, solids, and liquids that can be stimulated are called the *lasing medium*. The medium typically is placed in an optical cavity between two mirrors that are configured to bounce the stimulated photons back and forth. The result of many stimulated emissions and reflections is a narrow, intense beam of laser light that is allowed to escape the optical cavity (Fig. 1–9).

In order for lasing to occur, there must be a greater number of electrons in the excited state than in the ground state. As mentioned earlier, this inverted population is created by infusing the lasing medium with electrical or light energy from an *excitation source*. Gases are easy to excite with electrical energy. A common example is the fluorescent light bulb. Crystals or other solids can be excited, or pumped, with light energy from a flashlamp similar to a photographic strobe light.

Because the lasing medium generally consists entirely of a single element, the photons released are all the same size and exactly match the photons required to stimulate the metastable electrons. Thus, laser light is monochromatic because it has one wavelength. Some lasers contain compounds or mixtures of elements and therefore have more than one lasing wavelength. However, the resulting light is produced at a particular wavelength and is still monochromatic. Laser light also is highly directional, or *collimated*, which means that it spreads very little as it travels. This is determined largely by the distance between the two mirrors in the laser cavity. Much like the difference between a bullet fired from a pistol versus a rifle, the longer the length of the laser cavity, the less the divergence, or spreading, of the beam that occurs over distance (Fig. 1–10).

Laser light energy is measured in watts (W), just as electrical energy is measured in volts (V). The amount of light delivered by a laser to a defined area is called *power density*. Power density is also sometimes referred to as *energy density, fluence, irradiance,* or *dose rate* and is usually measured in watts per square centimeter (W/cm^2).

Power density can be illustrated by using a magnifying glass to focus sunlight (Fig. 1–11). If the magnifying glass is held so that a large spot on a leaf is illuminated, the sun's photons are spread over a wide area (e.g., $1 \ W/cm^2$), and nothing happens. However, if you move the glass to focus the sun's light on a very small spot, you create an area of intense energy (e.g., $100 \ W/cm^2$) that causes the leaf to smolder. By focusing the spot, you increase the power density of the sun's photons.

Your electric bill each month shows you how much electrical energy you have used and for how long. Your energy usage is measured in ampere-hours (Ah). In lasing, the length of time you expose a particular tissue to

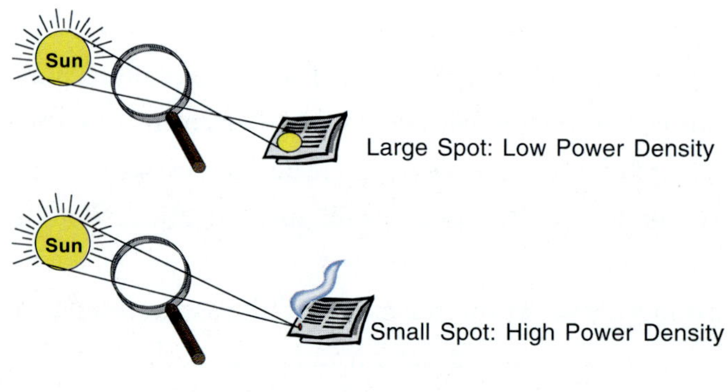

Figure 1–11. Power density/dose rate.

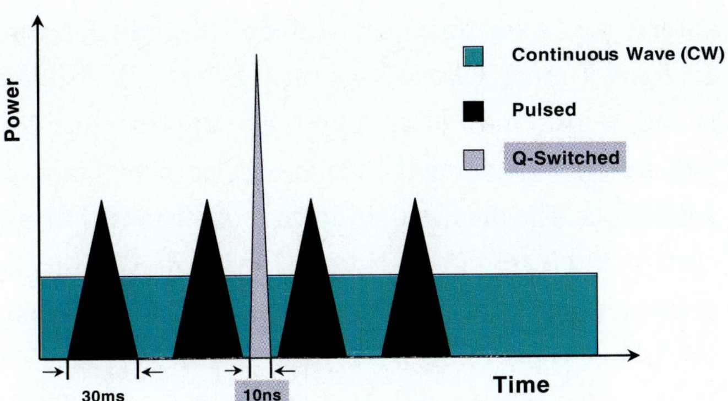

Figure 1–12. Laser emission.

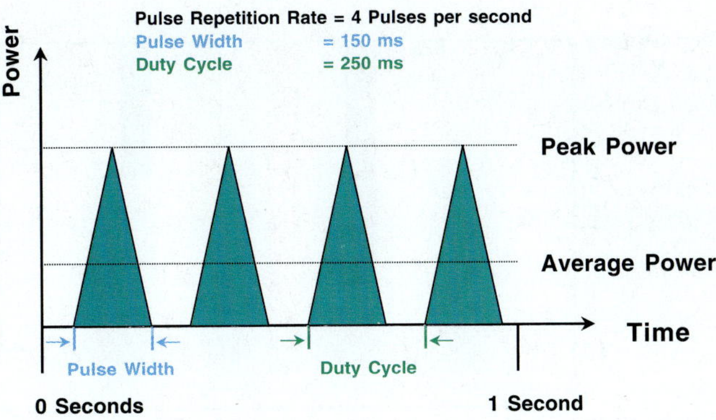

Figure 1–13. Pulse profile.

light, or the total dose of light, is measured in watt-seconds, called *joules* (J). One joule is equal to 1 watt shining on a tissue for 1 second.

Lasers can be divided into two broad groups, *continuous wave* (CW) and *pulsed*. The light of CW lasers undergoes little or no fluctuation over time. The light of pulsed lasers undergoes regular fluctuations. Superpulsing takes place when extremely high power is generated over an extremely short time interval, as in a Q-switched laser (Fig. 1–12).

Continuous wave laser output is measured in power, and pulsed laser output is measured in power over time, usually in joules. One hundred joules equals 100 W for 1 second or 10 W for 10 seconds. In pulsed lasers, the *pulse repetition time* (PRT) is the time interval between the peaks of two consecutive laser pulses. The *pulse repetition rate* (PRR) is the number of pulses per second and is inversely proportional to the PRT (Fig. 1–13).

Extremely high peak powers can be achieved by allowing the photons inside a laser cavity to build by using fully reflecting mirrors at both ends. A mechanically, optically, or electronically gated mirror within a laser cavity can release photons in a fraction of a millisecond. This process is called *Q-switching* and can generate gigawatt $(1 \times 10^9 \text{ W})$ pulses with pulse widths in the nanosecond range. These ultrashort pulses can produce 300°C tissue temperatures in nanoseconds. This causes a rapid thermal expansion that shatters the target (e.g., tattoo pigment) into extremely small particles that can be removed by macrophages in the patient's tissues.

The shock wave to tissue that results from this rapid thermal expansion is also referred to as the *photoacoustic effect*.

TISSUE INTERACTION

Light energy affects tissue in several different ways. The goal of lasing usually is to have the laser light absorbed into a specific target tissue. However, parts of the laser light are also reflected and scattered, and some can even be transmitted through and beyond the *target tissue* (Fig. 1–14). These other forms of incidental light must be assessed carefully in terms of patient safety (see Chapter 3).

The color of a tissue is determined by the wavelength (color) of light it reflects. A red tissue such as blood reflects the red portion of the visible light spectrum and absorbs the rest, and darker tissues absorb a larger portion of the visible light spectrum, much the way a dark automobile is hotter to the touch than a lighter car in a sunny parking lot.

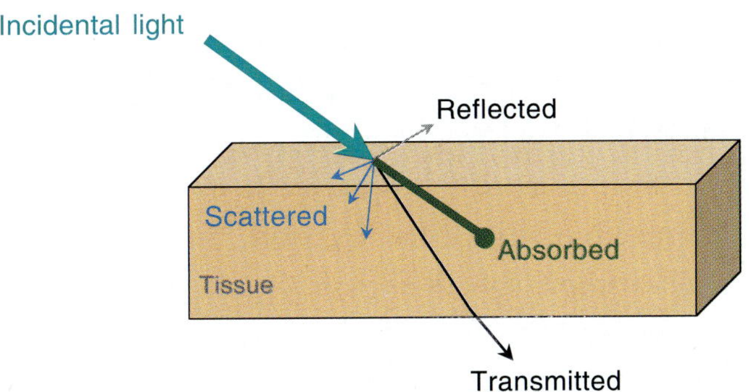

Figure 1–14. Light interaction with tissue.

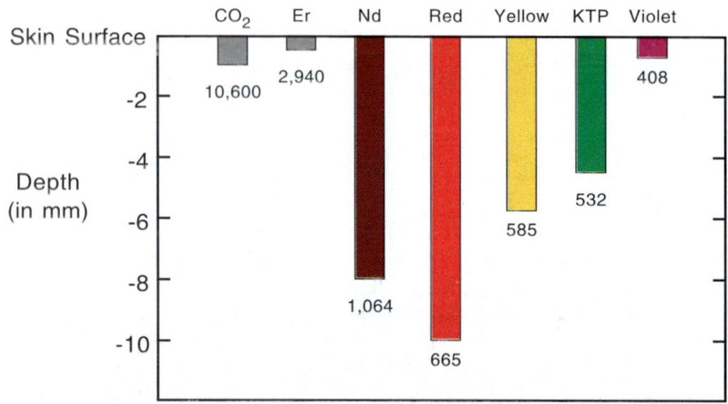

Figure 1–15. Tissue penetration by wavelength.

Most of the light energy of surgical lasers is absorbed by the target tissue, creating heat. The amount of heat generated determines whether target tissue is vaporized, carbonized, or coagulated or if the proteins are denatured. Different wavelengths are absorbed differently by various tissues. Tissues also absorb their complementary color. For example, the green output of an argon or potassium-titanyl-phosphate (KTP) laser is absorbed more into tissues of its complementary color, red. Thus, hemoglobin has an affinity for the light of these lasers, and the absorbed photons can heat blood enough to shrivel blood vessels or even vaporize vascular lesions. In addition, the variable absorption of different tissues means that certain wavelengths penetrate tissues more deeply than others (Fig. 1–15). For example, red light, with its longer wavelength, transmits the best through most tissue. Shining a flashlight (white light) through your fingers creates a red transillumination because all the other visible wavelengths are absorbed in the first few millimeters of tissue.

FIBER OPTICS

Laser light commonly is delivered to patients through thin strands of glass, called *fiber optics*. These fiber-optic strands transmit light throughout their length and do so very efficiently, with the wavelengths covering the UV, visible, and IR portions of the electromagnetic spectrum, between 200 and 1300 nm. Standard fibers used in laser surgery have a core diameter between 200 and 1000 μm (0.2 and 1 mm). Once a laser beam enters a fiber-optic strand, it loses most of its collimated (aligned) qualities and diverges on exiting the strand, similar to the beam of a flashlight. The predicted divergence of a standard fiber-optic strand is around 45 degrees. Thus, power density is greatest in a center spot on the target tissue, and it falls off toward the edges of the target tissue in a Gaussian distribution. Handpieces with lens systems are commonly employed to control the divergence to address specific surgical needs. Some handpiece systems allow for easy attachment of different tips to further modify beam divergence. Tips are usually made of quartz or sapphire and can minimize or maximize tissue penetration as well as target power density.

Some lasers, such as the CO_2 laser, produce wavelengths that are outside the range that can be handled by standard fiber optics. These beams are commonly delivered to patients by means of hollow tubes and mirrors. The mirrors are located in articulating joints and counterweights, allowing the tube assembly to be manipulated with relative ease. An area of new development involves liquid fiber optics, but at present, their relatively large diameter makes them less practical in a surgical setting.

GAS LASERS
CARBON DIOXIDE LASER

Similar to the way a household microwave oven (i.e., radiofrequency generator) resonates water molecules to create steam, a CO_2 laser, with a beam at 10,600 nm, instantly turns water molecules into vapor, creating intense heat and steam. The absorption of this energy causes cells to burst, inducing tissue destruction, heat coagulation, and local sterilization of the surgical site. Temperatures up to 10,538°C (19,000°F) can be obtained with the focused beam of a standard 60-W CO_2 surgical laser.

Nearly all the CO_2 laser's energy (99%) is absorbed by water in tissue. Because most human tissues consist primarily of water, the laser's energy is absorbed very quickly and its penetration into tissue is very shallow, on the order of less than 1 mm. Continued lasing and very high power densities yield only a few more millimeters of tissue penetration. This very visible effect is a great comfort to surgeons using the CO_2 laser as a tool, and the CO_2 laser is commonly called the "what-you-see-is-what-you-get" laser.

Historically, most work with the CO_2 laser has been done in the CW mode. Electrons in the lasing medium (CO_2) are excited by either electrical or radio waves and produce a CW output. In more modern CO_2 laser systems, rapid, high-energy pulsing of the output can be achieved. A break between high peak pulses lasting only milliseconds allows thermal relaxation of tissue, thereby controlling collateral heat damage to adjacent tissues and reducing carbonization of the surgical site. Coagulation is best done in CW mode because the lateral thermal spread shrivels the capillary beds.

Argon Laser

The argon laser was the first laser used in medicine. Its earliest use was for the treatment of vascular defects of the retina. The medical argon laser emits a visible blue-green beam at 488 and 514 nm; both wavelengths lase efficiently. Since the output of the argon laser is in the visible spectrum, fiber optics are used to conduct light to the patient. However, lasing lines in the UV spectrum have also been developed in research laboratories.

As mentioned earlier, green light is readily absorbed by hemoglobin. As a result, the vascular effects of the argon laser are profound, even at low energy densities. Vascular anomalies, such as port-wine-stain hemangiomas and telangiectasias, can be quickly eradicated with this laser. However, the output of the argon laser is also absorbed by the tissue pigments melanin and carotene, and complete blanching of skin around treated lesions is a common complaint. As laser technology evolved, other wavelengths were tested that provided better cosmesis than the argon laser for cutaneous vascular anomalies. These wavelengths were achieved with the dye laser.

SOLID-STATE LASERS
Yttrium-Aluminum-Garnet Lasers

The yttrium-aluminum-garnet (YAG) laser is known as a *solid-state laser* because a crystal, as opposed to a gas such as CO_2, is used as the lasing medium. Garnet is a silicate crystal, and it is used as a "seed" to grow a larger crystal that incorporates the two periodic elements yttrium and aluminum in a laboratory. While the crystal is growing, atoms of other elements can be evenly broadcast throughout the crystal. This process is called *doping*.

Neodymium:Yttrium-Aluminum-Garnet Laser

The neodymium:yttrium-aluminum-garnet (Nd:YAG) laser has neodymium atoms doped throughout the crystal. It is difficult to send electricity through a solid object, so the neodymium atoms are excited by light energy from continuous or pulsed lamps. Stimulated emission occurs, and the photons build up between two mirrors on each side of the Nd:YAG crystal. Neodymium is easy to excite and creates an IR beam with a wavelength of 1064 nm. Since 1064 nm is close to the visible light spectrum, it is referred to as *near-IR*. In contrast, the 10,600-nm wavelength of the CO_2 laser is called *far-IR*.

The Nd:YAG laser's 1064-nm beam falls well within the transmission capabilities of standard fiber optics. On delivery, the laser energy is absorbed by pigment-carrying bodies within tissue, as well as by proteins. In contrast, the laser energy is almost completely transmitted through water. Thus, the Nd:YAG laser may be used at both an air–tissue and a water–tissue interface, whereas a CO_2 laser may be used only at an air–tissue interface.

Nd:YAG lasers transmit thermal energy more deeply than CO_2 lasers and can be used to coagulate deeper and larger blood vessels. For hemorrhagic disorders of the skin, the Nd:YAG laser can be used through fiberoptic handpieces and, with its increased power, can coagulate larger vessels than the CO_2 or argon laser. The contact probe may also be used selectively to reach individual vessels. The Nd:YAG laser has been in use for over 30 years.

Erbium:Yttrium-Aluminum-Garnet Laser

Other elements can be doped on the YAG crystal to yield other wavelengths. Erbium can be doped into the crystal (Er:YAG laser) to produce a beam at 2.94 μm (2940 nm), in the mid-IR region. This wavelength is absorbed by water molecules and can be transmitted via special fiber optics. Typical pulse durations are in the 300-microsecond range, with repetition rates around 15 Hz. Superficial tissue effects can be achieved with power densities of 0.06 to 1.0 J. The advantage of this laser is that tissue water vaporization can be delivered through fiber optics with less tissue penetration than the CO_2 laser.

POTASSIUM-TITANYL-PHOSPHATE LASER

The potassium-titanyl-phosphate (KTP) laser is a frequency-doubled YAG laser. The KTP crystal lasing medium vibrates when light passes through it, and this doubles the oscillating frequency of the beam. Frequency is the inverse of wavelength, and, therefore, the YAG laser's 1064-nm beam is halved to create an emerald green beam at 532 nm. The wavelength of the KTP laser is similar to that of the argon laser, but the beam is produced much more efficiently. The tissue effects in skin are similar, but greater power can be achieved with a much more cost-effective and user-friendly system.

The KTP laser output is pulsed, but the rate is so fast that little difference is observable from the tissue effects of CW lasers. An array of fiber optic handpieces, scanning mirrors, and transcutaneous probes allows for an eclectic choice of beam delivery methods.

RUBY LASER

The synthetic ruby is a transparent crystal of corundum (Al_2O_3) doped with approximately 0.05% trivalent chromium ions in the form of Cr_2O_3. The aluminum and oxygen atoms of the corundum are inert; the chromium atoms constitute the lasing medium. The ruby lases at two wavelengths, 692 and 694 nm, the latter being dominant. The ruby laser is a Q-switched laser that is

"pumped" by a flashlamp, and typical pulse durations are 20 to 50 nanoseconds with a power density of up to 10 to 15 J/cm^2. The wavelengths produced lie on the border of visible and IR light and are absorbed primarily by the pigment melanin. They are also well absorbed by blue, black, and green tattoo pigments. In laser tattoo removal, the ink, when blasted by an ultrashort burst of photons, is disrupted and is usually removed from the dermis by macrophages.

DIODE LASERS

Diodes are "sandwiches" of metals and nonmetals that tend to either take on or give off electrons. When electric current is passed through the first layer of a diode, atoms can be excited and their electrons passed to the next layer. The excited atoms emit photons while returning to ground state, and, if several layers of material are used, vast numbers of photons can be created (Fig. 1–16).

Diode, or semiconductor, lasers are probably the most cost-effective and efficient lasers built to date. The first semiconductor laser was constructed using galena, a mineral consisting of lead sulfide, and the electric connections were so small that they resembled the whiskers of a cat. The laser was then often referred to as the "cat's whisker" laser.

Diode lasers emit light in a divergent fan, not in the classic narrow beam of some other lasers. However, small, inexpensive optical systems can be designed to replicate the narrow beam, as is commonly done with

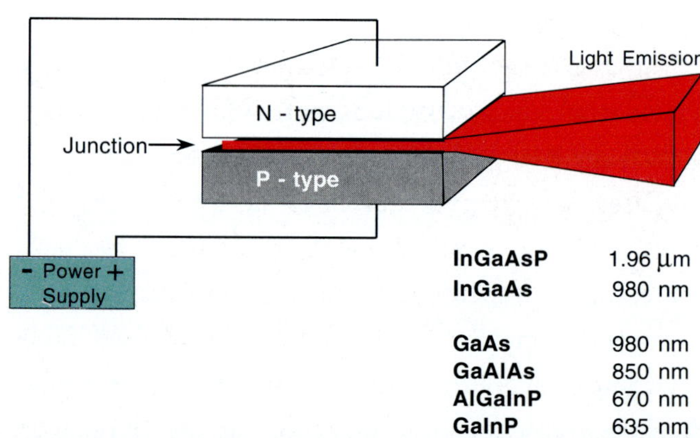

Figure 1–16. Diode/semiconductor lasers.

laser pointers. The typical pencil-sized laser pointer is an aluminum-gallium-indium-phosphide (AlGaInP) sandwich with a wavelength of 670 nm. Some pointers use other materials, which shift wavelengths to 635, 650, and 675 nm.

If diodes of different metals and materials are used, other wavelengths can be obtained from the longer visible wavelengths (orange–red) up to the mid-IR. Research into perfecting shorter-wavelength diodes (e.g., blue, violet, UV) continues, at the urging of the computer industry. Red diode lasers currently read and write information onto optical compact discs (CDs). If blue diodes (i.e., shorter wavelength) were to be used, three to four times the information could be stored on a single CD. If violet or ultraviolet diodes are developed, truly mind-boggling amounts of data could be stored and accessed on a single CD.

Infrared diode laser systems, in the 800- to 1100-nm range, have been used for thermal tissue destruction. The advantage of these systems is their small size, low cost, and interchangeability. A single power supply can have different handpieces, yielding different wavelengths for specific surgical applications.

DYE LASER

Specific wavelengths can be achieved with various gas and solid-state lasing media, but from time to time a wavelength is needed that cannot be produced by conventional means. Dye lasers use gas or solid-state lasers to fluoresce, or optically "pump," an organic or inorganic dye. The resulting fluorescence can be quite strong, and when it is captured in a series of strategically placed mirrors, a laser beam can be produced. Dye lasers typically have lasing wavelength bands that can be tuned from 20 to more than 100 nm in width. For example, an argon-pumped tunable dye laser using rhodamine 6G can produce light from the green into the orange spectrum, or about 560 to 625 nm. By tuning the dye laser to 585 nm, yellow-orange light is produced. This color light

is strongly absorbed by oxyhemoglobin, by a factor of almost 2 times greater than the argon laser's 488- and 514-nm lines.

Solid-state lasers such as the KTP laser also have been used successfully to pump dyes and make the tunable systems more user-friendly. Flashlamps, or strobes, can also be used to fluoresce dyes. Short pulses, measured in joules, can be used to obtain high peak powers and these short bursts of light facilitate thermal relaxation of the skin.

Dye laser systems are typically large and expensive and are known to be very difficult to operate. However, an adroit laser engineer or technician can facilitate several different medical applications by retuning the dye laser to different wavelengths. Treatment of vascular lesions and pigmented cutaneous lesions such as melasma are popular dermatologic applications of flashlamp systems because they can be eradicated effectively by slightly changing the wavelength.

PHOTODYNAMIC THERAPY

Photodynamic therapy (PDT) employs light-activated drugs to kill cells. The drugs can be tailored to be preferentially retained in certain cells, such as cancer cells or other atypical cells. O. Raab first documented a photodynamic effect in 1900, and H. von Tappeiner published results of the first treatments soon thereafter, using eosin and sunlight to treat skin cancers. It was not until the early 1970s that T.J. Dougherty used laser technology to more precisely deliver the drug-activating light. Since then, PDT has been used to treat a wide variety of afflictions, both neoplastic and nonneoplastic.

Photodynamic therapy uses light energy to excite the atoms in the molecules of a drug contained in a tissue. In addition to giving off photons, atoms can also transfer their stored energy to other molecules, such as oxygen. Excited oxygen species, such as singlet oxygen and other radicals, are short-lived but highly toxic to cells. The release of these highly charged oxygens initiates a cascade of intra- and extracellular events resulting in local necrosis.

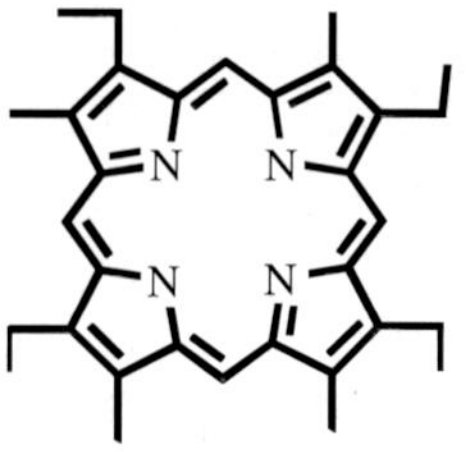

- **4 Pyrrole rings**
  - (Tetrapyrrole)
  - Each ring
    - 4 Carbon atoms
    - 1 Nitrogen atom
- **Nitrogens**
  - Face inward
  - Bind cations
- **Aromatic**
  - System stable due to arrangement of electrons

Figure 1–17. Porphyrins.

Many PDT drugs involve a tetrapyrrole, or a porphyrin ring (Fig. 1–17). Porphyrin rings are stable aromatic molecules that have alternating single and double bonds creating a supply of available electrons. At the center of the ring, four nitrogen atoms face inward and can bind to a cation. Outside the ring, various iso- and exocyclic rings can be chemically engineered. Both changes can modulate the absorption spectrum and pharmacokinetics of the compound.

In PDT, a specific number of photons are needed to cause the tissue effect, but the light is used solely to catalyze the drug, not to burn or vaporize tissue. The amount of light required to activate a PDT drug in a lesion is relatively low. A typical light dose is 200 J/cm^2. As mentioned earlier, 200 J (200 watt-seconds) is equal to the energy of a 100-W light bulb turned on for 2 seconds. During treatment, the rate of light delivery is slower, so tissue temperature is not elevated. The standard fluence for a PDT light treatment is 150 mW/cm^2. Treatment duration is calculated as the total dose divided by the fluence, so 200 J/cm^2 ÷ 150 mW/cm^2 would be a 1333-second treatment, or 22 minutes and 13 seconds.

Because red light penetrates deeply into most tissues, most PDT drugs are tailored to be activated by this wavelength of light. The laser systems used for PDT historically have been large-ion (argon or nitrogen) pumped dye lasers, which are less than ideal. The use of KTP lasers to pump organic dyes has made a significant impact on the ease of PDT light treatments. Very recently, diode lasers (2+ W) have been developed. They are about the size of a personal computer, run off standard wall current (110 or 220 V), and are air-cooled. These lasers have computerized feedback systems that control the output of the diode and can measure and calculate the power density and duration (called *dosimetry*) for treating lesions.

Because PDT drugs are light-sensitive, patients are photosensitive for a period of time after injection. The drugs are easily activated by visible wavelengths of sunlight, and significant sunburn can result if patients fail to take measures to protect themselves from bright light sources. In the early days of PDT, drugs produced photosensitivity lasting 1 to 3 months; with newer drugs, photosensitivity lasts from 2 to 4 weeks. Research into very-short-acting drugs with little to no photosensitivity is currently being conducted.

With regulatory approval in the United States and other countries, PDT is becoming an accepted modality for cancer treatment, and research is rapidly progressing on a variety of nononcologic applications.

THE FUTURE

Research and development of smaller, more efficient, and more cost-effective laser systems will continue for many years. The basic physics of lasers will not change, but the growth potential for new wavelengths and new applications is essentially unlimited.

BIBLIOGRAPHY

Dougherty TJ, Weishaupt KR, Doyle DG. New methods of cancer treatment. In: Devita VT, Hellman S, Rosenberg SA, eds. *Cancer Principles and Practice of Oncology.* Philadelphia: JB Lippincott; 1982:1836–1844.

Einstein A. Zur Quantentheorie der strahlung. *Physiol Z.* 1917; 18:121–128.

Fine S, Maiman TH, Klein E, et al. Biological effects of high peak power radiation. *Life Sci.* 1964;3:209–222.

Goldman L, Dreffer R, Rockwell RJ, Perry E. Treatment of port-wine marks by argon laser. *J Dermatol Surg Oncol.* 1976; 2:385–388.

Gordon JP, Townes CH, Zeigler HJ. The master-new type of amplifier, frequency standard, and spectrometer. *Physiol Rev.* 1955;99:1264–1274.

Greenwald J, Rosen S, Anderson RR, et al. Comparative histological studies of the tunable dye (at 577 nm) laser and argon laser: the specific vascular effects of dye laser. *J Invest Dermatol.* 1981;77:305–310.

Keller GS. Laser treatment of vascular skin lesions: which laser, when, why, and how? *Facial Plast Surg Cutaneous Laser Surg.* 1989;6:175–179.

Keller GS, Razum NJ, Doiron DR. Photodynamic therapy for non-melanoma skin cancer. *Facial Plast Surg Cutaneous Laser Surg.* 1989;6:180–184.

Maiman TH. Stimulated optical radiation in ruby. *Nature.* 1960; 187:493–494.

Raab O. Über die wirkung fluoreszierender stoffe auf infusoria. *Z Biol.* 1900;39:524–526.

Razum NJ, Balchum OJ, Profio AE. Skin photosensitivity: duration and intensity following hematoporphyrin derivative intravenous injection. *Photochem Photobiol.* 1987;46: 925–928.

Schawlow AL, Towns CH. Infrared and optical lasers. *Physiol Rev.* 1958;112:1940.

Tappeiner HV, Jesionek A. Therapeutishe versuche mit fluoreszierenden stoffe. *Muench Med Wochenschr.* 1903;47: 2042–2044.

CHAPTER 2

Laser Systems and Instrumentation for Aesthetic Surgery

MICHAEL SLATKINE AND CLIFFORD E. MORROW

Currently, more than 8000 lasers worldwide are used in cosmetic and aesthetic surgical procedures in hospitals, physicians' offices, and ambulatory surgical centers. The rapid advancement of laser technology has fostered revolutionary advances in skin resurfacing and rejuvenation, treatment of vascular lesions, hair removal and restoration, skin depigmentation, and endoscopic plastic surgery.

Each type of laser has unique features that determine its appropriateness for specific aesthetic surgical procedures. Generally these features involve the wavelength of the light produced by the laser and the pulse duration (time of exposure) and area of tissue interaction (spot size) of the laser beam. For example, lasers that produce long infrared wavelengths (e.g., carbon dioxide [CO_2] and erbium:yttrium-aluminum-garnet [Er:YAG] lasers) vaporize extremely thin layers of skin. This has allowed unprecedented fast, accurate, and controlled techniques of skin resurfacing. Lasers that produce wavelengths in the visible part of the spectrum (e.g., potassium-titanyl-phosphate [KTP], dye, ruby, and alexandrite lasers) penetrate more deeply into the skin, and the laser light is selectively absorbed by chromophores, such as oxyhemoglobin in small blood vessels, melanin in hair shafts and follicles, and tattoo ink in the epidermis and dermis, without damaging surrounding structures. This has resulted in newer, noninvasive methods to treat telangiectasias, spider veins, and to some extent small leg veins, as well as methods to remove unwanted hair, excessive pigmentation, and tattoos. In addition, some lasers can create very confined tissue coagulation effects by controlling the time duration of the laser action (e.g., superpulsed CO_2 laser). The result is highly controlled skin or blood vessel contraction and control of necrosis and/or hemostasis depth.

Figure 2–1 presents the optical absorption coefficients of the three most important biological substances in aesthetic laser surgery and shows where the various lasers fit

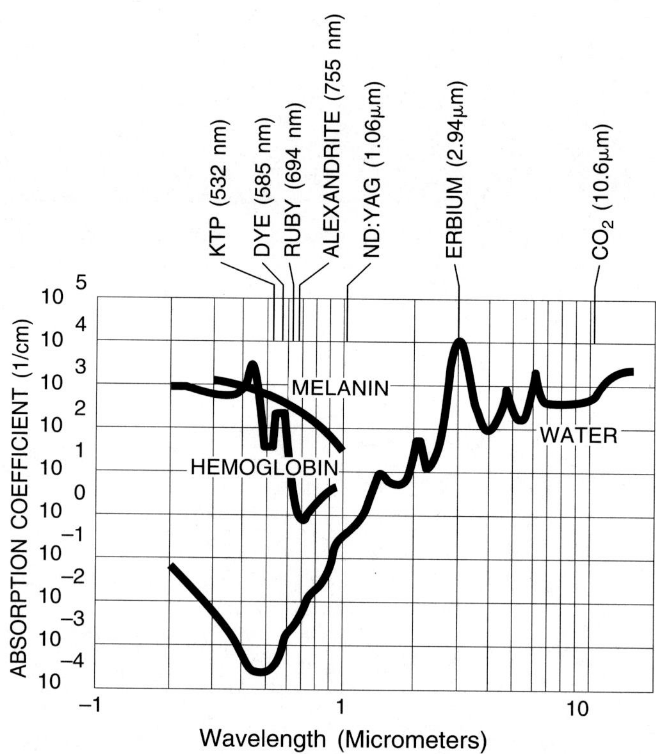

Figure 2–1. Optical absorption spectrum of three important biological chromophores.

in this scheme. The CO_2 laser beam (10,600-nm [10.6-μm] wavelength) penetrates 30 μm into water. As a result, CO_2 laser tissue effects are shallow (although not shallower than 30 μm) and nonselective. The Er:YAG laser beam (2940-nm [2.94-μm] wavelength) penetrates 3 to 10 μm into tissue. This provides an even more superficial tissue effect that can be limited to the epidermis (5–20 μm). The yellow-dye laser beam (585-nm wavelength) is only slightly absorbed by skin connective tissue, thus penetrating only a few millimeters into tissue. However, high oxyhemoglobin absorption makes this laser an ideal tool for selective coagulation of blood vessels. The ruby (694 nm) and alexandrite (755 nm) laser beams are barely absorbed by blood vessels and connective tissue but are rather highly absorbed by melanin. Therefore, these lasers are used to remove unwanted pigment and hairs.

This chapter reviews the operating principles of the major laser systems currently used in aesthetic surgery, with particular focus on the types of laser–tissue interactions on which each procedure is based and the key accessories needed for success (Table 2–1).

SKIN RESURFACING AND REJUVENATION

Facial skin rejuvenation currently is performed with two different types of lasers. The CO_2 laser, in pulsed or continuous-wave (CW) mode, is used to resurface deep wrinkles and for long-lasting results. The Er:YAG laser is used to eliminate very fine and superficial wrinkles and rejuvenate areas with extremely thin skin, such as the hands and neck.

CARBON DIOXIDE LASER

The CO_2 laser is by far the most popular tool for skin resurfacing. Over 4000 CO_2 laser systems have been installed worldwide, and more than 1 million facial rejuvenation procedures have been performed during the past 5 years with great success and safety.

Char-Free Tissue Vaporization

Because of the high water content of the epidermis and relatively high water content of the dermis, the typical depth of penetration of the CO_2 laser beam into skin is 30 μm.[1] Absorption of laser energy by skin first produces an elevation in surface temperature, and this is followed by (1) vaporization of tissue water, which results in tissue ablation and the creation of a crater, and (2) conduction of heat into subjacent tissue.

Slow deposition of CO_2 laser energy produces thermal conduction into skin and leads to deep coagulation, possibly resulting in scar. However, fast deposition of CO_2 laser energy, at a fluence threshold level of 5 J/cm^2 and a pulse duration of less than 0.5 millisecond,[2,3] results in tissue vaporization (ablation) with minimal subjacent thermal damage (40–100 μm) and no char (Fig. 2–2). The thermal relaxation time of a 30-μm tissue layer (equal to the depth of penetration of the CO_2 laser) is 0.5 millisecond. This ability to attain a 5 J/cm^2 fluence threshold in an extremely controlled and homogeneous manner over large areas of the face forms the basis of CO_2 laser rejuvenation.

Skin Resurfacing

Skin resurfacing for the removal of fine rhytids was first performed by Fitzpatrick and Goldman[4] and Weinstein[5] with the Ultrapulse CO_2 laser and by Keller and Lask[6,7] with the Surgipulse 150XJ Laser (Sharplan/Surgilase, Allendale, NJ). These lasers were operated in a high-energy pulsed mode, typically at an energy level of 400 to 500 mJ. The 0.5- to 1-millisecond, 400-W peak power

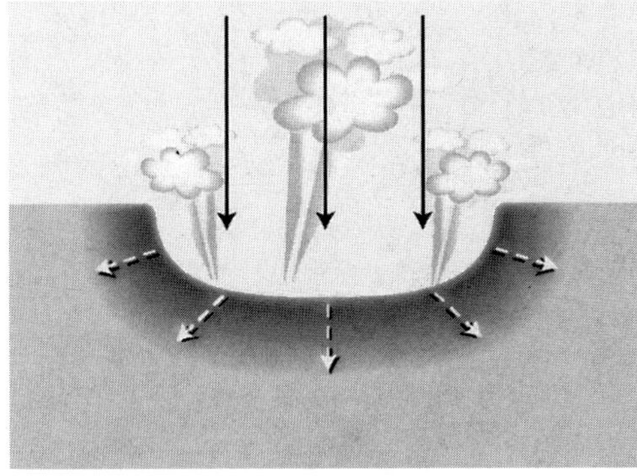

Figure 2–2. Thermal effect of quick energy delivery. Over 5 J/cm^2 causes vaporization of tissue, which is expelled. Less than 1 millisecond (thermal relaxation time of tissue) does not allow surrounding tissue to heat, resulting in a very thin, coagulated collagen and elastin protein tissue layer that heals without scarring.

Table 2–1. Major Laser Systems and Accessories for Aesthetic Procedures

Procedure		Tissue Interaction	Laser System				Typical Result	Possible Postoperative Adverse Effect(s)
Type	Specific		Laser	Accessory	Wavelength	Typical Parameters		
Skin resurfacing	Wrinkle removal—deep and superficial rhytids	Nonselective superficial (30–100 μm) vaporization;	Focused CW CO_2	Flashscanner (FeatherTouch)	10.6 μm	F = 200 mm P = 30 W T = 0.1 s 10 mm scan	Long-term elimination of deep and superficial wrinkles	Typically 2–4 months' erythema
		Energy > 5 J/cm^2, dwell time < 1 ms 40–70μm necrosis	Defocused CO_2 pulsed (Surgipulse/Ultrapulse)	Defocusing or collimated handpiece Computerized pattern scanner	10.6 μm	E = 400–500 mJ T < 1 ms spot size = 3 mm scan size ~ 15 mm	Long-term elimination of deep and superficial wrinkles	Typically 2–4 months' erythema
Facial rejuvenation	Very superficial skin freshening—"lunchtime peeling"	Nonselective—extremely superficial vaporization (5–30 μm); Energy < 1.5 J/cm^2 dwell time 200 μs, 5–20 μm necrosis	Defocused Er:YAG	Defocusing handpiece for painting	2.94 μm	5–15 J/cm^2 spot 35 mm 20 pps scan size ~ 10 mm	Fine wrinkles and pigmented skin resolved	Typically up to 2–3 weeks' erythema
	Rejuvenation of Asian skin, mainly pigmented			Computerized pattern scanner			Good combination with CO_2	
Vascular lesions	Treatment of port-wine stain, telangectasia	Selective photothermolysis	Pulsed dye	Fiber and defocusing handpiece	585 nm (yellow)	~ 10 J/cm^2, 5 mm spot, ~ 1 mS, 1 pps	Long-term elimination of vascularity	2–3 weeks' purpura
	Thin leg veins Diameters < 0.5 mm	Thermal relaxation time ~ 1.5 ms	CW frequency doubled Nd:YAG (KTP)	Fiber and focusing optics, painting, focusing optics and scanner	532 nm (green)	3–5 W 200 μm spot; 2.5 ms dwelling time	Long-term elimination of very thin and superficial vascularity	No purpura
			Intense flashlamp (Photoderm)	Contact flashlamp	Filtered lamp, ~600 nm	~ 10 J/cm^2 8 × 20 mm spot > 10 ms		Hyperpigmentation if filter not properly selected

F = focal length of handpiece lens; P = power; T = dwell time; E = energy; pps = pulses/sec.; ns = nanosecond; mS = microsecond; μm = micrometer

Hair removal		Melanin-based selective photothermolysis	Long-pulse ruby	Fiber or articulated arm + defocusing optics	694 nm	~ 25 J/cm², 7 mm spot, 1 ms, 1 pps	Multiple treatment, 10% growth 4–8 months after last treatment	Transient: redness, possible hypopigmentation, possible superficial burn
			Long-pulse alexandrite	Fiber + defocusing handpiece	755 nm	25 J/cm² 7 mm spot 2, 4, 10 ms 5 pps		
			Intense flashlamp	Contact light guide	Filtered infrared	40 J/cm² 8 × 30 mm 10 ms		
		Follicle-staining lotion-based photothermolysis	Q-switched Nd:YAG	Articulated arm	1.06 μm	10 J/cm² 5 mm 20 ms 5 pps	Multiple treatments, regrowth reported	
Tattoo removal and pigmented lesions	Removal of blue, black, green tattoos, treatment of pigmented lesions	Selective photothermolysis of protein encapsilated ink particle	Q-switched ruby	Articulated arm	694 nm	4–10 J/cm² 4 mm 20–40 ns 1 pps	Multiple treatments, permanent results	Transient tissue whitening, painful
	Removal of red and dark tattoos (not blue and green), treatment of pigmented lesions		Q-switched alexandrite		755 nm	4–10 J/cm² 4 mm 20–40 ns 1–10 pps		
			Frequency doubled Q-switched Nd:YAG	Articulated arm	532 nm	4–10 J/cm² 4 mm 10 ns 1–10 pps		
Hair transplantation	Preparation of recipient holes for micrografts in large sections	Nonselective vaporization of tissue, char free, short dwelling time, 40 μm thermal damage	Focused high-power CO$_2$	Focusing handpiece and flashscanner	10.6 μm	40–80 W 0.1 s	More natural results with micrografts	2 weeks' delayed growth when compared with nonlaser treatments
Endoscopic surgery	Forehead muscle release, facelifting	Nonselective tissue incision, good hemostasis, minimal thermal damage	CO$_2$ pulsed	Flexible waveguide and curved sheath	10.6 μm	400 mJ 10 W average 1 mm diameter	Excellent char-free incision, highly controlled	

laser beam was defocused to a spot size of 2 to 3 mm, thus attaining the char-free threshold of 5 J/cm^2.

The Surgipulse laser differs from the Ultrapulse laser by incorporating a brief cessation during the lasing phase. This allows removal of vapors from the laser pathway and provides better tissue cooling. Results with both lasers, however, are impressive.

To increase the speed of treatment and provide better control of beam overlap, a galvanometric computerized scanner can be added to the laser. Figure 2–3A shows a single scan pattern with a pulsed laser. However, the scanner can be adjusted to generate a variety of shapes to accommodate different facial zones (Fig. 2–3C).

Similar results can be achieved with a smaller, less expensive CW CO_2 laser known as the CO_2 *flashscanner*.[7–11] Figure 2–4 illustrates the operating principles of the flashscanner (SilkTouch or FeatherTouch, Sharplan). The optomechanical scanner consists of two orthogonally vibrating mirrors and a focusing lens. Reflection of the CO_2 laser beam between the mirrors causes the beam to deviate from its original direction by an angle θ. The microprocessor-controlled mirrors are programmed to vary θ spatially and nonlinearly to generate a rapidly collapsing spiral curve on tissue with a constant tangential linear velocity (see Fig. 2–3B). It is this constant tangential velocity that results in homogeneous tissue vaporiza-

tion. A focusing lens of focal length F is attached to the mirror assembly. This allows the CO_2 laser to generate a tight focal spot that rapidly and homogeneously spiral scans a round area of diameter $2F \tan \theta_{max}$ on tissue at the focal plane. The skin resurfacing handpiece uses a focusing lens with a focal length of 125 to 260 mm that provides selectable treatment areas of 2 to 15 mm in diameter. Square, rectangular, and various other geometric scan shapes are also available (Fig. 2–3C).

Rapid movement of the CO_2 laser beam over the tissue ensures a 0.3-millisecond duration of exposure for individual sites within the area. As mentioned earlier, this is shorter than the thermal relaxation time of skin tissue for a laser beam depth of penetration of 30 μm. When the CO_2 laser is operated at power level between 7 and 60 W, depending on the focal length, a fluence threshold of 5 J/cm^2 is attained at each focal spot in the scan pattern. The FeatherTouch flashscanner has been installed in close to 2000 facilities, and excellent results are the rule.

Recently, Ross et al[12] presented an analysis of the shallow residual effects on skin tightening of CO_2 lasers versus nonlaser skin resurfacing. The three physiologic steps in the process of long-term skin rejuvenation (tissue vaporization, skin contraction, and collagen remodeling) were measured quantitatively through the use of skin dot tat-

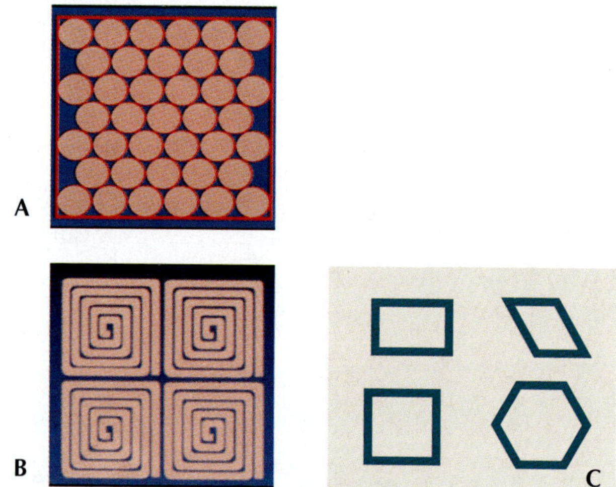

Figure 2–3. Some CO_2 laser scan patterns: (A) pattern generated by a computerized pulsed scanner; (B) spiral scan generated by a CW CO_2 flashscanner; (C) patterns generated by CO_2 laser scanners.

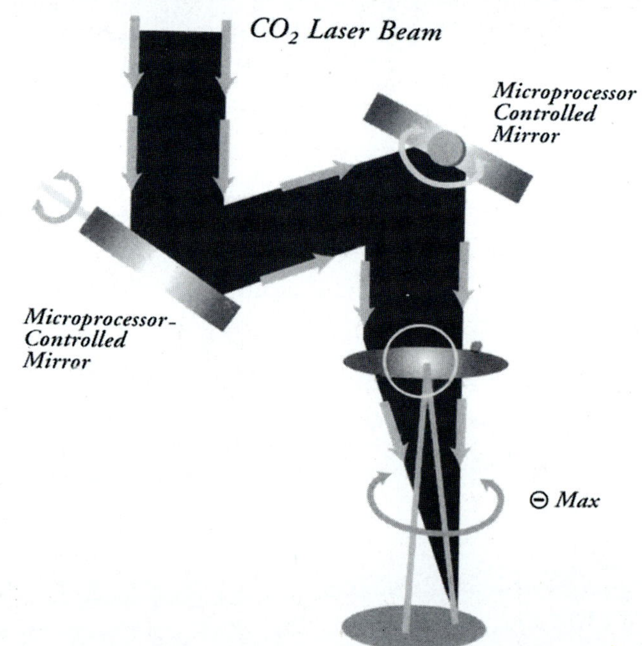

Figure 2–4. Operating principles of the CO_2 flashscanner.

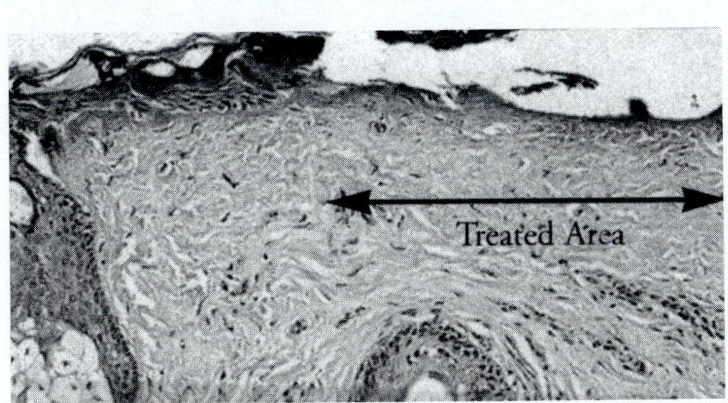

Figure 2–5. Histology of skin treated with the SilkTouch flashscanner, one pass (3 μm of residual thermal damage).

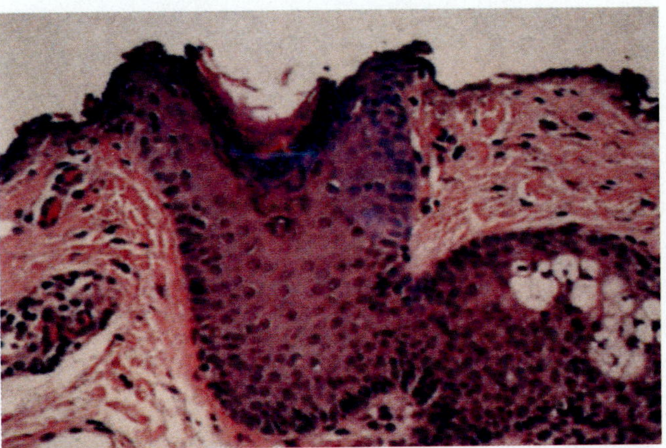

Figure 2–6. Skin histology following an Er:YAG laser treatment.

tooing. The results show up to 25% skin contraction with the CO_2 laser, an improvement over nonlaser techniques.

Skin resurfacing has also been used in other rejuvenation processes, such as scar removal and recently also for the preparation of dermal implants to treat facial depressions.[13] Another recent development in CO_2 laser rejuvenation is the development of dual-mode scanners that combine a computerized pulsed scanner with a CW flashscanner in a single system (XJ Scanner, Surgilase).

ERBIUM:YAG LASER

The Er:YAG laser is a pulsed system that produces a 2940-nm wavelength light beam. Pulse duration is between 200 and 300 microseconds. Energy levels range from 0.5 to 3 J per pulse. However, depth of tissue penetration depends on fluence (energy per square centimeter), not on energy level. Thus, the Er:YAG laser nonselectively ablates skin layers from 5 to 30 μm deep at fluences of 5 to 15 J/cm^2. These fluences are attained with collimated beams that are 3 to 5 mm in diameter. Because of this shallower skin penetration, the threshold for char-free tissue vaporization with the Er:YAG laser is 1.5 J/cm^2, as compared with 5 J/cm^2 for a CO_2 laser. The collateral thermal necrosis range for the Er:YAG laser is between 5 and 20 μm, which in skin resurfacing results in considerably shorter postoperative healing and erythema as compared with the CO_2 laser.[14,15]

An important difference between Er:YAG and CO_2 laser-tissue interactions is the consistency of vaporization depth for multilayer treatment. Vaporization with the

CO_2 laser produces a residue of desiccated tissue that has a slight effect on the next level of vaporization. The Er:YAG laser does not produce coagulation, thus leaving wet tissue and allowing continuous vaporization. Figures 2–5 and 2–6 show the histology of skin specimens treated with the CO_2 and Er:YAG lasers, respectively.

The Er:YAG laser is often operated in a "painting" mode (free-hand painting of tissue) or in a computerized pulsed scanning mode that covers tissue in a much more homogeneous way. Although the painting mode is convenient for single-layer "lunchtime peeling" procedures in which a few overlaps of lasing spots or gaps are not critical, the scanning mode is widely considered the technique of choice for treating areas with thin skin, such as the neck and hands, or for treating deeper rhytids. The Er:YAG scanners have variable overlap-density parameters (mostly −30 to +30%), which allow control of gaps between round treatment areas. The speed of treatment with the Er:YAG laser depends on the average power level (currently up to 20 W), and this is a multiple of the pulsed energy level and repetition rate (which can be as high as 20 pulses per second with current systems).

TREATMENT OF VASCULAR LESIONS

The effective noninvasive treatment of a wide range of vascular lesions has been made possible by the discovery of selective photothermolysis with lasers emitting in the visible part of the electromagnetic spectrum.[16] Selective thermolysis involves absorption of specific wavelengths of light energy by chromophores in tissue. The chromophores in vascular lesions are hemoglobin and oxyhemoglobin, which selectively absorb wavelength-specific light in the range of about 500 to 1000 nm. Recently, spectrally filtered high-intensity flashlamp (nonlaser) sources have also been used successfully in the treatment of larger-diameter blood vessels.[17,18]

PULSED DYE LASER

The most widely used laser in the treatment of vascular lesions is the pulsed dye laser, which operates at a wavelength of 585 nm.[19–22] This laser has a pulse duration of up to 1.5 milliseconds. Selective photothermolysis with a pulsed dye laser shrinks or eliminates blood vessels as a result of the sequence of events in Box 2–1.

As a general rule of thumb, optimal pulse duration T for the treatment of vascular lesions is given by

$$T = d^2/4K$$

where d is the diameter of the vessel into which the heat diffuses and K is the thermal diffusivity of the tissue $\left(1.3 \times 10^{-3} \text{ cm}^2/\text{second}\right)$.

As can be seen from this equation, the thermal relaxation time of tissue is proportional to the square of the depth or vessel diameter. This equation is also used to set the dwell time of scanning CW lasers employed in the treatment of vascular lesions. One such laser is the CW frequency-doubled neodymium:yttrium-aluminum-garnet (Nd:YAG) laser, operated at 532 nm. This laser can be used in conjunction with a fast scanner[23] to treat large port-wine stains. Dwell time should be submilliseconds. Figure 2–7 shows the operating principles of a pulsed dye laser for the treatment of blood vessels, whereas Figure 2–8 shows the operating principles of a frequency-doubled laser.

NONLASER FLASHLAMPS

Photothermolysis of very large blood vessels requires a pulse duration that is much longer than 1 millisecond. In fact, it should be rather close to 30 milliseconds. More-

over, the light energy should be further shifted to the red range, close to 595 nm. For this purpose, the PhotoDerm flashlamp (ESC Sharplan, Norwood, MA) produces a 595-nm beam of light with a pulse duration of up to 30 milliseconds. Flashlamps are nonlaser light sources that emit a very broad spectrum of light. However, various color filters can be used to match the light to the wavelength-specific chromophore in the tissue to be treated. As mentioned, the pulse duration can also be varied to match the diameter of the blood vessel to be treated. As with lasers, flashlamp pulse duration can be calculated using the equation already given on this page.

Box 2–1. Treatment of Vascular Lesions with the Pulsed-Dye Laser

1. A laser beam $\left(8–15 \text{ J/cm}^2\right)$ approximately 5 mm in diameter is fired at the vascular lesion. (The lesion may be telangiectasia, where individual tiny vessels are clear, or port-wine stain, where a large area is excessively red as a result of diffused vascular tissue.)

2. The laser beam penetrates the skin while being strongly scattered by the connective tissue.

3. Scattered laser light that coincidentally hits blood vessels is absorbed by hemoglobin and oxyhemoglobin all across the vessel diameter of a few hundred microns. (Yellow light penetrates about 600 μm into blood, whereas green light, such as that generated by a frequency-doubled Nd:YAG laser, penetrates only 200 μm. Thus, the Nd:YAG laser is an ideal tool for the treatment of very thin and superficial vascular lesions.)

4. The temperature of the blood vessel is elevated to over 60°C for approximately 1 millisecond (the pulse duration of the laser), which results in blood vessel endothelial contraction. The surrounding tissue is not heated because the laser pulse duration has been tailored to be close to the thermal relaxation time of the blood vessel.

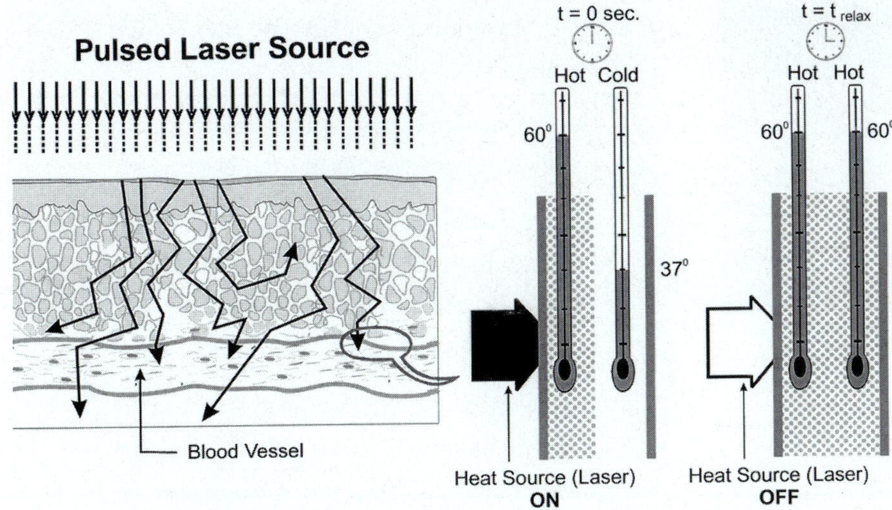

Figure 2–7. Operating principles of photothermolysis.

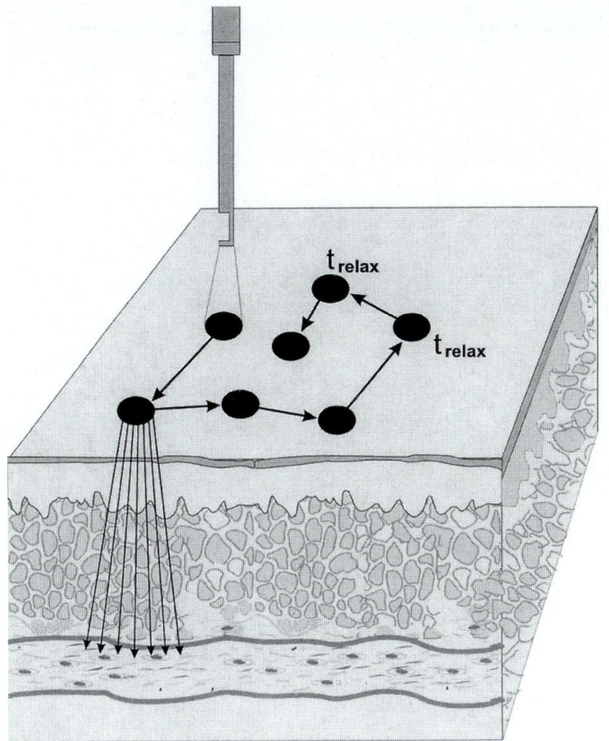

Figure 2–8. Treatment of vascular lesions with a fast scanner and small spot size.

HAIR REMOVAL

The concept of using selective photothermolysis to remove hair was first presented by Zaias in 1990.[24] Deep penetration of laser energy into the skin enables scattered radiation to impinge on hair shafts and follicles and be absorbed selectively by melanin, hair's primary chromophore (Fig. 2–9). A zone of thermal necrosis limited to the follicle results from the short pulse duration and limited energy of the laser. The procedure is fast and achieves long-lasting depilation in many fewer sessions than needed with electrolysis.

Results with both ruby and alexandrite lasers, as well as flashlamps, are excellent.[25–28] The procedure requires two to three treatments, followed by a few touch-ups, because only hairs in the anagen phase of their growth cycle are long enough and capable of absorbing the necessary laser energy for destruction. The time between treatments depends on the inflammatory response of the

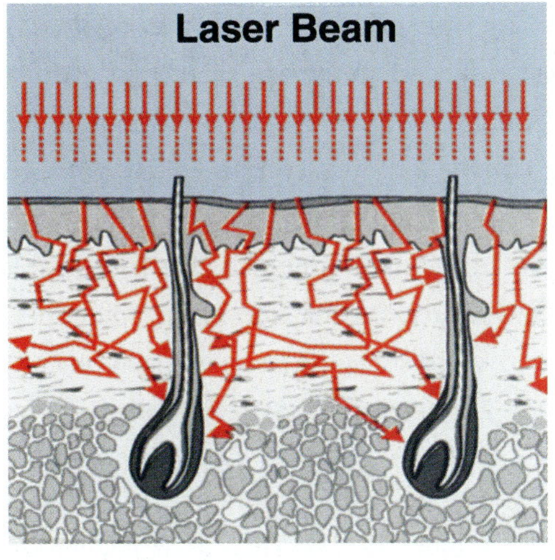

Figure 2–9. Operating principles of laser hair removal.

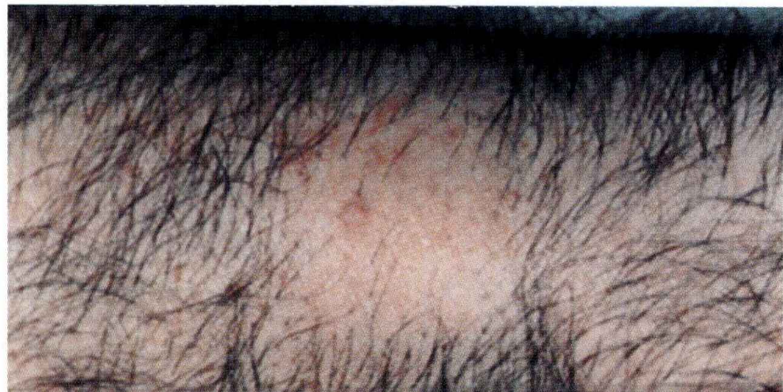

Figure 2–10. Hair removal (2–year follow up after last treatment).

treated site. Figure 2–10 shows a result 2 years after a second treatment with a ruby laser.

HAIR FOLLICLE COAGULATION

To obtain effective photothermolysis of the entire follicle, including the bulb and the bulge (a condition believed necessary for long-lasting hair removal), the laser energy should penetrate at least 3 mm into the skin and be selectively absorbed by melanin (not oxyhemoglobin). Thus, the alexandrite and ruby lasers are clearly the lasers of choice. They are currently popular in dermatology clinics in their Q-switch modes (20–30-nanosecond pulse duration) for tattoo removal and the treatment of various pigmented lesions.[29,30] However, because hair follicles typically have a diameter of 30 to 100 μm and a thermal relaxation time of a few milliseconds, these lasers should be used for hair removal in their free-running mode with sufficient energy for follicle coagulation.

The laser parameters necessary to fully coagulate a hair follicle depend on the hair shaft color, diameter, and depth. A statistical Monte Carlo computer simulation of the scattering of a ruby laser beam in the vicinity of a hair shaft leads to the conclusions in Box 2–2 and Figure 2–11. An additional prerequisite for follicle ablation is light skin, because the melanin in the epidermis of dark skin selectively absorbs the laser light and precludes penetration of the laser energy into the dermis.

EPIDERMAL HEAT SINK

Even in very light skin, potentially damaging epidermal heating may occur unless an appropriate method of heat sinking is applied to the skin. This involves application of

Box 2–2. Determinants of Effective Hair Follicle Coagulation

1. The temperature of an irradiated follicle decreases rapidly with hair shaft depth.

2. Internal scattering of laser energy in the skin requires a minimum spot size on the skin of approximately 3 to 4 mm because further reduction in spot size would not increase energy density inside the tissue.

3. The energy density (fluence) necessary to fully coagulate a follicle (T $\approx$ 60°C) with a 50-μm-diameter black hair shaft that is 3 mm deep is 20 J/cm^2 with a spot size of 5 mm. A lighter hair would need a higher energy density. The diameters of hairs taken from the arm in a number of treated volunteers ranged between 30 and 70 μm. Other hairs, including bikini line hairs (a frequently requested target of laser hair removal), are usually thicker. As a result, a laser generating a fluence of 20 to 40 J/cm^2 with a spot size of 4 to 7 mm and a pulse duration of 1 millisecond or more is adequate for hair removal.

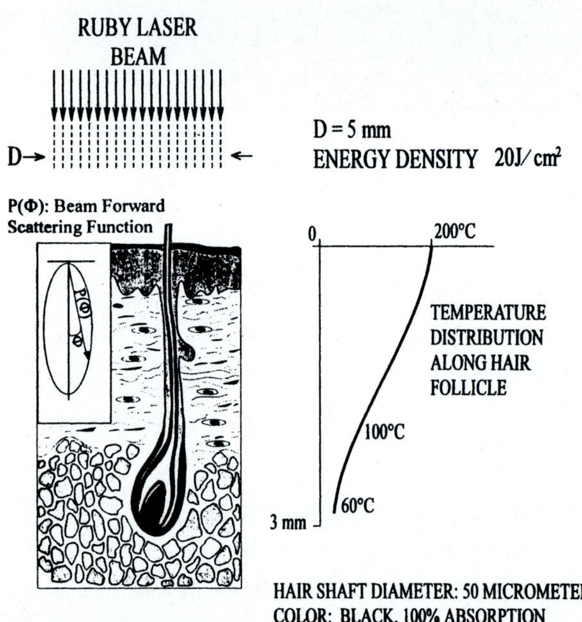

Figure 2–11. Temperature distribution along a laser-irradiated hair follicle (computer simulation).

a transparent room-temperature gel to the treatment site during the procedure to cool the epidermis, which has a thermal relaxation time of 1 millisecond. The resulting cooling considerably reduces immediate posttreatment inflammation and erythema and also potentially prevents epidermal damage in patients with darker skin types.

A thin laser beam aligning sheet (grid) is placed on top of the cooling gel before firing to enable the proper positioning of the laser beam and homogeneous coverage of the skin (Fig. 2–12). The grid is particularly useful because the laser beam does not leave any visible marks on the skin. The laser is operated at a repetition rate of 1 to 5 pulses per second depending on its type, thus covering a 12- to 70-cm^2 surface area in about 1 minute. The laser energy is always kept at the maximum level, while spot size is adjusted to obtain the proper fluence.

An alternative heat sink technique was developed recently in conjunction with a 3-millisecond pulsed ruby laser. This technique uses a low-temperature flowing liquid enclosed in a container that is in contact with the skin. In addition, the device slightly enhances radiation density in the targeted follicles.

TATTOO REMOVAL AND THE TREATMENT OF PIGMENTED LESIONS

Laser removal of tattoos also employs the concept of photothermolysis, on a nanosecond time scale. The operating principles of laser tattoo removal are depicted in Fig. 2–13. A pulsed laser emitting wavelengths in the visible part of the spectrum is used. The laser energy penetrates the epidermis as well as the upper papillary dermis layer and is selectively absorbed by the variously colored tattoo ink particles. For blue, green, and black ink particles, a ruby or alexandrite laser (red) is used, because their light is maximally absorbed by these colors. For red ink particles, a frequency-doubled Nd:YAG laser (green) is used.

In tattoos, the ink particles are embedded in a protein envelope. As the particles absorb laser energy, they heat up and explode the protein envelope shattering the particles. Then the much smaller particles are removed by phagocytosis. Most tattoo ink particles are a few microns in size and have a thermal relaxation time of a few nanoseconds. Thus, the lasers used for tattoo removal are operated in Q-switch mode, which generates a pulse duration of 10 to 40 nanoseconds.

Energy densities for tattoo removal range between 4 and 10 J/cm^2, with minimal spot sizes of 3 to 4 mm. Treatment is always associated with tissue whitening (due to collagen envelope blasting). Multiple treatments (three to eight) are necessary at intervals of every few weeks to allow phagocytes to clear the debris.[29,30]

The treatment of pigmented lesions is very similar to tattoo removal, although pigments are localized mostly in the epidermis only.[31] Recently, the Er:YAG laser has gained wide acceptance for the treatment of pigmented lesions, particularly in Asian patients, in conjunction with facial rejuvenation.

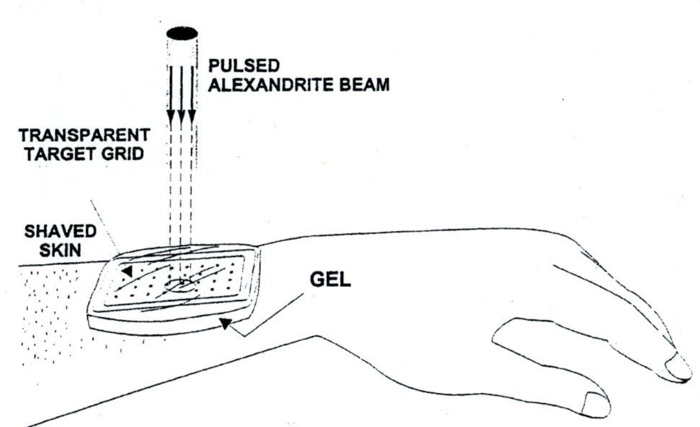

Figure 2–12. The use of heat sink gel and targets for homogeneous skin cover.

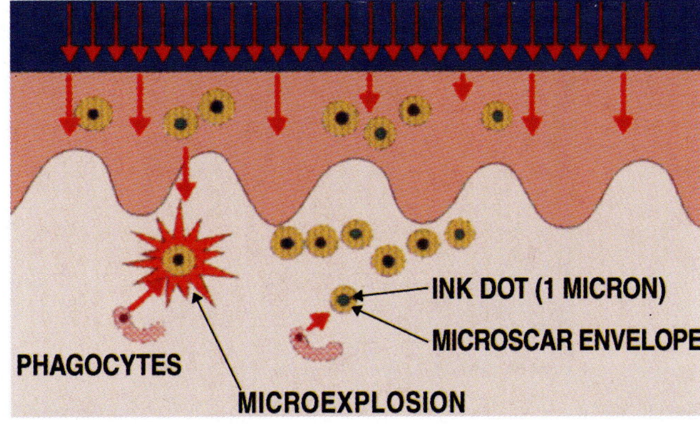

Figure 2–13. Operating principles of tattoo removal with a Q-switched laser.

HAIR TRANSPLANTATION

Laser-assisted hair transplantation has been performed on a few thousand patients with great success over the past 2 years.[32–36] The laser is used mainly to prepare micrograft recipient holes (0.6–0.9 mm) in large sessions. Use of a laser to create such small-diameter holes makes hair transplantation easier and faster and results in very natural-looking growth. Large-diameter minigrafts ($\geq$ 1.5 mm) are usually prepared mechanically.

The laser most frequently used for hair transplantation is a high-power CO_2 laser (such as the Sharplan/Surgilase 150XJ) in conjunction with a flashscanner. Hole diameters are adjusted between 0.6 and 1.2 mm. The laser is operated for a pulse duration of 0.1 second at 45 to 100 W. A typical recipient hole prepared by a CO_2 laser is shown in Fig. 2–14. The depth of thermal necrosis is only 40 μm because of the less than 1-millisecond dwell time of the laser beam on the tissue.[35] This amount of thermal damage allows nutrients to feed the implanted graft and also minimizes bleeding during the procedure. Figure 2–15 shows a laser-prepared site prior to grafting. Growth is usually delayed by 2 weeks when compared with mechanical graft preparation.

LASER ENDOSCOPY

Minimally invasive laser endoscopy in cosmetic surgery is an evolving technique first proposed by Keller in 1990 and used mainly in forehead muscle release,[37,38] face lifting, and to some extent abdominal surgery. Its very high potential is based mainly on the current availability of thin, flexible, hollow waveguides that efficiently transmit CO_2 laser energy. The laser is used at an energy level of 250 to 400 mJ and an average power of 20 to 50 W. The subcutaneous incisions are performed under endoscopic vision, which is advantageous to the patient postoperatively.

OPTICAL WAVEGUIDE TECHNOLOGY

The operating principles of optical hollow fibers[39,40] are depicted in Fig. 2–16. The laser beam is coupled via a focusing lens to the center of a thin metallic tube. The flexible tube is coated with a dielectric silver iodine or silver bromide film, reflective at grazing incidence. This optical coating is highly reflective at a wavelength of 10.6 μm (10,600 nm). Multiple reflections of the laser beam off the waveguide walls enable the trapped optical radiation to propagate along the fiber and produce a 1-mm spot at a distance of 1 mm from the distal end of the fiber. The optical beam divergence is 30 degrees, thus enabling slight defocusing by pulling back the fiber.

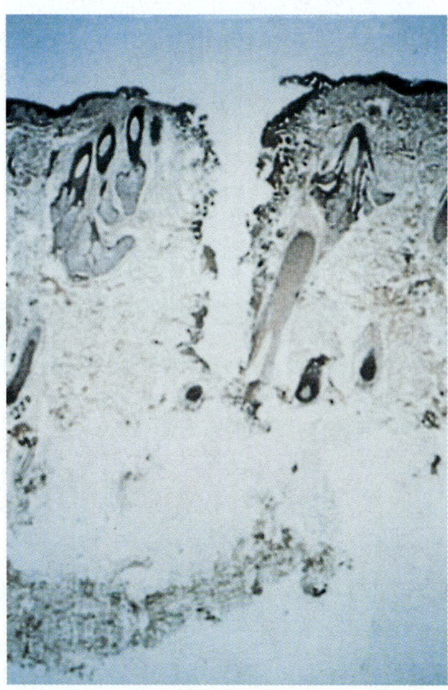

Figure 2–14. Histology of a hair transplantation recipient hole created by a high-power flashscanner CO_2 laser.

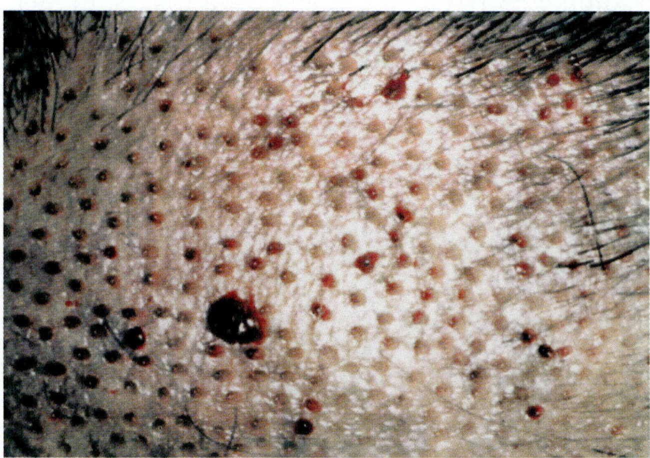

Figure 2–15. Preparation of hair transplantation recipient holes with a CO_2 flashscanner laser.

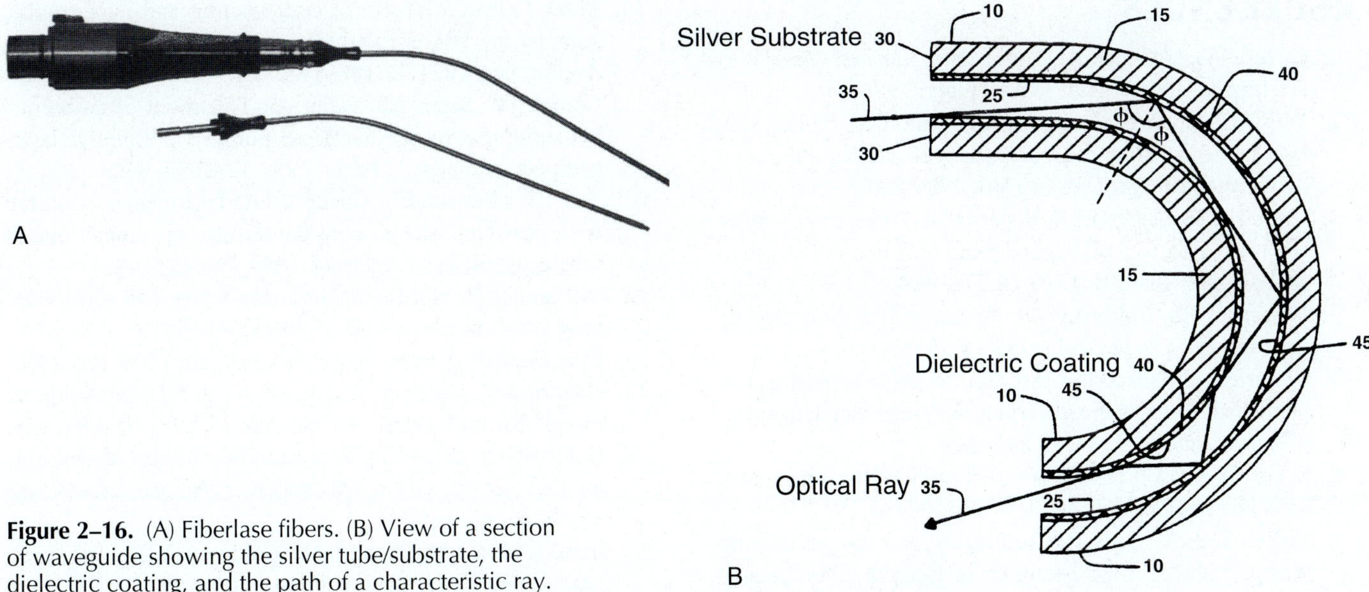

Figure 2–16. (A) Fiberlase fibers. (B) View of a section of waveguide showing the silver tube/substrate, the dielectric coating, and the path of a characteristic ray.

Airflow through the fiber is synchronized with laser activation so that the walls of the fiber do not heat up and the optical channel is kept clean of debris. Hollow fibers used for forehead surgery are slightly curved and can efficiently transmit laser radiation generated in the Surgipulse mode (transmissivity, 90%). Consequently, when the approximately 10-cm fibers are used in the near-contact mode (spot size, 1 mm), peak power densities of 200 W/mm^2 are attained on tissue with a CO_2 laser that generates pulses of 350 W peak power and pulse durations of 300 microseconds in the Surgipulse mode. This is high enough to produce char-free ablation. Longer fibers used in flexible endoscopy have a transmissivity closer to 80%.

BLEPHAROPLASTY

Blepharoplasty is performed with a non-scan-mode focusing handpiece with a traditional CO_2 laser in incisional mode. Focal length is 50 to 125 mm, and average power level is 5 to 7 W. Laser-assisted blepharoplasty is especially useful in conjunction with the transconjunctival technique because of the excellent hemostasis provided by the laser.

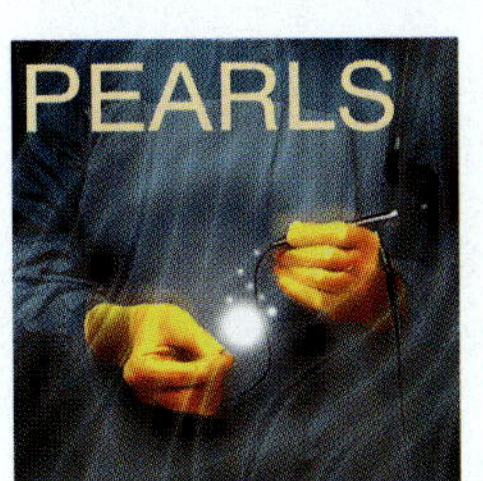

- Although using the painting mode with the Er:YAG laser is convenient for single-layer "lunchtime peeling," the scanning mode is widely considered the technique of choice for treating areas with thin skin, such as the neck and hands, and for treating deeper rhytids.

- Photothermolysis of very large blood vessels requires a pulse duration that is much longer than 1 millisecond, and the light energy should be further shifted to the red range. Flashlamps with various color filters can match the light to the chromophore (hemoglobin), and the pulse duration also can be varied to match the diameter of the blood vessel to be treated.

- Use of a laser with a flashscanner to create multiple small-diameter holes makes hair transplantation easier and faster and results in very natural-looking growth. There is no need to unplug residual tissue from the recipient hole.

- The small amount of thermal damage resulting from laser hair restoration allows nutrients to feed the implanted graft and also minimizes bleeding during the procedure, therefore there is less need for vasocontriction.

REFERENCES

1. Carruth JAS, McKenzie AL. *Medical Lasers: Science and Clinical Practice*. Bristol, Great Britain: Adam Hilger; 1986.
2. Walsh JT, Flotte TJ, Anderson RR, Deutsch TF. Pulsed CO_2 laser tissue ablation: effect of tissue type and pulse duration on thermal damage. *Lasers Surg Med.* 1989;8:108–118.
3. Green HA, Domankevitz Y, Nishioka NS. Pulsed carbon dioxide laser ablation of burned skin: in vitro and in vivo analysis. *Lasers Surg Med.* 1990;10:476–484.
4. Fitzpatrick RE, Goldman MP. Advances in carbon dioxide laser surgery. *Clin Dermatol.* 1995;13:35–47.
5. Weinstein C. Ultrapulse carbon dioxide laser removal of periocular wrinkles in association with laser blepharoplasty. *J Clin Laser Med Surg.* 1994;12:205–209.
6. Keller GS, Cray J. Laser assisted surgery of the aging face. *Facial Plast Surg Clin North Am.* 1995;3:319–341.
7. Lask G, Keller G, Lowe N, Gormley D. Laser skin resurfacing with the SilkTouch Flashscanner for facial rhytides. *Dermatol Surg.* 1995;21:1021–1024.
8. Chernoff G, Slatkine M, Zair E, Mead D. SilkTouch: a new technology for skin resurfacing in aesthetic surgery. *J Clin Laser Med Surg.* 1995;13:97.
9. Kauver ANB, Geronomus RG, Waldorf HA. Char-free tissue ablation: a comparative histopathological analysis of new carbon dioxide (CO_2) laser systems (abstract). *Lasers Surg Med.* 1995;16(Suppl 7):50.
10. Hruza GJ. Skin resurfacing with lasers. Fitzpatricks *J Clin Dermatol.* 1995;3:38–41.
11. Slatkine M, Mead D. Laser facial rejuvenation. US patent 5 611 795. 1997.
12. Ross EV, Greveling, Naseet GS, Skrobal M, Grevelink JM, Anderson RR. Dermal collagen shrinkage and remodeling following CO_2 laser resurfacing. *Lasers Surg Med.* 1996; Suppl 8:38.
13. Abergel RP, Schlaak CM, Garcia LD, Slatkine M, Mead D, Peng SK. The laser dermal implants: a new technique for preparation of autologous dermal grafts using SilkTouch laser technology. *Am J Cosmet Surg.* 1996;13:15–18.
14. Khatri K, Ross EV, Grevelink J, Anderson R. Comparison of Er:YAG and CO_2 lasers in wrinkle removal. *Lasers Surg Med.* 1997;Suppl 9:37.
15. Kaufman R, Beier Ch, Ochsendorf F, Hibst R. Er:YAG ablation of pigmented skin lesions. *Lasers Surg Med.* 1997; Suppl 9:37.
16. Anderson RR, Parrish RR. Selective photothermolysis: precise microsurgery by selective absorption of pulsed radiation. *Science.* 1983;230:524–527.
17. Eckhouse S. US patent 5 405 368.
18. Weiss RA, Weiss MA. New treatment for telangiectasia and venulectases: status of intense pulse light therapy. *Dermatol Surg.* 1996;22:7–11.
19. Geronemus RG. Treatment of spider telangiectases in children using the flashlamp-pumped dye laser. *Pediatr Dermatol.* 1991;8:61–63.
20. Alster TS. Improvement of erythematous and hypertrophic scars by the 585 nm flashlamp-pumped tunable dye laser. *Ann Plast Surg.* 1994;32:186–191.
21. Garden JM, Bakus AD, Paller AS. Treatment of cutaneous hemanigomas by the flashlamp-pumped pulsed dye laser: prospective analysis. *J Pediatr.* 1992;120:550–560.
22. Tan OT, Sherwood R, Gilchrest BA. Treatment of children with port-wine stains using the flashlamp-pumped pulsed tunable dye laser. *N Engl J Med.* 1989;320:416–421.
23. McDaniel DH, Mordon S. Hexascan: a new robotized scanning laser handpiece. *Cutis* 1990;45:300–305.
24. Zaias N. Method of hair depilation. US Patent 5 059 192. 1991.
25. Grossman M, Anderson R. Damage to hair follicles by normal mode ruby laser pulse. *J Am Acad Dermatol.* 1997;35:889–894.
26. Goldberg DJ, Littler CM, Wheeland RG. Topical suspension-assisted Q-switched Nd:YAG laser hair removal. *Dermatol Surg.* 1997;23:741–745.
27. Lask G, Elman M, Slatkine M, Waldman A, Rozenberg Z. Laser assisted hair removal. *Dermatol Surg.* 1997;23:737–739.
28. Finkel B, Eliezri Y, Waldman A, Slatkine M. Pulsed alexandrite laser technology for hair removal. *J Clin Laser Med Surg.* 1997;15:225–229.
29. Reid WH, McLeod PJ, Ritchie A, Ferguson PM. Q-switched ruby laser treatment of black tattoos. *Br J Plast Surg.* 1983;36:455–459.
30. Anderson RR, Margolis RJ, Watanabe S, Flotte T, Hruza GJ, Dover JS. Selective photothermolysis of cutaneous pigmentation by Q-switched Nd:YAG laser pulses at 1064, 532, 355 nm. *J Invest Dermatol.* 1989;93:28–32.
31. Goldberg D. Benign pigmented lesions of the skin: treatment with the Q-switched ruby laser. *J Dermatol Surg Oncol.* 1993;19:376–379.
32. Grevelink JM, Brennick JB. Hair transplantation facilitated by CO_2 laser enhanced flashscanner. Operative techniques in head and neck surgery. *Head Neck Surg.* 1994;5:278–280.
33. Villnow M, Slatkine M, Strobele B, Mead D. Megasession hair transplantation with a CO_2 laser flashscanner technology. *J Clin Laser Med Surg.* 1995;13:259.
34. Unger WP. Laser hair transplantation II. *Dermatol Surg* 1995;21:759–765.
35. Smithdeal CD. Carbon dioxide laser assisted hair transplantation. The effect of laser parameters on scalp tissue—a histologic study. *Dermatol Surg.* 1997;23:835–840.
36. Vila-Rovira R, Schleifer R. Recipient hole histologic study in CO_2 laser assisted hair transplantation. 5th Annual Meeting of the International Society for Hair Restoration Surgery. 1997; Barcelona, Spain.
37. Keller G. Method of laser cosmetic surgery. US patent 5 370 642. 1994.
38. Keller G, unpublished paper on endoscopy.
39. Morrow CE, Gu G. Fiberlase: a monolithic hollow waveguide. *SPIE Proceedings.* 1994;2131:18.
40. Gu G, Morrow CE. Reimaging and concentrating CO_2 laser beam from Fiberlase: a high-efficiency flexible hollow waveguide. *SPIE Proceedings.* 1996;2677:103.

CHAPTER 3

Laser Safety

JULENE E. CRAY

As lasers and related technology such as intense pulsed light sources proliferate, physicians who have cosmetic practices or who aspire to ward off the financial constraints of managed health care have had to broaden the scope of the topic of laser safety amid much confusing and inconsistent information from various sources. This chapter examines the regulatory agencies, standards, and guidelines relating to laser safety and provides some practical rules of thumb designed to protect patients, staff, and physicians involved with laser and light source technology. This chapter also addresses some of the related issues facing physicians in the new millennium, such as laser treatment by nonphysicians.

REGULATORY AGENCIES, STANDARDS, AND GUIDELINES

Physicians frequently instruct their staff members to become credentialed, certified, or licensed in the safe use of lasers. When staff members begin to search for this "diploma," the confusing semantics begin. Currently, there are no national, state, or local certification or licensing agencies to qualify the competency of surgeons, nurses, or technicians in the safe use of lasers.[1] Insurance companies and state medical boards, therefore, occasionally make uneducated and uninformed policies. Laser manufacturers inadvertently use the terms *credentialed* and *certified* loosely to describe the training provided to their customers. Any person (medical or nonmedical) who attends a workshop or training course sponsored by an agency or company receives a certificate of attendance, but these entities have no authority to license or credential. Rarely, especially in training sessions provided by laser companies, are there pretests, goals and objectives, adequate hands-on instruction, or posttests to guide and assess the educational progress of the participants.

The American National Standards Institute (ANSI) is the only nationally accepted, nonregulatory, nongovernmental agency that provides guidelines for the safe use of lasers in any setting—hospital, office, clinic, surgery center, or mobile unit. The ANSI standard Z136.3, *American National Standard for the Safe Use of Lasers in Health Care Facilities*, is the definitive source for implementing safety policies and procedures in virtually any laser program. The goal of this standard is to provide guidance for the safe use of lasers for diagnostic and therapeutic uses in health care environments. Although the standard is lengthy and comprehensive, implementation of its provisions is not difficult. It is used by the Occupational Safety and Health Administration (OSHA) and accreditation organizations such as the Joint Commission on the Accreditation of Healthcare Organizations (JCAHO). It is also used frequently as an exhibit reference during litigation.[2] Box 3–1 lists the addresses of ANSI and other

Box 3–1. Laser Safety Resources

American National Standards Institute (ANSI)
11 West 42nd Street
New York, NY 10036
212-642-4900

Laser Institute of America
(Secretariat for the ANSI Standard Z136.3)
12424 Research Parkway
Orlando, FL 32826
800-345-2737
407-380-1553

American Society for Laser Medicine and Surgery (ASLMS)
2404 Stewart Square
Wausau, WI 54401
715-845-9283

Occupational Safety and Health Administration (OSHA)
Bureau of National Affairs
1231 25th Street, NW
Washington, DC 20037
202-452-4200

Conference of Radiation Control Program Directors (CRCPD)
205 Capitol Avenue
Frankfort, KY 40601
502-227-4543
(Provides information on individual state requirements)

Association of Operating Room Nurses (AORN)
2170 South Parker Road, No. 300
Denver, CO 80231
800-755-2676

groups involved in laser safety. It should be noted that some of these other sources, such as the American Society for Laser Medicine and Surgery, also have practice guidelines and recommendations that are helpful in developing and implementing laser safety in a practice.

An important governmental agency is the Food and Drug Administration (FDA), which is involved in the classification of the lasers. In 1976, Congress directed the FDA (through the Medical Device Amendments to the FFDCA) to classify all medical devices[3] (Table 3–1).

The Center for Devices and Radiological Health (CDRH), a division of the FDA, regulates medical and radiation devices. This division's *Federal Laser Product Performance Standard* requires laser products to comply with adequate safety-related control features, labeling, and instructions for use.[4] This standard uses a class I to IV scheme, and most, if not all, medical lasers fall into the class IV category for laser hazard evaluation (see Table 3–1).

With the recent development of intense pulsed light nonlaser devices for laser-like applications (e.g., vascular anomalies, pigmented lesions, tattoo removal, and hair removal), the scheme employed to classify a system in

an office practice becomes significant in determining who can legally use these lasers and light sources. The intense pulsed light sources are not lasers because they are not monochromatic and the light is not collimated. Thus, even though the intense pulsed light (IPL) sources are considered class-II medical devices by the FDA, as are lasers, they are not categorized in the CDRH laser classification scheme. As a result, there has been much confusion about the safety of IPL devices as compared with true laser systems. For example, lasers *require* eye protection, whereas eye protection is only *recommended* for IPL sources. Furthermore, the states that have ruled on the issue of who can legally treat have only referred to lasers in their rulings thus far.

PRACTICAL SAFETY PRECAUTIONS
OCULAR SAFETY

The eye is the part of the human body most vulnerable to damage from a laser beam and may be exposed to either direct or reflected laser light. Lasers in the visible range of the electromagnetic spectrum can cause retinal damage,

Table 3–1. Classification Systems

FDA Medical Device Classification (Medical Device Amendments to the FFDCA)

Class	Definition	Examples
I	Devices subject to general controls	Crutches, stethoscopes
II	Devices subject to a performance standard to ensure safety and effectiveness	Lasers, intense pulsed light sources, syringes, chest tubes
III	Devices for life support and implants	Cardiac catheters

Federal Laser Product Performance Standard Classification

Class	Definition	Hazard	Control Measures
I	Very-low-power laser systems	Safe to vision	Warning sign at access panel of laser
II	Visible light-emitting lasers that do not have enough power to injure someone accidentally	Retinal injury if viewed directly for $>$ 0.25 seconds	Protective housing, warning signs
IIIa	Medium-power lasers— visible light—does not cause injury if viewed directly	Retinal injury if energy focused in the eye	Engineering controls, protective eyewear, administrative controls, warning signs
IIIb	Medium-power lasers that can cause accidental injury if viewed directly	Not safe for brief viewing of direct beam or scattered specular radiation	Same as class IIIa
IV	Most medical lasers, high-power lasers that produce a hazardous diffuse reflection resulting in a skin hazard	Not safe for brief viewing of direct or scattered radiation	Same as class IIIa

whereas those in the ultraviolet and infrared ranges can cause corneal damage. In two independent studies, one by the FDA based on a review of 134 laser accidents recorded from 1984 to 1989 and another from Rockwell based on a review of 272 laser accidents occurring between 1964 and 1994, eye injuries were the most common injury and constituted 75 and 73% of all injuries, respectively.[5] Yet, eye injury is completely preventable if the proper protection is provided for patients and staff members.

The ANSI sets forth guidelines that specify the design and safety features of protective eyewear for physicians, staff members, and patients. Included are such specifications as the required optical density of the material and the permissible occupational exposure limits. Everyone in the laser suite must wear the appropriate wavelength-specific eyewear. Glasses or goggles that lack permanent labels indicating appropriate wavelength and optical density should *never* be considered adequate protection. Moreover, protective eyewear should be located outside the door to the laser suite so that anyone entering the room may also have protection. In addition, patients and all personnel should be instructed never to look directly into the laser beam or at laser light being scattered from reflective surfaces.

Many eyewear manufacturers offer an entire range of appropriate glasses and goggles for laser safety. Frequently, glasses and goggles are supplied along with the laser. In addition, prescription lenses can also be ground into the safety eyewear.

When a patient undergoes cutaneous laser surgery of the periorbital region, he or she must wear appropriate eye shields in place of protective glasses or goggles. It is important for the eye shield to fit securely and to cover the entire orbit to prevent ocular injury from laser energy. Many of the eye shields commercially available today are not designed for laser use. Plastic eye shields and corneal protectors, especially those made in darker colors, should not be used because they may actually facilitate significant laser damage to the eye.[6]

The ANSI's *American National Standard* also recommends all health care personnel who are working with the laser systems have a baseline eye examination before starting work, immediately after a suspected abnormal laser exposure to the eye, and at the termination of work with lasers.

ENVIRONMENTAL SAFETY
Preoperative Safety

A laser safety checklist is an excellent guide for preparation before a laser procedure. It is essential to set up all equipment in a manner that is conducive to ease of use and safety. A laser safety officer, as defined by the *American National Standard*, should be appointed. Sometimes this is the physician by default if he or she has not designated a person from the office staff. The laser safety officer is ultimately responsible for all facets of safe use of the laser.

A laser warning sign should be posted at every entrance to the laser suite. The *American National Standard* recommends the sign be consistent with suggested regulations. The sign should be removed after the laser procedure is completed. In addition, all windows to the outside of the room, whether to a street or to an internal hallway, should be covered from the inside with a shade or dark towel to block any transmission of the laser beam.[7]

When the laser is not in use, the key should be removed and kept in a secure location to prevent unauthorized use of the laser. The laser system and ancillary equipment should be checked to ensure they are working properly before bringing the patient into the room. This may require checking the alignment of the laser beam for some wavelengths.

All standard electrical precautions and fire precautions should be maintained. Sterile water or saline should be available in the room to douse a small fire if necessary. A fire extinguisher should also be readily accessible.

Intraoperative Safety

Patients should *never* be prepped with flammable solutions such as alcohol or chlorhexidine gluconate (e.g., Hibiclens). If the procedure involves working around the hairline, there should be no remnants of flammable hair products such as hairspray or gel. Appropriate eye shields should be applied to the patient. The patient's teeth should also be protected from enamel damage by a stray laser beam.

The laser system should be put on standby whenever the laser is not being aimed at the target tissue. One staff member in the room should be designated to make sure that the standby switch is on. Clear communication is essential between the operator and the person at the laser. Sometimes this is the same person. The foot pedal should be used only by the person directing the laser beam. In addition, the laser foot pedal should be isolated to prevent accidental firing of the laser. If another foot pedal is in close proximity, this increases the risk of an accidental firing.

If the patient requires general anesthesia, only nonflammable anesthetic gases should be used. The anesthesiologist should be well aware of all the necessary precautions used to prevent airway fires. Drapes and gowns should be flame retardant. The area surrounding the target site should be kept clear of dry 4 × 4's and other flammable materials or reflective instruments, as well being surrounded by wet towels or wet 4 × 4's. Proper smoke evacuators should be in place, and masks should be worn during laser procedures in which plume is created.

Postoperative Safety

Once the procedure is completed, the patient's eye shields should be removed. If scleral shields are used, an eye-wash solution should be administered to help remove the ocular lubricant. Dressings or ointments are applied, if needed, and any instructions or precautions should be reviewed with the patient before the patient is discharged.

The laser equipment should be cleaned, the handpieces removed, and smoke evacuator filters disposed of properly (see section on smoke evacuation). The safety checklist should be completed and signed. The laser log book also should be completed for the particular parameters of the case. It should be noted that the Safe Medical Devices Act of 1990 makes it mandatory for health care personnel to report device-related adverse events to the manufacturer and to the FDA.[8]

Smoke Evacuation

The amount of laser plume formed during a procedure depends on the type of application to tissue, the wavelength of the laser being used, the duration of exposure, the power of the energy, and the technique. There have been numerous studies over the past 10 years with varying results as to the presence of viable biologic materials in laser plumes. However, recent studies conclude that laser vapors can contain infectious viruses, viral genes, or viable cells and may promote the spread of infections or tumor cell dissemination.[9] Medical personnel working with lasers are exposed to the risk of inhaling the laser plume if proper smoke evacuation and filter systems are not used appropriately. A high-volume smoke evacuation system must be used, and the tip of the suction device should be placed within 1 cm of the area being lased. The use of close-fitting laser masks that filter out particles smaller than 0.1 μm can greatly reduce the risk of respiratory exposure to the plume. In addition, universal precautions for blood-borne material should be followed in the management of the laser plume. All disposable tubing and filters should be discarded in a red biohazard waste receptacle.

ADMINISTRATIVE ISSUES

A successful and comprehensive laser safety program takes planning and the involvement of the entire staff, from the person answering the phone to the physician. Accidents can only be prevented by an educated staff and an administrative policy that supports continual efforts toward a safe laser environment. Laser safety and training programs are outlined in detail in the *American National Standard*. The training should provide staff members with a complete understanding of all the requirements for the safe use of lasers.

Policy and procedures should be written and enforced by a designated laser safety officer, whether there is one laser in the practice or five. Establishing control measures, implementing a safety protocol, instituting a medical surveillance program, and identifying action items to ensure a safe laser environment are all imperative administrative tasks.

LASER TREATMENT BY NONPHYSICIANS

Since 1994, laser and light source hair removal has been increasingly seen in the cosmetic and medical arenas. This has presented new challenges to practitioners and regulators alike. Laser manufacturers opened laser hair-removal spas staffed with nonmedical technicians who perform laser (class-IV) treatments without a physician on site. Physicians have started appealing to their medical boards for some type of control and regulatory directives. Because most state medical boards admittedly are reactive and not proactive, this situation was not addressed until very recently. More than two thirds of the states still have not taken a position on who can legally treat patients with a laser. For example, in New Jersey, only licensed physicians are allowed to do hair removal with lasers; in California, registered nurses, physician assistants, and licensed physicians can legally do the procedure; and in Arizona, there has been no ruling.

In some states, if nurses use lasers for any application (e.g., removal of spider veins, tattoos, pigmented lesions, or hair) without the appropriate documentation required by the state nursing board and are involved in a medical/legal dispute, they could be fined for practicing medicine without a license in some states (a misdemeanor that can include a $1000 fine and/or 6 months in jail). The physician in whose practice this occurs could be charged as an accomplice, and his or her license could also be in jeopardy. It is imperative that any person in a practice who treats with a laser adhere to state regulations, that is, scope of practice, licensing requirements, standardized procedures, etc. For example, a registered nurse in California can treat with lasers provided the Standardized Procedure Guidelines found in the California Administrative Code, Chapter 14, Article 7, Sections 1470–1474 are signed and adhered to by both the nurse and the physician.[10] Medical assistants may not use lasers because they are not specifically included in the "technical supportive services" section of the regulations (Title 16, California Code of Regulations, Section 1366).[5]

Also extremely important in this equation is the physician's malpractice insurance carrier, which can determine who is covered under the physician's policy. It is essential to know if the person doing the treatments is outside his or her scope of practice. An insurance company cannot insure someone who is illegally practicing outside the scope of his or her license. For instance, an X-ray technician may be treating leg veins with a laser—under the physician's supervision and with a letter from the insurance company that states that it will cover the technician for the use of lasers. However, under the "scope of practice" in the license or certification that the state grants the technician, there may be no mention of the word *laser*. This issue remains complex, and solutions are constantly changing throughout the United States. Health practitioners cannot ignore the importance of this issue in the overall success and safety of their laser programs.

CONCLUSION

Physicians and their staffs have an enormous responsibility with regard to the safe use of laser systems in their practices. Ongoing education through networking and workshops, teamwork, and communication are vital to the overall success of a laser program. As technology advances at almost overwhelming rates, health providers will continue to be challenged to keep laser safety a priority. Every person involved in a laser program must "take ownership" and be committed to the safest laser environment possible.

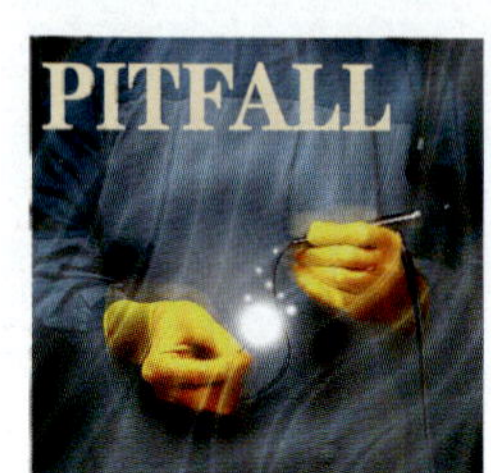

- Currently, there are no national, state, or local certification or licensing agencies to qualify the competency of surgeons, nurses, or technicians in the safe use of lasers. Anyone who attends a workshop or training course sponsored by an agency or company receives a certificate of attendance, but these entities have no authority to license or credential.

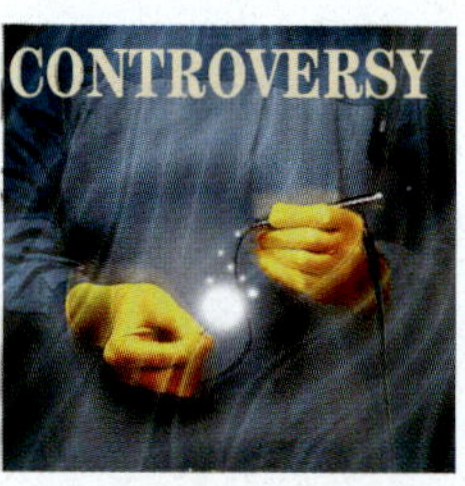

- There has been much confusion about the safety of intense pulsed light (IPL) devices as compared with true laser systems. For example, lasers *require* eye protection, whereas eye protection is only *recommended* for IPL sources. Furthermore, states that have ruled on the issue of who can legally treat have only referred to *lasers* in their rulings thus far.

- There is no unanimous decision about whether laser plumes contain viable biological materials. Recent studies conclude that laser vapors can contain infectious viruses, viral genes, or viable cells and may promote the spread of infections or tumor cell dissemination. Universal precautions for blood-borne material should be followed in the management of the laser plume.

- Laser manufacturers have opened laser hair-removal spas staffed with nonmedical technicians who perform laser (class-IV) treatments without a physician on site. Many states still have not taken a position on who can legally treat patients with a laser.

REFERENCES

1. Pfister J. Education and credentialing in laser surgery. In: Arndt K, Dover J, Olbricht S, eds. *Lasers in Cutaneous and Aesthetic Surgery.* Philadelphia: Lippincott-Raven; 1997:446–472.

2. Smalley P. Laser safety management: hazards, risks, and control measures. In: Alster T, Apfelberg D, eds. *Cosmetic Laser Surgery,* 2nd ed. New York: Wiley-Liss; 1999:305–319.

3. American National Standards Institute. Z136.3, *American National Standard for the Safe Use of Lasers in Health Care Facilities, Section E3, Medical Devices,* 1996.

4. American National Standards Institute. Z136.3, *American National Standard for the Safe Use of Lasers in Health Care Facilities, Section 1.2.2,* 1996.

5. Arndt K. Hazards associated with the use of lasers. In: Arndt K, Dover J, Olbricht S, eds. *Lasers in Cutaneous and Aesthetic Surgery.* Philadelphia: Lippincott-Raven; 1997:402–406.

6. Ries W, Clymer M, Reinisch L. Laser safety features of eye shields. *Lasers Surg Med.* 1996;18:309–315.

7. Ball K. *Lasers: The Perioperative Challenge.* St. Louis: Mosby; 1990.

8. Cray J, Pica-Furey W, Kulick M. Laser safety for aesthetic procedures: surgical and nonsurgical. In: Kulick M, ed. *Lasers in Aesthetic Surgery.* New York: Springer; 1997:1–16.

9. Zeigler B, Thomas C, Meier T, et al. Generation of infectious retrovirus aerosol through medical laser irradiation. *Lasers Surg Med.* 1998;22:37–41.

10. Bradford T. No standardized procedure—go to jail! *Forum J.* 1995;2:1–6.

Selective Photothermolysis

PAUL C. LEVINS

Advances in laser theory and practice over the past two decades have brought many types of lasers to the attention of patients and physicians. More recently, the scientific principles of laser therapy have been applied to new and exciting areas such as skin resurfacing and hair removal.

This chapter briefly surveys the history, reviews the relevant scientific principles, and outlines laser applications in various relevant fields: skin resurfacing, vascular lesions, hair removal, pigmented lesions, and photodynamic therapy. The importance of the theory of selective photothermolysis is emphasized as the key element moving laser surgery from a "slash-and-burn" approach to an elegant method of selective destruction of targeted tissue.

HISTORICAL BACKGROUND

Lasers (light amplified by stimulated emission of radiation) were first envisioned by Einstein and brought to fruition after the production of radar and the maser, which was a precursor to the laser that used microwave energy instead of light. Maiman reported the first working laser, a ruby laser at 694 nm, in 1960.[1]

Clinical impetus for the medical applications of lasers was provided by the late Dr. Leon Goldman, who pioneered use of the ruby laser first on cadaver skin, later on convicts, then later on willing patients.[2] Other lasers were then developed, including the continuous-wave (CW) carbon dioxide (CO_2) laser by Patel and the argon ion laser that emitted light mainly at 488 and 514 nm, wavelengths strongly absorbed by blood. This led to the use of the CW argon laser for the treatment of vascular lesions, specifically birthmarks such as port-wine stains (PWSs) and other vascular malformations and hemangiomas (now the preferred nomenclature).[3]

The immediately recognized clinical issue that led to development of the theory of selective photothermolysis was the scarring that occasionally happened after CW or shuttered argon laser treatment, especially in the pediatric population. Thus, in 1981 Anderson and Parrish[4] published a theoretical and clinical construct in which they identified a chromophore (oxyhemoglobin), chose a wavelength of light (577 nm) that absorbed selectively over other chromophores (melanin), and selected a pulse width (versus CW irradiation) that was appropriate for the diameter of the vessel.

Elegantly modeling human skin with the PWS as the ultimate clinical target, Anderson and Parrish worked through theoretical, animal, and normal human skin models before finally establishing parameters that led to the clearing of PWSs in humans using pulsed laser light without scarring. Publishing in *Science* in 1983, they named this construct *selective photothermolysis*.[5]

BASIC PRINCIPLES

Selective photothermolysis is based on skin optics, the presence (or absence) of biological chromophores (i.e., molecules or substances that absorb electromagnetic radiation, more specifically in this case radiation in the visible spectrum, commonly known as light), and the proper selection of pulsed or continuous laser energy to be selectively absorbed, leading to destruction of the target tissue(s). The key characteristics of most lasers are monochromaticity, coherence, brightness, and occasionally high power. Laser media include chemical, electrical, optical, or semidiode sources. The key breakthroughs were understanding the chromophore absorption spectrum–laser wavelength connection and the concept of the thermal relaxation time of biological structures.[6]

Chromophore Absorption and Laser Wavelengths

The relationship between the range of chromophore absorption and laser wavelength is relatively self-explanatory: red objects reflect red light but absorb other wavelengths. As long as competition from competing chromophores is minimized, then the target object can be destroyed without damaging surrounding tissue such as the epidermis, dermis, collagen, elastin, dermal appendages, and fat. Melanin is the chief chromatophore of skin, but it also includes carotenoids, porphyrins, urocanic acid, and occasionally exogenous pigments. For example, to successfully lase a specific area of skin that is heavily melanized (e.g., a mole), it is necessary to select a wavelength that is absorbed by melanin but not the other chromophores to avoid collateral damage in the surrounding skin.

Because the depth of penetration of light depends on wavelength (short wavelengths scatter more; longer wavelengths do not and penetrate more deeply), theoretical and, later, clinical data were generated that precisely localized the depth of penetration of light into and through human skin. The next breakthrough was realizing that the temporal and spatial localization of the absorption of photons (leading to heat production) could be used to selectively destroy targets of known absorption spectra, depth, and size. This was based on the law of Grotthus-Draper, which states that only absorbed pho-

tons create biological effects, whether photothermal, photochemical, or photomechanical.

Thermal Relaxation Time

From this realization emerged the concept of *thermal relaxation time*. This is the concept that if adequate photons, and therefore heat, are delivered faster than it takes for 50% of the heat energy to dissipate to surrounding structures, then targeted structures are quickly heated and destroyed without damage to nontargeted structures. This was an advantage over the early CW laser beams that slowly heated targeted structures and then, by default, nontargeted structures, leading to scarring, pigmentary changes, and other unwanted effects.

Through a series of experiments, researchers, including the Anderson and Parrish group at the Wellman Photomedicine Research Laboratories, have worked out the putative thermal relaxation times for various subcellular organelles (e.g., melanosomes), cells (melanocytes), vessels (venules), skin (epidermis), and appendages (hair).[4,7] As an experimental and clinical construct, the theory of selective photothermolysis has revolutionized and revitalized the world of cutaneous laser surgery and reinvigorated the pioneering work of Leon Goldman.

CURRENT CLINICAL APPLICATIONS

Following is a brief survey of the current clinical applications of selective photothermolysis, which compartmentalizes the laser realm by type of treatment or lesion rather than by laser system—although both approaches offer advantages. Understanding lasers by medical (i.e., dermatologic) diagnoses mirrors historical development and is the approach used here.

Skin Resurfacing

The theory of selective photothermolysis, combined with the clinical efforts of experienced laser physicians such as Laurence David and Gary Lask, led to approaches to ablating skin that was sun-damaged and precancerous, sun-damaged, or aging (e.g., solar elastosis and rhytids, encompassing intrinsic and extrinsic aging). Various CO_2 lasers, including the CW, "chopped beam" CW, and pulsed and ultrapulsed versions, as well as further developments such as the erbium:yttrium-aluminum-garnet (Er:YAG) laser, have led to multiple competing laser systems—each of which promises different, albeit efficacious, results.[8–10]

More data and clinical experience are needed before establishing optimal parameters for the ablation of solar elastosis, rhytids, and other aspects of cutaneous aging without resultant scarring. Although studies support ~ 1 millisecond as the thermal relaxation time of skin (i.e., epidermis), further sophisticated analyses are necessary before arriving at reproducible, safe, and effective parameters.

Vascular Lesions

The theory of selective photothermolysis is most dominant in the treatment of lesions containing hemoglobin and its variants (e.g., oxyhemoglobin, deoxyhemoglobin). Port-wine stains in all age groups are best treated by pulsed dye lasers emitting 577 to 595 nm, with pulse widths ranging from 450 microseconds to 1.5 milliseconds. Depending on pulse width, energy fluences range from 4 to 12 J/cm^2. Multiple treatments using contiguous, nonoverlapping pulses have resulted in eventual complete clearing of lesions. Adverse effects are generally minimal and transient, including purpura lasting for 7 to 14 days, occasional hyper- or hypopigmentation, and, extremely rarely, true scarring.[11–13]

Analogously, facial telangiectasias can be treated similarly in one or two treatments with complete resolution. Enlarged vessels below the umbilicus, however, remain problematic, and various pulsed laser and nonlaser light sources have been used to eradicate "leg veins," ranging from small, red telangiectatic mats to larger, bluish phlebectasias. Drawbacks include pigmentary change, lack of efficacy, and the need for multiple treatments. Additional rigorous, controlled studies are needed.

Hair Removal

The latest test of the theory of selective photothermolysis is laser hair removal (although some systems use nonlaser pulsed high-intensity light sources; see Chapter 25). Because some of the cells of the hair follicle contain melanin, they are logical targets for laser ablation. All lasers are capable of ablating hair—the variables are how long the effect lasts, the side effects, and the risk of pigmentary changes.

Several laser and nonlaser systems have been reported to ablate hair with minimal adverse effects. Multiple, randomized, controlled studies are required to determine the optimal methods of permanent or nonpermanent laser hair removal.[14,15]

Pigmented Lesions and Tattoos

Pigmented lesions encompass a wide variety of cutaneous hyperpigmented lesions: nevomelanocytic nevi (generally not accepted as amenable to laser treatment in the United States currently), lentigines, hamartomas, melasma, postinflammatory hyperpigmentation, tattoos, and assorted other hypermelanotic lesions. Lentigines respond well to the therapies listed here for tattoo removal (as well as to cryotherapy), but the preferred modality is the 532-nm neodymium:YAG (Nd:YAG) laser at 3 J/cm^2.[16]

In general, tattoos respond quite well to nanosecond-domain pulses (Q-switched) of green (532 nm), red (694 nm), or infrared (1064 nm) laser radiation, as well as alexandrite (755 nm) and pulsed green (510 nm) laser radiation; rarely, nonspecific CO_2 thermal ablation can produce cosmetically acceptable scars, replacing the offending tattoo.[17]

Miscellaneous Lesions

Miscellaneous lesions such as striae, scars, and verrucae have all been treated with pulsed dye lasers, sometimes relying on the theory of selective photothermolysis (e.g., striae, scars) and sometimes relying on nonspecific thermal ablative effect (e.g., verrucae).[18] Again, individual case reports and small series are promising, but larger studies with scientific controls are needed to establish efficacy.

PHOTODYNAMIC THERAPY

The theory of selective photothermolysis again plays a role in determining the appropriate source of radiation (laser energy at 633 nm versus broad-spectrum visible light) based on chromophore targets and depth of lesion targeted. Photodynamic therapy offers a viable option for many malignancies superficial enough to absorb energy from laser and nonlaser light sources. See Chapter 34 for more detailed information about this type of therapy using light energy.

CONCLUSION

Selective photothermolysis is a theoretical and practical laser construct that has been experimentally and clinically successful in skin resurfacing and hair removal, as well as in the treatment of vascular and pigmented lesions and tattoos. To date, the theory of selective photothermolysis has certainly broadened and enhanced the world of lasers first envisioned by Albert Einstein and subsequently made into reality by the work of physicians and researchers the world over. However, further studies are needed to fully explore the potential as well as the limitations of the theory of selective photothermolysis.

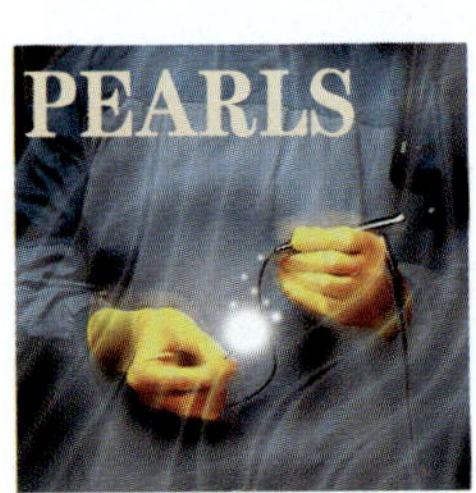

- The occasional scarring after CW or shuttered argon laser treatment of children was one of the clinical issues that led to the development of the theory of selective photothermolysis.
- A laser's ability to deliver wavelengths quicker than a tissue's thermal relaxation time reduces collateral damage and represents a huge advantage over the early CW lasers that slowly heated targeted structures and then, by default, nontargeted structures.
- The theory of selective photothermolysis is most dominant in the treatment of lesions containing the chromophore hemoglobin and its variants (e.g., oxyhemoglobin, deoxyhemoglobin).

- All lasers are capable of ablating hair, but lasers vary in how long the effect lasts, side effects, and risk of pigmentary changes.

REFERENCES

1. Maiman T. Stimulated optical radiation in ruby. *Nature.* 1960;187:439.
2. Goldman L, et al. Pathology of the effect of the laser beam on the skin. *Nature.* 1963;197:912.
3. Mulliken, Young, et al. *Vascular birthmarks: hemangioma and malformations.* Philadelphia: W.B. Saunders; 1988.
4. Anderson R, Parrish J. Microvasculature can be selectively damaged using dye lasers: a basic theory and experimental evidence in human skin. *Lasers Surg Med.* 1981;1:263.
5. Anderson R, Parrish J. Selective photothermolysis: precise microsurgery by selective absorption of pulsed radiation. *Science.* 1983;220:524.
6. Dierickx C, et al. Thermal relaxation of port-wine stain vessels probed in vivo: the need for 1–10 millisecond laser pulse treatment. *J Invest Dermatol.* 1995;105:709.
7. Anderson R, et al. Selective photothermolysis of cutaneous pigmentation by Q-switched Nd: YAG laser pulses at 1964, 532, and 355 nm. *J Invest Dermatol.* 1989;93:28.
8. Bernstein L, et al. The short- and long-term side effects of carbon dioxide laser resurfacing. *Dermatol Surg.* 1997;23:519.
9. Khatri K, et al. Comparison of erbium:YAG and CO_2 lasers in skin resurfacing. *Lasers Surg Med Suppl* 1997;9:37.
10. Ross E, et al. Long-term results after CO_2 laser resurfacing: a comparison of scanned and pulsed systems. *J Am Acad Dermatol.* 1997;37:709.
11. Tan O, et al. Treatment of children with port-wine stains using the flashlamp-pulsed tunable dye laser. *N Engl J Med.* 1989;320:416.
12. Grevelink J, et al. Pulsed laser treatment in children and the use of anesthesia. *J Am Acad Dermatol.* 1997;37:75.
13. Van der Horst C, et al. Effect of the timing of treatment of port-wine stains with the flash-lamp-pumped pulsed dye laser. *N Engl J Med.* 1998;338:1028.
14. Grossman M, et al. Damage to hair follicles by normal-mode ruby laser. *J Am Acad Dermatol.* 1996;35:889.
15. Dierickx CC, Grossman MC, Farinelli WA, Anderson RR. Permanent hair reduction after ruby laser exposures. *Arch Dermatol.* 1998;134:837–842.
16. Kilmer S, et al. Treatment of epidermal pigmented lesions with the frequency-doubled Q-switched Nd:YAG laser: a controlled, single impact, dose-response, multicenter trial. *Arch Dermatol.* 1994;130:1515.
17. Taylor C, et al. Treatment of tattoos by Q-switched ruby laser: a dose response study. *Arch Dermatol.* 1990;126:893.
18. Hruza G. Laser treatment of warts and other epidermal and dermal lesions. *Dermatol Clin.* 1997;15:487.

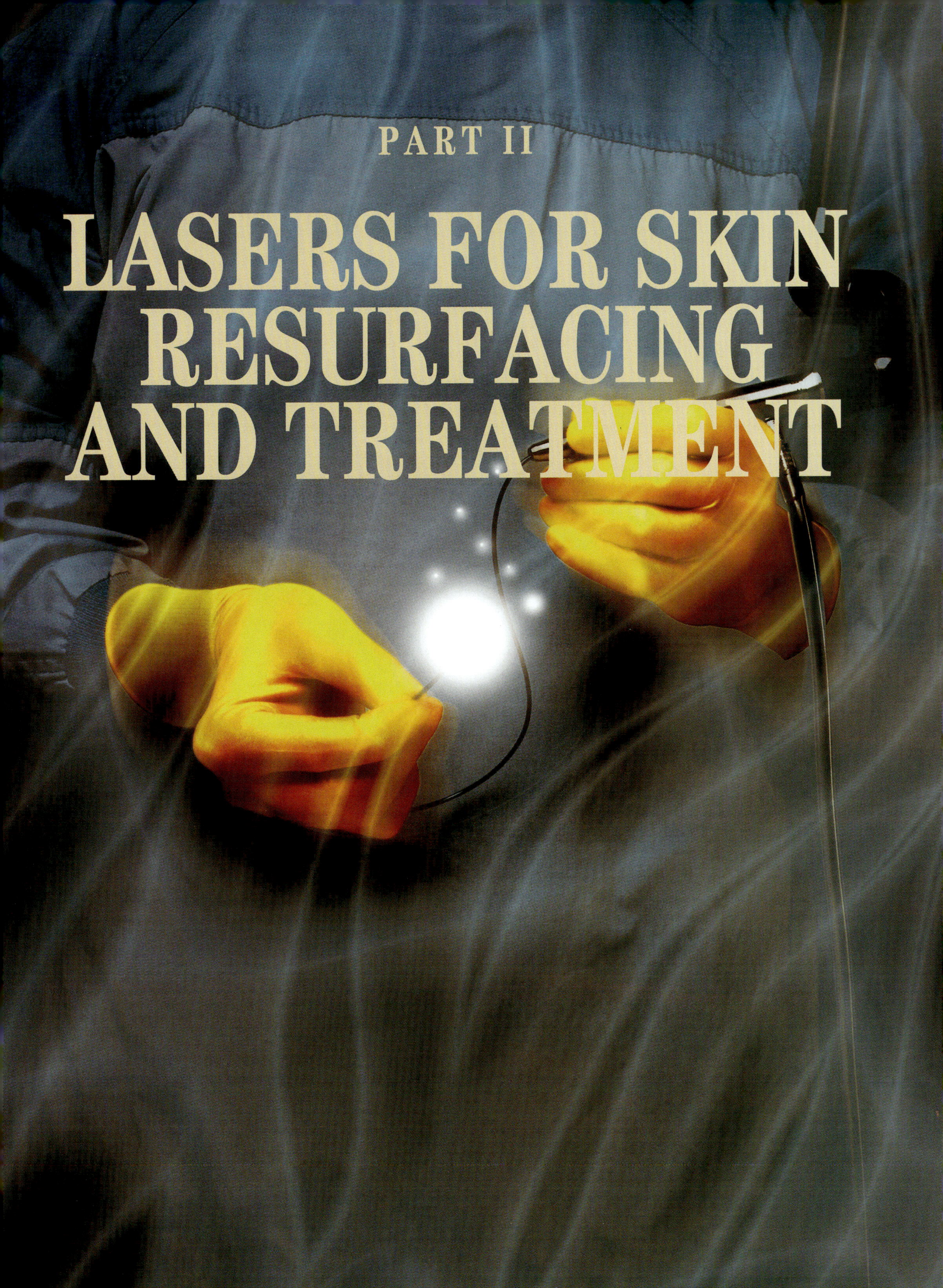
PART II
LASERS FOR SKIN RESURFACING AND TREATMENT

CHAPTER 5

Laser Resurfacing: An Overview

GREGORY S. KELLER AND VICTOR G. LACOMBE

Laser resurfacing inspires physicians and patients more than any other laser application. Although not without complications, laser skin rejuvenation has developed into an effective modality for both tightening the skin and restoring skin texture. Although the desire to rejuvenate aging skin dates back to ancient times (Cleopatra used abrasion techniques and chemical peel solutions to maintain her beauty), using laser light to restore aging skin is also the first completely new resurfacing technique to emerge in thousands of years.

Of course, there are many nonmedical uses for lasers, and more are being developed every day, but it is in medicine that lasers realize their greatest potential. In skilled hands, lasers enable us to rejuvenate even severely damaged skin with predictable results (and a predictable incidence of complications). The effective use of lasers, however, requires knowledge of skin, medicine, technique, and pre- and postoperative care.

Laser resurfacing began in the 1970s with continuous wave (CW) carbon dioxide (CO_2) laser systems. Originally, these systems were used for "laserbrasion" of tattoos, actinic chelitis, and hyperkeratoses, as well as for the vaporization of small lesions such as syringomas and warts. During the 1970s and 1980s, CO_2 laser systems were tried for the treatment of aging skin, but the results were variable and inconsistent.

By the early 1990s, newer high-energy pulsed CO_2 lasers and "flash scan" technology were used by gynecologists for ablative procedures and by otolaryngologists for laser-assisted uvulapalatoplasty procedures. Subsequently, dermatologists began to use these systems for rapid lesion ablation and abrasion of skin. The aesthetic use of these instruments by dermatologists, plastic surgeons, and facial plastic surgeons for wrinkle removal, acne scar repair, and facial skin rejuvenation soon followed.[1–12]

Improvements in laser instrumentation occurred simultaneously with the aging of the baby-boomer generation that had experienced early sun exposure in an atmosphere with a diminished ozone layer. Many of the members of this generation were and are eager to retard the aging process. As a result, the first generation of high-energy CO_2 resurfacing lasers received overwhelming acceptance by patients and physicians alike.

The use of laser systems for skin exfoliation and rejuvenation quickly eclipsed all other medical uses of lasers. Most manufacturers of laser systems rushed to produce high-energy CO_2 resurfacing lasers, most of which are capable of achieving acceptable results.

Although laser resurfacing techniques are relatively simple compared with chemical peeling and dermabrasion and do not produce hypopigmentation as consistently, many physicians who entered the field of laser resurfacing did not have experience with chemical peeling or dermabrasion, nor did they have experience with laser systems. As in other types of surgery, with the increasing numbers of laser resurfacing cases came complications such as scarring, hypopigmentation, hyperpigmentation, prolonged erythema, nonhealing wounds, and infections.

From these complications came modifications in techniques and lasers that were designed to avoid these problems while maintaining a high degree of treatment efficacy. This second generation of lasers and techniques uses laser scanners, newer laser types [Erbium:yttrium-aluminum-garnet (Er:YAG), FeatherTouch, nanosecond CO_2], and lighter resurfacing methods that strike a balance between superb results and avoidance of complications.

Adjunctive techniques are used with laser resurfacing to diminish the amount of laser energy or number of laser "passes" that are delivered to an area. For instance, botulinum toxin (e.g., Botox) can be used to paralyze rhytids that are caused by muscle contraction (e.g., crow's feet). A lighter resurfacing with a newer-generation laser can then tighten and/or smooth the skin. Alternatively, a filler substance (such as Isologen—autologous fibroblast injections) can be used to fill acne scars or perioral rhytids. The laser then can be used to further smooth and freshen the skin.

The future holds promise for even greater improvements in laser resurfacing. Several laser systems are now available for treatment of the skin dermis without injury to the epidermis. One of the primary advantages of these new systems is that they require no recovery time. While they are reported to result in a degree of skin contraction, thus far these systems have produced minimal efficacy in terms of removing wrinkles and altering skin texture. Their promise, with improvements, is to provide a method of resurfacing all patients, even those with darker skin pigmentation.

CO_2 LASER RESURFACING
SCIENTIFIC PRINCIPLES

Treatment strategies and second-generation CO_2 laser systems are derived from scientific principles that need to be completely understood by the laser surgeon if he or she is to use the machinery safely and to its best advantage. Most properties and tissue effects of any laser system can be understood in terms of the wavelength, pulse, delivery spot size, and repetition rate of the laser. Box 5–1 summarizes common laser terminology.

Box 5–1. Laser Terminology

Power = watts (W)

Power density = W/cm^2

Energy = joules (J) = watts $\times$ time (s)

Energy density = J/cm^2

Ablation threshold = 5.5 J/cm^2 (for a CO_2 laser)

Pulses/second = hertz (Hz)

The CO_2 lasers emit laser light at a wavelength of 10,600 nm. This wavelength is highly absorbed by tissue water. When laser light is absorbed by tissue, the light energy is absorbed mainly by tissue water and converted into localized heat. The skin tissue targeted by the laser must be heated to approximately 100°C for it to be vaporized (the desired result). A crater of vaporization is created where the laser beam strikes. Next to this crater, a zone of thermal injury is produced as the heat from the laser dissipates into the surrounding tissue. Where tissue is not heated sufficiently for vaporization to occur, thermal damage of a reversible or irreversible nature results.

Because most tissue contains large amounts of water, the CO_2 laser has a shallow penetrance. The tissue water in the superficial layers of skin absorbs the laser energy before it can penetrate very deeply. This shallow penetrance is the reason that the CO_2 laser is a relatively precise surgical tool compared with lasers that penetrate more deeply [e.g., the neodymium (Nd):YAG, KTP (potassium titanyl phosphate), ruby, and alexandrite lasers]. Vaporization of the targeted tissue occurs at the surface where the laser is aimed.

The *pulse* of a laser can be described in terms of its energy (or power output), delivery time, repetition rate, and delivery spot size. Variations in these parameters are what makes each manufacturer's machine different.

The total *power output* of a laser is described in watts. An allocation of this total power is delivered in a focused beam of a given diameter. In a laser that is turned on for a fairly long period of time (CW), the amount of power delivered to a given spot over that time period is its *power density* (W/cm^2).

The longer that a given power (wattage) of laser light is delivered, the greater the energy density the spot receives. Thus 1 watt delivered over 1 second results in 1 joule of energy density. This concept can be expressed mathematically as follows: joules (J) = watts (W) $\times$ time (t). The "energy" that results is the power multiplied by the time in which it is delivered.

The density of energy delivered in a given laser pulse can be expressed mathematically in joules per square centimeter (J/cm^2). To produce a larger spot size with the same energy density delivered over the same time period requires that the power be increased by the square of the previous spot size. It requires four times the power to obtain 16 J/cm^2 of energy density with an 8-mm-diameter spot than with a 4-mm-diameter spot $\left[16/\left(\frac{1}{2}d\right)^2 \times \pi\right]$. As the need for a larger diameter laser spot increases, a more powerful (and more expensive) laser is required, but this allows a given area of skin to be treated more quickly.

This is important because tissue ablation depends on the energy density delivered. Tissue "perceives" laser light in the form of energy density and reacts accordingly. The *ablation threshold* for skin is the amount of energy density required to vaporize skin with a minimal amount of thermal damage. The ablation threshold for skin using the CO_2 laser is approximately 5.5 J/cm^2. To perform predictable skin resurfacing with a minimal amount of thermal damage, a laser must achieve this ablation threshold.

There is also a time factor involved. Large amounts of power delivered over short time periods cause less damage than small amounts of power delivered over long time periods, despite the fact that they result in the same energy. For instance, 1 W of power delivered over 1 second will cause more tissue injury than 1 kW of power delivered over 1 millisecond, despite the fact that both combinations result in 1 J of power.

The optimal time period for laser light delivery to any tissue is related to its *thermal relaxation time* (the period of time required for the target tissue to release 50% of its absorbed heat). The temperature of the skin surrounding the vaporized area must decrease rapidly after its exposure to the laser in order to avoid thermal damage. For skin, the thermal relaxation time is thought to be under 1 millisecond, although longer times have been used successfully by some manufacturers (e.g., Laserscope, Luxar). Shorter laser light delivery times (in the nanosecond range) are thought to further reduce thermal damage. The short-pulsed CO_2 (Tru-Pulse) laser uses this operating principle.

Most high-power, high-energy pulsed lasers use 3- to 5-mm spots to deliver approximately 7 to 10 J/cm^2. In contrast, flash scanning (as popularized by Sharplan) is a technique whereby a very small laser spot (0.1–0.2 mm) is scanned at a very rapid rate over a given area. The flash scanner, using a tiny spot (a 0.1-mm spot requires 90 times less power than a 3-mm spot to achieve a given energy density), enables a normal CW laser to achieve the energy levels of a larger, more expensive machine.

High-energy pulsed lasers deliver energy in "pulse packages," and manufacturers often describe a single pulse of their laser's energy in terms of the pulse package without specifying the delivery time. A high-energy pulsed laser setting may be in millijoules or joules. Because tissue effects are most related to energy density, it is often useful to convert this "pulse energy" into energy density. This allows comparisons of the tissue effects of various lasers. The conversion formula for pulse energy to energy density is

Pulse energy$/0.00785 \times$ (spot diameter)^2 = energy density

or

$$J/0.00785 \times d^2 = J/cm^2.$$

Because each of these pulses contains a specific amount of energy, the only way to increase the power delivered to a tissue is to increase the number of pulses delivered per unit time. In this event, watts become a measure of the rate of energy delivery as well as a measure of power: $W = J/cm^2/s$. A laser set at 3 W repeats pulses faster (and delivers more of its power to tissue) than one set at 1 W. The operator can appreciate this by listening to the increase in the laser's staccato, machine-gun–like delivery rate.

The *duty cycle* of a laser is the percentage of time that the laser is turned on during a pulse cycle. The laser *delivery rate* is the number of pulses delivered per unit time. Pulse delivery rates may be expressed in terms of pulses per second, or hertz (Hz). A delivery rate of 1 pulse/s = 1 Hz. A faster delivery rate enables a surgeon to resurface a given area more quickly. A laser of greater total power will be able to deliver faster pulses and can produce a larger spot size (beam diameter) of a given energy at a similar delivery rate than a less powerful laser. A larger beam diameter (e.g., 10 rather than 3 mm) per pulse at the same delivery rate is another factor that allows the surgeon to complete a resurfacing job in an area of the face or neck more quickly.

TISSUE EFFECTS

Unavoidably, the CO_2 laser thermally damages tissue around the boundaries of tissue that it vaporizes. The spread of thermal damage beyond the zone of vaporization (or ablation) is termed the *scatter of heat. Forward scatter* (into the tissue away from the operator), *side scatter*, and *backscatter* (toward the operator) are all terms used to describe the direction of heat spread.

This zone of thermal injury is thought to be an important part of the dynamic reaction of heat-induced inflammation and repair within the skin tissue that the laser initiates. Collagen shrinkage and an immediate heat-induced tissue contraction result and can be seen without magnification.

The spread of thermal damage produces two zones of coagulation. Next to the zone of vaporization is a zone of tissue that is irreversibly damaged. Adjacent to this is a zone of tissue that is reversibly damaged and has the potential to recover. Before reepithelialization and resolution of crusting, the zone that is irreversibly damaged must be extruded from the wound. Before resolution of erythema, the zone of irreversible thermal damage must heal, and the resulting inflammatory reaction must resolve. Zones of injury that are reversibly damaged can necrose if they become hypoperfused or

infected. If the inflammatory reaction is prolonged— because of infection, hypersensitivity, individual skin reaction, or extension of thermal damage from vigorous treatment—complications such as scarring, hyperpigmentation, hypopigmentation, and prolonged erythema may result.

A laser wound, like any other wound, goes through phases of inflammation, proliferation, and remodeling. During the stage of inflammation, platelets secrete growth factors that attract macrophages and neutrophils. These cells clean up debris, and the macrophages secrete transforming growth factor-beta (TGF-β) to attract fibroblasts. Fibroblasts secrete collagen and extracellular matrix. This is the beginning of the proliferative phase. In addition to the effects of collagen formation, reepithelialization occurs from progenitor cells in hair follicles and sweat glands.

Activated fibroblasts continue to produce new collagen (neocollagenesis) for 3 months after laser resurfacing. This may explain the continued contraction of the skin that is seen even after wound healing appears to be complete. Neocollagenesis results in an increased deposition of collagen in the Grenz layer of the dermis.

Despite this, the tightening and contraction of skin that occurs with laser resurfacing are not fully explained. Immediate and long-term skin contracture may occur by different mechanisms. Many authors attribute immediate skin contraction to heat-induced collagen shrinkage. Collagen shrinkage and denaturation are known to occur at tissue temperatures above 55°C. The skin surrounding the vaporized area undergoes a sufficient heat transfer after high-energy laser treatment to reach 55°C, and an immediate skin contraction is seen that has been attributed to collagen shrinkage.[13] Long-term skin contraction appears to be due to dynamic, laser-induced cellular reactions. The long-term increase in type-1 collagen and elastic tissue and the rearrangement of abnormal cytologic architecture in "laser-braded" tissues are probably the result of these cellular reactions. Recently, Smith et al[14] have demonstrated that a superficial laser abrasion of skin with atypia produced by nitrogen mustard resulted in a remodeling of skin. New fibroblasts and myofibroblasts, clearly different from the old fibroblasts, produced a restoration of normal skin architecture associated with an increase in smooth muscle actin, factor XIIIa, and vimentin-positive cells in the papillary dermis.

Two distinct types of contraction occur after laser abrasion of tissue.[15] The initial skin contraction occurs immediately perpendicular to the relaxed skin tension lines (much like the folding of an accordion). Later, a more powerful contraction (13–16%) occurs perpendicular to the relaxed skin tension lines.

GENERAL PRINCIPLES OF RESURFACING

While specific methods of resurfacing with specific lasers are covered in subsequent chapters, certain principles of resurfacing are common to all laser systems. First and foremost, contemporary resurfacing is a balance between achieving optimal results and avoiding complications (Table 5–1). Laser surgeons have specific goals for specific treatments, such as the restoration of a more youthful texture to skin, the resolution of rhytids, the elimination of age spots and keratoses, and the flattening of acne pits and scars.

Laser surgeons also endeavor to avoid such complications as scarring, dyschromias (i.e., hyperpigmentation and hypopigmentation), undesirable alterations in skin texture (e.g., focal thinning, thickening, and unevenness), prolonged erythema, herpetic and bacterial infections, hypertrophic scars, hypersensitivity reactions, and postinflammatory telangiectasias. Erythema that is prolonged beyond the usual duration (4–6 weeks) or that is

Table 5–1. Potential Complications of Laser Resurfacing

Desired Results	Potential Complication(s)
Wrinkle removal	Dyschromias
Skin texture rejuvenation	Scar
Age spot removal	Skin texture abnormalities
Keratoses resolution	Prolonged erythema
Acne pit improvement	Infection

firmer or a deeper red than usual seems to be a central element of these complications. (Prolonged erythema implies prolonged inflammation, as a result of either infection, allergic reaction, host response, or overzealous resurfacing. It can be an early warning of the onset of scarring or postinflammatory hyperpigmentation.)

Minimizing complications requires careful preoperative management that takes into account all predisposing factors. Patient selection should be rigorous, and as many patients with potential for complications as possible should be weeded out. The preoperative discussion of risks and benefits should be extensive and individually based.

Conservative perioperative treatment techniques are the trend in laser resurfacing. Less energy and fewer passes are used today than in years past. Adjunctive treatments such as botulinum toxin, collagen, and Isolagen are used to modify lines, wrinkles, scars, and pits so that the laser resurfacing can be more conservative.

Postoperative care arguably is the most important part of laser resurfacing, once the decision to treat has been made. Watchful follow-up to detect potential complications is an extremely important part of patient care, implying frequent physician visits during the immediate postoperative phase. Box 5–2 shows the triad for successful laser resurfacing.

Box 5–2. Triad for Successful Laser Resurfacing

Preoperative selection
Perioperative technique
Postoperative care

PREOPERATIVE MANAGEMENT

The first phase of preoperative management is patient selection. The conventional wisdom that a surgeon's income is made by the patients that he or she treats—while his or her reputation is made by the patients that he or she refuses—is nowhere more true than in laser resurfacing. Patients who are at higher risk for complications should only be treated with their clear understanding and documented consent regarding the risks and benefits of

Table 5–2. Case Selection

Conditions Favorable for Resurfacing	Conditions Unfavorable for Resurfacing
Rhytids	
Static rhytids	Dynamic rhytids
Skin laxity	Structural laxity
Acne	
Shallow pits	Deep pits
Stretchable pits	Ice picks
	Accutane
Skin Pigmentation	
Fitzpatrick I–II	Fitzpatrick IV–VI
Deep rhytids	Asians
(makeup accentuates)	Melasma
	Hyperpigmentation

surgery. See Table 5–2 for factors that affect preoperative patient selection.

Realistic expectations on the part of the patient and physician are essential. Advertising and publicity in newspapers and other media have led many patients to expect more from laser resurfacing than can ever be achieved, especially with reasonable risk.

Rhytids

An important part of patient evaluation is the establishment of the type and quality of the rhytids. "Wrinkles at rest," or *static rhytids*, respond quite well to laser resurfacing (with the exception of rhytids on the chin). We believe that chin rhytids are difficult to treat to the point of disappearance without producing skin texture changes. A moderate resurfacing followed by the addition of filler material such as collagen or Isolagen can give excellent results.

"Wrinkles in motion," or *dynamic rhytids*, that occur with or are accentuated by muscle contraction, particularly around the periocular and glabellar areas, usually are not completely eradicated. To eradicate dynamic rhytids with laser resurfacing alone implies the use of extremely aggressive—and therefore risky—resurfacing.

Botulinum Toxin   Concomitant or preoperative treatment with botulinum toxin applied to the periocular and glabellar areas to change a dynamic rhytid into a static rhytid is an extremely useful technique. Less laser energy and fewer passes are required to treat the now static rhytid than would have been required were the rhytid not deactivated by the botulinum toxin.

Prior to injecting the botulinum toxin, the patient must be told that the treatment will need to be repeated every 4 to 6 months for the rhytids to remain adynamic. A eutectic mixture of local anesthetics (EMLA cream, Astra Pharmaceuticals) is then placed over the areas to be treated, and ice is applied to help prevent bruising and to alleviate pain. A vial of botulinum toxin is then diluted with 3 mL of diluent so that each 0.1 mL contains approximately 0.33 units of botulinum toxin. For glabellar lines, the patient is then asked to frown, and 0.1 mL of the dilute solution are placed in each corrugator fold and in the procerus above brow level. Usually 12 to 15 units are used (0.4–0.5 mL). For periocular lines, the patient is asked to smile. Each orbicularis fold is injected with 0.1 mL of the dilute solution. Approximately 9 to 15 units are injected (0.3–0.5 mL). The injections are placed just lateral to the bony orbital rim, below the brow, and above the malar eminence to avoid the zygomatic and levator muscles.

Resurfacing versus Surgery   The question of whether a patient should have a surgical procedure or whether laser resurfacing will suffice is often debated. This decision is based on whether the rhytid is due to skin wrinkling and aging or there is structural sagging and "folds." A modest degree of skin contraction and a great deal of skin rejuvenation can be achieved with the laser. Dramatic results can be achieved in patients with loose skin, sun damage

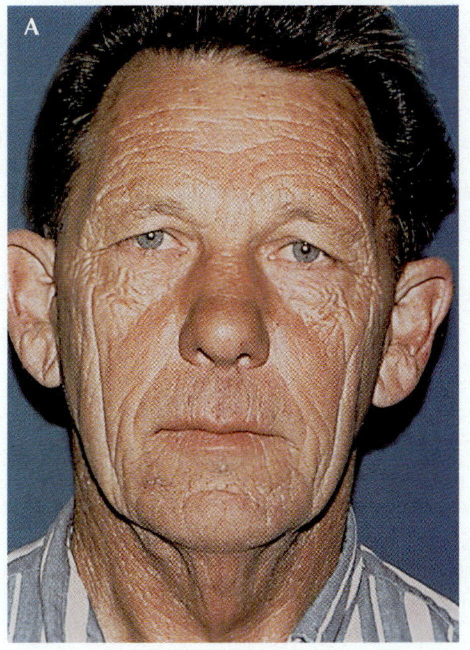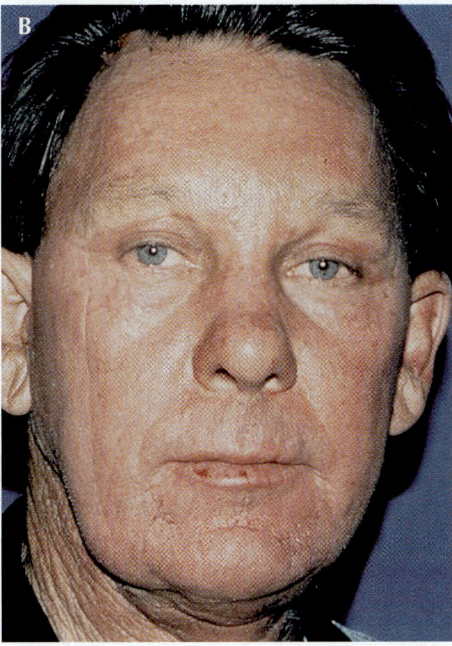

Figure 5–1. (A) Preoperative view of patient undergoing CO_2 laser skin resurfacing. The patient has severe sun damage. (B) Postoperative result. Dramatic results are achieved routinely in patients such as this. (From Keller G, Rawnsley J, Cutcliffe B, Watson J. Erbium:YAG and carbon dioxide laser resurfacing. *Facial Plast Surg Clinics North Am.* 1998;6:167–181.)

(Fig. 5–1), or rhytids (Fig. 5–2). Patients with mild to moderate *skin laxity* rhytids (wrinkles, not folds or sagging structures) are good candidates for resurfacing.

Patients with *structural laxity* rhytids or folds generally will be disappointed with laser resurfacing. Nasolabial folds, fallen malar pads, jowls, platysma muscle bands, neck sagging, brow ptosis, and other structural components of facial aging are best treated with surgical correction. Patients with both structural laxity and skin laxity often require combination treatment with skin resurfacing and surgery. In addition, patients with severe skin laxity also may require rhytidectomy to excise some skin, followed by laser resurfacing to further tighten and rehabilitate the skin.

Whether to perform the surgical treatments sequentially or simultaneously is a matter of debate. If performed sequentially, the surgeon must decide whether to perform the rhytidectomy or the resurfacing first. Most

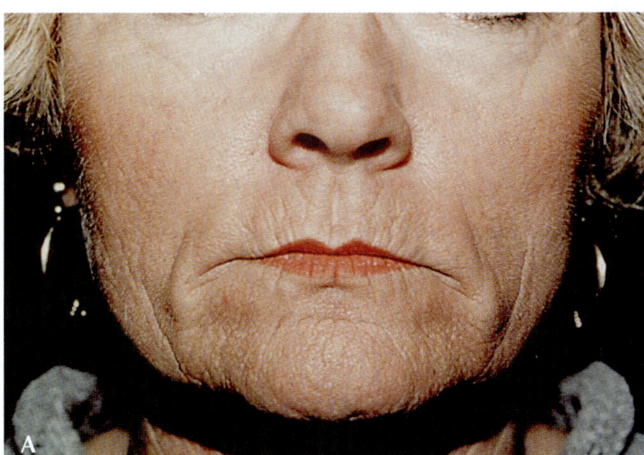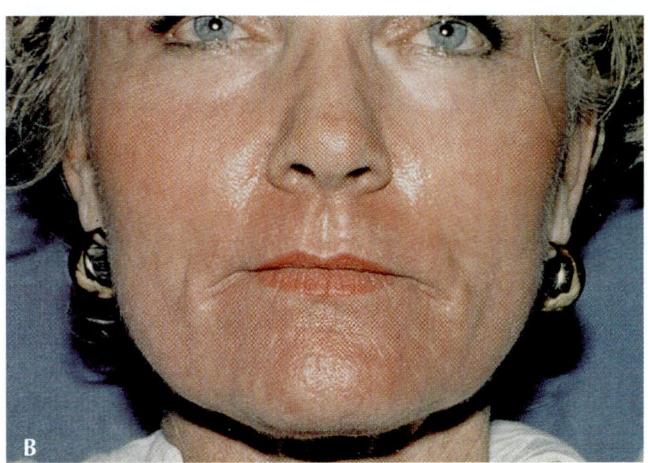

Figure 5–2. (A) Preoperative view of patient undergoing CO_2 laser skin resurfacing. The patient is an ex-smoker with perioral rhytids. (B) Postoperative result. While there is a dramatic improvement in the perioral rhytids, some rhytids are left.

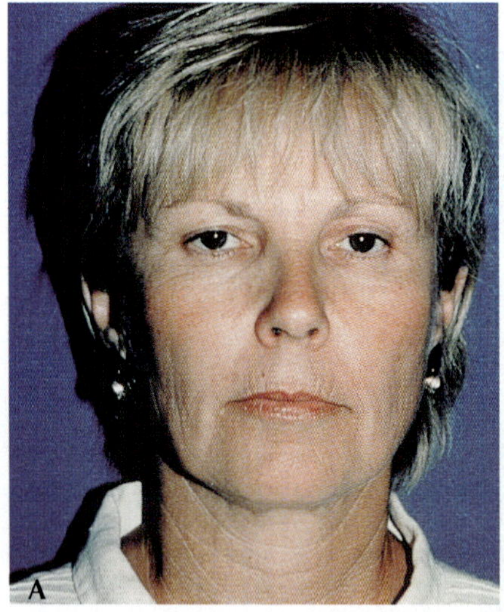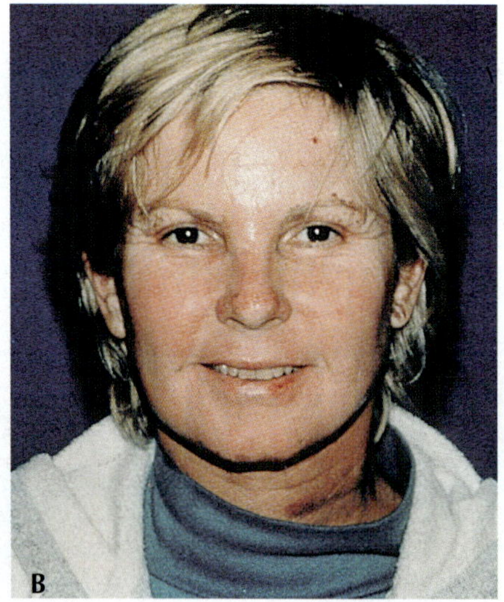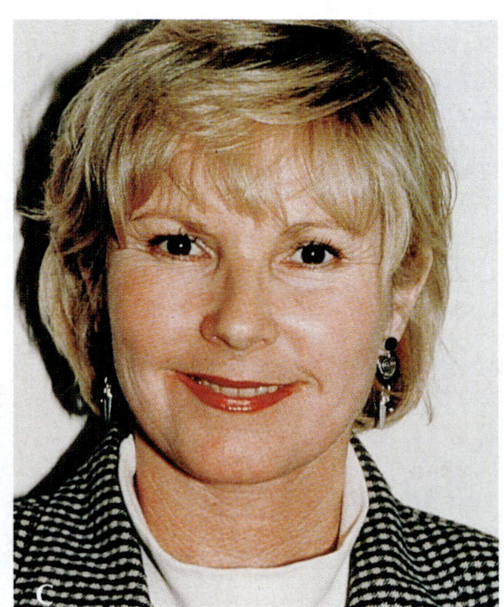

Figure 5–3. (A) Preoperative view of patient undergoing CO_2 laser skin resurfacing and simultaneous neck lift. She has skin laxity of the face that is more significant than her structural laxity. In addition, she has structural laxity of the neck. (B) Postoperative result at 3 weeks. (C) Postoperative result at 6 months. Full-face laser resurfacing and structural neck lift are commonly performed together.

surgeons will "set the structure" and perform rhytidectomy prior to rehabilitating the skin with the laser. This provides the surgeon with the opportunity to tighten the skin further and eliminate rhytids, as well as to recondition the skin after the rhytidectomy. There is no reason, however, not to resurface the skin first and then perform rhytidectomy.

Many surgeons will not resurface facial skin over an area where they have lifted, despite many articles reporting the safety of simultaneous resurfacing and rhytidectomy. Some surgeons, however, will resurface the central face during a rhytidectomy, particularly if the area has had a deep plane lift or if the area to be resurfaced has not been undermined.[15,16] We agree with published articles that report that conservative resurfacing (central) may be performed but carries an increased risk and requires a prolonged healing period.[17] One rationale for the increased risk is that resurfacing of a skin flap releases mediators of inflammation that cause increased flap edema and decreased microvasculature in the flap. Because of these concerns, we use the Er:YAG laser for this purpose.

Generally, the forehead may be resurfaced over an endoscopic forehead lift. The forehead is usually undermined subperiosteally, resulting in an extremely resilient segment of elevated skin, muscle, and periosteum. Areas of the face and neck that are not lifted may also be resurfaced. An example of this is the combination of a segmental neck lift with a full-face laser resurfacing (Fig. 5–3).

Acne

Acne pits and scars are improved with laser resurfacing. The Er:YAG laser may be preferable to the CO_2 laser because the Er:YAG laser has an absorption peak at about 2990 nm, which is specific for collagen and scar. Treatment with this laser can improve acne scars by about 40 to 60%. Combination treatment with autologous fibroblast injections can improve this result to 80%. The fibroblasts are best injected postoperatively, although excellent results can be obtained with pretreatment with autologous fibroblasts followed by resurfacing. Ice pick scars generally are not improved with either laser or autologous fibroblasts. These must be removed with an 0.8- to 2-mm punch prior to or simultaneously with resurfacing.

Accutane for acne treatment reduces the number of sebaceous elements and hinders reepithelialization after laser resurfacing. Most surgeons wait for at least a year after discontinuance of Accutane prior to resurfacing. We also evaluate the status of the patient's sebaceous elements by asking whether he or she sweats in the facial area with exercise or has skin that is consistently dry. If there is doubt as to whether the patient has regenerated sufficient sebaceous elements to reepithelialize the laser wound, laser resurfacing is postponed. We also make sure that any active acne has been controlled prior to laser resurfacing. The fact that acne is quiescent preoperatively does not guarantee that an outbreak will not complicate the postoperative period, although it provides a good indication.

Skin Pigmentation and Dyschromias

A patient's skin type is classified by the Fitzpatrick rating (Table 5–3). Patients with Fitzpatrick skin types III to VI are considered by most surgeons to be at greater risk for dyschromias than patients with Fitzpatrick skin types I and II. The higher the skin type, the more prone the patient is to develop hyperpigmentation and hypopigmentation.

Asian patients are extremely prone to dyschromias, as are patients of Spanish descent. Most of these patients will develop hyperpigmentation after laser resurfacing. While most, but not all, episodes of postinflammatory hyperpigmentation are transient and eventually will respond to topical treatment modalities, many are either long lasting or permanent. Furthermore, patients with Fitzpatrick

Table 5–3. Fitzpatrick Skin Types

Type	Skin Characteristics
Type I	White, never tans, always burns
Type II	White, sometimes tans, usually burns
Type III	White, tans at average rate, sometimes burns
Type IV	Moderate brown, tans with ease, rarely burns
Type V	Dark brown, tans very easily, very rarely burns
Type VI	Black, tans very easily, does not burn

skin types IV to VI who develop postinflammatory hyperpigmentation eventually may develop delayed permanent hypopigmentation up to a year and a half after the initial treatment.[18]

In our practice, patients with type I and II skin and patients with lighter type III skin are considered candidates for CO_2 or Er:YAG laser resurfacing. Patients with darker type III skin and type IV skin are not considered good candidates for such laser resurfacing. Patients with darker skin types must be willing to wear cover-up makeup after laser resurfacing if a dyschromia should occur. A reasonable darker-skinned candidate for laser resurfacing is an older woman who has rhytids that are so deep that makeup only accentuates the rhytids (Fig. 5–4). Such patients often wear makeup at all times. Flattening

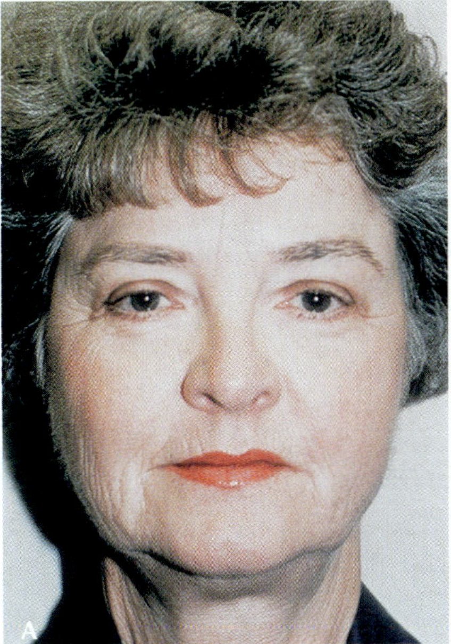
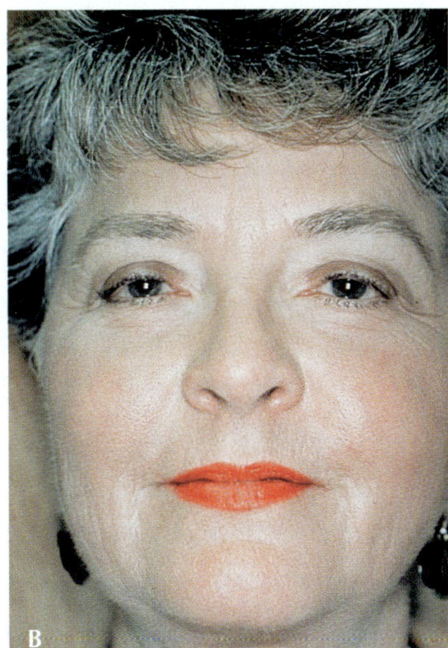

Figure 5–4. (A) Preoperative view of patient undergoing CO_2 laser skin resurfacing. Her rhytids are accentuated by her makeup. (B) Postoperative result. Note that the patient's appearance with makeup is markedly enhanced.

of the rhytid will enable the patient to look better while wearing makeup, even in the event of a permanent dyschromia. Discussion of the risks and benefits of laser resurfacing with these patients is essential.

Patients with melasma and those with previous episodes of hyperpigmentation related to hormone shifts or the use of birth control pills are at increased risk for dyschromias following laser resurfacing. A careful history is essential to screen for these patients. A history of such incidents as hyperpigmentation following an acne out-break or hypopigmented spots following trauma will alert the surgeon to potential problems.

When in doubt about whether to resurface a patient, a test spot is reasonable. A test spot of about 2×2 cm is not entirely predictive of whether dyschromia will occur, but it can demonstrate how inflamed the patient's skin will become in response to the laser's thermal challenge.

PRETREATMENT

Pretreatment in laser resurfacing is a matter of debate. Very few studies are available that document conclusively the benefit of any form of pretreatment, with the exception of pretreatment for herpetic breakout. Because of the lack of consensus, it seems difficult to advocate pretreatment as a "standard of care." In our practice, we use pretreatment with skin agents and sunscreens to help "train" the patient to maintain his or her skin and to establish a lifelong program of aftercare. We do not refuse to treat a low-risk patient who has not undergone pretreatment because of a lack of desire, money, or time. Nor have we noted a difference in complications or results between our pretreated patients and those not undergoing pretreatment.

Herpetic Infection

One study that documents the need for pretreatment is a cohort study performed by Perkins et al.[19] These authors indicated that patients with a negative history of herpetic infection (cold or canker sores) had a 6.6% chance of developing herpetic infection without pretreatment. With a positive history of herpetic infection, 50 to 100% of patients presenting for resurfacing developed herpetic infection without pretreatment. These authors advocate using 2400 mg of acyclovir per day beginning 48 hours preoperatively and continuing for 14 days.

We have seen two episodes of breakthrough herpetic infection in postoperative resurfacing patients who were taking acyclovir and one breakthrough herpetic infection in a postoperative patient taking valacyclovir. These patients responded to famaciclovir, which has a longer half-life (20 hours) and better absorption. No scarring resulted, but one of these patients had erythema that lasted for 4 months. Most physicians use some form of prophylactic treatment for herpes. Acyclovir, valacy-clovir, and famaciclovir are all acceptable modes of pretreatment therapy.

Bacterial Outbreaks

The use of systemic antibiotics to prevent bacterial out-breaks is a matter of debate. Apfelberg[20] has surveyed plastic surgeons and has documented that 60% use prophylactic antibiotics, and 40% do not. In this same survey, Apfelberg documented that 90% of plastic surgeons used prophylactic antiviral therapy. We use prophylactic antibiotics on a routine basis. With resistant streptococcal and staphylococcal infections in the community, the benefits for us of preemptive treatment seem to outweigh the risks.

Acid Treatments and Melanin Suppresive Agents

Pretreatment of the skin with retinoids, glycolics, and other light acid treatments, as well as melanin suppressive agents, is also a matter of active debate.[1,3,9,10,20–24] Advocates of pretreatment believe that it enhances skin healing by increasing fibroblast activity and skin vascularity to the area treated.[23] They also feel that by thinning the stratum corneum and reducing the potential for hyperkeratotic change, fewer laser passes may be required, thus producing less thermal injury.

Dyschromias

Proponents of pretreatment to prevent dyschromias use Kligman's formula (Retin-A, hydroquinone, and hydrocortisone in equal parts), glycolics with hydroquinones, or "pigment creams" (consisting of kojic, lactic, salicylic, and azelaic acids). They feel these treatments prevent hyperpigmentation by "shutting down the melanosome" in its tyrosine cycle that produces melanin. Detractors of pretreatment believe that the effective penetration of pretreatment agents is only intraepidermal. According to their arguments, the melanosomes that are shut down are only those in the epidermis, and these are removed with the first pass of the laser.[25] Detractors also suggest that increasing the vasculature to the skin with retinoids may cause more postoperative telangiectasia and erythema, in addition to "irritating the skin" preoperatively. Some also believe that the laser treatment itself stimulates fibroblasts to a maximal degree.

CONTRAINDICATIONS

Many conditions, habits, or skin characteristics place patients at increased risk for complications of laser resurfacing (Box 5–3). These conditions need to be evaluated preoperatively, before a decision is made on whether the patient is an acceptable candidate for the procedure. A severe form of any one relative contraindication or the presence of several contraindications usually will disqualify a patient. If a patient with a relative contraindication is accepted for resurfacing, the procedure should be performed conservatively.

Relative Contraindications

Patients who have received chemotherapy, radiation to the skin, or previous dermabrasion or chemical peeling (particularly if they have atrophic skin) have relative contraindications for laser resurfacing. People who smoke marijuana or tobacco and people with diabetes also have diminished wound-healing capacities and must be evaluated carefully. People who tend to form hypertrophic

---

Box 5–3.   Contraindications to Laser Resurfacing

Relative Contraindications

   Previous chemotherapy

   Previous irradiation to the skin

   Previous resurfacing procedures

   Smoking

   Diabetes

   Hypertrophic scarring

   Active acne

   Unstable personality

   Dyschromia

   Skin hypersensitivities

   Dissatisfaction with aesthetic surgery

   Eyelid laxity

Absolute Contraindications

   Systemic lupus erythematosus

   Scleroderma

   Keloids

   Recent Accutane use

   Unwillingness to use sun protection and sun avoidance

   Unwillingness to assume resurfacing risks

---

scars present a relative contraindication for laser surgery, but patients who have hypertrophic scars in body areas that are prone to hypertophic scars (e.g., breast, sternum) may be accepted if they otherwise scar normally. People with active uncontrolled acne, unstable personality types, dyschromias, skin hypersensitivities (to makeup, sunscreens, or topical treatments), and those who are unhappy with previous aesthetic surgery also represent relative contraindications to laser surgery.

When in doubt as to whether to treat a patient with a relative contraindication, the use of a test spot is helpful. A 2 $\times$ 2-cm test patch will not be entirely predictive of the overall laser result but can give some information about how a patient's skin will react to resurfacing.

Absolute Contraindications

Absolute contraindications for laser surgery at our clinic include patients who have systemic lupus erythematosus or scleroderma and those who form keloids. We do not resurface patients who are unwilling, reluctant, or nervous about assuming the risks of resurfacing. Another absolute contraindication to laser surgery is a patient's refusal or reluctance to protect herself or himself from the sun for a period of 6 months following laser resurfacing.

PERIOPERATIVE MANAGEMENT

At present, many types of CO_2 laser resurfacing systems are available. They differ greatly in their pulse widths, energy delivery systems, pulse energies, and manner of application. Most of these systems are covered individually in subsequent chapters. However, one major recent advance in perioperative laser care is the laser scanner. Laser scanners allow the laser surgeon to apply laser energy with uniformity and speed. These machines produce a pattern of laser pulses or energy (e.g., a square or a rectangle) that can be tailored to fit a given area of the face.

Most scanning systems can be set to overlap pulses to varying degrees. The degree of overlap is referred to as the density of the scan (Fig. 5–5). Usually 0% density implies no overlap, or laser spots that are barely touching.

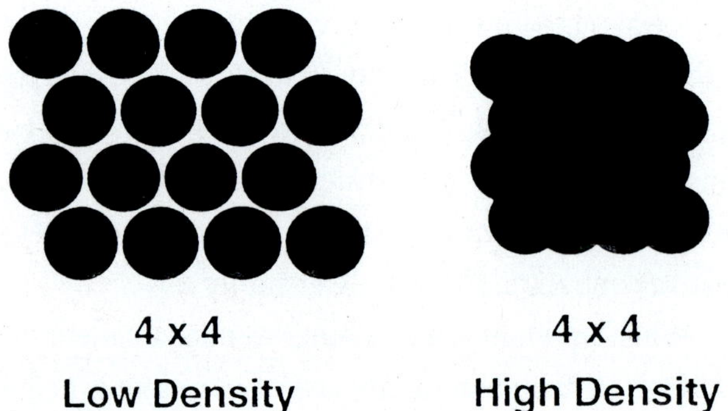

Figure 5–5. Automated laser scanners can vary the density of laser delivery spots. (From Keller G, Rawnsley J, Cutcliffe B, Watson J. Erbium:YAG and carbon dioxide laser resurfacing. *Facial Plast Surg Clinics North Am.* 1998;6:167–181.)

Increasing the density of the scan increases the thermal damage delivered to an area.

When using a laser scanner, the surgeon is careful to place each scan pattern immediately adjacent to the preceding pattern. Although usually inconsequential, overlapping of scan patterns with the CO_2 laser can produce areas of increased thermal energy in the overlapped area, resulting in erythema or scarring.

Most surgeons use multiple passes of the laser to treat a given area. After a laser pass, the treated area is wiped with a moist sponge to remove residual debris. Each pass of the laser affects the skin to a degree depending on the particular type of laser used. Generally, the first laser pass will remove all or most of the epidermis. The second pass usually reaches the upper papillary dermis, and the third pass reaches the midpapillary dermis. With each successive pass, the amount of tissue vaporized per pass decreases, and the amount of tissue coagulated per pass increases. After three or four passes, the tissue becomes visibly desiccated, and subsequent passes produce only thermal damage. Very little vaporization or tissue ablation occurs. At this point, the laser treatment is terminated.

Other endpoints of laser treatment are the disappearance of a rhytid or a texture abnormality or chamois color. If either of these endpoints is seen prior to tissue desiccation, treatment is terminated. The chamois color may indicate that the reticular dermis has been reached and that further treatment may produce scarring.

Wrinkle disappearance is usually the object of treatment, so there is no point to proceeding further than necessary. It is not necessary, however, to see the wrinkles disappear during the perioperative period to produce wrinkle clearing after healing is complete. The thermal injury that the CO_2 produces results in inflammatory changes that subsequently tighten the skin further. Because of this thermal injury and subsequent inflammation, the depth of injury (in contrast with dermabrasion) does not reliably correlate with the degree of tightening and rejuvenation. Injury to the midpapillary dermis generally produces changes in all but the most severe rhytids. Box 5–4 lists the endpoints for cessation of treatment.

> **Box 5–4. Endpoints for Cessation of Treatment**
>
> Tissue desiccation
> Chamois color
> Wrinkle disappearance
> Preset number of passes

More passes are delivered to the shoulders of a rhytid or acne scar than to the furrow or pit. Two to four passes to a rhytid's shoulder and one or two passes to the surrounding area are used depending on skin thickness and the degree of actinic change.

More passes or higher energies are required to treat thicker or actinically damaged skin than thin skin without severe damage. Higher energies (particularly on the first pass) increase the ablation depth. More passes extend the area of coagulation.

Specific Areas of Treatment

In the lip, the treatment area is extended over the lip surface. If treatment is terminated at the vermilion border, the rhytids that extend into the lip will remain and appear out of place.

In the eye area, one or two passes are required. After the first pass, the tissue is wiped. Then areas with rhytids are selectively spot treated on the shoulder of the rhytid. Whether to treat the skin over the tarsus is a matter of debate. Advocates of tarsal treatment feel that it produces an even appearance to the lasered eyelid. We believe the tarsal skin is so thin that it is not subject to a great deal of actinic damage and that the ultimate appearance is no different with or without treatment of this area. In fact, treatment of this area can produce a scleral show.

Prior to treatment, elasticity of the eyelid is measured with a "snap" test. A poor return of the eyelid may indicate that an incipient ectropion is possible. In such situations, canthal tightening or suspension is usually necessary. Malar bags, if present, are treated aggressively with two to three passes to the thicker skin below the eyelid.[26] One to three re-treatment sessions may be necessary to remove the bag. Nonetheless, treatment of malar bags with the laser is one of the few modalities that work, short of direct excision with resulting scar. Feathering treated areas is usually necessary. Lower energies that are still above the ablative threshold of skin $(5.5\ J/cm^2)$ are used to taper the laser treatment over the mandible and nontreated areas of skin.

Treatment of the neck with the CO_2 laser is controversial. Neck skin is thinner than facial skin and has fewer sebaceous glands and other epithelial regenerative elements. As a result, the neck is considered a hazardous area to resurface. The senior author (GSK) has seen patients with neck scarring from relatively benign laser treatments such as a pulse dye laser treatment for port-wine stains. While many authors feel that treatment of neck skin with the CO_2 laser is safe,[27,28] Fitzpatrick and Goldman[29] recently have reported a high incidence of scarring with CO_2 laser treatment. As a result, we have adopted the policy of not treating the neck with the CO_2 laser. Box 5–5 provides some treatment tips.

> **Box 5–5. CO_2 Laser Treatment Tips**
>
> Treat selectively (i.e., use a greater number of passes to the rhytid or acne scar shoulder)
> Extend one pass onto vermilion of lip
> Do not treat the tarsal plate
> Evaluate eyelid with a "snap" test
> Treat malar bags assertively
> Avoid treatment of the neck and chest with the CO_2 dioxide laser

POSTOPERATIVE CARE AND MANAGEMENT

Postoperative care and management of laser resurfacing patients are at least as important as the perioperative treatment. Careful monitoring of the patient by both the laser practitioner and the staff is often more time consuming than the actual laser treatment.

Pain

If not given before the laser treatment, regional nerve blocks for the infraorbital, submental, supraorbital, supratrochlear, zygomaticotemporal, and zygomaticofrontal nerves are administered. These treatments help diminish postoperative pain in the first 2 hours postoperatively.

The patient's face is also cooled in the immediate postoperative period. This cooling may be accomplished with ice bags, a package of frozen vegetables, refreezable "blue ice," or recirculating closed-system facial masks (Polaris). Cooling diminishes the immediate pain associated with resurfacing.

Ointments and Dressings

After laser treatment, the wound is occluded to maintain a moist environment for wound healing. Either ointments or wound dressings may be used for this purpose.

A number of ointments are available. Many of these, however, can cause hypersensitivity reactions in postoperative laser patients. It is essential to make sure that these ointments do not contain fragrances, aloe, vitamins, or other sensitizing agents. Antibiotic ointments are particularly likely to cause hypersensitivity reactions, but almost any ointment is capable of triggering an acute erythematous reaction. Vaseline and Crisco (soybean oil) seem to cause the least number of hypersensitivity reactions in our patients. Both are inexpensive and effective. On the negative side, Vaseline is so occlusive that milia can result, and Crisco is messy.

Koch et al[30] recently evaluated various wound dressings and discovered no differences in effectiveness. In this study, a significantly quicker healing time, less erythema, and less pain were seen when a closed dressing was used than when emollient ointments were applied without a dressing. Other authors have emphasized an increased incidence of wound infections with dressings that are not porous. Our personal preference is to use a porous Teflon burn dressing that is applied immediately after laser resurfacing is finished. The dressing is covered with Crisco and held in place with stockinet.

Postoperative care from days 1 to 3 aims at promoting reepithelialization and preventing infection. With occlusive dressings such as Vigilon, this may mean removing the dressing, showering or washing with mild soap, and replacing the dressing for 48 hours. With emollient ointments, similar washing and reapplication of the ointment may be required. In patients with porous Teflon dressings, we begin Burow's solution soaks on day 2 or 3 and frequent showering or washing, followed by reapplication of soybean oil as an ointment (Crisco). This regimen is continued until reepithelialization is complete or the dressing separates from the skin. Burow's solution helps to prevent infection by skin acidification and diminishes pruritus.

Proponents of Silastic dressings often lift these dressings and bathe the wound with a vinegar solution. These dressings are associated with a 4 to 6% incidence of infection. However, infection may also occur with other dressings or with ointments as well. Dressings such as Flexan or Duoderm have adhesives that cause them to adhere to the skin until epithelialization occurs. Removal of these dressings can disrupt the fragile new epidermis. Once the epidermis has re-formed, it is kept moisturized. Hundreds of moisturizing agents are available, and selection is an individual choice made by the patient and the practitioner.

Topical Agents

The skin is hypersensitive during the postoperative phase, and any topical agents (including sunscreens, makeup, and moisturizers) applied to the skin should be hypoallergenic (fragrance-free, etc.). We have the patient test the agent in the office by applying the agent to a small area. The area of application is then gradually expanded as it becomes apparent that there is no skin reaction. Makeup may be applied after reepithelialization is well established. Sun precautions (e.g., sunscreen, sun avoidance, and hats) should be continued for 3 to 6 months.

Erythema is the leading characteristic of the time period immediately following reepithelialization. It should be mild (pink) and last from 3 to 6 weeks depending on the type of laser used, the depth of laser resurfacing, and the avoidance of complications.

Complications and Adverse Effects

The senior author (GSK) has had the opportunity to care for a number of patients referred with problems. The following represents our approach to the care of these patients. Other reviews of complications are worthwhile for the reader.[31–34]

Laser resurfacing has advanced a great deal in recent years. Improvements in CO_2 laser systems and conservative treatment techniques have made resurfacing safer and more reproducible. Although complications are numerous, they are usually self-limiting, and many can be classified as adverse effects of laser treatment. There is a relatively low incidence of severe complications.

Erythema

Erythema is a side effect of laser resurfacing that occurs in 100% of patients. Prolongation or an increase in the intensity of normal erythema, however, is a warning sign for the clinician (Fig. 5–6).

In the immediate postoperative period, an increase in the intensity of erythema around the laser-treated area is often an indication of hypersensitivity or infection. Hypersensitivity to topical substances is one of the most common causes of severe erythema in the postoperative period (Fig. 5–7). Often the laser practitioner did not prescribe the substance leading to the topical sensitivity, but the patient selected it, or a holistic healer, aesthetician, or other person may have prescribed the substance (often aloe or other herbs).

Treatment consists of discontinuing the offending substance, ruling out infection, and administering topical (low-dose) or systemic steroids. If the erythema is prolonged or severe and infection has been ruled out, a brief dose of systemic steroids, such as is prescribed in a Medrol dose pack, is helpful. Erythema is usually a self-limited inflammatory process, but patients must be reassured constantly. The use of hypoallergenic makeup with sunscreens allows the patient to feel more confident about her or his appearance in public. The makeup is applied in small areas at first to assess whether the patient (who is now hypersusceptible to topical agents) will develop hypersensitivity to it. Avoidance of all topical agents, except for those prescribed by the physician, is emphasized. Sun avoidance during this period is especially important to avoid an inflammatory response. All skin treatments (such as facials) are postponed until healing is complete.

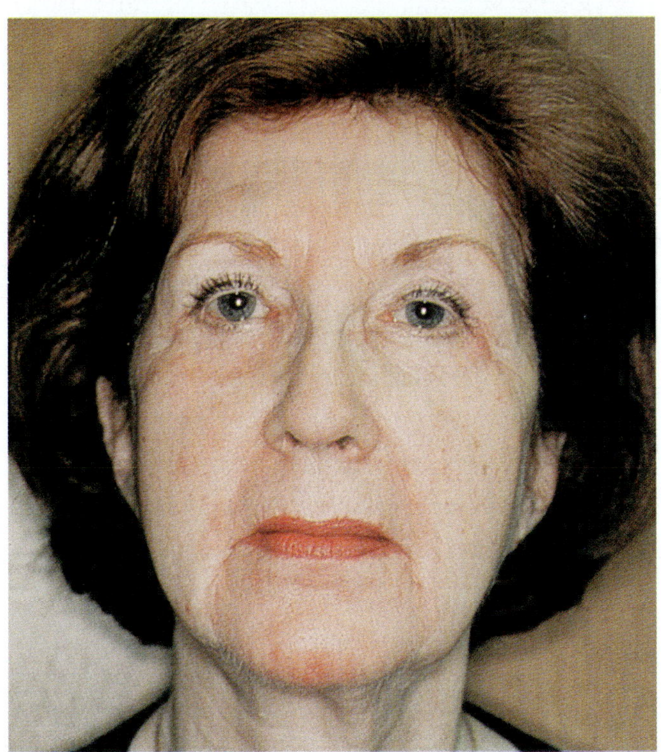

Figure 5–6. Patient with prolonged erythema lasting 4 months.

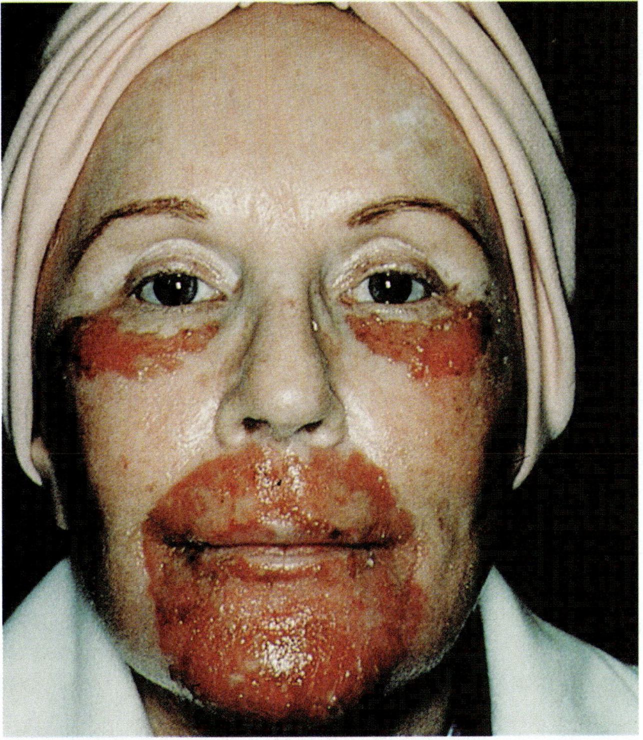

Figure 5–7. Patient with a severe hypersensitivity reaction to aloe vera.

If there are local areas of thickened, erythematous skin, an impending hypertrophic scar is suspected. Treatment of this condition is described below.

Hyperpigmentation

Hyperpigmentation is often preceded by erythema and may be considered to be postinflammatory hyperpigmentation. Hyperpigmentation is an adverse effect that occurs consistently in patients of Asian and Latin descent. It is more prevalent in darker skin types, and all such patients should be apprised preoperatively of their potential to develop this problem.

Any patient can develop hyperpigmentation, however. A previous history of postinflammatory hyperpigmentation is helpful to assess the potential risk. The effects of hormones on an individual patient's skin should also be assessed. There is no conclusive evidence that pretreatment with topical agents prevents hyperpigmentation.

Hyperpigmentation usually appears after erythema resolves. The first line of treatment for this complication is prevention. The patient must remain covered when exposed to sunlight in the postoperative period. Even sunlight exposure through glass should be avoided. It is important to delay topical treatment for hyperpigmentation until all erythema has resolved because the treating agents may produce further inflammation and restart the cycle of erythema and further postinflammatory hyperpigmentation.

Initially, after resolution of all erythema, we test a small area of the hyperpigmentation with a hydroquinone cream. If there is no reaction to the cream, treatment of larger areas follows.

After epithelialization is complete and stable, treatment of the hyperpigmented areas may extend to include kojic, azelaic, and glycolic acid solutions. Hydroxyquinones may be continued if the patient is not susceptible to onchrynosis. Sunlight avoidance and protection remain important aspects of treatment.

Hypopigmentation

Hypopigmentation is normally a delayed reaction to laser resurfacing, usually appearing between 4 and 12 months after resurfacing. This complication may be seen in all skin types. However, hypopigmentation may be relative. That is, the laser may restore a youthful skin color and texture in one area, while adjacent areas that are sun damaged may have a permanent hyperpigmented or yellow, keratotic appearance. Light peels with a glycolic acid or a combination of kojic, lactic, salicylic, and azelaic acids of the adjacent areas may help blunt the contrast. In some instances, patients with hypopigmentation may have experienced a cycle of prolonged erythema and hyperpigmentation prior to the hypopigmentation. Postoperatively, their skin may have appeared normally pigmented for a period of time.

The mechanism for hypopigmentation is unkown. Laws et al[35] noted that melanosomes in a patient with hypopigmentation had melanocytes that were concentrated under a layer of scar tissue. On histologic sections, they noted no difference in the numbers of melanocytes from these hypopigmented areas when compared with areas with normal pigmentation.

A repeat light resurfacing may cause a release of these melanocytes or stimulate an ingrowth of melanocytes from peripheral areas. We have not seen consistent repair of hypopigmented skin with repeat resurfacing, although isolated patients have responded. Exposure to sunlight, ultraviolet light, or psoralen-ultraviolet-light therapy may be helpful if the Wood's light demonstrates melanocytes in the dermis. Usually, however, hypopigmentation is a permanent and stable condition.

In properly selected patients, hypopigmentation is now less prevalent than with chemical peeling with melanocytic agents such as phenol. It also occurs more rarely than with dermabrasion. It may have an increased incidence in patients who have been resurfaced with lasers, chemical peels, and dermabrasion previously or in patients who have had radiation to the skin.

Scarring

Like many other complications of laser resurfacing, scarring often is preceded by erythema. If there are local areas of erythematous, thickened skin, the treating practitioner should suspect an impending hypertrophic scar. Such scars may occur in areas of scanner overlap, where the coagulative necrosis may have been more severe than expected. In this case, the areas of hypertrophic scar might mimic the scanner pattern. Other causes of hypertrophic scar formation are overtreatment, infection, intrinsic disease processes, chronic inflammation, previous resurfacing, and idiopathic causes.

If the practitioner suspects an impending hypertrophic scar, a fluorinated steroid ointment is used for 1 week. Silicone patches are used at night, and silicone gel is used during the day. After the wound closes, flash pump dye laser treatment to the area can be extremely helpful. If the erythematous area thickens, Kenalog injections are considered. Most lesions respond to 2.5 to 10% injections, but greater concentrations may be required. Atrophic areas of scar or texture change usually respond well to autologous fibroblast injections (Isolagen). Generally, three injections are required to each area.

Infection

Bacterial or fungal infection occurs infrequently. Intense erythema, crusting, yellowish or green discharge, and premature lateralization of the dressing are the usual signs of infection occurring between the second postoperative day and reepithelialization. Immediate Gram stains, potassium hydroxide smears, cultures, fungal and herpes stains and cultures (as determined by clinical findings), and treatment are indicated. If the infection occurs in the presence of prophylactic antibiotics, infection with *Pseudomonas* or resistant staphylococcal or streptococcal organisms should be suspected. Such infections, particularly with *Pseudomonas*, are seen more commonly with nonporous, occlusive dressings. If infection is suspected, the dressing should be removed and the area cleansed with mild soap and/or Burow's solution. Medication should be prescribed according to the results of the smears and cultures.

If there are pustules, occlusive milia, acne outbreaks, and yeast infections need to be differentiated from each other. Milia are tiny epidermal cysts that are often attributed to the use of thick occlusive ointments. Nanni and Alster[34] have reported an incidence of milia of 14% in laser resurfacing patients. Unroofing of larger lesions

with a 20-gauge needle is effective. Smaller lesions tend to resolve spontaneously or with application of standard dilute glycolic acid home skin care products.

Acneiform outbreaks manifest larger pustules and reddened papules. We have found azithromycin to be an effective treatment. Topical antibiotic solutions usually are avoided during the immediate postoperative period because of the tendency of the skin to develop hypersensitivity to these topical solutions.

Cutaneous candidiasis can be difficult to differentiate from acne with pustule formation. These lesions are usually small pustules with a reddened base that are grouped together. A potassium hydroxide prep is helpful for diagnosis. Diflucan is used for treatment.

Herpes simplex infections present in a variety of ways. Herpetic vesicles, punctate erosions, and excessive crusting can all represent herpes. Cultures and smears are helpful for diagnosis. Pain is often the hallmark of herpetic infections. Pain presenting without an obvious cause should be assumed to be herpetic until proven otherwise. Prophylactic treatment of herpes was described earlier. Antiviral prophylaxis is recommended for all laser resurfacing patients. Breakthrough infections are treated with maximal-dose treatment. Intravenous acyclovir may be indicated for severe, disseminated herpes (Fig. 5–8).

In addition, it is important to note that immunocompromised patients and people with diabetes are more susceptible to infections. As mentioned previously, these patients have a relative contraindication for surgery.

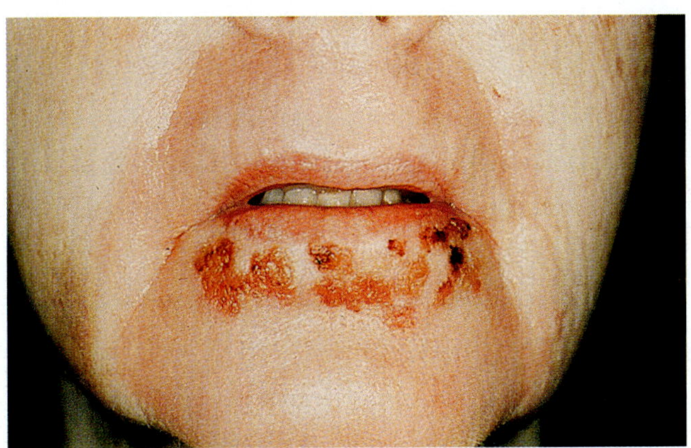

Figure 5–8. Patient with a breakthrough herpes simplex infection.

Lower Eyelid Retraction

Postoperative ectropion of the lower eyelid is seen rarely because a snap test is performed preoperatively to assess eyelid function. Laxity of the lid is best treated with a suspension procedure. Lower eyelid retraction can occur after laser resurfacing. Usually this will improve with massage, taping, and time. If it does not, various surgical procedures (e.g., SOOF lifts, mucosal grafts, and suspension procedures) are available to correct this disorder.

OTHER COMPLICATIONS

Telangiectasias are not uncommon following laser resurfacing. They may be treated with a flash pump dye or other vascular lesion laser. One unusual complication the senior author has had the opportunity to review is a spontaneous outbreak of multiple keratoacanthomas. In addition, transepidermal elimination of elastic fibers was reported by Richert and Bridenstine.[36] It is unlikely that most practitioners will encounter either of these problems.

ERBIUM:YTTRIUM-ALUMINUM-GARNET LASER RESURFACING

Although the CO_2 laser is an extremely effective skin resurfacing tool, the residual thermal damage that is produced along with skin ablation results in erythema as an adverse effect, which can be troubling to the patient. As a result, a search for a surgical laser that can produce precise skin ablation without the coagulative tissue necrosis produced by the CO_2 laser has resulted in the development of the Er:YAG laser.

SCIENTIFIC PRINCIPLES AND TISSUE EFFECTS

The Er:YAG laser emits light at 2940 nm. This wavelength coincides with the maximal absorption peak of water. The absorption of Er:YAG laser light in water is 10 to 12 times greater than the absorption of CO_2 laser light. Because of its increased absorption in tissue water, the Er:YAG laser energy (at an energy level of only 1.5 J/cm^2 vs. 5.5 J/cm^2 by the CO_2 laser) produces an extremely shallow ablation crater with minimal thermal injury. Box 5–6 summarizes the physics and tissue effects of the Er:YAG laser.

Box 5–6. Er:YAG Laser Physics and Tissue Effects

Ablation threshold $= 1.5$ J/cm^2

Increased energy $=$ increased ablation (2.5 μm for each J/cm^2 over the ablation threshold to 25 J/cm^2)

Increased number of passes and/or density of the scanner $=$ increased skin contraction with slightly increased coagulation

---

The Er:YAG laser's wavelength coincides with an optimal collagen absorption peak at 3000 nm, which means it is selectively absorbed by collagen. Miller[37] has noted that in all laser resurfacing, ablation competes with coagulation. Unlike the CO_2 laser, with the Er:YAG laser, tissue ablation predominates over coagulation (thermal injury). Because of this predominance, the Er:YAG laser can continue to ablate tissue into the dermis. True dermal ablation not due to thermal coagulation is therefore possible with this laser.

The Er:YAG laser both has a small zone of thermal injury and directly ablates collagen in the dermal tissue. As a result, the Er:YAG laser, with high energy and multiple passes, can ablate tissue all the way through the dermis and into the subcutaneous tissue. Because of its selective absorption by collagen, this laser can also be used to ablate scar tissue. After the epidermis is removed, the amount of ablation that can be achieved with the CO_2 laser is limited. After two to four passes, additional passes only result in further thermal injury (coagulation).

The Er:YAG laser is an extremely precise surgical tool owing to its predominance of ablation over coagulation. Light intraepidermal resurfacing can be done with one pass that produces minimal, if any, thermal injury. Each additional pass can produce a calibrated amount of damage that can extend as deep into the dermis as required. Only a minimal amount of increased coagulation is produced per laser pass until the number of passes increases to an extreme beyond clinical practicality.

Increase in the Er:YAG laser's energy also produces a precise increase in ablation depth per pass. Hohenleutner et al[38] noted that each joule per square centimeter increase in Er:YAG laser energy over the ablation threshold produces 2.5 μm of ablation in skin. This relationship remains linear until 25 J/cm^2 of laser energy is reached. From 1.5 to 25 J/cm^2, any thermal injury that is produced remains minimal. Above 25 J/cm^2, the amount of ablation per pulse diminishes and coagulation increases.

Because of the lack of coagulative thermal injury, the Er:YAG laser allows for quicker healing with less erythema than the CO$_2$ laser. Thus, the Er:YAG laser can be used for younger patients and darker-skinned patients (patients with Fitzpatrick skin type III and greater). Even without a great deal of coagulative thermal injury, the Er:YAG laser produces skin contraction. Our interdisciplinary group's studies on pig skin at the University of California–Los Angeles have shown that this contraction does not depend on energy per pulse but rather on the number of passes and the energy density of the scanner[15] (Fig. 5–9). The energy per pulse affects the depth of tissue ablation per pulse but not the amount of skin contraction that is achieved.

After Er:YAG laser resurfacing, the initial contraction of skin is perpendicular to the relaxed skin tension lines

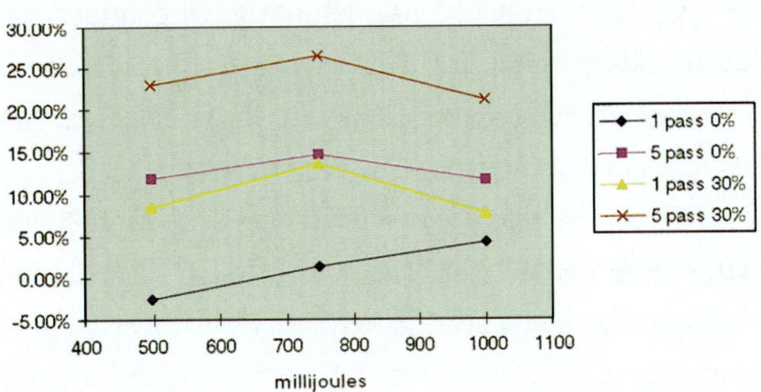

Figure 5–9. Skin contraction from the Er:YAG laser is directly related to energy density of the scanner and the number of passes. Laser power energy affects ablation depth but, with the density of the scanner and the number of passes remaining the same, has little effect on skin contraction. (From Keller G, Rawnsley J, Cutcliffe B, Watson J. Erbium:YAG and carbon dioxide laser resurfacing. *Facial Plast Surg Clinics North Am.* 1998;6:167–181.)

and is weaker than that produced by the CO$_2$ laser. Longer-term skin contraction, however, was equivalent for both lasers when similar depths of injury were seen (Fig. 5–10). However, the amounts of thermal injury and erythema were diminished with the Er:YAG laser. The healing time was also shortened with the Er:YAG laser compared with

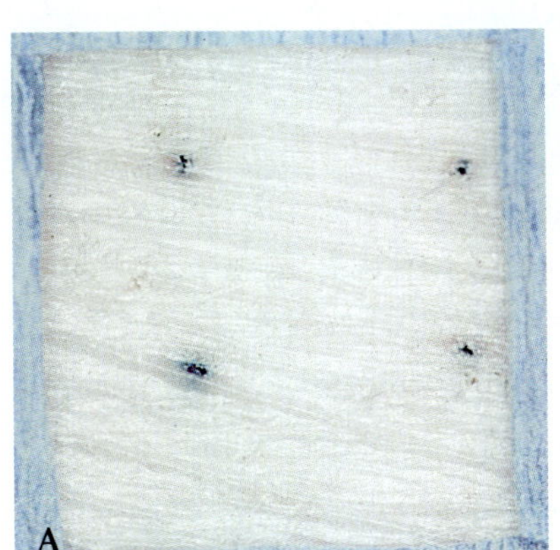
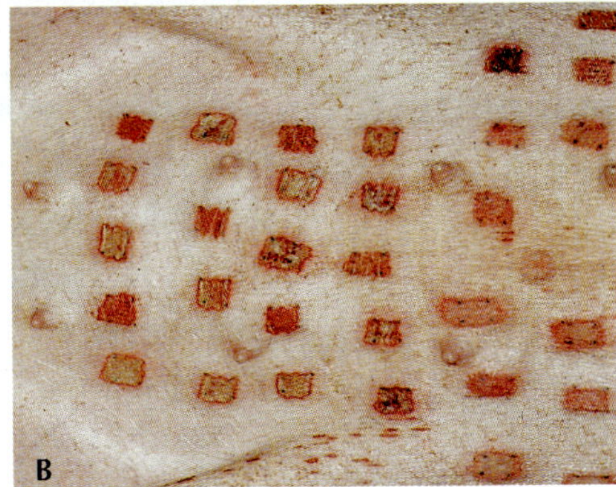
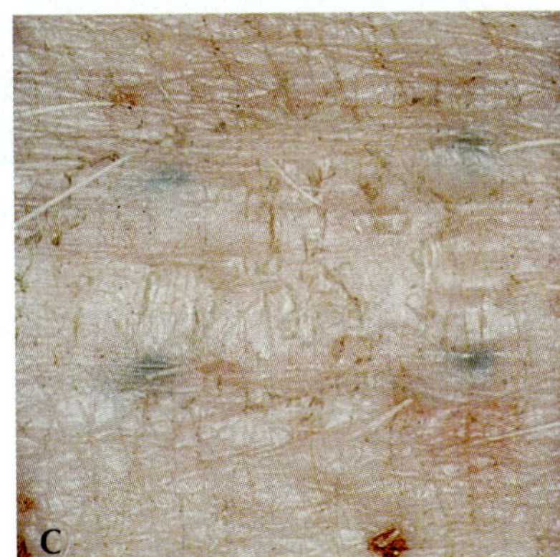
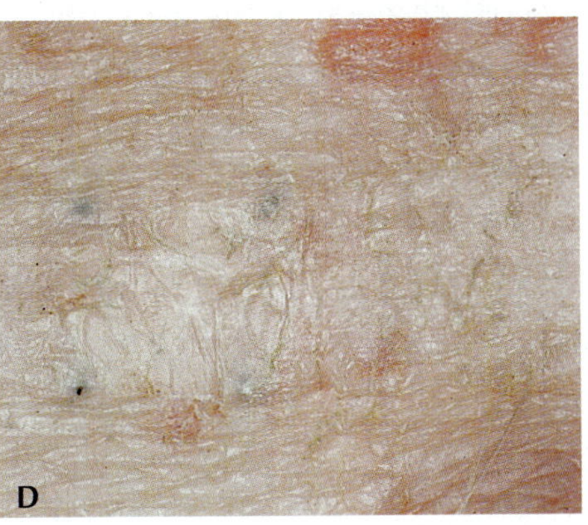

Figure 5–10. (A) Tattooed square of pig skin before laser resurfacing. (B) Laser-treated squares of pig skin. Different laser energies, scanner densities, and numbers of passes were used for each square. (C) Short-term contraction occurred perpendicular to the relaxed skin tension lines, producing a rectangular shape. (D) Longer-term skin contraction occurred both perpendicular and parallel to the relaxed skin tension lines, producing a return to a square shape. (From Keller G, Rawnsley J, Cutcliffe B, Watson J. Erbium:YAG and carbon dioxide laser resurfacing. *Facial Plast Surg Clinics North Am.* 1998;6:167–181.)

the CO_2 laser. Hughes[39] haa demonstrated contraction of human skin with the Er:YAG laser and noted contraction of forearm skin in patients treated with the Er:YAG laser similar to that resulting from CO_2 laser treatment.

We believe that use of a scanner is even more helpful with the Er:YAG laser than with the CO_2 laser. Slight overlapping of the scan patterns helps to overcome the tendency of the center of the spot to be "hotter" than the more peripheral portions. The scanner pattern, by overlapping the "skirt" (peripheral portion) of the laser beam, tends to equalize the amount of energy received by the entire surface. This is true whether the beam pattern is Gaussian or collimated because of beam dynamics.

By increasing the scanner overlap to 10 to 30%, a slight increase in heat, sufficient to prevent pinpoint bleeding, can be produced. The scan patterns may be overlapped slightly as well, particularly on the second scan. Because the Er:YAG laser produces minimal coagulation of tissue, overlapping of each scan pattern produces no lines of demarcation.

Scanning allows more uniformity than beam treatment in our opinion. However, excellent clinical results can be obtained with both scanner and beam systems. The following remarks on clinical use of the Er:YAG laser are made with the Sharplan-ESC laser in mind; it is the machine with which we are most experienced.

CLINICAL USE OF THE ERBIUM:YTTRIUM-ALUMINUM-GARNET LASER

Many different treatment approaches and methods are employed with the Er:YAG laser.[40–45] Several of these are described in subsequent chapters. Our preferred techniques for resurfacing with this laser are described below.

The Er:YAG laser is our choice for treatment of the aging face (with the exception of perioral lines), scars, skin rejuvenation in younger patients, melasma, periocular rhytids, neck skin, and small dermatologic lesions. The CO_2 is our choice for treatment of perioral rhytids and removal of larger dermatologic lesions (e.g., rhinophyma; see Box 5–7).

Box 5–7. Lasers of Choice for Specific Conditions

Er:YAG Laser
  Facial and periocular rhytids
  Younger patients
  Scars (e.g., rhinophyma)
  Small dermatologic lesions (e.g., syringoma, lentigo, milia, trichoepithelioma)
  Neck resurfacing
  Acne scars
CO_2 Laser
  Perioral rhytids
  Larger dermatologic lesions

Preoperative and postoperative care is similar to that for the CO_2 laser. Treatment of complications, though they are diminished in number and extent, is also similar to that for the CO_2 laser. The Er:YAG laser has no definitive endpoints. Pinpoint bleeding is cited, but it may occur before wrinkle effacement is complete, thereby compromising the procedure.

Light Resurfacing

Light resurfacing is used for patients with mild sun- and age-induced skin damage without significant rhytids (lines, not wrinkles). Light resurfacing is also useful for neck skin. Patients who are candidates for light resurfacing are often younger and have only mild lines (not wrinkles). Treatment is directed toward early changes of sun- and age-related skin changes (e.g., pigmented areas, skin coarseness, keratotic changes).

One or two passes are performed with a scanner density of 0 to 10% (barely touching laser spots). These passes are applied to the areas selected for resurfacing. An energy density of 5 to 8 J/cm^2 is used. If a "lunchtime" laser peel is desired, 2.0 to 2.5 J/cm^2 is used with a 0% energy density. One pass is made over the entire face to achieve the same result as microdermabrasion or light peels.

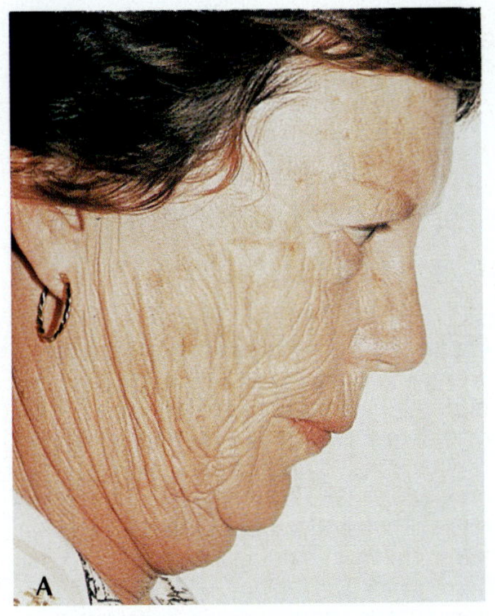
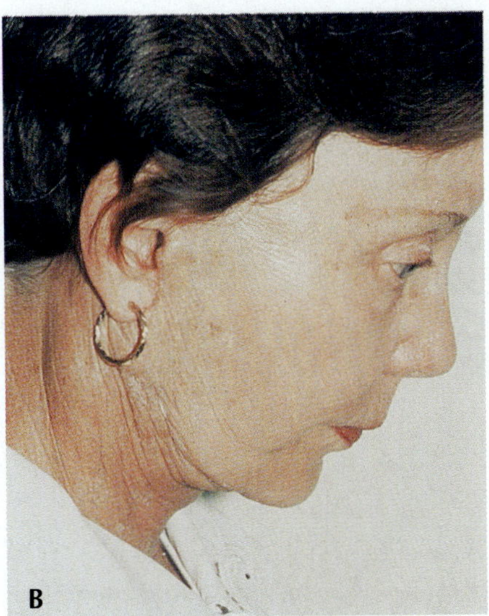

Figure 5–11. (A) Preoperative view of patient undergoing simultaneous light Er:YAG laser skin resurfacing to the central face and deep plane rhytidectomy. The patient is a nonsmoker in good health who insists on simultaneous resurfacing and rhytidectomy, as was recommended to her by another surgeon. (B) Postoperative result 5 months later. One or two passes at 15 J/cm^2 and 10 to 20% scanner density were used on the central two thirds of the face. Her postoperative period was probably prolonged by about 1 week. She is about to undergo light neck resurfacing (one pass to her lower neck and two passes to her upper neck). She had decided previously against two-step rhytidectomy and resurfacing but has decided to resurface the neck after seeing the favorable result of facial resurfacing.

Light to moderate resurfacing with the Er:YAG laser may be used, in very specific situations (e.g., extreme photodamage, nonsmoker, healthy skin), to resurface the central face and forehead of a patient receiving a deep plane face lift. For this, only one or two passes are used in the central areas that are undermined (Fig. 5–11).

Because of the lack of a thermal component to the laser injury, treatment is often not described as painful. Frequently, only a topical anesthesia, such as EMLA or Topicaine, is used. If the topical anesthesia is not effective, nerve blocks, infiltrative anesthesia, or MAC may be used.

Moderate Resurfacing

Moderate resurfacing is used for patients with moderate lines and wrinkles. Often skin contraction is desired in these patients in their middle years (although they may be younger if they are smokers or sun worshippers) (Figs. 5–12 and 5–13). They also may have sun spots and keratoses.

The various settings are determined by the patient's skin, the clinician's experience, the laser used, and other factors. For the surgeon new to Er:YAG resurfacing, it is recommended to start at the lower range of settings until experience is gained.

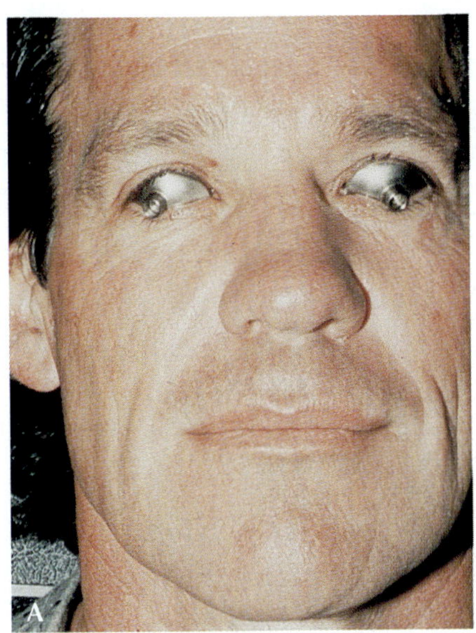
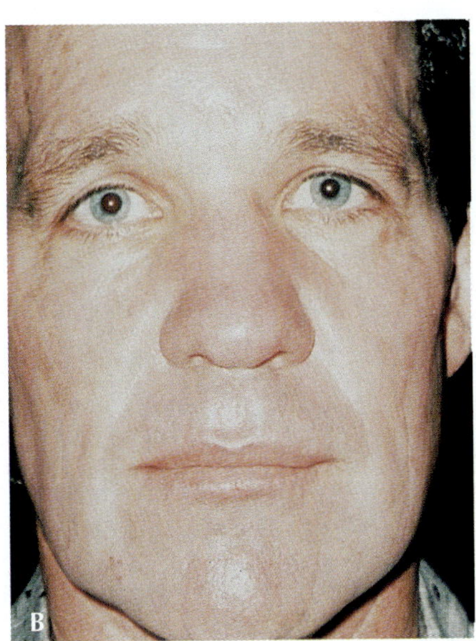

Figure 5–12. (A) Preoperative male patient for moderate Er:YAG laser skin resurfacing. He has mild rhytids and sun-induced skin change. (B) Postoperative results 10 days later. After one or two passes at 15 J/cm^2 with a 30% scanner density, he is able to return to work without makeup (which he would not wear).

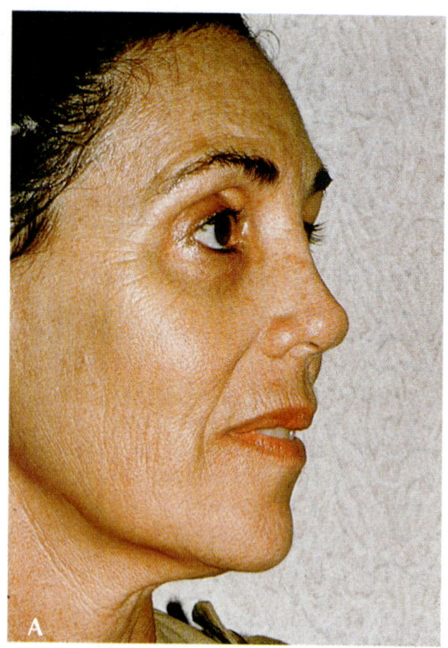
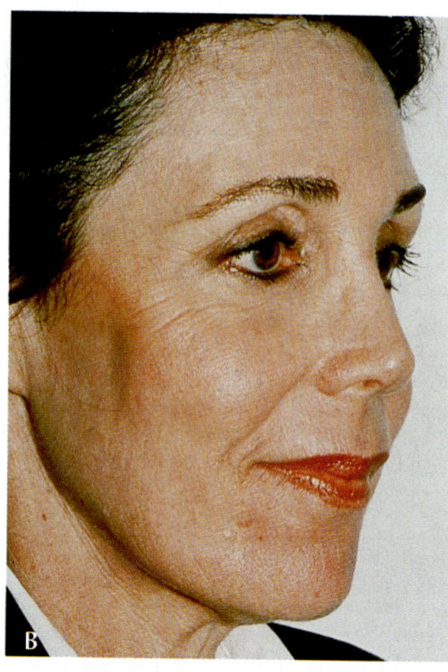

Figure 5–13. (A) Preoperative view of woman with Fitzpatrick skin type IV undergoing moderate Er:YAG laser resurfacing. She objects to the cheek rhytids and would like some skin contraction. She has only a short recovery time. (B) Postoperative result 8 months later. The moderate resurfacing (two passes at 15 J/cm² with 30% density) has produced skin contraction and diminished cheek rhytids. She had only transient mild hyperpigmentation.

Usually one or two passes with a 3-mm handpiece at 5 to 8 J/cm² on a beam setting are done on the shoulders of the rhytid, followed by two or three passes with the scanner. The scanner is used with 10 to 30% energy density at 5 to 15 J/cm².

Two passes with the laser scanner produces injury that ablates the epidermis and may (depending on energy settings) extend into the upper papillary dermis. Ablation of the epidermis is all that is attempted for sun-damaged skin that is treated in the central portion of a deep plane face lift. Extension into the upper papillary dermis is helpful for mild photoaging. Three to four passes produces injury that extends to the upper to middle papillary dermis, depending on the settings. This is appropriate for resurfacing patients with significant sun-induced changes.

Heavy Resurfacing

Heavy resurfacing is used for deeper rhytids. The 3-mm handpiece is used in beam mode to treat the rhytid shoulders with two to five passes at 5 to 15 J/cm². The entire area is then treated with three passes at 5 to 15 J/cm² using the laser scanner with a 10 to 30% overlap.

Often these patients have heavy perioral rhytids. Our approach at present is to treat the perioral rhytids with

the CO_2 and to treat the rest of the face with the Er:YAG laser. We then use the Er:YAG laser to perform one pass on the areas that have been treated with the CO_2 laser. This treatment approach theoretically reduces the zone of thermal injury produced by the CO_2 laser by partially ablating the thermal injury zone with the Er:YAG laser.

Other authors[46–48] advocate using the Er:YAG laser for all resurfacing, citing the advantages of diminished erythema and quicker recovery. We, as others,[49] feel that for difficult rhytids, the Er:YAG laser is actually more dangerous than the CO_2 laser. For deep rhytids, the Er:YAG laser must be taken to a depth that is dangerous for scarring; leaving fewer skin elements to assist wound healing. The CO_2 laser, by contrast, is somewhat self-limited in its ablation depth, producing results with thermal injury. The inexperienced laser surgeon may be better served by a laser (CO_2) that is relatively safe, albeit causing erythema of longer duration, than a laser that requires an increased depth of injury in a bloody field.

Acne Scars

The Er:YAG laser is the treatment of choice for acne scars (other than those of the ice pick variety). The shoulders of the scar are taken down with the 3-mm spot in the beam mode $\left(5-15 \text{ J/cm}^2\right)$ using two to four passes. Autologous fibroblasts[49] (Isolagen) are then injected into the pit of the scar, either during the procedure or subsequently.

Facial Scars

Scars that are not reddened and that extend above the surrounding skin are taken down using the Er:YAG laser with a 3-mm spot in a similar manner to that described for acne scars. The shoulders of depressed posttraumatic scars are treated similarly. Autologous fibroblasts are injected into depressed or atrophic areas. Reddened hypertrophic scars are treated with silicone patches and gel, topical or injectable steroids, and the flash pump dye laser.

Small Lesions

Skin tags are vaporized with a 2-mm spot. Xanthelasmas and syringomas are "unroofed" and vaporized with topical anesthesia. The Er:YAG laser is used at a setting of 5 to 15 J/cm^2. In general, lesions smaller than 2 to 3 mm may be vaporized with the laser without scarring.

Combination Treatment

Many surgeons have treated the face with the CO_2 laser followed by a single pass with the Er:YAG laser to remove a portion of the zone of thermal injury that the CO_2 laser produces. As described above, we use this method to treat deep perioral rhytids. Recently, Goldman and Fitzpatrick[50] have studied this method of treatment by performing side-by-side studies with the Er:YAG laser and combination treatment. Half the face was treated with the Er:YAG laser alone, and the other half was treated with the CO_2 laser followed by removal of the thermally damaged zone with one pass of the Er:YAG laser. They found no difference in healing times and erythema between the two treatment modalities. They also treated pigskin and performed posttreatment biopsies. The zone of thermal necrosis induced by CO_2 laser treatment was markedly reduced when an Er:YAG laser pass was used.

Other physicians have used the Er:YAG laser to remove the epidermis, followed by CO_2 laser treatment to the dermis. We have used the Er:YAG laser in this manner and have noted decreased erythema as compared with CO_2 laser treatment alone. However, we noted no advantage over Er:YAG laser treatment alone when sun- and age-related skin changes were treated. With deep rhytids, the combined laser treatment seemed to offer no advantage over CO_2 laser treatment alone.

LASER RESURFACING WITHOUT EPIDERMAL ABLATION

Undoubtedly, the future of laser resurfacing lies in minimally invasive laser treatments. If we could treat rhytids and shrink skin without ablating the epidermis, perform laser treatment without a burn type of injury, and treat all skin types, we would have advanced our field years ahead of where it is today. In fact, several laser systems are able to affect the dermis without epidermal ablation. The Nd:YAG laser, operating at 1320 nm, has been used recently with an epidermal cooling apparatus for this purpose.[51] Dermal damage with new collagen deposition into the dermis has been documented histologically in the face of an intact epidermis. Unfortunately, to date, rhytid resolution has been neither complete nor long lasting. Clinical improvement on a modest scale has been reported. Further information on this laser system is contained in Chapter 15.

A diode laser system with an innovative contact probe delivery system has been used to perform similar dermal wounding in the face of an intact epidermis.[52] Investigators using these systems have reported skin contraction occurring after laser treatment. Other laser systems that are in common use for other purposes have been used to cause dermal wounding without epidermal ablation. The Q-switched Nd:YAG laser with and without carbon potentiation has been reported to affect rhytids,[53,54] as has the flash pumped dye laser.[55]

The fact that any effect on rhytids can be achieved with these systems is impressive. The degree to which these effects are temporary and due to the tissue edema these lasers produce still needs to be defined. Permanent effects can only be achieved with collagen deposition and remodeling. Hopefully, these systems can be developed to a high degree of effectiveness. There is certainly a need for laser systems that are useful for resurfacing but produce no side effects or complications.

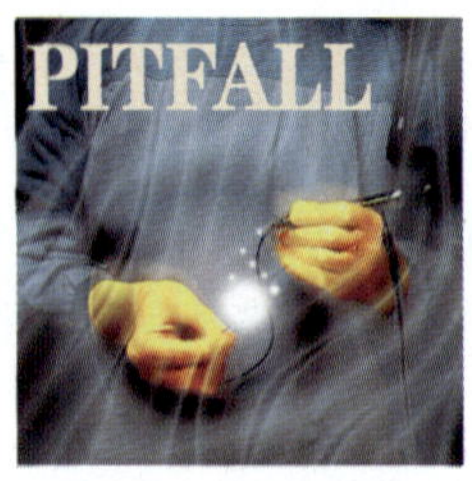

- Although laser resurfacing techniques are relatively simple, many practitioners who initially entered the field of laser resurfacing did not have experience with laser systems. With the increasing numbers of laser resurfacing cases came complications such as scarring, hypopigmentation, hyperpigmentation, prolonged erythema, nonhealing wounds, and infections.

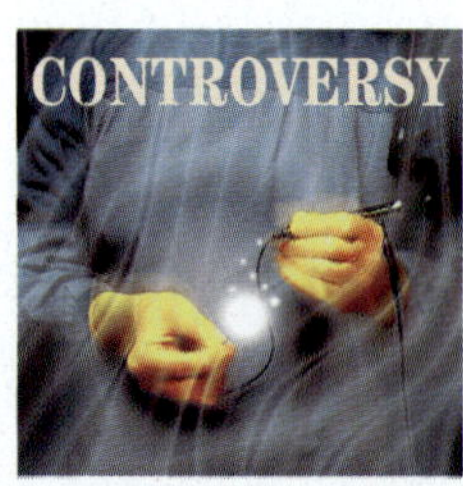

- Many surgeons will not resurface facial skin over an area where they have lifted, despite evidence of the safety of simultaneous resurfacing and rhytidectomy. Conservative resurfacing (central) may be performed but carries an increased risk and results in a prolonged healing period.
- Very few studies are available that document conclusively the benefit of any form of pretreatment (except for herpes). Because of the lack of consensus, it seems difficult to advocate pretreatment as a "standard of care."
- While many authors feel that treatment of neck skin with the CO_2 laser is safe, there have been reports of a high incidence of scarring with CO_2 laser treatment.
- Some advocate using the Er:YAG laser for all resurfacing, citing the advantages of diminished erythema and quicker recovery. Others feel that for difficult rhytids, the Er:YAG laser is actually more dangerous than the CO_2 laser.

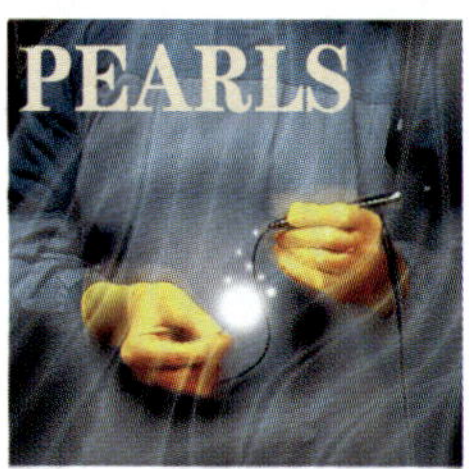

- When in doubt about whether to resurface a patient, a test spot is reasonable. A test spot of about 2×2 cm is not entirely predictive of whether dyschromia will occur, but it can demonstrate how inflamed the patient's skin will become in response to the laser's thermal challenge.
- One endpoint of laser treatment is a chamois color. The chamois color may indicate that the reticular dermis has been reached and that further treatment may produce scarring.
- Vaseline and Crisco (soybean oil) seem to cause the least number of hypersensitivity reactions in our patients. Both are inexpensive and effective, but Vaseline is so occlusive that milia can result, and Crisco is messy.

REFERENCES

1. Lask G, Keller G, Lowe N, et al. Laser skin resurfacing with the SilkTouch flashscanner for facial rhytids. *Dermatol Surg.* 1995;21:1021–1024.
2. Lowe NJ, Lask G, Griffin ME, et al. Skin resurfacing with the ultrapulse carbon dioxide laser: observations on 100 patients. *Dermatol Surg.* 1995;21:1025–1029.
3. Goodman GJ. Facial resurfacing using a high-energy short pulse carbon dioxide laser. *Aust J Dermatol.* 1996;37:125–132.
4. David L, Ruiz-Esparza J. Fast healing after laser skin resurfacing: the minimal mechanical trauma technique. *Dermatol Surg.* 1997;23:359–361.
5. Fitzpatrick R, Goldman MP, Satur NM, et al. Pulsed carbon dioxide laser resurfacing of photoaged facial skin. *Arch Dermatol.* 1996;132:395–402.
6. Ho C, Nguyen Q, Lowe NJ, Griffin ME, Lask G. Laser resurfacing in pigmented skin. *Dermatol Surg.* 1995;21:1035–1037.
7. Weinstein C, Alster TS. Skin resurfacing with high energy, pulsed carbon dioxide lasers. In: Alster TS, Apfelberg DC, eds. *Cosmetic Laser Surgery.* New York: John Wiley & Sons; 1996:9–27.
8. Chernoff G, Schoenrock L, Cramer H, et al. Cutaneous laser resurfacing. *Int J Aesthetic Restor Surg.* 1995;3:57–68.
9. Bernstein LJ, Kauvar ANB, Grossman MC, Geronemus RG. Scar resurfacing with high-energy, short-pulsed and flashscanning carbon dioxide lasers. *Dermatol Surg.* 1998;24:101–107.
10. Alster TS, West TB. Resurfacing of atrophic facial acne scars with CO_2 laser. *Dermatol Surg.* 1995;21:151–155.

11. Koch J. CO_2 laser-assisted skin resurfacing: current practices. *Am J Cosmet Surg.* 1998;15:27–35.

12. Trimas SJ, Ellis DAF, Metz RD. The carbon dioxide laser: an alternative for the treatment of actinically damaged skin. *Dermatol Surg.* 1997;23:885–889.

13. Fitzpatrick RE, Tope WD, Goldman MP, et al. Pulsed carbon dioxide laser, trichloroacetic acid, Baker-Gordon peel, and dermabrasion: a comparative clinical and histologic study of cutaneous resurfacing in a porcine model. *Arch Dermatol.* 1996;132:469–471.

14. Smith KJ, Skelton HG, Graham JS. Increased smooth muscle actin, factor XIIIa, and vimentin-positive cells in the papillary dermis of carbon dioxide laser-debrided porcine skin. *Dermatol Surg.* 1997;23:891–895.

15. Keller G, Rawnsley J, Cutcliffe B, Watson J. Erbium:YAG and carbon dioxide laser resurfacing 1998. *Facial Plast Surg Clinics North Am.* 1998;6:167–181.

16. Morrow D, Morrow L. Carbon dioxide laser-assisted laser facelift. *Am J Cosmet Surg.* 1992;9:177–180.

17. Bisaccia E, Sequeira M, Magidson J, Scarborough D. Surgical intervention for the aging face. Combination of mini-face-lifting and superficial carbon dioxide laser resurfacing. *Dermatol Surg.* 1998;24:821–826.

18. Guyuron B, Michelow B, Schmelzer R, et al. Delayed healing of rhytidectomy flap resurfaced with CO_2 laser. *Plast Reconstr Surg.* 1998;101:816–819.

19. Perkins SW, Sklarew EC. Prevention of facial herpetic infections after chemical peel and dermabrasion: new treatment strategies in the prophylaxis of patients undergoing procedures of the perioral area. *Plast Reconstr Surg.* 1996;98:427–433.

20. Apfelberg DB. Summary of the 1997 ASAPS/ASPRS laser task force survey on laser resurfacing and laser blepharoplasty. *Plast Reconstr Surg.* 1998;101:511–518.

21. Duke D, Grevelink J. Care before and after laser skin resurfacing: a survey and review of the literature. *Dermatol Surg.* 1998;24:201–206.

22. Alster T, West T. Effect of topical vitamin C on postoperative carbon dioxide laser resurfacing erythema. *Dermatol Surg.* 1998;24:331–334.

23. Geronemus R, Alster T, Brandt F, et al. Table talk. *Dermatol Surg.* 1998;24:121–130.

24. Beasley D, Jones C, McDonald WS. Effect of pretreated skin on laser resurfacing. *Lasers Surg Med.* 1997;9(suppl);43.

25. Apfelberg DB. Perioperative considerations in laser resurfacing. *Int J Aesthetic Restor Surg* 1997;5:21–28.

26. West T, Alster T. Effect of pretreatment on the incidence of hyperpigmentation following cutaneous CO_2 laser resurfacing. *Dermatol Surg.* 1999;25:15–17.

27. Baker SS. CO_2 Laser blepharoplasty, ptosis correction, and treatment of festoons. In: Alster TS, Apfelberg DC, eds. Cosmetic Laser Surgery. New York: Wiley-Liss; 1999:135–138.

28. Rosenberg G. Full face and neck resurfacing. *Plast Reconstr Surg.* 1997;100:1846–1854.

29. Fitzpatrick RE, Goldman MP. Resurfacing of photodamage of the neck using the ultrapulse CO_2 laser. *Lasers Surg Med.* 1997;20(suppl 9):33.

30. Koch RJ, Newman JP, Goode RL. Closed dressings after laser skin resurfacing. *Arch Otolaryngol Head Neck Surg.* 1998;124:751–757.

31. Kilmer SL. Laser resurfacing complications: how to treat them and how to avoid them. *Int J Aesthetic Restor Surg.* 1997;5:41–45.

32. Bernstein LJ, Kauvar ANB, Grossman M, Geronemus RG. The short- and long-term side effects of carbon dioxide laser resurfacing. *Dermatol Surg.* 1997;23:519–525.

33. Sriprachya-Anunt S, Fitzpatrick RE, Goldman M, Smith S. Infections complicating pulsed carbon dioxide laser resurfacing for photoaged facial skin. *Dermatol Surg.* 1997;23:527–536.

34. Nanni CA, Alster TS. Complications of carbon dioxide laser resurfacing: an evaluation of 500 patients. *Dermatol Surg.* 1998;24:315–320.

35. Laws RA, Finley EM, McCollough ML, Grabski WJ. Alabaster skin after carbon dioxide laser resurfacing with histologic correlation. *Dermatol Surg.* 1998;24:633–636.

36. Richert S, Bridenstine J. Transepidermal elimination of elastic fibers after carbon dioxide laser resurfacing: a report of two cases. *Dermatol Surg.* 1998;24:275–278.

37. Miller ID. The erbium laser gains a role in cosmetic surgery. *Biophotonics Int.* May/June 1997:38–43.

38. Hohenleutner U, Hohenleutner S, Baumler W, et al. Fast and effective skin ablation with an Er:YAG laser: determination of ablation rates and thermal damage zones. *Lasers Surg Med.* 1997;20:242–247.

39. Hughes PS. Skin contraction following erbium:YAG laser resurfacing. *Dermatol Surg:* 1998;24:109–111.

40. Ziering C. Cutaneous laser resurfacing with the erbium YAG laser and the char-free carbon dioxide laser: a clinical comparison of 100 patients. *Int J Aesthetic Restor Surg.* 1997;5:29–37.

41. Weinstein C. Computerized scanning erbium:YAG laser for skin resurfacing. *Dermatol Surg.* 1998;24:83–89.

42. Kye YC. Resurfacing of pitted facial scars with a pulsed Er:YAG laser. *Dermatol Surg.* 1997;23:880–883.

43. Kaufmann R, Hibst R. Pulsed erbium:YAG laser ablation in cutaneous surgery. *Lasers Surg Med.* 1996;19:324–330.

44. McDaniel DH, Ash K, Lord, et al. The erbium:YAG laser: a review and preliminary report on resurfacing of the face, neck, and hands. *Aesth Surg.* 1997;17:157–164.

45. Teikemeier G, Goldberg DJ. Skin resurfacing with the erbium:YAG laser. *Dermatol Surg.* 1997;23:685–687.

46. Khatri K, Ross V, Grevelink J, Anderson R. Comparison of erbium:YAG and CO_2 lasers in wrinkle removal. *Lasers Surg Med.* 1997;21(suppl 9):37.

47. Fleming D. Controversies in skin resurfacing: the role of erbium. *J Cutan Laser Ther.* 1999;1:15–21.

48. Adrian RM. Pulsed carbon dioxide and erbium-YAG laser resurfacing: a comparative clinical and histologic study. *J Cutan Laser Ther.* 1999;1:29–35.

49. Watson D, Keller G, Lacombe V, et al. Autologous fibroblasts for treatment of facial rhytids and dermal depressions. *Arch Facial Plast Surg.* (In Press).

50. Goldman M, Fitzpatrick R. Presented at American Academy of Cosmetic Surgery Annual Meeting; January 31,1999; Los Angeles, CA.

51. Lask G, Lee P, Seyfeadeh M, et al. Nonablative laser treatment of facial rhytids. *SPIE Proceedings.* 1997;2970:338–349.

52. Muccini JA, O'Donell FE, Fuller T, et al. Laser treatment of solar elastosis with epithelial preservation. *Lasers Surg Med.* 1998;23:121–127.

53. Goldberg D, Metzler C. Skin resurfacing utilizing a low-fluence Nd:YAG laser. *J Cutan Laser Ther.* 1999;1:23–27.

54. Goldberg DJ, Whitworth J. Laser skin resurfacing with the Q-switched Nd:YAG laser. *Dermatol Surg.* 1997;23:903–907.

55. Kilmer SL, Chotzen VA. Pulsed dye laser treatment of rhytids. *Lasers Surg Med.* 1997;9(suppl):17.

CHAPTER 6

Cutaneous Laser Exfoliation

W. GREGORY CHERNOFF

Cutaneous laser exfoliation has gained widespread acceptance among specialists offering rejuvenation and general skin care. This acceptance has spurred the development of improved delivery systems that provide precise and selective control of tissue exfoliation. Laser systems employed in ablative exfoliation include the erbium:yttrium-aluminum-garnet (Er:YAG) laser and the carbon dioxide (CO_2) laser; nonablative, nonexfoliating lasers include the 1320-nm YAG laser and the 980-nm diode laser. However, it is essential that those who use these systems for rejuvenation acquire a working knowledge of the histologic aspects of laser exfoliation. Moreover, regardless of the system used, practitioners must have a working knowledge of both laser physics and tissue biophysics to achieve good results (see Chapters 1 and 5). This chapter examines the correlations revealed by histologic studies between clinical treatment endpoints, depth of exfoliation, postoperative erythema, and rhytid resolution. Failure to understand and respect these correlates can lead to undesirable results and scarring in the rejuvenation patient population. The chapter concludes with a brief discussion of the approach to treatment of rejuvenation patients.

ABLATIVE EXFOLIATION

To achieve precise skin exfoliation, one must maximize tissue ablation and minimize residual thermal damage, that is, reduce the amount of heat conducted to surrounding tissue. This balance revolves around a concept known as *thermal relaxation time*. The thermal relaxation time is the maximum amount of time a tissue can absorb energy of a specific wavelength with less than 50% conduction to the surrounding tissue. This has been calculated for a number of chromophores and serves as the basis of successful therapeutic regimens for multiwavelength laser therapy. The thermal relaxation time for the epidermis is approximately 1 millisecond (10^{-3} second), or 1000 microseconds (10^{-6} second). This is calculated based on tissue water as the primary chromophore. Studies have shown, however, that thermal relaxation time for the dermis is more likely dependent on absorption of energy by collagen.[1–19]

CARBON DIOXIDE LASER

In the late 1960s, Fitzpatrick outlined the principle of selective photothermolysis using the CO_2 laser to vaporize specific layers of skin. He noted that the infrared (IR) energy produced by the CO_2 laser at 10,600 nm had a high absorption coefficient for water. Water therefore is the principal chromophore for the CO_2 laser.[8,20] Because of this, the CO_2 laser became a mainstay of cutaneous exfoliation. Application of improved delivery systems, including superpulsed, ultrapulsed, and rapid-scanning technology, allowed for predictable vaporization of the epidermis and dermis with acceptable levels of residual thermal damage. Each of the CO_2 laser delivery systems produces different levels of skin penetration with variable depths of ablation and surrounding thermal damage.[21-24]

The predictability of CO_2 laser systems yielded improved efficacy over conventional forms of exfoliation such as chemical peels and dermabrasion. Chemical peels, whose origins date back centuries, had been the workhorse of aesthetic procedures. However, variations in the type and concentration of acid used, in preoperative skin preparation, and in contact time with the skin had always limited their predictability and safety. In dermabrasion, excessive bleeding during the procedure made visualization of treatment endpoints difficult, resulting in an increased risk of scarring and hypopigmentation. Furthermore, aerosolization of blood posed a significant risk of viral transmission from patient to patient and from patient to medical personnel.

The energy density (fluence) needed for ablation of the skin (both epidermis and dermis) with the CO_2 laser has been calculated to be 5.5 J/cm^2. Thus, the number of watts required to produce a 1-cm^2 spot with sufficient energy to surpass the thermal relaxation threshold of skin with a pulse duration of 1 millisecond would be 5000 W (fluence = power × pulse duration ÷ spot size).[1-3] To reduce this high power requirement, different technologies and lasing strategies have been developed. High-peak-energy, short-exposure-time CO_2 lasers allow for selective and precise tissue exfoliation with lower power (wattage) requirements. The pulses are grouped with short pauses to protect the tissue from excessive thermal damage. These lasers, when coupled with computer-controlled scanning devices that can deliver the pulses rapidly over a large area, yield more rapid treatment times at lower power.

Other delivery systems for CO_2 laser exfoliation use orthogonally rotating mirrors that create a spiral scan. A 0.1- to 0.25-mm focused beam is rapidly scanned over a circular or oval pattern. The "dwell" time over an area and the speed of the scan are calculated by a computer to impart the desired amount of laser energy.[7,8]

The CO_2 laser has been studied using lower fluences in an effort to yield Er:YAG laser–like results. By dropping energy density below 100 to 125 mJ/cm^2 with a spot size of 2.25 mm and performing one pass, Er:YAG laser–like effects could be achieved. Used in this way, the CO_2 laser produced less residual thermal damage, which equates with decreased erythema that persists for a shorter period of time.

Erbium:Yttrium-Aluminum-Garnet Laser

As technology developed, it was found that the Er:YAG laser, emitting a beam of IR energy at 2940 nm, had 10 to 12 times greater absorption by water, yielding increased precision of skin ablation over the CO_2 laser. This higher absorption by water reduces laser energy scattering in the surrounding tissue and subsequent collateral thermal damage. The epidermis and dermis therefore can be ablated serially with the Er:YAG laser with minimal accumulative thermal damage. Thus, the Er:YAG laser is useful for exfoliating superficial epidermal lentigines but is limited in terms of tissue shrinkage per pass when compared with the CO_2 laser. This has clinical importance with regard to rhytid resolution.[16-19]

The Er:YAG laser results in 10 to 12 times greater water absorption than the CO_2 laser at 10,600 nm. In addition, because of the selective absorption of its energy by collagen, the Er:YAG laser also causes tissue ablation with minimal tissue desiccation. Thus, with a typical pulse duration of 250 to 350 microseconds, which is less than the thermal relaxation time of skin at 1 millisecond, the energy density for the ablation of human skin by the Er:YAG laser has been calculated to be 1.6 J/cm^2, as compared with 5.5 J/cm^2 for the high-energy, short-pulsed CO_2 laser. Therefore, the Er:YAG laser produces 10 to 40 μm of tissue ablation with as little as 5 μm of residual thermal damage (proportional to the parameter used).[25-28] In contrast, the high-energy, short-pulsed CO_2 laser produces 80 to 120 μm of tissue ablation but with 50 to 60 μm of irreversible thermal tissue necrosis and an additional 50 μm of thermal damage. With the

Table 6–1. Average Thickness of the Skin in Different Facial Zones

Facial Zone	Epidermis (μm)	Dermis (μm)	Dermis and Epidermis*	Hypodermis (μm)	Total
Mental	149	1375	1524	1020	2544
Forehead	202	969	1171	1210	2381
Upper lip	156	1061	1217	931	2148
Lower lip	113	973	1086	829	1915
Tip of nose	111	918	1029	735	1764
Neck	115	138	253	544	797
Cheek	141	909	1050	459	1509
Glabella	144	324	468	223	691
Eyelids	130	215	345	248	593

*Important skin layers for resurfacing (see text and Fig. 14–10 this volume).

Er:YAG laser, more passes are required to achieve the same level of penetration into the dermis as the high-energy, short-pulsed CO_2 laser. At comparable levels of tissue ablation, however, the Er:YAG laser produces significantly less thermal damage. The downside, however, is the need for a higher number of passes to achieve similar ablation depths. In addition, the Er:YAG laser is not a coagulating laser, so bleeding occurs in the course of treatment when vascular networks are crossed. This can result in the same negative effects as dermabrasion in terms of treatment endpoints and risk to patients and personnel.

HIERARCHY OF MODALITIES

A natural hierarchy of therapeutic modalities arises when comparing these systems. Patients with superficial lentigines or superficial sun-induced damage can benefit from Er:YAG laser exfoliation more so than from CO_2 laser exfoliation, which yields prolonged erythema. Patients desiring maximal reduction of static rhytids, however, would benefit more from CO_2 laser exfoliation because the greater thermal ablation and deeper penetration stimulate an increased collagen remodeling response per pass, thus increasing the rhytid reduction.[29–32]

Table 6–2. Safety Ratio: Dermis/Dermis and Epidermis

Rank and Area	Ratio	Percentage
Low Safety Ratio		
1. Neck	138/253	54.5
2. Eyelids	215/345	62.3
3. Glabella	324/468	69.2
Moderate Safety Ratio		
4. Forehead	929/1171	79.3
5. Cheek	909/1050	86.6
High Safety Ratio		
6. Upper lip	1061/1217	87.2
7. Nasal tip	918/1029	89.2
8. Lower lip	973/1086	89.6
9. Mentum	1375/1524	90.2

COMPARATIVE HISTOLOGIC AND CLINICAL RESULTS

No matter which of these laser systems is used to ablate tissue, excessive thermal injury or coagulative necrosis that extends into adnexal structures will result in scarring. To prevent this, it is important for treating practitioners to have a good working knowledge of the average thicknesses of the epidermal and dermal layers in various zones of the face (Tables 6–1 and 6–2). Figures 6–1 through 6–3

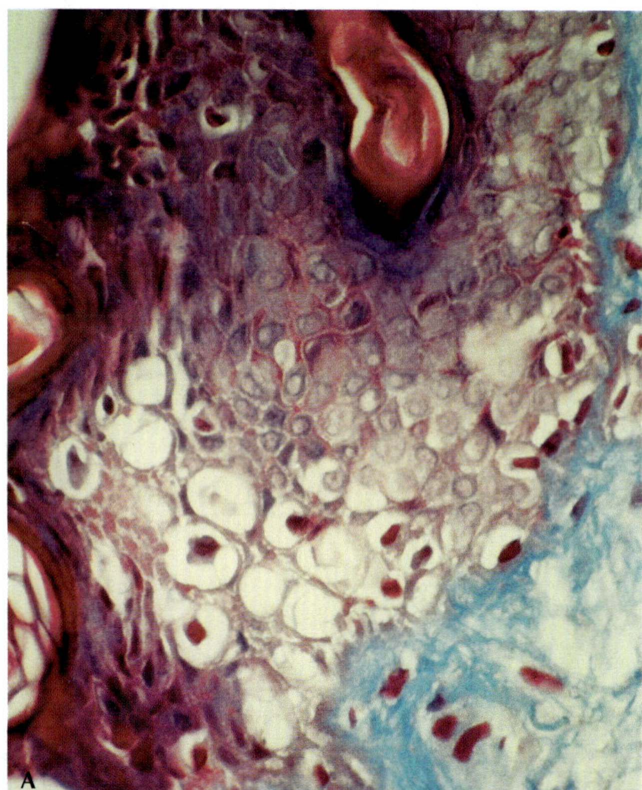
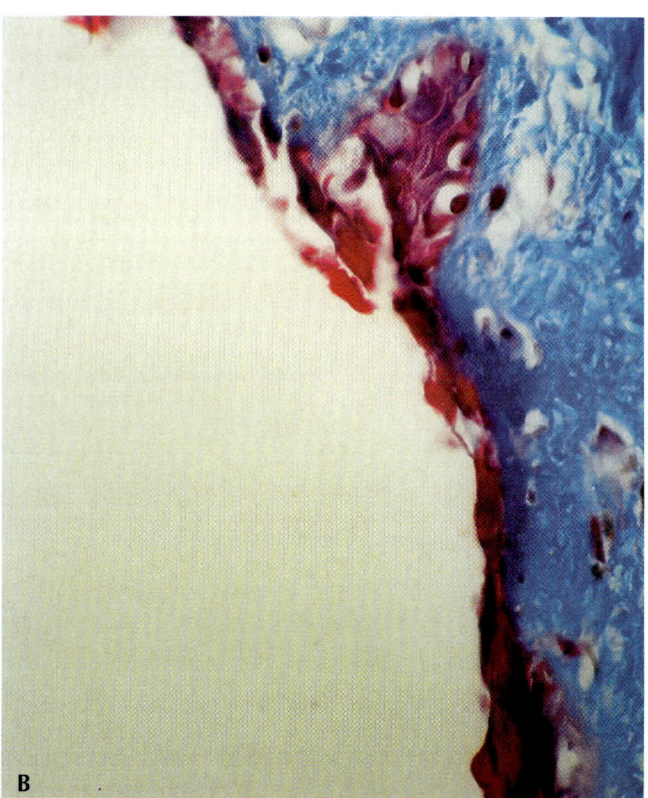

Figure 6–1. (A) Control, trichrome stain. (B) After one pass with the Er:YAG laser at 3 J/cm². Note that 20 μm of exfoliation and 5 μm of residual thermal damage are seen.

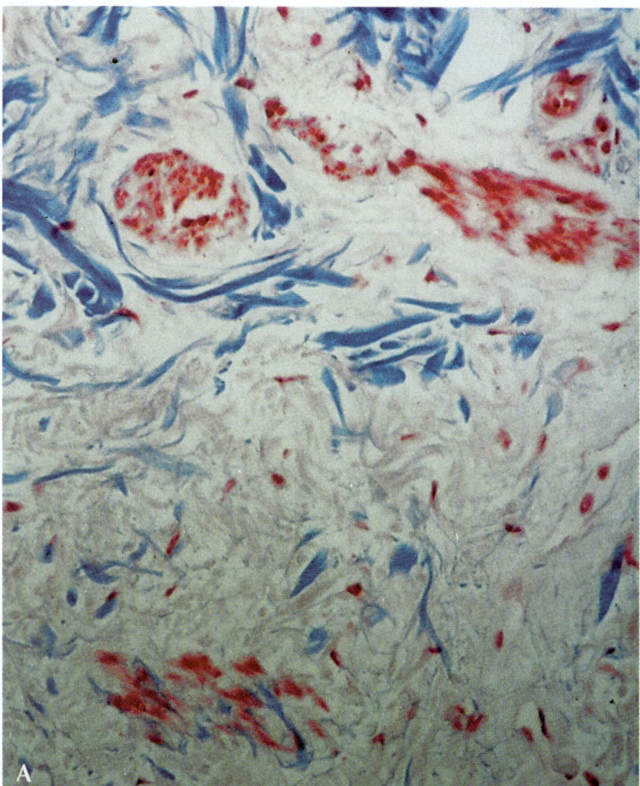
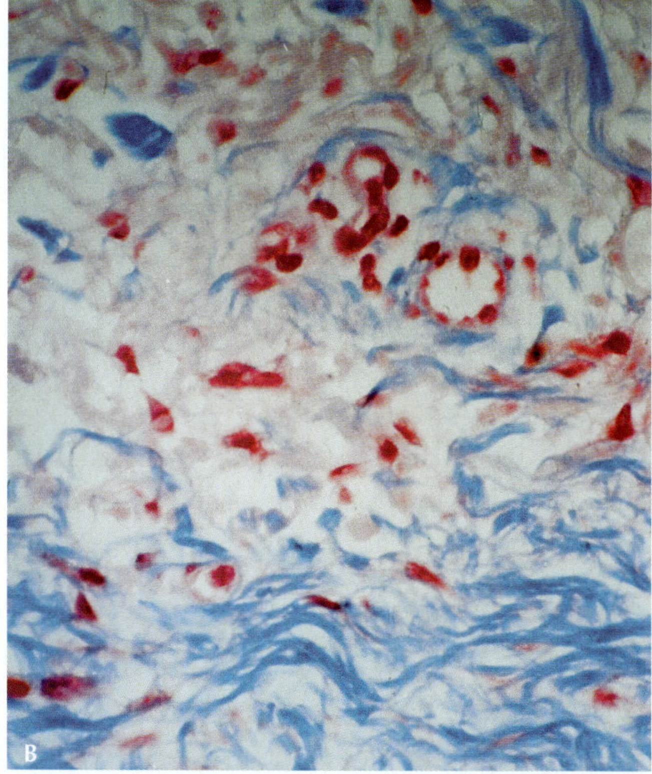

Figure 6–2. (A) Control. (B) One year after Er:YAG laser exfoliation. Note the collagen contraction and neocollagen formation.

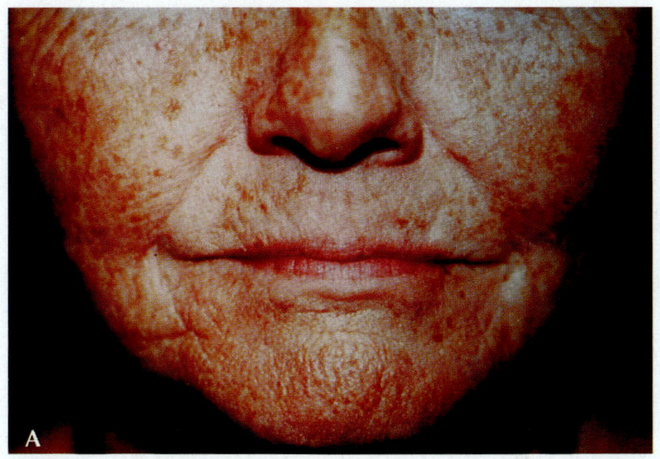

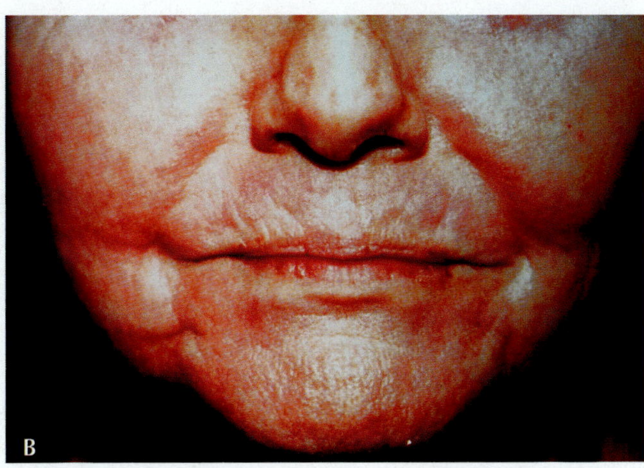

Figure 6–3. (A) Preoperative appearance. (B) Appearance 10 days after Er:YAG laser exfoliation.

illustrate these average thicknesses and should be kept in mind when treating patients with conditions ranging from superficial lentigines to rhytids and scars. Box 6–1 lists lesions that are appropriate for laser exfoliation, lesions that probably should not be exfoliated with the laser, and contraindications to laser exfoliation.

Representative Results

Figure 6–1 presents representative results achieved with the Er:YAG laser. Figure 6–1A provides a preoperative control view, whereas Figure 6–1B shows the results after one pass of the Er:YAG laser. Note the minimal exfoliation and minimal residual thermal damage. Figure 6–2 shows the amount of collagen contraction visible 1 year after Er:YAG laser exfoliation. Figure 6–3 is representative of the clinical results achievable with the Er:YAG system. Note that the superficial epidermal lentigines have been meticulously removed.

Figures 6–4 through 6–6 illustrate the comparable CO_2 laser results. Figure 6–4A is a preoperative control view, and Figure 6–4B shows the result after one pass at 150 mJ/cm^2. Notice the increased depth of exfoliation, as well as the increased residual thermal damage. Figure 6–5 illustrates the collagen contraction and neocollagen formation at 1 year. Figure 6–6 shows a typical patient result at 6 months.

Box 6–1. Skin Changes Treatable by Laser Resurfacing
Photo damage
Uneven pigmentation
Atrophic wrinkles
Early redundant skin
Actinic keratosis
History of superficial facial skin cancers
Traumatic scars
Mild to moderate acne scars

Overly Aggressive Exfoliation

Figure 6–7A shows a biopsy specimen from an Er:YAG laser exfoliation that was too aggressive. Note the accumulation of thermal damage. This resulted in clinical scarring, as seen in Fig. 6–7B.

Figure 6–8A shows another specimen from a CO_2 laser exfoliation that was too aggressive. This treatment produced coagulative necrosis that extended into the adnexal structures and left a residual open wound that had to heal from the peripheral edges. The wound took 6 months to heal, and the patient ended up with scarring and hypopigmentation, as seen in Figure 6–8B.

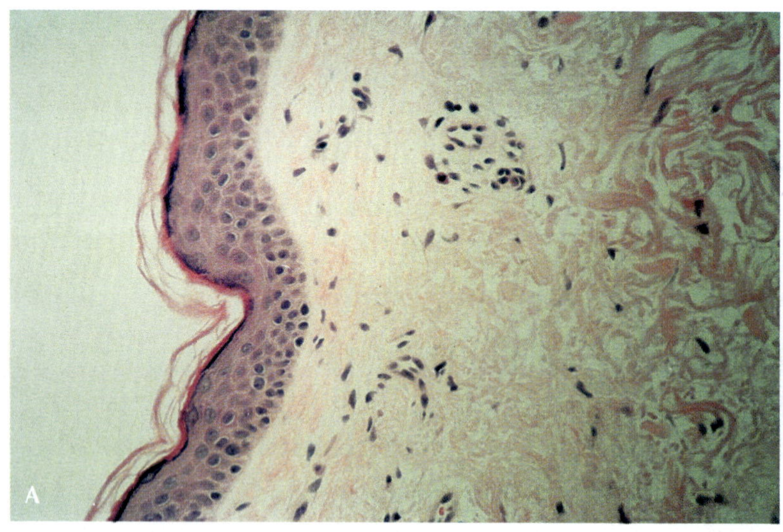

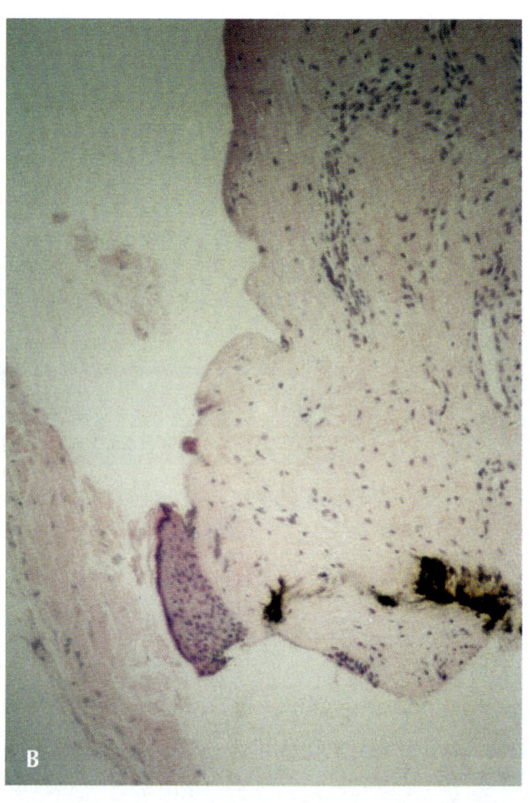

Figure 6–4. (A) Control, H&E stain. (B) After treatment with the CO_2 laser at 150 mJ/100 W, density level 3, one pass. Note the 50 μm of exfoliation and 20 μm of residual thermal damage.

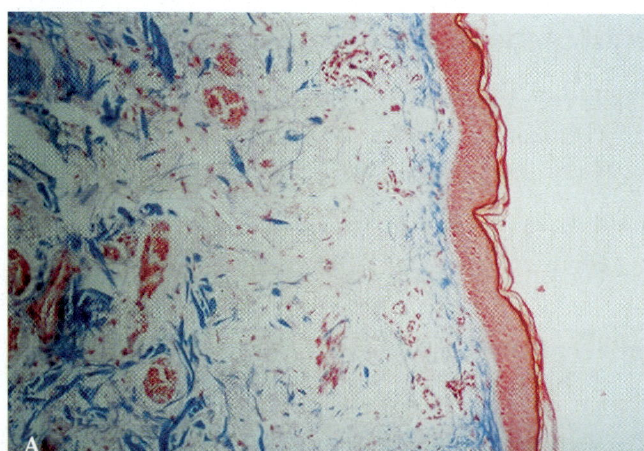

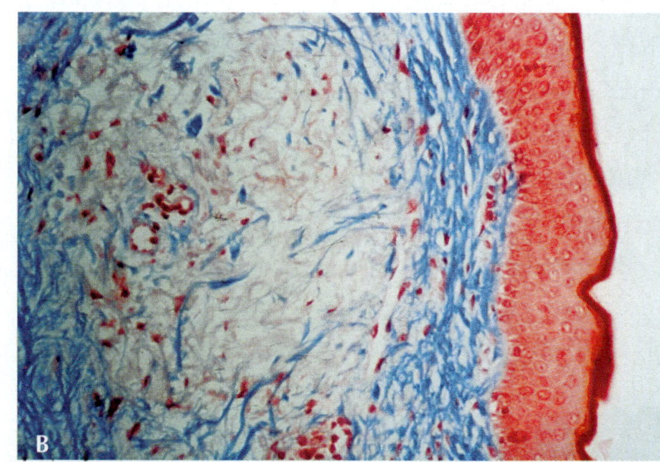

Figure 6–5. (A) Control. (B) One year after CO_2 laser exfoliation.   Note increased collagen contraction and neocollagen formation.

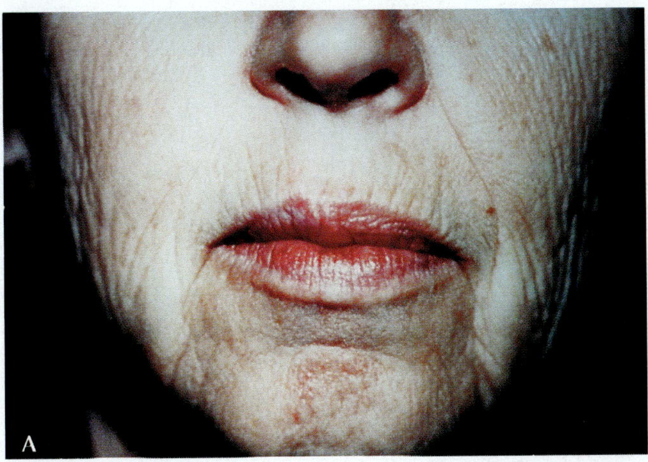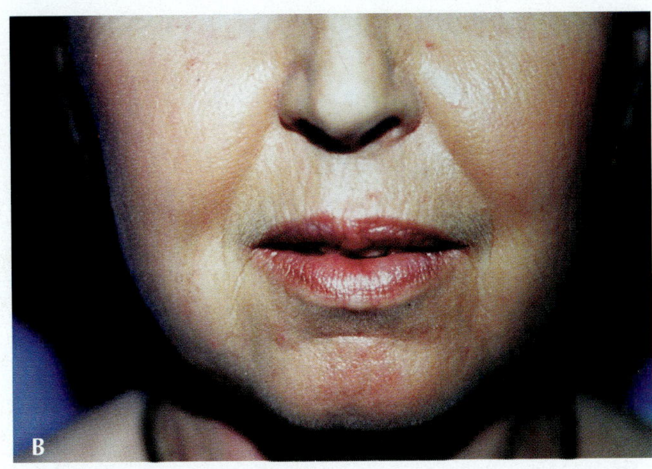

Figure 6–6. (A) Preoperative appearance. (B) Appearance 6 months after CO_2 laser exfoliation.

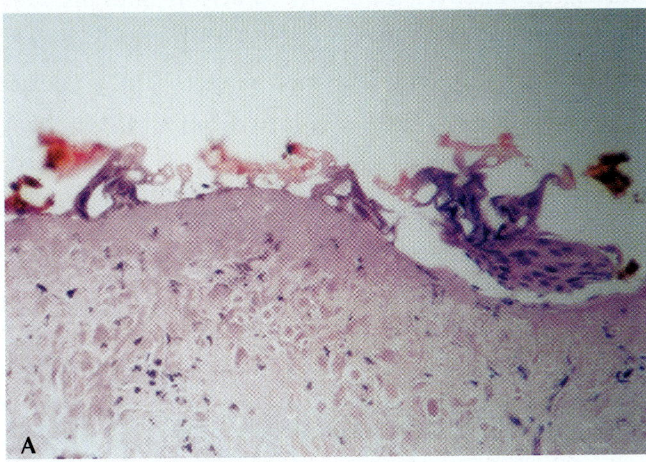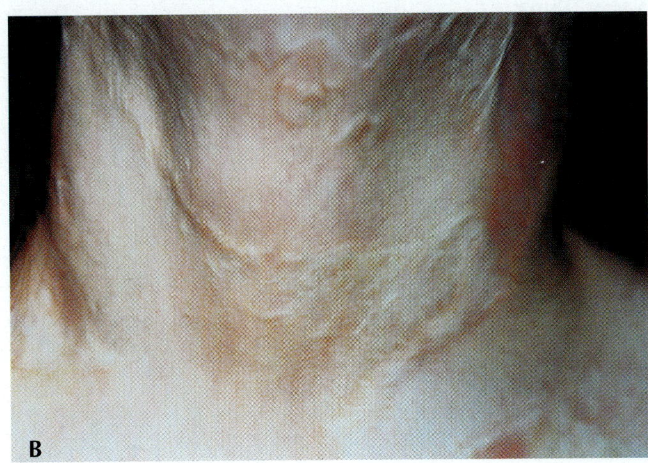

Figure 6–7. (A) After treatment with the Er:YAG laser at 3 J/cm^2, with a 3-mm spot size, seven passes. Note the residual thermal necrosis. (B) Resulting scarring.

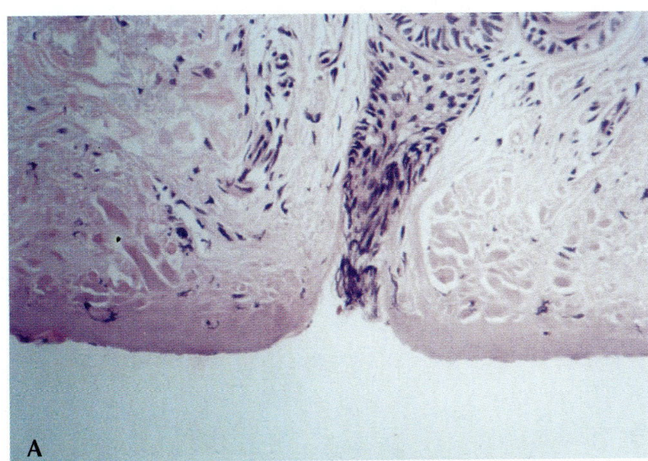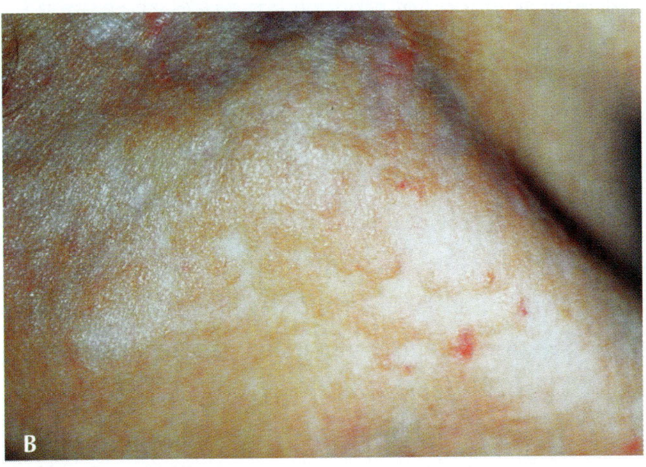

Figure 6–8. (A) After treatment with the CO_2 laser at 300 mJ/100 W, with a 2.25-mm spot size, three passes. Note the residual thermal necrosis. (B) Resulting scarring.

Table 6–3. Fitzpatrick Classification of Skin Type

Type	Hair Color	Skin Color	Eye Color	Reaction to Sun
I	Red	Light	Blue-green	Burns, never tans
II	Blonde	Light	Blue	Burns, may tan
III	Brown	Medium	Brown	Burns, then tans
IV	Brown-black	Moderate brown	Brown-black	Tans
V	Black	Dark brown (Asian)	Dark	Tans
VI	Black	Black (African)	Dark	Tans

LASER AND PATIENT SELECTION

SKIN TYPE

Several factors are helpful in selecting the appropriate laser fluence for each patient. One such factor is the Fitzpatrick skin type (Table 6–3). This classification is used to predict skin reactivity to thermal exposure based on pigment content and reaction to sun exposure. Patients with Fitzpatrick skin types I and II are more prone to postoperative erythema. Patients with higher skin melanin content (Fitzpatrick skin types V and VI) are more likely to show pigment abnormalities following therapy. However, such patients have greater resistance to sun-induced photoaging because of the higher melanin content of their skin. For these patients, treatment with the Er:YAG laser is thought to be a better choice than the CO_2 laser because of its lower likelihood of producing pigmentary changes.

SKIN THICKNESS AND PHOTO DAMAGE

Another factor in selection is skin thickness (Table 6–4). Patients with areas of thicker epidermis and dermis, irrespective of the cause, will require higher fluences or more passes with either laser. In addition, the laser should be used to feather the surrounding skin areas to avoid abrupt lines of demarcation.

The degree of sun-induced photo damage and the patient's age also have a direct impact on the degree of skin aging. Ultraviolet light changes both the epidermis and the dermis over time. The epidermis thickens, and this becomes apparent clinically as an increase in keratoses. The rete ridges, however, retract. With a thicker epidermis, higher fluences will be required to exfoliate this layer prior to reaching the dermis to stimulate collagen remodeling. However, with increased sun exposure over time, both the papillary and the reticular dermis become thinner.

AGE

The dermal appendages also decrease with age. This is important because these appendages are necessary for

Table 6–4. Absolute Thickness of the Dermis*

Rank and Area	Thickness of Dermis (μm)
1. Neck	138
2. Eyelids	215
3. Glabella	324
4. Cheek	909
5. Nasal tip	918
6. Forehead	969
7. Lower lip	973
8. Upper lip	1061
9. Mentum	1375

*For thin dermis, less energy should be used after the first pass of the laser.

skin regeneration after deep exfoliation. With age, the collagen may thicken but become less organized. Changes in collagen organization and compaction parallel to the skin surface are apparent over time with exfoliation accomplished with either the Er:YAG or CO_2 laser. Along with these collagen changes, increased elastin deposition occurs in the dermis. The collagen-elastin effects are considered responsible for effacing deeper wrinkles.

PATIENT EXPECTATIONS

As with any aesthetic procedure, the treating practitioner must determine that the patient has realistic goals and expectations for laser exfoliation, no matter which laser system is to be used. Both the Er:YAG and the CO_2 laser achieve their effects by generating sufficient heat energy within the dermis to both stimulate new collagen formation and cause contraction of existing collagen and elastin fibers. The net result is a softening of static facial rhytids. However, thermal effects are not the only mechanism involved, because rhytids can also be improved with both chemical peels and dermabrasion.

CONCLUSION

The postoperative erythema seen with laser therapy is directly proportional to the depth of exfoliation and the residual thermal damage. The resulting neovascularization is a normal part of wound healing that also contributes to the erythematous state. Known danger areas in which to avoid excessive or aggressive exfoliation are those with few adnexal structures to contribute to successful healing. Such areas should be treated with caution. However, to avoid significant postoperative hypertrophic scarring, treating practitioners must learn to correlate "per pass" clinical criteria with proven data derived from histologically examined specimens. Once this working knowledge becomes second nature, com-

plication rates of less than 1% should become the standard of care.

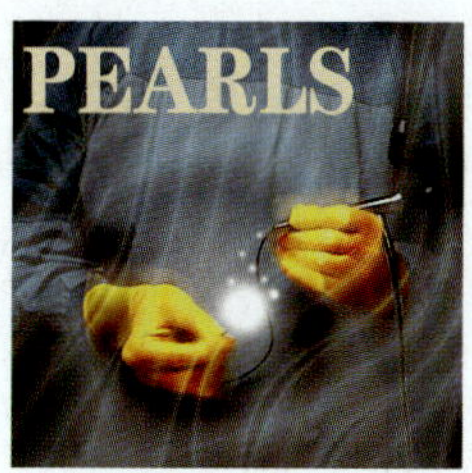

- To achieve precise skin exfoliation, one must maximize tissue ablation and minimize residual thermal damage.
- The predictability of CO_2 laser systems yields improved efficacy over conventional forms of exfoliation such as chemical peels and dermabrasion.
- The CO_2 laser has been studied using lower fluences in an effort to yield Er:YAG laser–like results. By dropping energy density, using a smaller spot size, and performing one pass, Er:YAG laser–like effects could be achieved. Used in this way, the CO_2 laser produces less residual thermal damage, which equates with decreased erythema that persists for a shorter period of time.
- The Er:YAG laser is absorbed more by water, yielding increased precision of skin ablation over the CO_2 laser and less laser energy scattering in the surrounding tissue and subsequent collateral thermal damage. Thus, the Er:YAG laser is useful for exfoliating superficial epidermal lentigines.
- At comparable levels of tissue ablation, the Er:YAG laser produces significantly less thermal damage than the CO_2 laser.

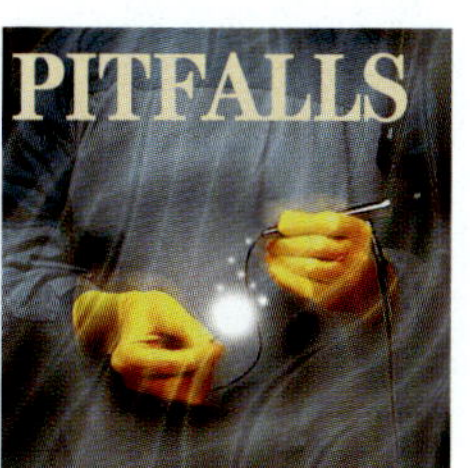

- More passes are needed with the Er:YAG laser to achieve similar ablation depths to those of the CO_2 laser.
- The Er:YAG laser is not a coagulating laser, so bleeding occurs in the course of treatment when vascular networks are crossed.
- Regardless of which laser system is used to ablate tissue, excessive thermal injury or coagulative necrosis that extends into adnexal structures will result in scarring.

REFERENCES

1. Anderson RR, and Parrish JA. Selective photothermolysis: precise microsurgery by selective absorption of pulsed radiation. *Science* 1983;220:524.
2. Walsh JT Jr., Flotte TJ, Andersonn RR, and Deutsch TF. Pulsed CO_2 laser tissue ablation: effect of tissue type and pulse duration on thermal damage. *Lasers Surg. Med.* 1988; 8:108.
3. Walsh JT Jr., and Deutsch TF. Pulsed CO_2 laser tissue ablation: measurement of the ablation rate. *Lasers Surg. Med.* 1988;8:264.
4. Weinstein C. Ultrapulse carbon dioxide laser removal of periocular wrinkles in association with laser blepharoplasty. *J Clin Laser Med Surg.* 1994;12:205.
5. Alster TS, and West TB. Resurfacing of atrophic scars with a high-energy, pulsed carbon dioxide laser. *Dermatol Surg.* 1995;22:151.
6. Waldorf HA, Kauvar ANB, and Geronemus RG. Skin resurfacing of fine to deep rhytides using a char-free carbon dioxide laser in 47 patients. *Dermatol Surg.* 1995;21:940.
7. Lask G, Keller G, Lowe NJ, and Gomley D. Laser skin resurfacing with the SilkTouch flashscanner for facial rhytides. *Dermatol Surg.* 1995;21:1021.
8. David LM, Sarne A, and Unger WP. Rapid laser scanning for facial resurfacing. *Dermatol Surg.* 1995;21:1031.
9. Alster TS, and Garg S. Treatment of facial rhytides with a high-energy, pulsed carbon dioxide laser. *Plast Reconstr Surg.* 1996;98:794.
10. Fitzpatrick RE, Goldman MP, Satur NM, and Tope WD. Pulsed carbon dioxide laser resurfacing of photoaged facial skin. *Arch Dermatol.* 1996;132:395.
11. Alster TS. Comparison of two high-energy, pulsed carbon dioxide lasers in the treatment of periorbital rhytides. *Dermatol Surg.* 1996;22:341.
12. Apfelberg DB. Ultrapulse carbon dioxide laser with CPG scanner for full-face resurfacing of rhytides, photoaging, and acne scars. *Plast Reconstr Surg.* 1997;99:1817.
13. Apfelberg DB. A critical appraisal of high-energy pulsed carbon dioxide laser facial resurfacing for acne scars. *Ann Plast Surg.* 1997;38:95.
14. Bernstein LJ, Kauvar ANB, Grossman MC, and Geronemus RG. Scar resurfacing with high-energy, short-pulsed and flashscanning carbon dioxide lasers. *Dermatol Surg.* 1998;24:101.
15. West TB, and Alster TS. Improvement of infraorbital hyperpigmentation following carbon dioxide laser resurfacing. *Dermatol Surg.* 1998;24:65.
16. Kye YC. Resurfacing of pitted facial scars with a pulsed Er:YAG laser. *Dermatol Surg.* 1997;23:880.
17. Teikemeir G, and Goldberg DJ. Skin resurfacing with erbium:YAG laser. *Dermatol Surg.* 1997;23:685.
18. Perez MI, Bank DE, and Silvers D. Skin resurfacing of the face with the erbium:YAG laser. *Dermatol Surg.* 1998;24:653.
19. Bass LS. Erbium:YAG laser skin resurfacing: preliminary clinical evaluation. *Ann Plast Surg.* 1998;40:328.
20. Fitzpatrick RE, Ruiz-Esparza J, and Goldman MP. The depth of thermal necrosis using the CO_2 laser: a comparison of the superpulsed mode and conventional mode. *J Dermatol Surg Oncol.* 1991;17:340.
21. Lanzafame RJ, Naim JO, Rogers DW, et al. Comparisons of continuous-wave, chop-wave, and superpulse laser wounds. *Lasers Surg Med.* 1988;8:119.
22. Alster TS, Kauvar ANB, and Geronemus RG. Histology of high-energy, pulsed CO_2 laser resurfacing. *Semin Cutan Med Surg.* 1996;15:189.
23. Alster TS, Nanni CA, and Williams CM. Comparison of four carbon dioxide resurfacing lasers: a clinical and histopathologic evaluation. *Dermatol Surg.* (In press).
24. Stuzin JM, Baker TJ, Baker TM, and Kligman AM. Histologic effects of the high-energy pulsed CO_2 laser on photoaged facial skin. *Plast Reconstr Surg.* 1997;99:2036.
25. Walsh JT Jr., Flotte TJ, and Deutsch TF. Er:YAG laser ablation of tissue: effect of pulse duration and tissue type on thermal damage. *Lasers Surg Med.* 1989;9:327.
26. Hibst R, and Kaufmann R. Effects of laser parameters on pulsed Er:YAG laser ablation. *Laser Med Sci.* 1991;6:391.
27. Hohenleutner U, Hohenleutner S, Baumaler W, and Landthaler M. Fast and effective skin ablation with an Er:YAG laser: determination of ablation rates and thermal damage zones. *Lasers Surg Med.* 1997;20:242.
28. Alster TS. Comparison of six erbium:YAG lasers for cutaneous resurfacing: a clinical and histopathologic evaluation. *Lasers Surg Med.* 1998;10(Suppl.):32.
29. Ross E, Naseef G, Skrobal M, et al. In vivo dermal collagen shrinkage and remodeling following CO_2 laser resurfacing. *Lasers Surg Med.* 1996;18:38.
30. Fulton JE, and Barnes T. Collagen shrinkage (selective dermaplasty) with the high-energy pulsed carbon dioxide laser. *Dermatol Surg.* 1998;24:3.
31. Ross EV, and Anderson RR. The Erbium Laser in Skin Resurfacing. In Alster TS and Apfelberg DB (Eds.), *Cosmetic Laser Surgery*, 2nd Ed. New York: John Wiley, 1999;57:84.
32. Alster TS. Laser Resurfacing of Rhytides. In Alster TS (Ed.), *Manual of Cutaneous Laser Techniques*. Philadelphia: Lippincott-Raven, 1997;104–122.

CHAPTER 7

Sharplan SilkTouch and FeatherTouch Flashscanners

VICTOR G. LACOMBE, KEITH E. BLACKWELL, AND GREGORY S. KELLER

The carbon dioxide (CO_2) laser has evolved significantly from the original continuous wave (CW) lasers used since the early 1970s for cutting and ablating skin and other tissues. These improvements have occurred largely through efforts to reduce the incidence of complications, such as scarring, hyper- and hypopigmentation, and skin textural changes that were prevalent when older CW lasers were used. The transformation of the CO_2 laser into a tool for aesthetic resurfacing has resulted in the development of more appropriate methods of energy delivery to the tissue. Current technology attempts to maximize ablative precision and minimize the undesired spread of thermal damage to surrounding tissue. Although debate continues about whether a certain degree of thermal energy transfer to collagen in the dermis is necessary for skin contraction and remodeling, there is agreement that char-free resurfacing is absolutely imperative and that overly aggressive lasing is worse than a conservative approach that may require several treatment sessions.

The two philosophies of laser energy application involve (1) a high-energy, pulsed laser or (2) a CW laser beam that is focused on a tiny spot and then rests for an extremely short time. The Sharplan SilkTouch and FeatherTouch flashscanners utilize the CW mechanism of action. Energy from the CO_2 laser is focused through a lens (F = focal length = 125 mm) into a 0.1-mm spot that is aimed by a microprocessor-controlled optome-chanical set of rotating mirrors that trace a collapsing spiral pattern on the target tissue surface. The diameter of the traced area ranges from 1 to 6 mm. The 0.1-mm spot is focused on the tissue for only 1 millisecond (less than the thermal relaxation time of skin), and the entire scan area is treated within 200 milliseconds. In this way, high energies can be delivered to tissue over a short period of time. The small spot size allows the laser system to operate with lower overall power requirements, and the rotating mirrors allow for rapid treatment of a reasonably sized area.[1]

At a typical operating power of 7 W and a 3-mm scan size, 70 μm of ablation and 75–150 μm of residual thermal damage can be expected with the first pass of the laser. Subsequent passes result in less ablation and relatively greater thermal injury secondary to tissue desiccation. Histologically, this depth has been demonstrated repeatedly.[2,3]

ACCESSORIES

The rapidity of treatment can be improved by adding a computerized pattern generator (CPG) that rapidly fires multiple repetitions of the scan area over a larger area. In this way, a large area can be treated with great precision and controlled degrees of overlap. For example, without a CPG, using a 0.2-second "on" time and a 0.4-second "off" time between repeat pulses with a 3-mm spot size requires a very long time to resurface an entire face.

Furthermore, the amount of overlap of each pulse depends on the freehand skill of the operator. However, a computer can aim the beam accurately and fire repetitive pulses in very rapid succession. The amount of overlap—0, 10, or 30%—can be programmed to occur with unparalleled precision.

The CPG is also available on the FeatherTouch flashscanner, which is a second-generation device from Sharplan. In addition to the CPG function, the FeatherTouch comes with a display screen that allows for easy programming of the CO_2 laser for CW cutting or aesthetic resurfacing and provides recommended settings. There is now a 260-mm handpiece that can be programmed to lase a 15 $\times$ 15-mm area in an extremely short time.

TREATMENT PROTOCOL

The FeatherTouch is quite user friendly and is geared toward the clinician who may or may not have much experience with lasers. Certainly, larger spot sizes require higher power settings, and the display panel recommends initial settings. The importance of test firing the laser prior to use on patients cannot be overstated because high wattage in a focused beam can cause serious tissue damage. The important thing to remember is that treating a patient with a laser is not technically demanding. However, selection of the appropriate candidate for treatment, the laser parameters, and the optimum number of passes requires judgment and varies from patient to patient, as well as from one anatomic area to another. Perioperative management is also extremely important in the overall treatment process. Much time and effort are required by the physician and his or her staff to counsel and care for the patient before and after the few minutes the laser is actually employed. Complications that result from improper treatment and poor perioperative management can be devastating. Therefore, the novice laser surgeon should be warned that the procedure is not as easy as an instructional video or afternoon workshop may indicate.

PATIENT SELECTION AND PREPARATION

Patient selection and counseling are perhaps the most important aspect of any laser resurfacing procedure. Ideally, patients should be fair-skinned (i.e., Fitzpatrick skin type I or II) and desire moderate reduction of fine lines and/or removal of sun damage or epidermal lentigines. They should expect 6 weeks or more of postoperative erythema and understand that sunscreen is mandatory for 6 months following treatment. Extensive education frequently is necessary for patients who expect the "miracle" of laser surgery to restore their youth, remove all wrinkles, and result in very little "down time."

Patients should comply with a preoperative skin regimen that includes retinoic acid or α-hydroxy acid and a bleaching agent, such as hydroquinone. Darker-skinned patients are urged to use bleaching agents for 2–4 weeks prior to treatment. An antiviral and antibiotic (usually cephalexin) are prescribed for 7 days after surgery.

PERIOPERATIVE TREATMENT

For periocular and perioral treatments, regional nerve blocks are often adequate for anesthesia. Occasionally, direct local infiltration of anesthesia is necessary. For full-face resurfacing, patients usually receive monitored anesthesia care with propofol and fentanyl. The areas to be treated are cleansed with alcohol and allowed to dry thoroughly before laser activation. Eye shields are employed routinely. After each pass of the laser, the areas are wiped gently but firmly with saline-soaked gauze to remove debris from the skin surface. Periocular regions are treated with an average of 5 W and the rest of the face with 7–8 W. Perioral furrows often require multiple passes aimed at the shoulders of the rhytids to achieve satisfactory results. Thinner skin (e.g., eyelids) certainly receives no more than two passes. A chamois color of the skin or a maximum of four passes is the usual endpoint of treatment. Touch-ups later are preferable compared with the risk of scarring from aggressive treatment.

POSTOPERATIVE TREATMENT

Postoperatively, the treated areas are covered with a porous Teflon semiocclusive dressing and then coated with Crisco vegetable shortening. The closed method of wound healing has been shown to decrease erythema and

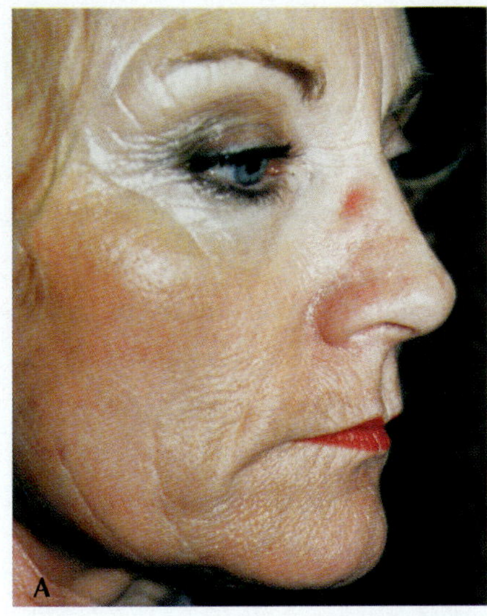
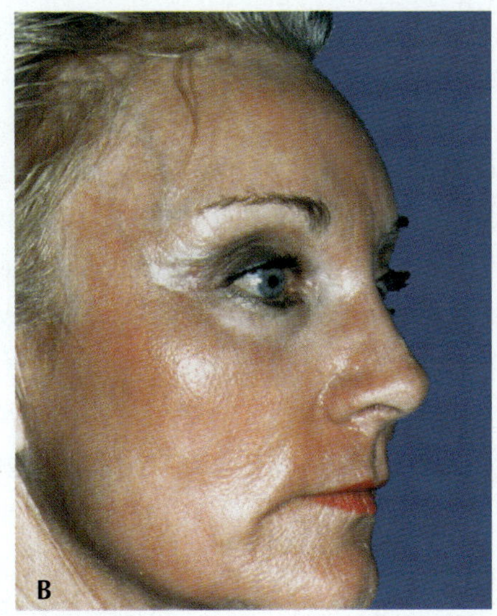

Figure 7–1. (A) A 55-year-old woman before full-face CO_2 laser resurfacing. (B) Postoperative result.

discomfort, as well as speed reepithelialization.[4] Patients are instructed not to use antibiotic ointments because sensitivity reactions are common. In addition, patients are reminded to report any persistent pain because this is probably a sign of infection. With continuous application of Crisco there is minimal crusting or scab formation, and healing is usually complete by 7–10 days. Thereafter, a mild moisturizer is recommended, and a 1% to 2% hydrocortisone cream can be applied to lessen erythema. Patients also receive at least one course of a Medrol (methyl prednisolone) dose pack.

Sunscreen and cosmetic camouflage may begin after 2 weeks if there are no complications, but cosmetics should be new because used brushes and compacts may harbor bacteria. Spot testing new brands or those used in the past is also recommended because skin sensitivity is very high at this point. Green-tinted cosmetics best conceal erythema and can be used under foundation or base normally worn by the patient. Erythema should decrease over the next 6 weeks or so, but some patients take up to 3 months to resolve completely.

CLINICAL RESULTS AND COMPLICATIONS

The SilkTouch and FeatherTouch flashscanners are very effective tools for CO_2 laser skin resurfacing. Studies have shown significant reduction in rhytids, as well as up to a 30% contraction of the skin.[5] Figures 7–1 and 7–2 show good results obtained with this laser system.

Persistent erythema can be seen in some patients even after sensitivity reactions, infection, and sun exposure

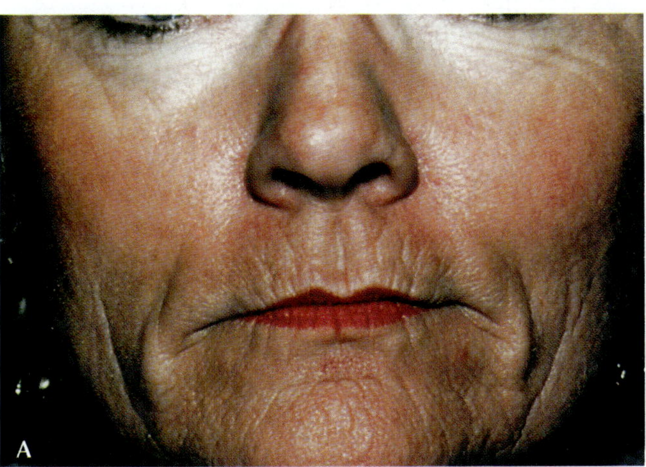
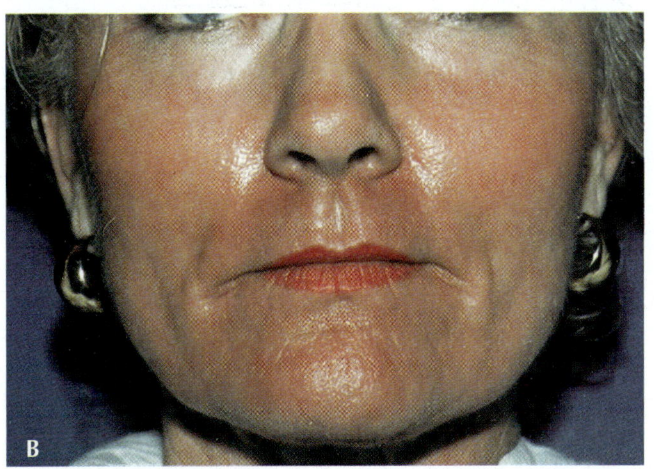

Figure 7–2. (A) A 55-year-old woman before CO_2 laser treatment of deep perioral rhytids. (B) Postoperative result.

have been ruled out. These patients can be helped with either topical steroid preparations or oral corticosteroid tapers.

Hyperpigmentation is common following laser resurfacing of patients with skin type IV or higher. This phenomenon is rarely permanent and can often be prevented or treated with bleaching agents such as 4% hydroquinone and sunscreen. Reassurance and time are the best medicine for these patients. The most dreaded complication is hypopigmentation, which can occur up to 1 year after initial treatment. Prolonged healing times, infection, and unusually persistent erythema or hyperpigmentation may signal that hypopigmentation will occur.

Scarring occurs primarily from resurfacing too deeply, resurfacing skin that has few adnexal structures, or lasing skin that has been scarred previously. The use of isotretinoin within 1 year prior to laser treatment also can result in scarring.[6] In light of complications such as these, the importance of conservatively using such a powerful tool becomes acutely obvious.

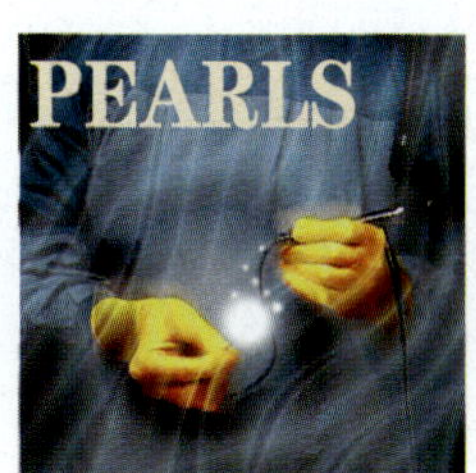

- The use of a microprocessor-controlled optomechanical set of rotating mirrors to trace a collapsing spiral pattern on the target tissue surface and the addition of a computerized pattern genera torallow a large area to be treated with great precision and controlled degrees of overlap without relying on the variable freehand skill of the operator.

- Although the FeatherTouch is quite user friendly, it is important to test fire the laser prior to use on a patient because high wattage in a focused beam can cause serious tissue damage. The procedure is also not as easy as an instructional video or afternoon workshop may indicate.

- As with other laser modalities, touch-ups are preferable to the risk of scarring from aggressive treatment.

- The closed method of wound healing using Crisco vegetable shortening has been shown to decrease erythema and discomfort, as well as speed reepithelialization. With continuous application of Crisco there is minimal crusting or scab formation, and healing is usually complete by 7–10 days.

REFERENCES

1. Chernoff G, Slatkine M, Zair E, et al. SilkTouch: a new technology for skin resurfacing in aesthetic surgery. *J Clin Laser Med Surg.* 1995;13:97–100.
2. Chernoff G, Schoenrock L, Cramer H, et al. Cutaneous laser resurfacing. *Int J Aesthetic Reconstr Surg.* 1995;3:57–68.
3. Lask G, Keller G, Lowe N, et al. Laser skin resurfacing with the SilkTouch flashscanner for facial rhytids. *Dermatol Surg.* 1995;21:1021–1024.
4. Koch RJ, Newman JP, Goode RL. Closed dressings after laser skin resurfacing. *Arch Otolaryngol Head Neck Surg.* 1998;124:751–757.
5. Keller G, Rawnsley J, Cutcliffe B, Watson J. Erbium:YAG and carbon dioxide laser resurfacing 1998. *Facial Plast Surg Clin North Am.* 1998;6:167–181.
6. Nanni CA, Alster TS. Complications of carbon dioxide laser resurfacing: an evaluation of 500 patients. *Dermatol Surg.* 1998;24:315–320.

CHAPTER 8

Surgipulse Laser Resurfacing

WILLIAM H. BEESON

Laser resurfacing has ushered in a new era in aesthetic facial surgery. In the past, chemical exfoliation was the primary treatment for sun-induced photoaging. Chemical peels were divided into superficial, medium, and deep categories based on the depth of wounding produced by a particular agent. This nomenclature has been carried over to laser resurfacing modalities.

By definition, a *superficial* chemical peel produces injury in the upper dermis and sometimes extends into the superficial papillary dermis. Dermal changes in superficial peels are generally minimal. A *medium-depth* peel induces histologic alterations in the upper reticular dermis and produces a wound depth of 0.45 to 0.60 mm. A *deep* peel extends into the reticular dermis with a wound depth of 0.6 to 0.8 mm.[1] This breakdown can serve as a benchmark for categorizing laser resurfacing techniques.

Use of the the carbon dioxide (CO_2) laser for resurfacing is not a new concept. Over recent decades, surgeons have used lasers increasingly and have refined the techniques for resurfacing. To date, the CO_2 laser has been the most popular laser for skin resurfacing. The histopathologic basis for its use has been to localize dehydration of the skin, limit the depth of tissue damage, and produce consistent attempts at penetration. This is an advantage over chemical exfoliation techniques, which may have a variable depth of penetration because of such factors as skin preparation, amount of peel solution applied, and application technique of the surgeon.

Coincident with their wider acceptance, CO_2 lasers have undergone significant technological advancements that have greatly improved clinical results. The extreme precision that can be obtained with the high-energy, ultrashort-pulse CO_2 laser has led to its use in treating a wide variety of cutaneous disorders. Currently, CO_2 lasers eclipse chemical exfoliation as the treatment of choice for photoaged skin.

High-energy CO_2 lasers are *gain-switching* lasers, which means that various waveforms can be created by switching the gain medium (also known as the lasing medium) that the power source "pumps" to create the laser beam. In the gain-switching mode, the power supply generates a high-power pulse of current that "overpumps" the lasing medium (gas mixture), producing a burst of optical power in excess of the laser's normal capacity. Typically, this burst is twice the normal output of the laser tube.

There are essentially two types of gain-switching lasers: those excited by alternating current (ac) and those excited by direct current (dc). Another advancement in CO_2 laser technology has been the development of *flash scanners*. These are microprocessor-controlled miniature optical-mechanical scanners that consist of two orthogonally vibrating mirrors and a focusing lens. Reflection of the laser light between the vibrating mirrors and through the lens causes the beam to deviate, generating a rapidly collapsing spiral curve on the tissues with a focus that is smaller than 0.2 mm in diameter. The time required to complete the spiral is approximately 0.2 seconds. Thus, a CO_2 laser with a 7:1 flash scanner can deliver approximately 400 mJ/cm^2 of energy to tissues.

It is important to have a sound comprehension of the pathophysiology of laser surgery. In essence, the light beam of a CO_2 laser is absorbed by a chromophore in the tissue, which for the CO_2 laser is water. When laser energy is absorbed by tissue water, the temperature of the tissue increases, which usually results in vaporization, or ablation, of the tissue proteins, with the heat being dispersed as steam and not as thermal trauma to tissues, according to a laser manufacturer (Sharplan Lasers, personal communication, 1997). If the tissue is heated without vaporization, tissue temperature increases dramatically to over 600°C, and charring can result. When this occurs, three zones of tissue damage result. The first is composed of carbonized eschar. Beneath this is an area of coagulative necrosis. And finally, there is a sheath of edema that surrounds the ablated site.

The amount of tissue vaporized is directly proportional to the power density of the laser. This is important because too much power produces a zone of damaged tissue in which the collagen is somewhat mummified, resulting in delayed healing of the dermis. If one can reduce this area of thermal damage, more rapid healing is seen and less scarring occurs. One way to do this is to use a shorter laser exposure with a very high power density. In this way, the same volume of tissue is vaporized as with a longer exposure, but at a lower power. This means that there is less thermal damage to the tissues. With high-energy gain-switching CO_2 lasers, surgeons now can achieve very high energy levels in very short periods of time in which each individual pulse of energy never exceeds 600 milliseconds, which is less than the thermal relaxation time of skin tissue.

SURGIPULSE XJ150 LASER

The Surgipulse XJ150 laser (Sharplan Lasers, Inc., Allendale, NJ) is an example of a high-energy, short-pulsed, dc CO_2 laser. The Surgipulse delivers precalculated, closely spaced pulse pairs that sum to the displayed energy. As noted earlier, the energy setting (power density) is critical to achieving the desired effects. The power setting on the Surgipulse laser reflects only the rate at which pulses are delivered. By manipulating the energy, power, and pulse-rate settings on the Surgipulse laser, the surgeon can obtain a wide variety of effects. Box 8–1 shows some of these relationships.

Box 8–1. Relationships between Energy, Power, and Pulse Rate on Surgipulse Laser

$$\frac{\text{Average power (watt continuous)}}{\text{Pulse rate (pulses/second)}} = \text{joules/pulse}$$

$$\frac{\text{Average power (watt continuous)}}{\text{Joules/pulse}} = \text{pulse rate (pulses second)}$$

$$\frac{\text{Joules/pulse}}{\text{Average power (watt continuous)}} = \text{pulse interval (second)}$$

Watts = joules/second. Note that one watt of power is the energy consumption rate of one joule per second[2].

HISTOPATHOLOGY

It is important for practitioners to make a histologic comparison of techniques and to use this information as the basis for selecting specific treatment modalities. An in vivo study using the high-energy, ultrashort-pulse CO_2 laser on human skin compared the histologic effects of this treatment modality with those of standard chemical exfoliation techniques.[2]

CO_2 Laser versus Chemical Exfoliation

In the first part of the study, specimens were examined at 1, 3, and 90 days after treatment with the CO_2 laser. On day 1, a moderately intense dermal infiltrate composed of mononuclear lymphocytes, neutrophils, and eosinophils was seen (Fig. 8–1). Partial or complete reepithelializa-

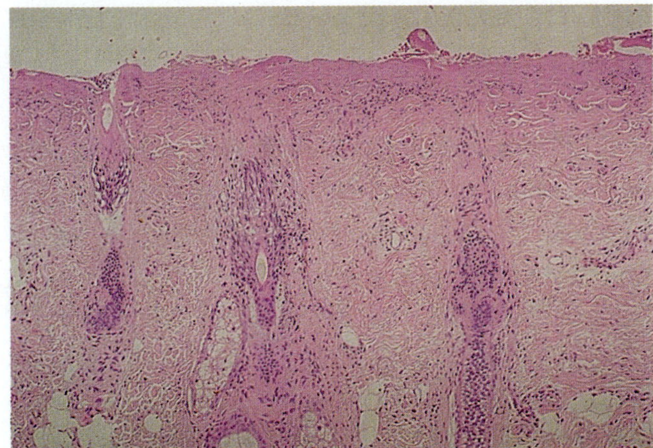

Figure 8–1. Appearance on postoperative day 1 following CO_2 laser resurfacing. Note the moderate dermal infiltrate.

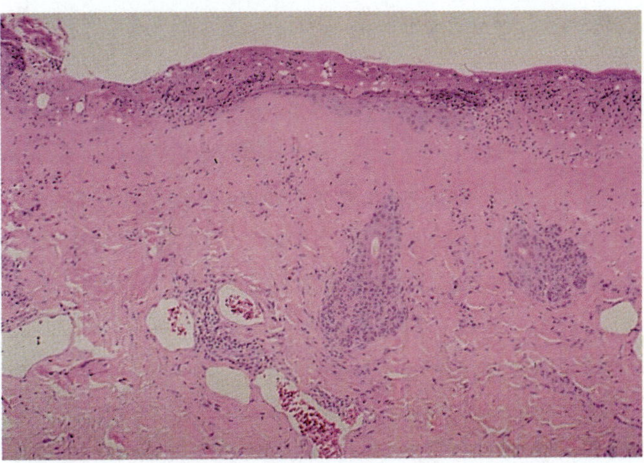

Figure 8–2. Appearance on postoperative day 3 following CO_2 laser resurfacing. Note that reepithelialization is almost complete.

tion occurred in over 78% of the specimens by day 3 (Fig. 8–2). Intact dermis with or without rete ridges was noted in all specimens on day 90 (Fig. 8–3). In the upper dermis, the repair zone consisted of dense, compact collagen bundles in parallel alignment with the epidermal surface. This band of collagen varied in thickness. Over half the specimens had regained a normal rete ridge pattern, and the remaining specimens demonstrated a flattened epidermis. The vast majority of specimens had a papillary dermal repair zone. Significant elastin fiber alteration was noted. Hematoxylin and eosine as well as acid orcein gemma stains helped to further delineate this papillary dermal repair zone. At higher magnifications,

the repair zone was noted to be almost completely devoid of elastin fibers. Normally, small elastin fibers are present perpendicular to the dermal surface. Abnormal elastin fibers were noted in the reticular dermis. A comparison in terms of energy setting, area of necrosis, and degree of fibrosis showed a direct correlation between energy level and degree of necrosis and fibrosis (Fig. 8–4).

In the second part of the study, the same protocol was used to provide a histologic analysis of various chemical exfoliation techniques. The specimens showed very superficial necrosis, and the remaining portions of the epidermis were normal with no alterations in the papillary dermis. This was true whether Jessner solution, resorcinol, 10 and

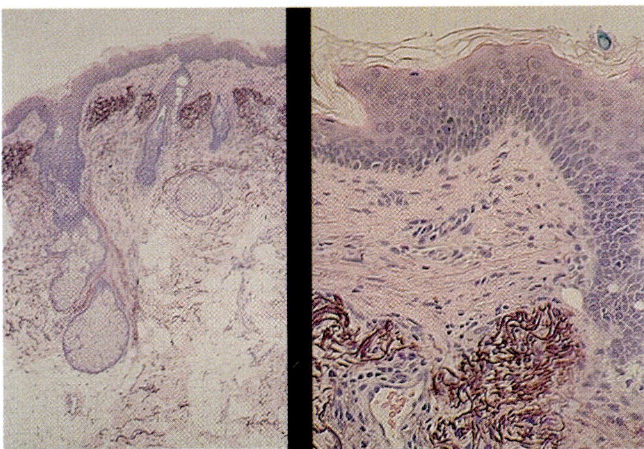

Figure 8–3. Appearance on postoperative day 90 following CO_2 laser resurfacing. Note the repair zone of dense, compact collagen and the normal rete ridge pattern.

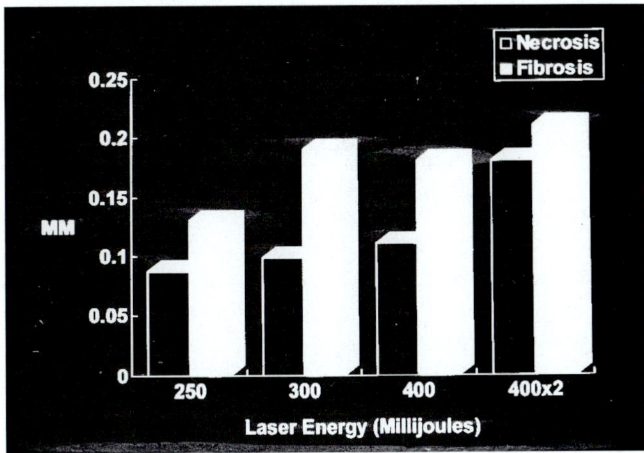

Figure 8–4. Comparison by energy setting, area of necrosis, and degree of fibrosis indicated a direct correlation between energy level and the degree of necrosis and fibrosis.

15% trichloroacetic acid (TCA), or 78% glycolic acid was used as the exfoliant. When a medium-depth peeling agent (88% phenol) was used, the histologic result was similar to that observed with laser resurfacing. There was necrosis of the epidermis and some alteration in the papillary dermis. By day 3, a partial reepithelialization was noted in some areas, whereas no reepthelialization was seen in other areas. A mixed dermal infiltrate was noted. At 90 days, the medium-peel specimens showed a very similar repair zone in the papillary dermis to that seen in the laser-treated specimens (Fig. 8–5). However, there was a significant inflammatory infiltrate in the upper reticular dermis not apparent in the laser-treated specimens.

If one looks at skin treated with a Baker-Gordon phenol peel with occlusion at 90 days, a repair zone and significant inflammatory infiltrates are noted. At higher magnification, the inflammatory infiltrates can be seen clearly, as well as a repair zone similar to that seen with laser resurfacing.

The conclusions reached in this study[2] were that the depth of laser injury approximated that of a medium-depth chemical peel. However, in the laser-treated patients, wound healing was much more rapid, and inflammatory infiltrates resolved much more quickly. It appeared that the subdermal repair zone of fibrosis accounted for the improved clinical appearance following laser treatment. However, the study showed that laser resurfacing is an

extremely technique-dependent procedure, because significant differences in tissue histology resulted from even minor variations in energy levels used or technique.

The reticular dermis seems to be a barrier to laser vaporization. Multiple passes beyond two may not deepen the laser wound appreciably but may increase the risk of complications. This may be due to the fact that, in deeper layers of the reticular dermis, collagen fibers are denser and retain less intracellular water. For this reason, less absorption by the primary chromophore of the CO_2 laser (i.e., water) occurs, and thus, more heat is transferred directly to the tissue.

In a clinical comparison of laser resurfacing versus phenol exfoliation, I have noted that patients appear to have less discomfort both during the treatment and postoperatively when laser resurfacing is used. Moreover, reepithelialization seems to be accelerated with laser use, with most individuals showing almost complete reepthelialization in 3 to 5 days, as opposed to 10 to 14 days when phenol exfoliation is used. A quicker resolution of erythema was also noted, as well as no dyschromia, following laser resurfacing. However, laser resurfacing was less effective than phenol exfoliation in eradicating the deepest facial rhytids with a single treatment. Two, and possibly three, laser resurfacings at appropriate treatment intervals subjectively provided 80% reduction of perioral rhytids when compared with a single phenol exfoliation. Brody[3] noted similar clinical findings. In a preliminary comparison between laser resurfacing and Baker-Gordon chemical exfoliation, he subjectively noted that laser resurfacing improved severe photodamaged skin by approximately 50%. The Baker-Gordon peel, however, eliminated the vast majority of rhytids in one treatment. In the treatment of Glogau photoaging type III of perioral skin, the laser may eliminate mild rhytids in one treatment with little risk of pigmentary change. The phenol-based peel eradicates the same rhytids but has a greater likelihood of producing hypopigmentation. In contrast, photoaging type IV skin with severe rhytids may required multiple "touch-ups" with the laser to obtain an adequate aesthetic result.[4] Box 8–2 presents a summary of the conclusions that can be drawn from these studies.

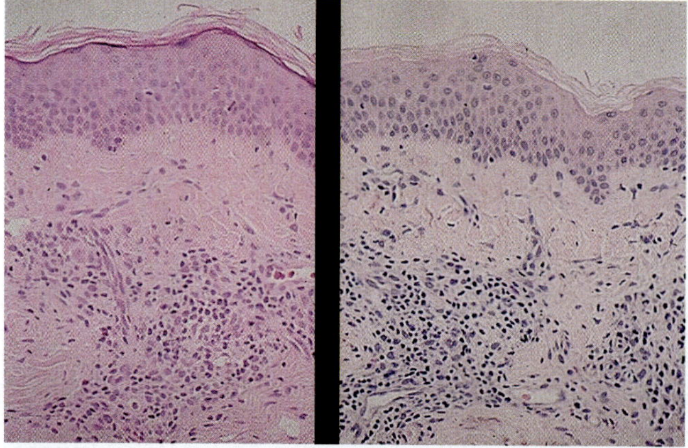

Figure 8–5. Comparison with a specimen treated with a Baker-Gordon phenol chemical peel with occlusion at 90 days shows a dermal repair zone similar to that seen with laser resurfacing.

> **Box 8–2. CO_2 Laser versus Phenol Peel**
>
> A. Histologic Effects of High-Energy, Ultrashort-Pulse CO_2 Laser on Human Skin
>
> - Depth of penetration approximates that of a medium-depth chemical peel.
> - Wound healing is rapid.
> - Subdermal repair zone of fibrosis accounts for improved clinical appearance.
> - Significant differences in tissue histology result from even minor variations in energy level used and practitioner technique.
> - Reticular dermis is a barrier to laser vaporization.
> - Multiple passes beyond two may not deepen the laser wound appreciably but may increase the risk of complications.
> - It is not clear whether the band of dermal damage seen on day 1 corresponds precisely to the thickness of new collagen seen on day 90.
>
> B. Advantages of Laser Resurfacing over Phenol Peel
>
> - Less patient discomfort
> - Quicker reepithelialization
> - Quicker resolution of erythema
> - No pigmentary changes
> - Safer (?)
> - Less effective eradication of deep rhytids with a single treatment

Stimulation of Tissue Growth Factors

There has been a debate about whether high-energy CO_2 laser treatment results in stimulation of tissue growth factors. Pogrel[5] reported accelerated wound healing with high-energy CO_2 lasers when compared with traditional scalpel incisions. However, other authors[6] have shown the levels of growth factors in CO_2 laser incisions and scalpel incisions to be no different. A recent study of high-energy CO_2 laser resurfacing has shown an interesting role for tissue growth factors in healing.[7] When the ultrashort-pulse CO_2 laser (Surgipulse XJ150) was compared with dermabrasion and chemical exfoliation in an in vivo comparative histologic analysis at 21 days, there appeared to be increased stimulation with the high-energy CO_2 laser.[8] Levels of transforming growth factors β_1 and β_2 (TGF-β_1 and TGF-β_2) were greater in specimens treated with the Surgipulse scanner than in specimens treated with the Silk-Touch (Sharplan Lasers) scanner. Both lasers demonstrated greater TGF-β_2 staining than did phenol exfoliation specimens. Specimens that demonstrated the highest levels of TGF-β_1 also demonstrated the strongest intensity of collagen. Thus, the ultrashort-pulse CO_2 laser (Surgipulse XJ150) may result in greater stimulation of tissue growth factors, which ultimately may lead to increased collagen deposition. Additional study is needed, however.

XJ DUAL-MODE SCANNER

A drawback of the Surgipulse XJ150 high-energy CO_2 laser is that it has a 3-mm spot size. Therefore, the laser can only be used to treat small- to medium-sized aesthetic units such as the perioral area, periorbital area, or localized rhytids. The recently developed XJ Dual-Mode Scanner (Sharplan Lasers) now allows large surface areas to be treated quickly by employing the high-energy, ultrashort-pulse modality (Fig. 8–6).

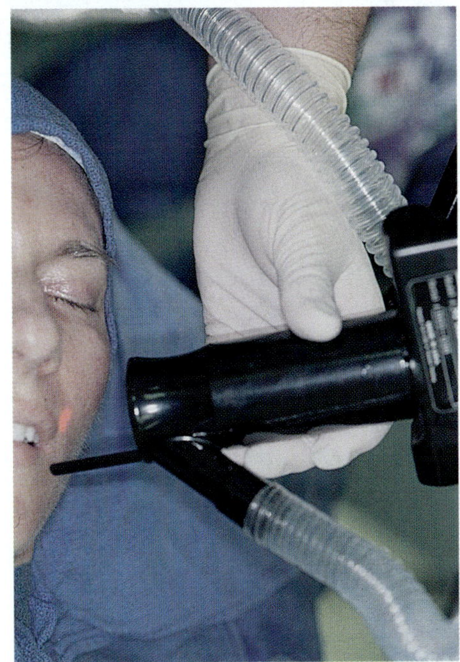

Figure 8–6. The XJ Dual-Mode Scanner allows expeditious resurfacing of large areas.

The XJ Dual-Mode Scanner is a closed-loop galvanometer-based scanner. Closed loop means that the positions of the mirrors reflecting the beam are continuously checked and adjusted so that beam delivery is precise and reproducible. In addition, because error signals and position are monitored continuously, the system controller can stop delivery of energy the very instant it is signaled. Open-loop systems do not have this feedback mechanism and can continue to deliver energy even if the galvanometer is not functioning within specifications. For this reason, closed-loop systems offer an increased level of protection for patients and precision for practitioners.

In the XJ scanner mode, the beam from the XJ Dual-Mode Scanner is collimated through a three-lens system to a 2-mm spot size on the target tissue. Both the pattern and the beam are collimated, so the pointer distance is not critical to achieving a proper pattern. The scanner will trace, with its HeNe beam, an outline of the area to be exposed when the laser is activated. The HeNe tracing can be adjusted to guide the placement of each pattern. On depression of the footswitch, the scanner reverts to the pattern delivery indicated by user settings while firing the laser in sequence with the scanner motions. Each spot position is checked before the laser is fired. Pulse deposition rates of up to 220 pulses per second can be produced. Maximum exposure areas are 20 × 20 mm for square configurations and a 25-mm diameter for round configurations. The peak power for this system is 400 W. The maximum energy per pulse pair is 400 mJ, with the maximum time on tissue for any single pulse being approximately 600 milliseconds.[9]

The scanner is made of lightweight molded plastic, which facilitates mobility. Suction can be attached directly to the unit, which facilitates evacuation of the laser plume and eliminates the need for a surgical assistant. The scanner is computerized, and functions are displayed on an LED screen. The computer computes the energy levels delivered to the tissue in joules per square centimeter as a result of the energy parameters selected by the surgeon. The pattern selected is displayed on the LED screen and can be manipulated easily using the touch-screen feature.

HISTOPATHOLOGY

As mentioned earlier, Geronemus and associates[8] reported a comparative histopathologic analysis of various lasers. They reported on elliptical specimens treated with one, two, or three passes using various lasers. The Coherent Ultra-Pulse 500 high-energy CO_2 laser (a radiofrequency laser) was used at 450 mJ/cm^2, with 4 W of power and a 3-mm spot size. The Surgipulse XJ150 high-energy CO_2 laser was used at 400 mJ/cm^2, with 10 W of power and a 3-mm spot size. The Silk Touch flash scanner was used at 8 W of power with a 0.2-second exposure and a 6-mm spot size. Essentially, there was little difference between the depth of penetration per pass between the SilkTouch flashscanner and the Surgipulse laser. With three passes, each penetrated to a depth of 150 μm. Three passes of the Ultra-Pulse 500 laser resulted in a penetration of approximately 70 μm.[8] This is supported by the histologic analyses reported of specimens treated with a Surgipulse XJ150 laser versus those treated with various chemical exfoliants.

PATIENT EVALUATION

To obtain the best and most consistent aesthetic results, the surgeon must know the limitations of the procedure and the expectations of each patient who seeks help. There is no substitute for experience in selecting patients for laser resurfacing. However, there are helpful guidelines. The ideal patient is a thin-skinned person with fair complexion and fine, generalized wrinkling. Such a person is less likely to undergo pigmentary changes. Patients with fine to moderate facial wrinkles, particularly in the perioral and periorbital areas, usually obtain excellent results with laser resurfacing. In addition, actinic keratosis and superficial acne scarring show a good response to laser treatment. The patient's skin type can be of paramount importance. Fitzpatrick's skin type classification system[10] provides a measure of pigmentary responsiveness of the skin to ultraviolet light (Table 8–1). When skin type is combined with eye color in the patient evaluation process, one is better able to predict the chance of pigmentary changes as a result of laser resurfacing. In

Table 8–1. Fitzpatrck's Classification for Sun-Reactive Skin Types

Skin Type	Color	Reaction to first summer sun exposure
I	White	Always burns, never tans
II	White	Usually burns, tans with difficulty
III	Light brown	Sometimes mild burn, tans average at/rate
IV	Moderate brown	Readily burns, tans with ease
V	Dark brown	Very rarely burns, tans very easily
VI	Black	Tans very easily

general terms, patients with Fitzpatrick skin types I to III are ideal for laser resurfacing. Patients with skin types IV to VI can undergo laser resurfacing but have a greater risk for transient pigmentary changes. See Box 8–3 for Glogau

---

Box 8–3. Glogau and Matarasso's Skin Classification System

Group I: Mild (usually 28–35 years of age)

No keratosis

Little wrinkling

No scarring

Uses little or no makeup

Group II: Moderate (usually 35–50 years of age)

Early actinic keratosis, slight yellow skin discoloration

Early wrinkling

Parallel smile lines

Mild scarring

Uses little makeup

Group III: Advanced (usually 50–65 years of age)

Actinic keratosis, obvious shallow skin discoloration
    with telangiectasias

Wrinkling present when at rest

Moderate acne scarring

Wears makeup always

Group IV: Severe (usually 60–75 years of age)

Actinic keratosis, skin cancers

Wrinkling, much cutis laxa of actinic gravitational and
    dynamic origin

Severe acne scarring

Wears makeup that does not cover but cakes on

---

and Matarasso's[11] classification system, which can also assist in patient selection.

It is important to analyze the face closely. Brody has pointed out that every cosmetic unit of the skin in the perioral, periorbital, cheek, forehead, and nasal areas should be individually assessed to determine which treatment modality is necessary for the best correction without undue risk (personal communication, August 1997). Many surgeons use a surface topography chart to indicate the exact location of facial scars, pigmentary changes, and cutaneous lesions, as well as the severity of rhytids in the various facial aesthetic units. Not only does this facilitate preoperative evaluation and procedure planning, but it is also an important medicolegal document.

If the periorbital area is to undergo laser resurfacing, additional preoperative documentation is indicated. It is important to document asymmetry in the periorbital tissues, visual acuity, eyelid function, elasticity of the lower eyelid area. The "lid snap" test should be performed preoperatively. If one can grasp the lower eyelid and pull it away from the globe more than 12 mm, the patient may be predisposed to the development of ectropion after laser resurfacing.

CONTRAINDICATIONS AND RISKS

Relative contraindications to laser resurfacing depend on the patient's skin type and medical history. Active herpes simplex infections should be allowed to heal prior to laser resurfacing. If there is a history of recurrent herpes simplex, pretreatment with oral acyclovir is advantageous. Recent studies indicate that such preparations should be given at the time of surgery and continued for 10 to 14 days postoperatively. This is based on the fact that herpetic lesions do not usually appear until reepithelialization has occurred, about 7 to 10 days after laser resurfacing. For this reason, it seems appropriate to treat for a longer course than has been advocated previously. In addition, recent studies by R.G. Deeter suggest that valacyclovir (Valtrex, Glaxo Wellcome, Triangle Park, NJ), 500 mg given twice daily, achieves higher levels in the bloodstream and is better tolerated by the gastrointestinal tract than acyclovir (Zovirax Glaxo Wellcome, personal communication, March 1996).

Patients at greatest risk for developing pigmentary problems following laser resurfacing include those who continue to have extraordinary occupational or recreational exposures to sunlight. They should be instructed to use a sunscreen with sun protective factor of at least 30 for approximately 3 months after laser resurfacing.

Scarring is probably the most feared complication associated with laser resurfacing. Patients with a history of hypertrophic scarring are at an increased risk for post-laser-resurfacing scarring and may not be appropriate candidates.

Because the pilosebaceous apparatus is of critical importance for adequate reepithelialization following laser resurfacing, patients with acne who have been treated recently with *cis*-13-retinoic acid (Accutane) are not appropriate candidates. At least 12 months should elapse before a patient who has been on Accutane undergoes laser resurfacing. If the physical examination reveals normal cutaneous topography, including the presence of an appropriate number of vellus hairs, treatment may be undertaken. If there is any question, a small biopsy should be performed for histologic evaluation.

Patients with a prior history of facial radiation as a treatment for acne should be evaluated carefully. If the result of the physical examination is satisfactory, such patients may be acceptable candidates for laser resurfacing. The absence of significant vellus hair on the face and the presence of numerous telangiectasias are indications of an increased risk for facial scarring.

Patients must also have realistic expectations to be appropriate candidates for laser resurfacing. The patient must understand that all rhytids or acne scarring cannot be removed. The realistic goal is to obtain improvement. Individuals who are preoccupied with minor facial wrinkling and slight skin textural changes need to realize that laser resurfacing will not arrest the aging process but will only provide improvement.

LASER SAFETY

In all laser procedures, the surgeon must ensure the safety of both the patient and the operating room staff. Because the human eye is extremely vulnerable to laser light, ocular hazards are of paramount importance. The eye has a natural protective mechanism, the blink reflex, that limits retinal exposure to irritants. The blink reflex occurs at a rate of every 0.25 second, but the intensity of some laser beams is so great that injury can occur before the protective lid reflex occurs. Because of the acoustic effects and heat flow, significant tissue damage can occur, resulting in severe visual impairment. When injury occurs to the cornea, it is usually superficial and involves the corneal epithelium. Reepithelialization occurs in 1 to 2 days, and total recovery of vision usually results. However, deeper penetration can result in corneal scars and permanent loss of vision.

EXPOSURE TO A REFLECTED BEAM

Ocular injury can occur from direct penetration of a focused beam. However, it is more likely for injury to result from accidental ocular exposure to a reflected beam. Protecting patients and staff from reflected laser beams can be difficult. The wavelength of a CO_2 laser beam is 10.6 μm, in the far-infrared spectrum, so it is invisible. A potentially hazardous reflection, therefore, can go unnoticed. For this reason, it is imperative that precautions be taken at all times when using the CO_2 laser.

Reflections occur most commonly from flat, metallic, mirror-like surfaces such as surgical instruments. Instruments with black anodized or abraded or roughened surfaces can reduce but not totally eliminate potential beam reflection. Roughening the surface is generally thought to be more effective than ebonizing the surface because it causes the beam to be diffused to a greater degree.[12]

Ordinary optical glass protects against all wavelengths shorter than 300 nm and greater than 2700 nm. Polycarbonate safety glass with side shields is suitable for use with CO_2 lasers if the power is below 100 W. Such glasses have an optical density of 4. While polycarbonate glasses may be adequate, there can be burn-through with higher-powered lasers. Thus, one would not want to focus the laser beam directly on the shield of safety glasses for any length of time.

During CO_2 laser resurfacing, moist gauze squares and moist towels are kept over the patient's eyes. For periorbital laser resurfacing, the eye being treated is protected with a metal eye protector, and the opposite eye is protected with moist gauze squares and a towel.

ACCIDENTAL FIRES AND BURNS

Accidental fires are a well-known hazard associated with laser treatment. Most laser fires result from ignition of surgical structures such as tubing, drapes, sponges, anesthetic gasses, or endotracheal tubes. Cutaneous fires are thought to ignite in an oxygen-rich environment because of melanin absorption, heat conduction, and light scattered by the epidermis. A fire can occur if laser energy is absorbed by melanin in the hair follicles or by other items in the surgical field. In addition, gauze, telfa pads, or surgical drapes can be ignited by direct or reflected laser beams. For this reason, surgical drapes should be moistened or nonflammable drapes should be used.

Female patients should be cautioned to remove all mascara and other makeup before undergoing periorbital laser resurfacing. Makeup, hairsprays, and alcohol-based colognes all have the potential for flammability. In addition, it is important to remember that petroleum-based ocular ointments may have potential flammability. Their avoidance is recommended.

Cutaneous injury from laser burns does occur. It results most frequently from inadvertent discharge of the laser. To minimize this potential, it is recommended that an assistant control the laser and place it on standby immediately after use. In addition, all other foot pedals should be removed from the area to prevent accidental misfiring of the laser.

NONBEAM LASER HAZARDS

In addition to the direct laser beam hazards to the eye and skin, several nonbeam laser hazards exist that need to be considered. These include electrical hazards, laser-generated airborne contaminants (laser plume), waste disposal of contaminated laser-related materials such as filters, and electromagnetic interference generated by the laser. Laser-generated airborne contaminants present a significant problem. Studies have shown the presence of gaseous compounds, bioaerosols, dead and live cellular material, and viruses in the laser plume. The laser plume can cause both ocular and upper respiratory tract irritation.[13] The unpleasant odors of the laser plume can cause discomfort to both the staff and the patient. The laser plume can cause ocular irritation and be even more of a problem for individuals who wear soft contact lenses because the particles can permeate the soft lenses and cause prolonged irritation.

A smoke evacuator is imperative when using a CO_2 laser. If the smoke evacuator is held 2 cm from the source of the laser plume, aerosolization of particles is minimal. The suction created by the laser evacuator and the diameter of the smoke evacuator tubing are important. This creates a vortex that removes the mutagenic debris and prevents aerosolization of carbonized particles. The plume components impregnate the tubing, which should be treated as biohazardous material. In most cases, commonly used operating room suction devices and suction tubing do not provide adequate evacuation of the laser plume during CO_2 laser resurfacing. While surgical masks may help to reduce plume exposure, their use alone is not adequate.

PREOPERATIVE PREPARATION

Preoperative and postoperative photographs are important to document the skin contour and tone. It is also important to use portrait lighting and ensure that lighting and photographic technique are uniform across both preoperative and postoperative views so that the result is clearly discernible. Typically, posteroanterior (PA), lateral, oblique, and close-up views of the perioral, periorbital, and malar areas are necessary. Whereas black-and-white photographs are used commonly in facial surgery for documentation, color photographs are needed to document laser resurfacing. The dyschromias and pigmentary changes that can occur as a result of laser resurfacing cannot be documented appropriately on black-and-white film.

PROPHYLACTIC DRUG THERAPY

I prefer to place patients on daily applications of tretinoin at least 2 weeks prior to laser resurfacing. This is based on research by Mandy[14] that showed accelerated reepithelialization with such treatments. In a study of over 100 patients who received pretreatment for at least 2 weeks with 0.05% tretinoin cream, healing, as evidenced by reepithelialization, was complete by 7 days, with most patients completely healed in 5 days. Patients who did not receive the tretinoin healed by 11 days, with none healing sooner than 7 days. No milia or postinflammatory hyperpigmentation was experienced by patients treated with tretinoin when the drug was resumed within 1 week of dermabrasion. In the group that received no tretinoin, milia and postinflammatory hyperpigmentation occurred in 28% postoperatively. In addition, Hevia et al[15] have shown that tretinoin accelerates wound healing. They concluded that pretreatment with 0.1% tretinoin for 2 weeks prior to TCA peel significantly increased wound healing and resulted in greater patient satisfaction with the result.

Patients with Fitzpatrick skin types IV to VI, as well as those who have previously demonstrated a tendency toward pigmentary changes, are pretreated with a hydroquinone prior to laser resurfacing. I use daily topical applications for approximately 6 weeks prior to laser resurfacing. The daily applications are reinstituted as soon as possible after reepithelialization and are continued for approximately 6 to 8 weeks. This markedly reduces the tendency for postinflammatory hyperpigmentation. However, these patients must be counseled that transient hyperpigmentation can occur despite pretreatment with hydroquinones and despite the use of appropriate sun precautions.

Patients with a previous history of herpetic lesions are placed on prophylactic valacyclovir (Valtrex), 500 mg twice daily, starting the day before surgery and continued for 10 to 14 days afterward. Patients are also given a cephalosporin (Keflex, Eli Lilly Pharmaceutical, Indianapolis, IN), 500 mg four times a day for 10 days. Goldman[16] has shown an approximately 8% incidence of bacterial infection following laser resurfacing when prophylactic antibiotics were not used. I frequently apply a moist dressing postoperatively, which is a potential medium for bacterial growth despite appropriate hygiene. For this reason, I feel that it is appropriate to use caution and institute prophylactic antibiotic treatment in laser resurfacing patients. In the early stages, an infection may be extremely difficult to identify. In addition, although rare, toxic shock syndrome has been reported following laser resurfacing (M. Goldman, personal communication, May 1998).

ANESTHETICS

Patient discomfort associated with laser resurfacing can vary widely. Many patients find that topical application of a eutectic mixture of local anesthetics (EMLA Cream, Astra Pharmaceuticals) applied 2 hours prior to treatment and combined with regional nerve blocks using 1% xylocaine with epinephrine 1:100,000 provides appropriate analgesia. While xylocaine diffuses quickly into soft tissues, the addition of a protolytic enzyme such as hyaluronidase (Wydase) in a 1:10 concentration can result in quicker dispersion of the anesthetic into the soft tissues. This is important because infiltration may cause a "ballooning effect" in the soft tissues that "ablates" the fine rhytids in the perioral or periorbital area. The use of xylocaine with hyaluronidase often allows local infiltration to be performed without adversely affecting the treatment process.

Other patients find laser resurfacing to be uncomfortable and prefer to undergo intravenous sedation. It is important to remember that oxygen and nitrous oxide should not be used with a CO_2 laser because of potential flammability. However, ultrashort-acting intravenous anesthetics such as propofol (Diprivan), fentanyl, and ketamine are useful in providing both analgesia and amnesia. When intravenous sedation is used, appropriate life-support systems must be readily available, and appropriate physiologic parameters should be monitored continuously.

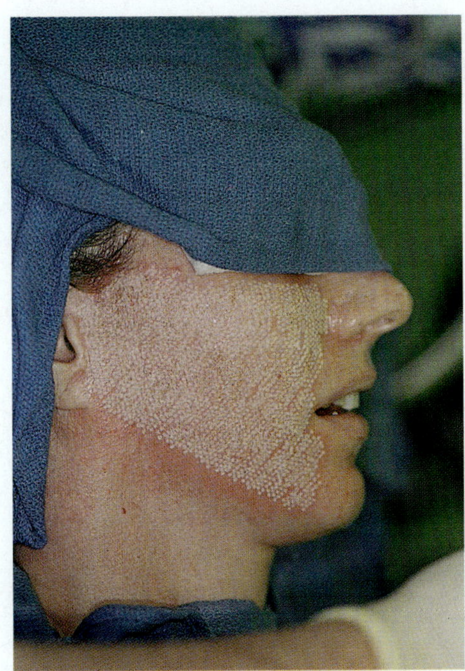

Figure 8–7. Malar area treated with a laser scanner. Great care is taken to avoid overlap of laser spot sizes.

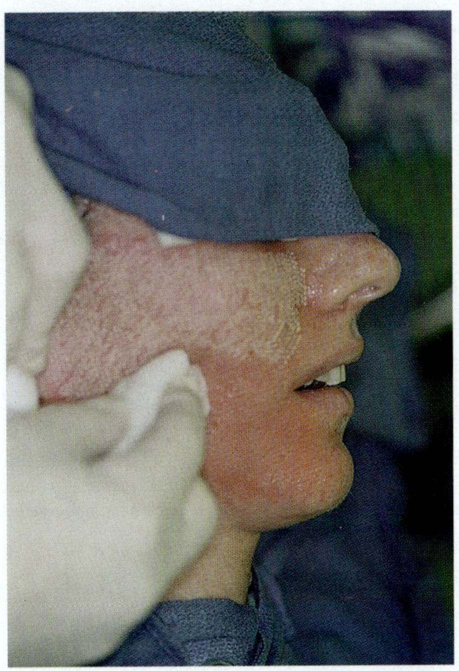

Figure 8–8. Saline-soaked gauze is used to gently remove debris following laser resurfacing.

SURGICAL TECHNIQUE

The face is divided into five aesthetic units: right malar, perioral, left malar, forehead, and periorbital-nasal areas. Laser resurfacing is performed on each aesthetic unit sequentially, with care being taken to avoid overlapping. The technique used is similar to that employed in a phenol-based peel.

Each aesthetic unit is treated in its entirety, avoiding overlap (Fig. 8–7). A setting of 350 mJ with 20% density is used to treat all areas except the periorbital tissues, which are treated at a setting of 300 mJ with 20% density. Moist saline-soaked gauze squares are used to remove debris (Fig. 8–8). This should be done gently to minimize additional tissue trauma. Removal is necessary to prevent a "heat sink" phenomenon, which results in more thermal irritation to tissues. The surface is then blotted with a dry gauze square.

Most areas are treated with a second pass (Fig. 8–9). Again, great care is taken to avoid overlapping of laser spot sizes. Debris is again removed with saline-soaked gauze (Fig. 8–10). Then the area is reevaluated under magnification. If rhytids or acne scarring persists, a third pass is possible. On rare occasions, a fourth pass may be used. Approximately 30% of the time, a third laser pass is employed. A fourth is used in less than 5% of patients.

The endpoint of treatment with laser resurfacing is gauged to be ablation of the rhytids, with a subjective limitation of three to four passes as the treatment limit. As noted previously, histologic studies have indicated that the depth of penetration into the reticular dermis is limited with increasing numbers of passes. Multiple passes can actually lead to increased dermal dispersion and tissue protein ablation as penetration into the reticular dermis increases. For this reason, I favor a conservative position, which is to limit the number of passes and relaser after dermal healing has progressed significantly (at least a 3-month interval and potentially longer based on the patient's skin type and texture).

THE NECK

As in phenol-based exfoliation, the neck is not treated. The pilosebaceous density in the neck is such that deep exfoliation, whether by chemical cauterants or laser vaporization, can lead to intractable scarring. However, the perimeter can be "feathered" with a single pass at the mandibular margin to avoid a frank line of demarcation

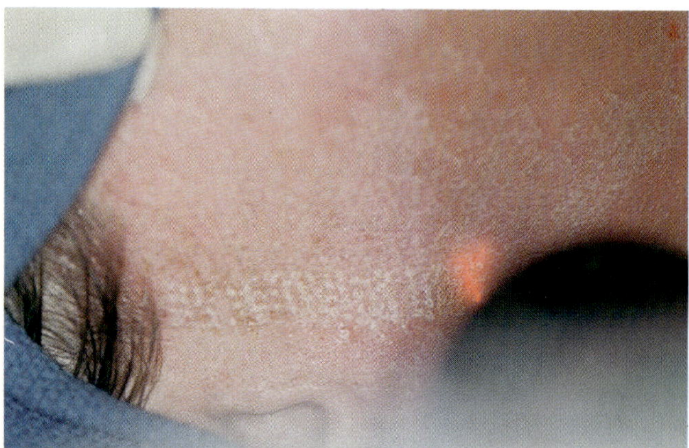

Figure 8–9. A second laser pass is used to treat the malar area. Again, great care is taken to avoid overlapping spot sizes. Note that delineation of the treated area is not as clear with the second pass as with the first.

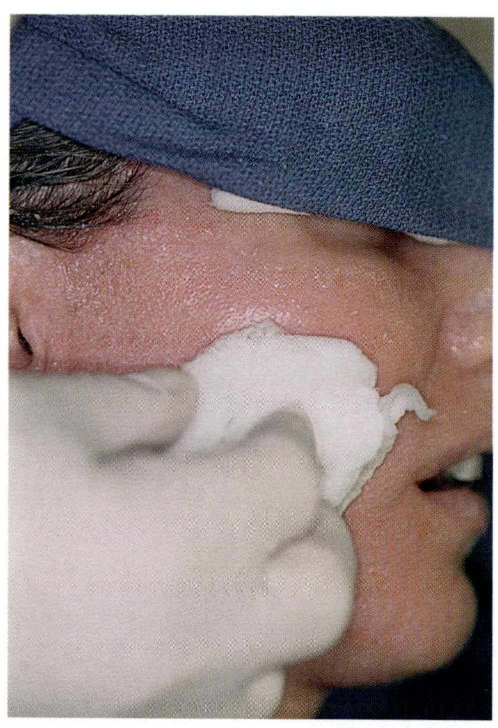

Figure 8–10. Saline-soaked gauze is used to remove debris.

between laser-resurfaced and nonresurfaced skin. I recommend holding the laser beam at an acute angle when feathering the margins. By using one pass at the periphery and two or three passes in other areas, a layering effect results that eases the transition between laser-resurfaced and nonresurfaced areas (Fig. 8–11). In some patients, a 25% TCA peel is used in the neck area. In such patients, it is essential to avoid applying the TCA to laser-treated areas.

Perioral Area

In the perioral area, laser resurfacing is carried on to the vermilion border (Fig. 8–12), as is done in a phenol-based peel. Perioral rhytids are very difficult to treat and frequently require multiple passes. Great care is taken to avoid allowing the laser beam to strike the dentition because irreversible discoloration of the tooth enamel can result. Some surgeons prefer to use a protective mouthpiece. I prefer not to use these appliances because they distort the perioral tissue and produce mechanical "ablation" of perioral rhytids.

Forehead

When treating the forehead area, the hair is moistened, and moist towels are used to protect the eyes. Care is taken to avoid lasering the hairline or eyebrows (Fig. 8–13). This is in contrast to the technique used with phenol-based peels, where the solution is blended into the hair-bearing areas. However, the laser vaporizes hair shafts, which can be a fire hazard and can also cause pseudoalopecia in that area.

Periorbital Area

When treating the periorbital area, I frequently use a light phenol (88% phenol) peel to treat periorbital rhytids when the rhytids are extremely deep or dyschromia is apparent in the lower lid skin. Otherwise, the laser is used. However, because the eyelid tissue is so delicate, reduced fluences are used; for example, 300 mJ with a 20% density is standard.

The eye to be treated is anesthetized with 2 drops of tetracaine (Fig. 8–14). A glass or metal Jaeger retractor is inserted under the lid to protect the globe. The retractor is always palpated digitally to ensure that the surface is smooth and free of any irregularities that could abrade the cornea. The retractor is also dipped in normal

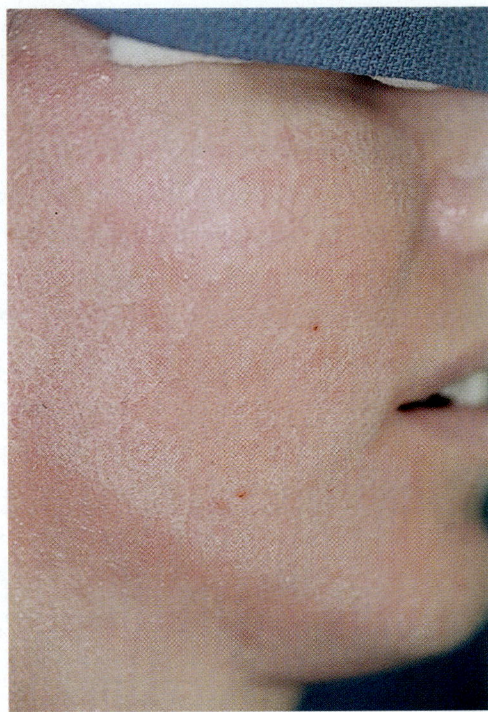

Figure 8–11. Layering effect is used along the mandible to avoid a frank line of demarcation between laser-treated and non-laser-treated areas.

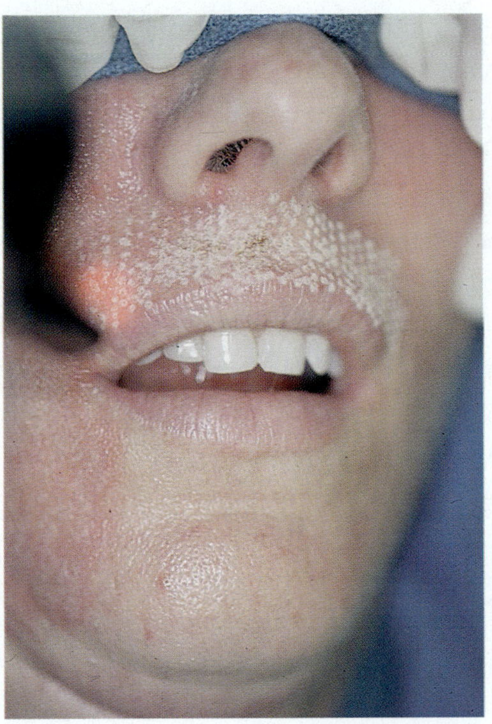

Figure 8–12. Treatment in the perioral area is carried on to the vermilion border. Great care is taken to avoid striking dentition with the laser beam.

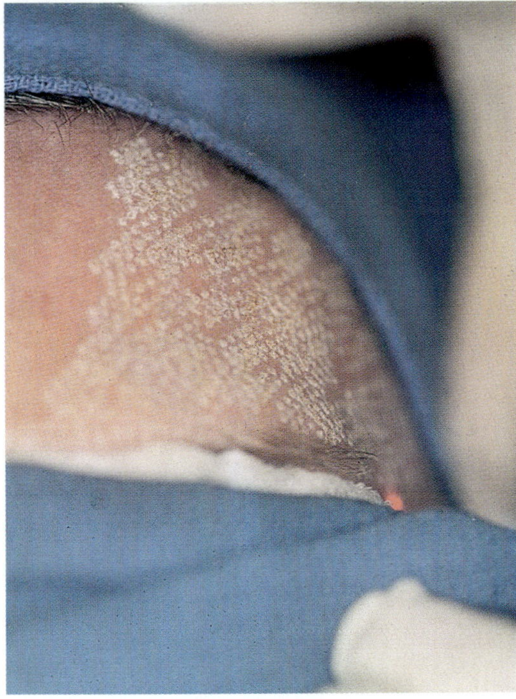

Figure 8–13. Saline-soaked towels are placed around the treatment site. Treatment in the forehead area avoids vaporization of eyebrows or hairline.

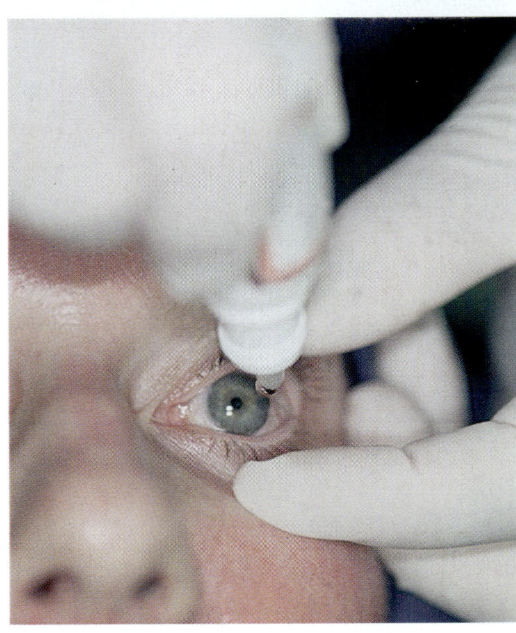

Figure 8–14. Tetracaine is used for anesthesia prior to placement of the eye shield.

saline to minimize abrasion. Petroleum-based ocular lubricants are not used because of their incendiary potential. An assistant uses an applicator stick to gently elevate the eyelashes out of the treatment field, and a finger is used to place the lower eyelid under general traction without ablating the fine rhytids (Fig. 8–15). Resurfacing is carried no closer than 3 to 4 mm from the ciliary margin to minimize edema and possible thermal irritation to the meibomian glands in the eyelid. Usually only one pass is necessary in the lower eyelid area. Multiple passes may be used to treat deep rhytids in the lateral canthal area, however. For the upper eyelid, treatment is carried down to the superior tarsal fold, but no further (Fig. 8–16).

At the end of periorbital laser resurfacing, it should be confirmed that there have been no changes in ocular status, and all areas are inspected to ensure proper treatment. An opened moist dressing with petrolatum is placed (Figs. 8–17 and 8–18). This is based on studies by Mybach and Rovee who demonstrated that the wound-healing sequence occurs more rapidly in cov-

ered wounds. Covering the wound keeps tissue fluid on the wound surface, in a liquid state, rather than allowing a deep crust to form, as happens in uncovered wounds. Crusting represents a mechanical barrier to epidermal migration. When hydration of the wound surface is maintained by topical ointments, no mechanical barriers are present, and migration of epithelial cells occurs on a plane with the uninvolved dermis. The rate of reepithelialization of these wounds is increased by 40%. While a variety of topical ointments have been advocated, I prefer petrolatum. It should be noted that the use of antibiotic ointments is associated with an extremely high rate of contact dermatitis in laser-resurfaced patients.

POSTOPERATIVE TREATMENT

At the end of the procedure, patients are discharged in the care of a responsible adult with both written and verbal instructions. Patients are seen the following morning and begin a regimen of frequent showering of the area

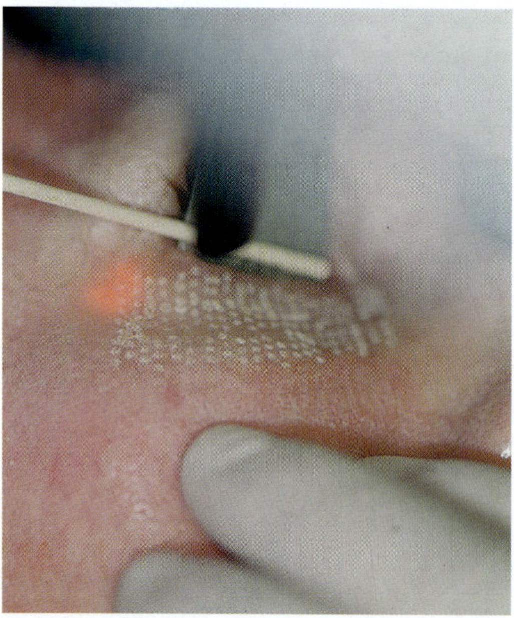

Figure 8–15. An eye shield used to protect the cornea. A swab is used to gently retract eyelashes from the treatment field. Resurfacing is carried to within 3 to 4 mm of the ciliary margin.

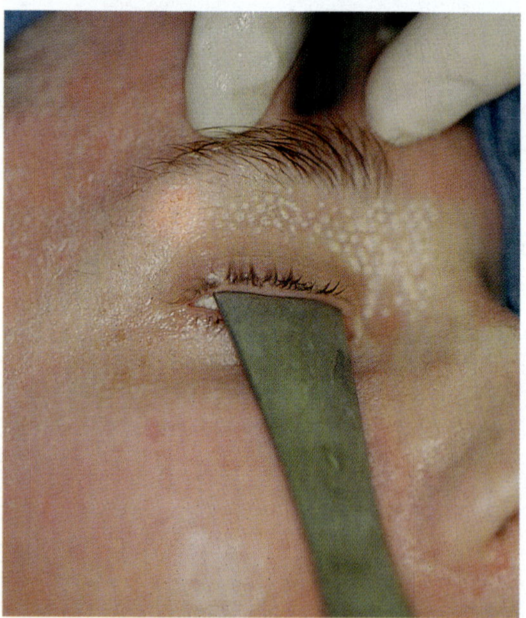

Figure 8–16. Laser resurfacing in the upper eyelid is carried down to the superior tarsal fold, but no further.

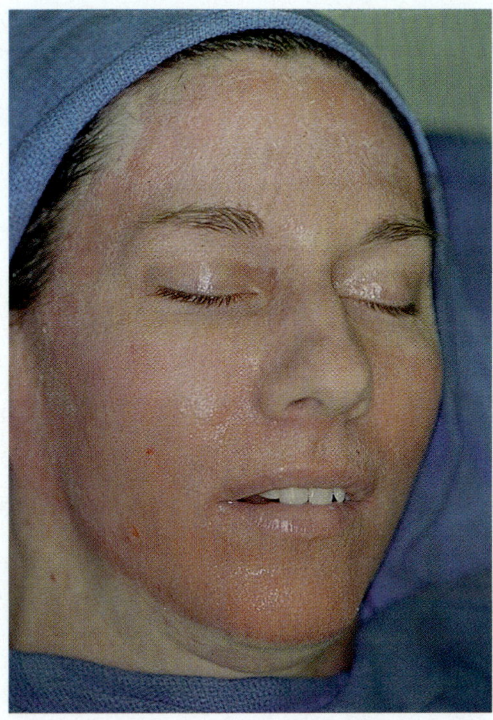

Figure 8–17. A patient after laser resurfacing and before application of dressing.

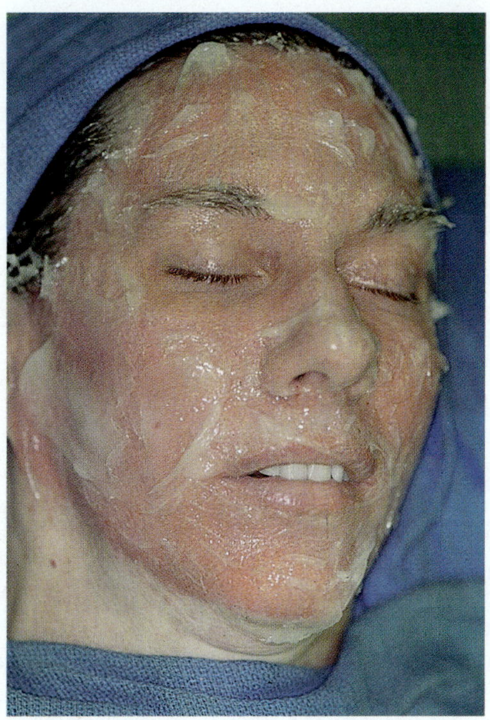

Figure 8–18. A thick layer of petrolatum is applied to laser-treated areas prior to patient release.

and application of petrolatum four to six times daily to laser-treated areas. Some discomfort may be noted following treatment. However, this is self-limited. Most patients describe this as a mild "prickling" sensation, and it requires no analgesia. Others find relief with Tylenol with codeine.

In most patients, reepithelialization is complete within 1 week, and makeup can be applied to the resurfaced area. Routinely, patients are started on a nonfluorinated steroid cream (Hytone cream $2\frac{1}{2}$%), to be applied at bedtime for 3 weeks. This accelerates resolution of erythema. It also eliminates the subclinical dermatitis that can occur when cosmetics, soaps, creams, or other lotions irritate the newly resurfaced skin.

The use of sun screens and sun precautions are recommended as soon as the skin has reepithelialized and should be continued for 3 to 6 months. Topical vitamin C lotion and tetranones are usually prescribed 1 month postoperatively and are continued indefinitely.

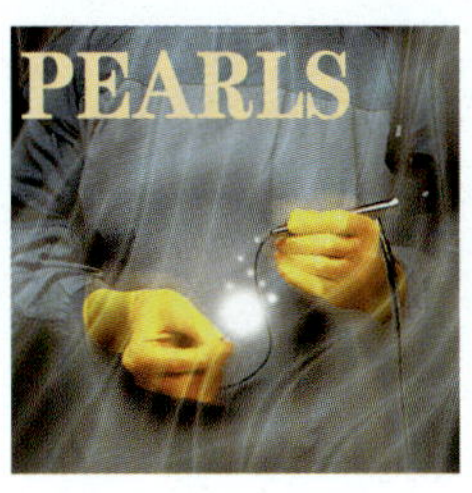

- CO_2 lasers have undergone significant technological advancements that have greatly improved clinical results. Currently, CO_2 lasers eclipse chemical exfoliation as the treatment of choice for photoaged skin.

- With high-energy, gain-switching CO_2 lasers, surgeons can achieve very high energy levels in periods of time shorter than the thermal relaxation time of skin tissue.

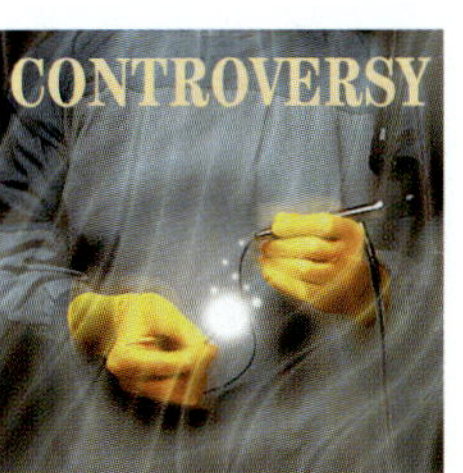

- There has been a debate about whether high-energy CO_2 laser treatment results in stimulation of tissue growth factors. There is accelerated wound healing versus scalpel incisions, but the levels of growth factors seem to be no different.

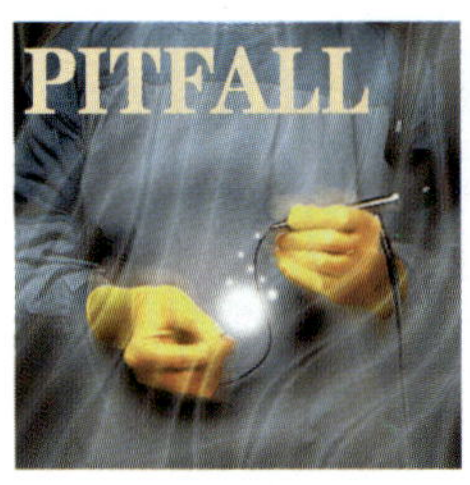

- A drawback of the Surgipulse XJ150 high-energy CO_2 laser is that it has a 3-mm spot size, which means it can only be used to treat only small- to medium-sized aesthetic units such as the perioral area, periorbital area, or localized rhytids.

REFERENCES

1. Fitzpatrick RE, Goldman MP, Sauter NM, et al. Pulsed carbon dioxide laser resurfacing of photo-aged skin. *Arch Dermatol* 1996;132:1395–1402.
2. Cotton J, Hood A, Gonin R, Beeson WH, Hanke CW. Histologic evaluation of pre- and post-auricular human skin following high-energy ultra-short carbon dioxide laser. *Ann Dermatol.* 1996;132:425–428.
3. Brody HJ. *Chemical Face Peeling.* St. Louis, MO: CV Mosby; 1997.
4. Alster TS, Kauver NA, Geronemus RG. Histology of high-energy pulsed carbon dioxide laser resurfacing. *Semin Cutan Med Surg.* 1996;15:189–193.
5. Pogrel MA. Profile of hyaluronidase activity distinguishes carbon dioxide laser from scalpel wound healing. *Ann Surg.* 1993;217:196–200.
6. Yu W. Expression of growth factors in early wound healing in rat skin. *Lasers Surg Med.* 1994;15:281–289.
7. Allen J. Laser resurfacing analysis of tissue growth factors. *Arch Otolaryngol Head Neck Surg.* Publication pending.
8. Geronemus RG, et al. Histologic comparison of carbon dioxide lasers - Surgipulse, SilkTouch, and Ultra-Pulse. Paper presented at: Annual Scientific Meeting of the American Society of Dermatologic Surgery and Oncology; May 1996; Hilton Head, SC.
9. Sharplan Lasers, Inc. Sharplan XJ Dual-Mode Scanner Operating Manual. Allendale, NJ.
10. Fitzpatrick T. The validity and practicality of some reactive skin types I–VI. *Arch Dermatol.* 1988;124:869–871.
11. Glogau RG, Matarasso SL. Chemical peels—trichloracetic acid and phenol. *Cosmetic Dermatol.* 1995;13:263–276.
12. Sliney DH. Laser safety. *Lasers Surg Med.* 1985;16:215–225.
13. Baggish MS, Elbarky M. The effect of laser smoke on the lungs of rats. *Am J Obstet Gynecol.* 1987;156:1260–1265.
14. Mandy SH. Tetranone in the preoperative and postoperative management of dermabrasion. *J Am Acad Dermatol.* 1986;15:878–879, 888–889.
15. Hevia O, Nemeth AJ, Taylor RJ. Tetranone accelerates healing after trichloracetic acid chemical peel. *Arch Dermatol.* 1991;127:678–682.
16. Goldman M. Third International Symposium on Cosmetic Efficacy; May 11, 1998; Cologne, Germany.

CHAPTER 9

Laser Resurfacing with UltraPulse Carbon Dioxide Lasers

PHILLIPA L. LOWE AND NICHOLAS J. LOWE

Carbon dioxide (CO_2) laser skin resurfacing for the treatment of facial aging skin was first introduced in the late 1980s with impressive results.[1,2] However, with the continuous-wave (CW) CO_2 laser, there is the risk of unwanted thermal injury to surrounding dermis and adnexal structures. Recent tecnological advances, such as rapidly pulsed lasers and flashcan techniques, allow more precise control of tissue ablation, thereby reducing the risk of scarring.[1–7] The UltraPulse CO_2 laser has been shown to be effective for treating aging facial skin. Laser resurfacing removes thin layers of old, damaged skin, which allows newly formed young, healthy skin to emerge.

Recent clinical and histologic comparisons of the pulsed CO_2 laser, medium-strength trichloroacetic acid peel, and dermabrasion show similar results, with the exception of Baker's phenol peel.[8] Healing after medium-strength trichloroacetic acid peel and dermabrasion resembled that after one to three passes with a pulsed CO_2 laser. Phenol-treated skin suffered deeper wounds and required longer recovery.

The CO_2 laser emits light at a wavelength of 10,600 nm. This light is absorbed by all biological tissue containing water—its target chromophore. Approximately 90% of the laser energy is absorbed within 30 μm of tissue, resulting in intracellular boiling at 100°C and vaporization. With the CW CO_2 laser, tissue becomes progressively desiccated, and heat accu-

mulates to 600°C. This excessive heat then conducts away from the treatment site, to a zone of thermal necrosis ranging in thickness from 200 μm to 1 mm. Such nonselective thermal damage can leave unwanted scars and discoloration.

ULTRAPULSE CO_2 LASERS

The UltraPulse 5000C is one type of pulsed laser system introduced by Coherent Medical. This laser produces high-energy pulses of very short duration to allow delivery of controlled skin ablation with a thermal injury depth of up to 70 μm. This laser has a pulse width of less than 1 millisecond and a pulse energy of up to 500 mJ. The energy is delivered through an articulated handle connected to a computer controlled pattern handpiece, which allows variable spot size, density of spot, and shape. When attached to the computerized pattern generator, the UltraPulse CO_2 laser delivers faster and more uniform skin resurfacing. This device allows small to large areas of the skin to be treated rapidly and with precision using various patterns.

Most studies have been performed on facial skin in patients with Fitzpatrick skin types I and II. There have been few reports on the use of lasers for the rejuvenation of photoaged neck skin. Moreover, neck skin is often considered to be an area of potential complication with such treatments as dermabrasion and chemical peels. In a recent study, 200 patients with facial photoaging and 40 patients with neck skin photoaging (Fitzpatrick skin types I, II, III, and IV) were treated. All patients illustrated in Figures 9–1 through 9–13 were treated with the Ultra-Pulse 5000 CO_2 laser with a computerized pattern-generator (CPG) handpiece. Energy settings between 225 and 300 mJ/cm^2 were used with a variety of density settings.

Facial photoaging was improved between 30 and 75% with one treatment. The degree of improvement after a single treatment continues to increase for 6 months to 2 years. Successful rejuvenation of neck skin was also achieved at 225 mJ low-density settings with the CPG and single laser passes without wiping of laser induced debris.

LASER PROTOCOL

Pretreatment

To obtain optimal results with laser skin resurfacing, carefully selected skin care regimens are needed both before and after treatment,[9,10] especially when treating darker-skinned patients.[9,10] Pretreatment consists of daily broad-spectrum sunscreens, a bleaching agent, such as hydroquinone or azelaic acid, and nightly application of tretinoin cream or glycolic acid cream. This regimen is usually started after the initial consultation, about 2 to 4 weeks prior to the procedure.

Technique

We used the UltraPulse 5000 CO_2 laser with CPG pattern 3 for most areas of the face or pattern 5 for periorbital and perioral skin. For the central and main areas of the face, the maximum size setting was 9 mm, with a density setting of either 5 or 6 W/cm^2, depending on the degree of photodamage. For subsequent laser pulses on the face, the settings were 250 mJ and 60 W with pattern 3 or 5 determined as above, with densities of 4 or 5 W/cm^2. For neck rejuvenation a single pass with the laser was used; laser energy settings of 250 mJ and

60 W were employed with pattern 3 and maximum size setting of 9 mm, with a density setting of 3 W/cm^2. For the face, vaporized skin was wiped after each pass, except the final pass, which was left unwiped. Vaporized skin on the neck was not wiped after using the single-low density laser setting.

Complications

Complications of laser surgery include infection, contact dermatitis, swelling, prolonged erythema, depigmentation, and scarring. Recurrent herpes infection can be prevented with prophylactic medication. A topical antibiotic is no longer recommended because of the common occurrence of contact dermatitis. Postoperative swelling, especially around the periorbital area, is managed with ice compresses. Prolonged erythema can last from several weeks to several months. Postinflammatory hyperpigmentation sometimes follows the erythema, so all patients with prolonged erythema are treated with a bleaching agent. Hyperpigmentation is most common in the infraorbital areas, where direct sunlight exposure may play a role. Hypopigmentation can also occur but tends to present 6 months to 1 year after the procedure, and probably is the result of overly aggressive laser resurfacing. Although laser skin resurfacing is precise, thermal damage accumulates with multiple passes of the laser, and hypertrophic scars have been reported. Scarring is related to the depth of resurfacing, as well as the location of treatment. The perioral area usually requires more passes, and a few cases of scarring have been reported.[10]

Results

For the treatment of facial photoaging, the results with the UltraPulse have been excellent. Thirty to 75% improvement was eventually achieved 12–24 months after a single laser treatment. A few patients have been successfully treated either completely or partially with a second laser treatment. In these patients, final improvement was

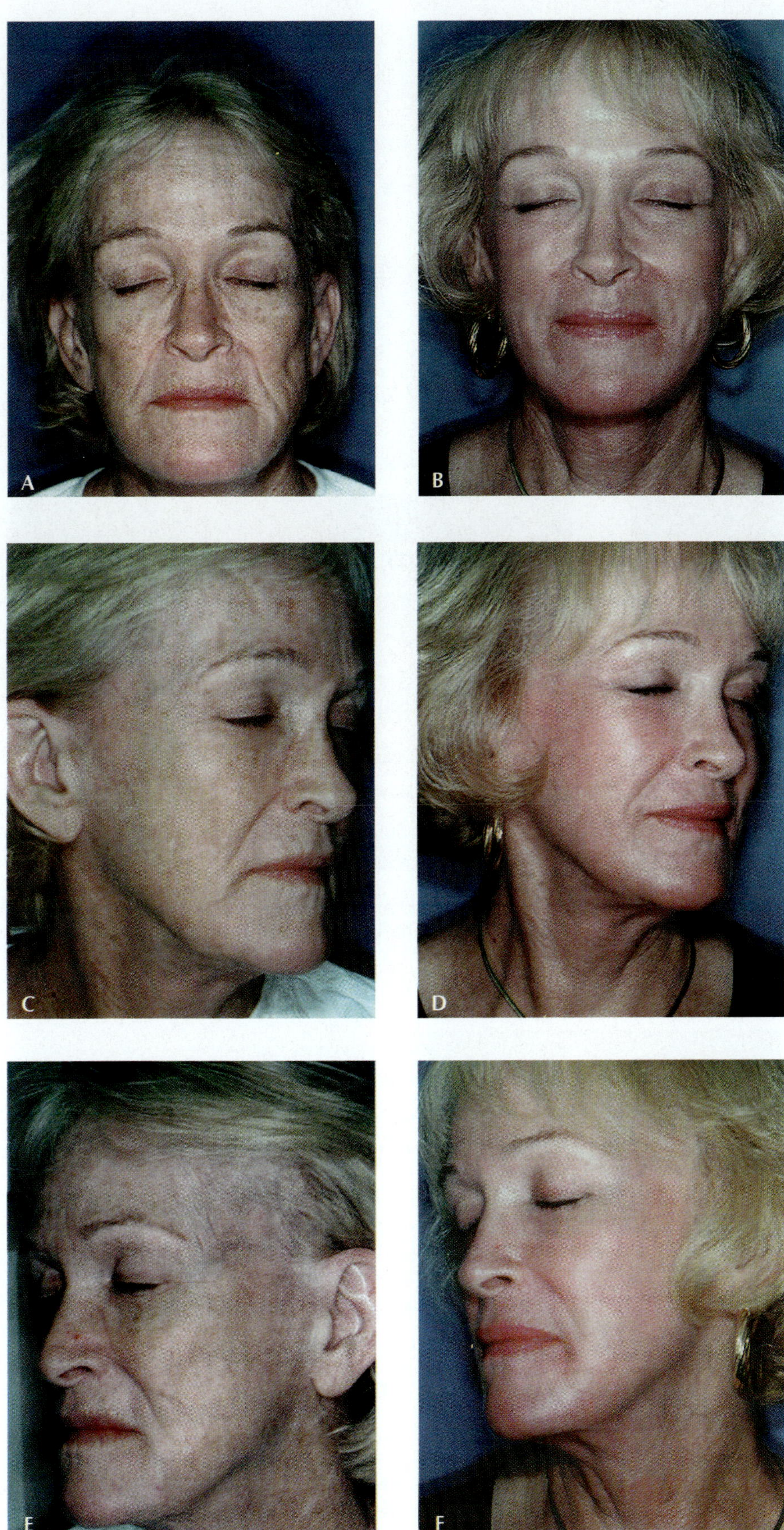

Figure 9–1. Severe photoaging. (A) Frontal, (C) right lateral, and (E) left lateral views before resurfacing. An 80% improvement is noted on (B) frontal, (D) right lateral, and (F) left lateral views 6 months after resurfacing of the face and neck. Two passes were done on the face: For the first pass settings were 300 mJ with a density of 5 and for the second pass, 250 mJ with a density of 4. One pass was done on the neck; the settings were 250 mJ with a density of 3.

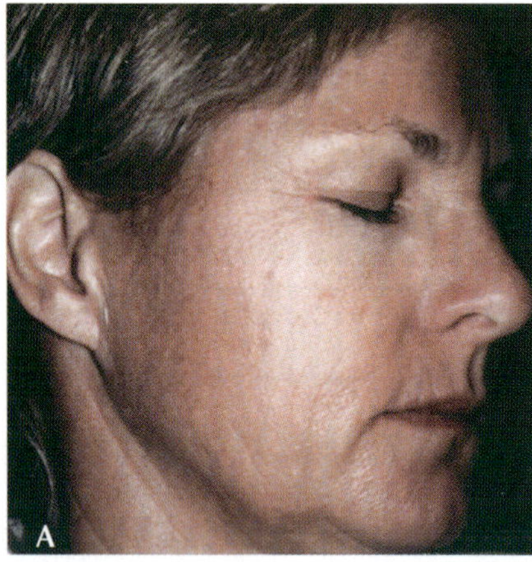 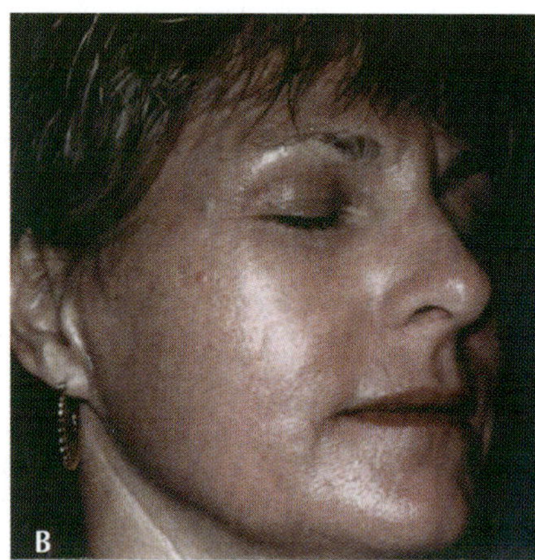

Figure 9–2. Moderate photoaging. (A) Before resurfacing, (B) A 60% improvement is noted 6 months after resurfacing. Two passes were done with settings at 300 mJ and 60 W with a density of 5.

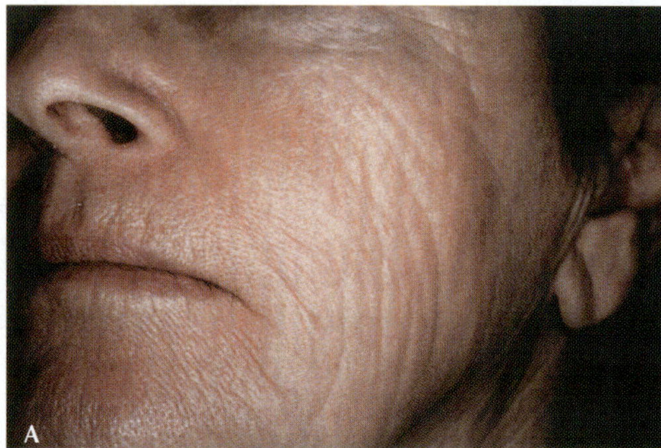 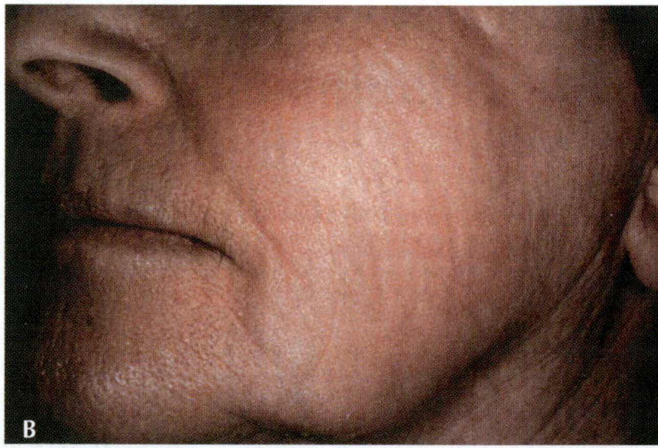

Figure 9–3. Severe photoaging. (A) Before resurfacing. (B) Twelve months after resurfacing. Two passes were made with settings of 300 mJ and 60 W with a density of 5. Density was set at 4 for a third pass on the cheeks.

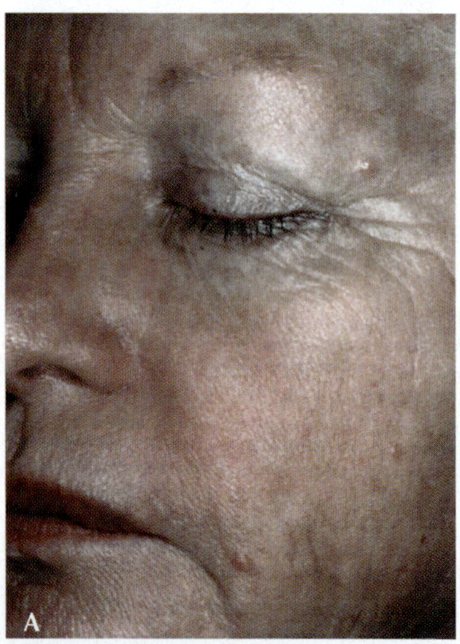 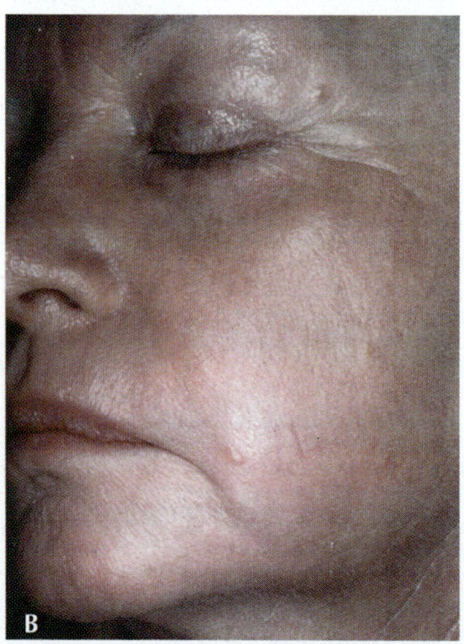

Figure 9–4. Moderate photoaging. (A) Before resurfacing. (B) Twelve months after resurfacing. Two passes were done. Settings for the first pass were 300 mJ and 60 W with a density of 5; settings for the second pass were 250 mJ and 60 W with a density of 4.

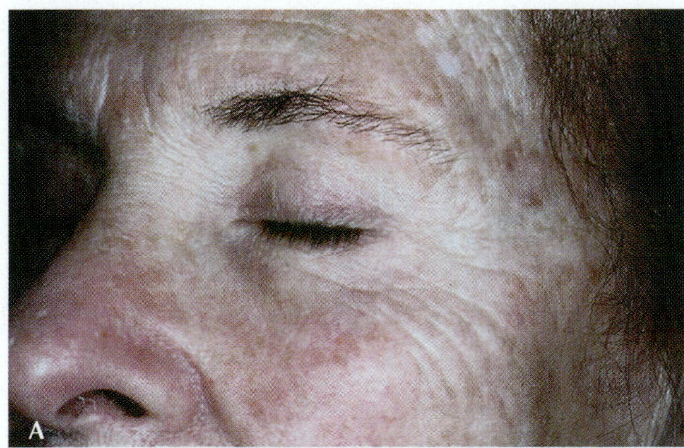
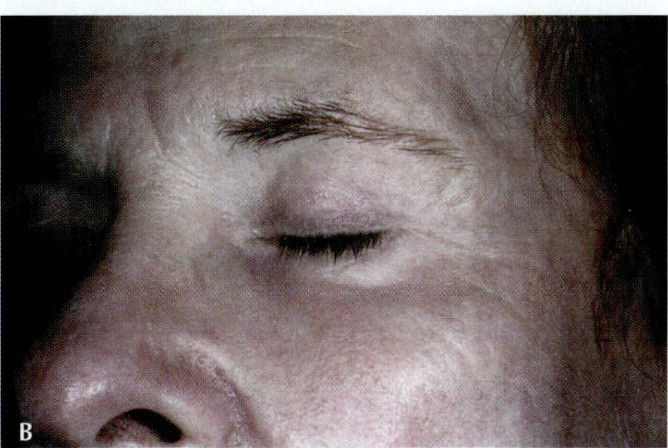

Figure 9–5. Moderate photoaging. (A) Before resurfacing. (B) A 70% improvement is noted 6 months after resurfacing. Two passes were done. Settings for the first pass were 250 mJ and 60 W with a density of 5; settings for the second pass were 225 mJ and 60 W with a density of 4. Botox® injections to the "crows feet" before and three months after laser treatment.

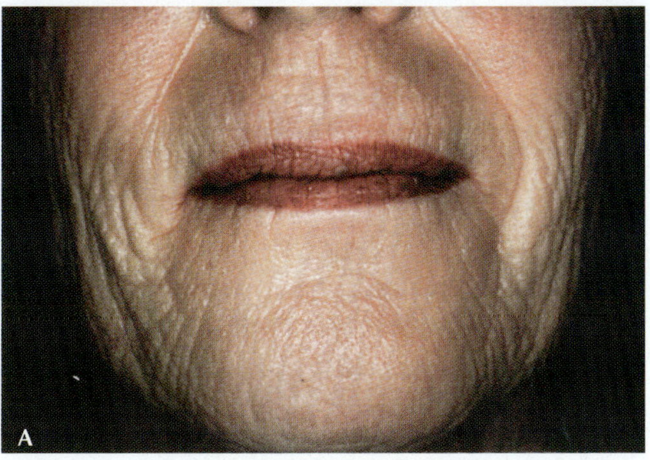
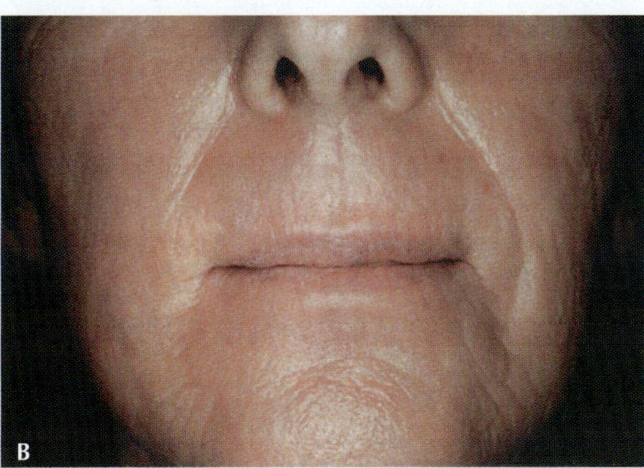

Figure 9–6. Severe photoaging. (A) Before resurfacing. (B) The posttreatment image was taken 18 months after the initial resurfacing and 6 months after a second treatment. Three passes were done for the first resurfacing; settings were 300 mJ and 60 W with a density of 5. Two passes were done for the second resurfacing; settings for the first pass were 300 mJ and 60 W with a density of 5 and settings for the second pass were 250 mJ and 60 W with a density of 4.

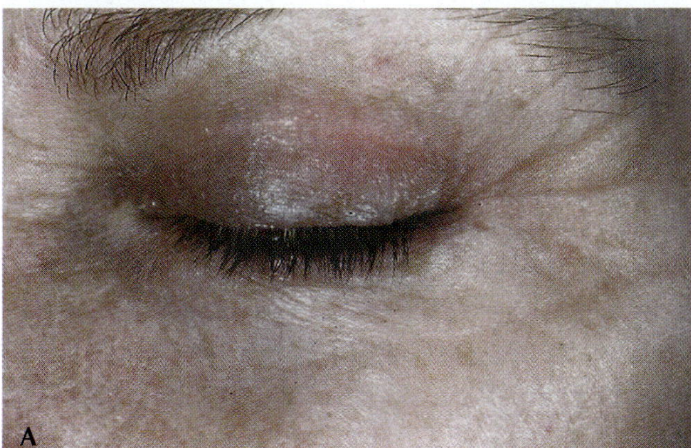
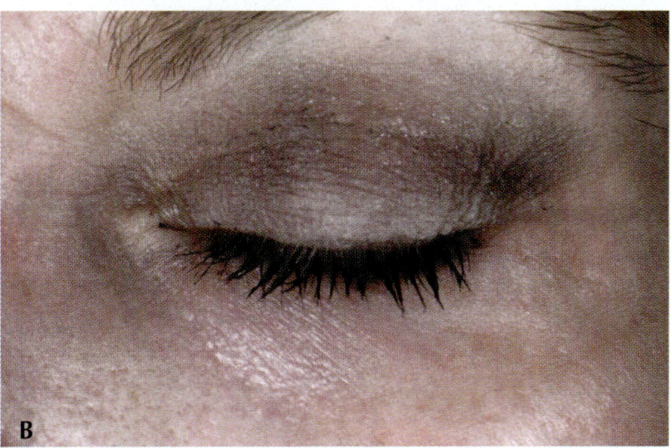

Figure 9–7. Moderate aging in the periorbital region. (A) Before resurfacing. (B) Six months after resurfacing. Two passes were done. Settings for the first pass were 300 W and 60 W with a density of 4; settings for the second pass were 250 mJ and 60 W with a density of 4.

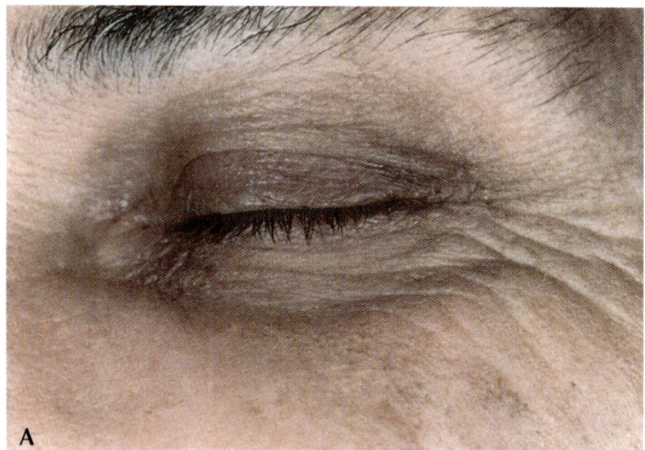

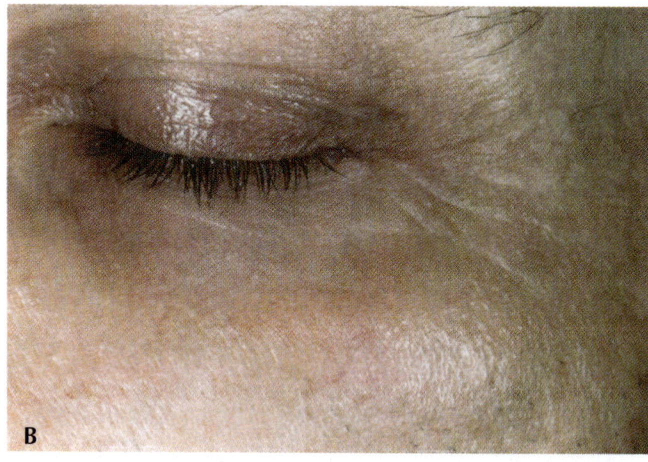

Figure 9–8. Moderate aging in the periorbital region. (A) Before resurfacing. (B) Twelve months after resurfacing. Two passes were done. Settings for the first pass were 300 mJ and 60 W with a density of 5; settings for the second pass were 250 mJ and 60 W with a density of 4.

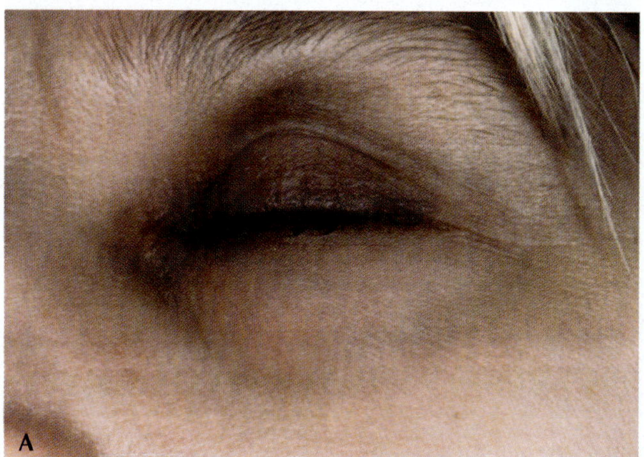

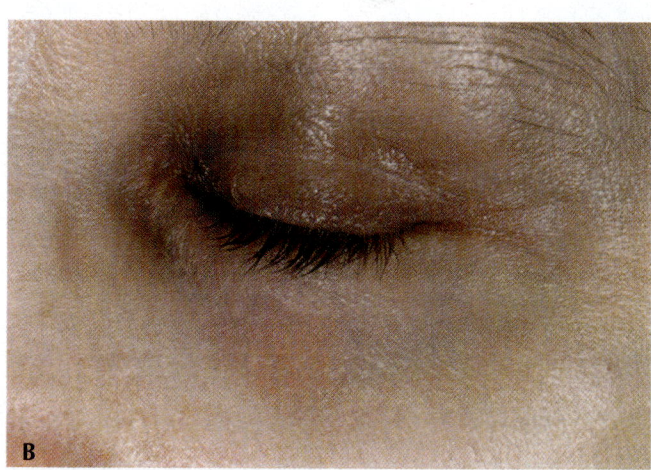

Figure 9–9. Mild aging in the periorbital region. (A) Before resurfacing. (B) A 50% improvement is noted 6 months later.

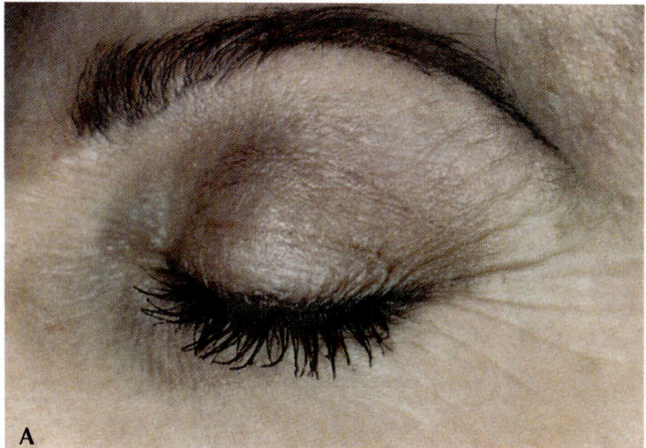

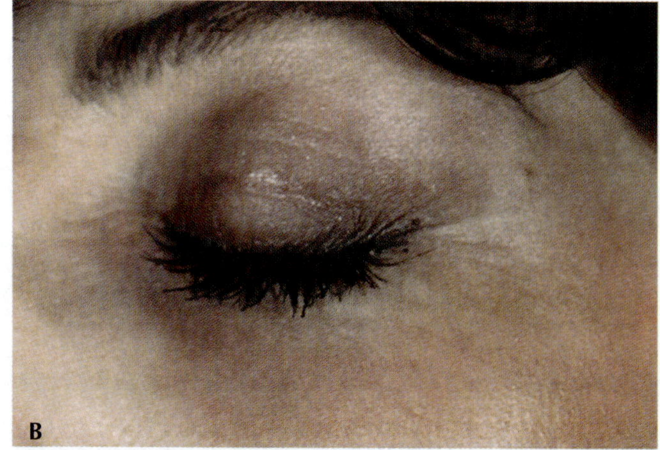

Figure 9–10. Mild periorbital lines. (A) Before resurfacing. (B) Twelve months after resurfacing. Two passes were done. Settings for the first pass were 250 mJ and 60 W with a density of 5; settings for the second pass were 225 mJ and 60 W with a density of 4.

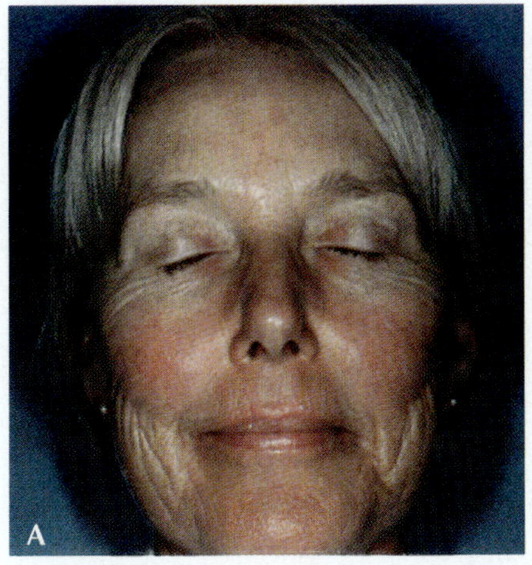
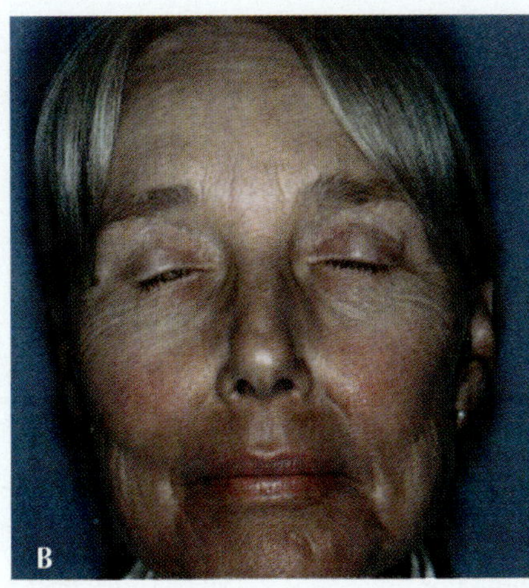

Figure 9–11. Moderate periorbital lines. (A) Before resurfacing. (B) An 80% improvement is noted 12 months after resurfacing. Three passes were done. Settings for the first pass were 300 mJ and 60 W with a density of 5; settings for the second pass were 250 mJ and 60 W with a density of 4; settings for the third pass were 250 mJ with a density of 4.

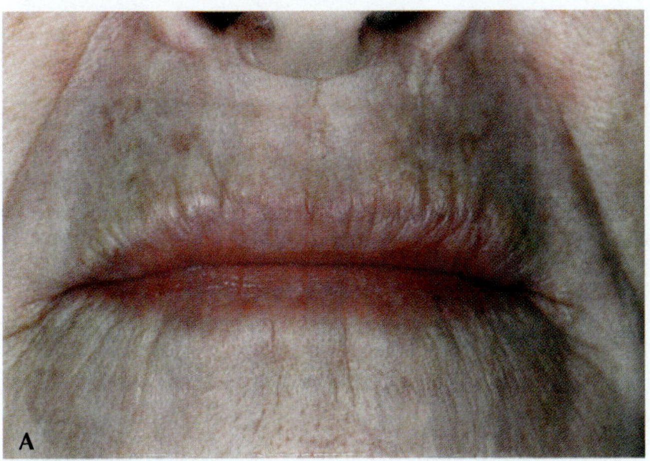
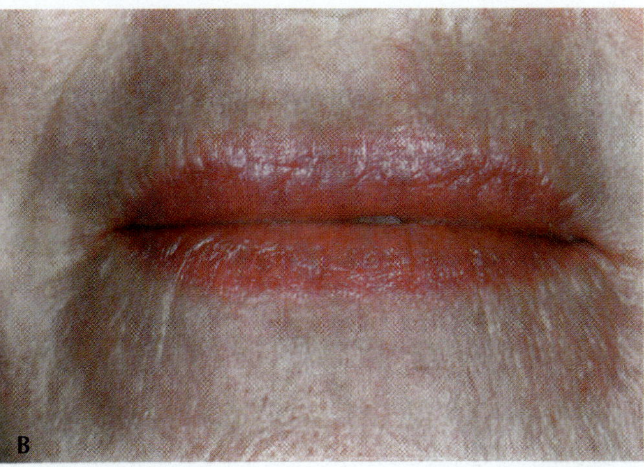

Figure 9–12. Severe perioral lines. (A) Before resurfacing. (B) An 80% improvement is noted 12 months after resurfacing. Three passes were done. Settings for the first pass were 300 mJ and 60 W with a density of 5; settings for the second pass were 250 mJ and 60 W with a density of 5; settings for the third pass were 250 mJ and 60 W with a density of 5. The patient also had a soft form implant to the upper lip at the time of resurfacing.

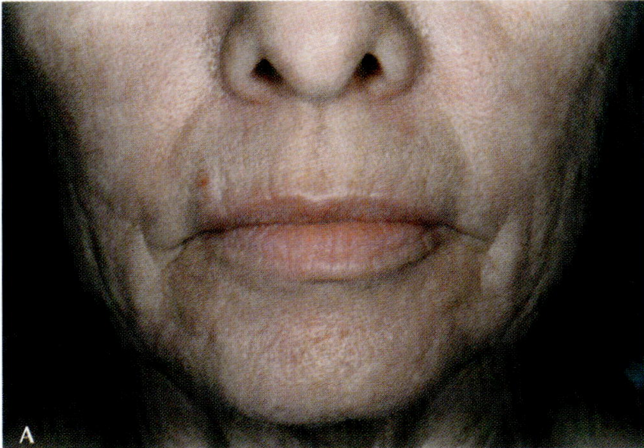
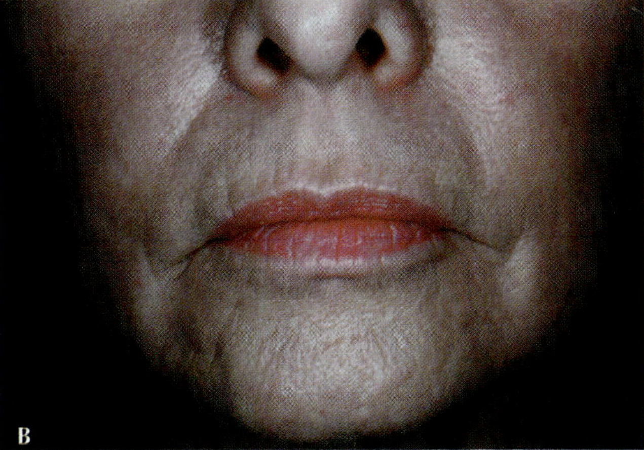

Figure 9–13. Moderate to severe photoaging. (A) Before resurfacing. (B) Twelve months after resurfacing of the perioral region and lower face. Two passes were done. Settings for the first pass were 300 mJ and 60 W with a density of 5; settings for the second pass were 250 mJ and 60 W with a density of 5.

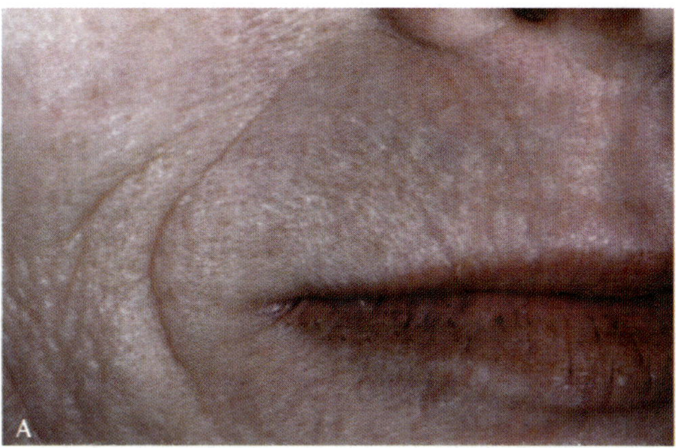

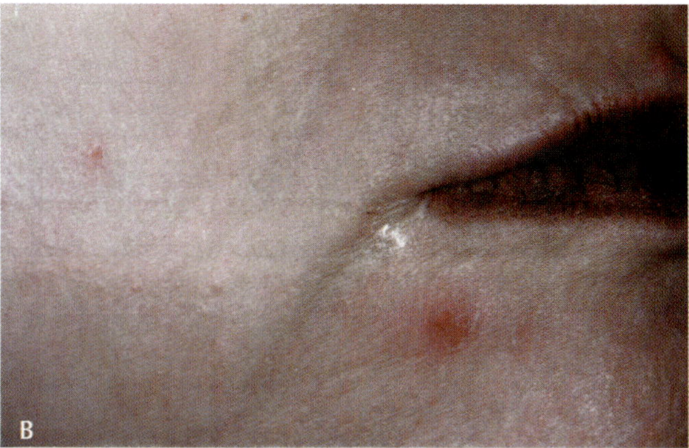

Figure 9–14. Severe photoaging. (A) Before resurfacing. (B) Acneform lesions and scattered telangiectasia are seen 3 weeks after resurfacing.

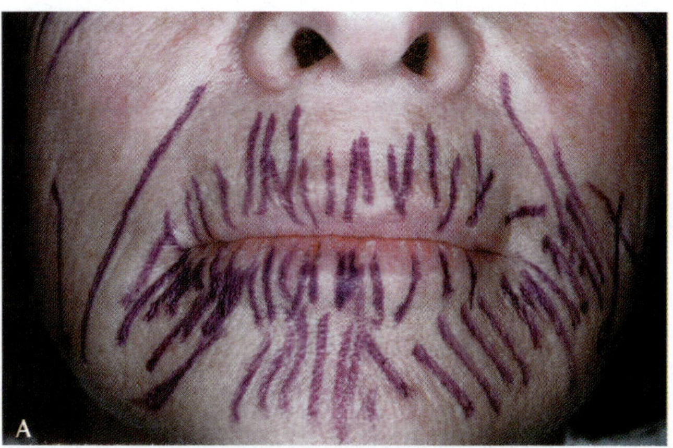

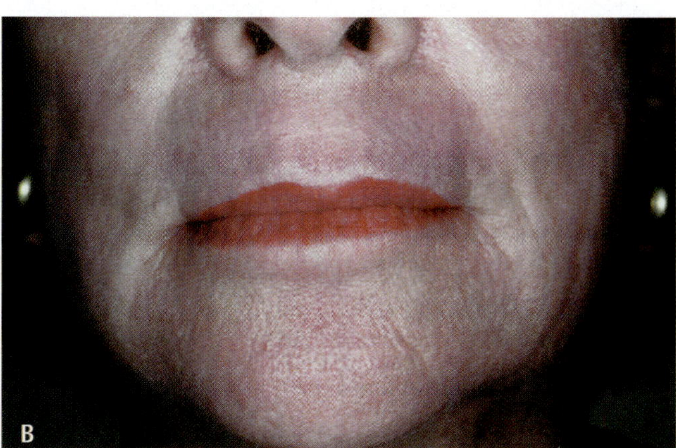

Figure 9–15. (A) Patient marked with gentian violet before treatment. (B) Erythema and mild skin whitening have developed 6 months later.

between 25 and 50% better than the first treatment response. In general, patients received fewer passes the second time than at their first treatment.

Global response following a single neck rejuvenation treatment varied between 40 and 75% improved. There is much greater risk for scarring on the neck than the face, and this risk increases the deeper the resurfacing in part due to the decreasing amount of adnexal structures. Temporary adverse effects (Figs. 9–14 through 9–16) were universal exudation, scaling, erythema, and discomfort. Complete reepithelialization was seen by 7 to 10 days with the parameters described. A smaller percentage of patients had post-laser erythema lasting up to 6 months. However, after the second month, erythema tended to be relatively mild and was often more pronounced during exercise or exposure to hot weather. Other clinicians used more aggressive neck resurfacing and had problems with scarring.

Skin resurfacing with the UltraPulse CO_2 laser has been confirmed as an effective mode of skin rejuvenation. It is important to use extreme caution in treating the neck with low density and a single pass with no wiping. Great care should be taken in treating the neck, and in some patients small test areas should be considered prior to the overall treatment of the neck.

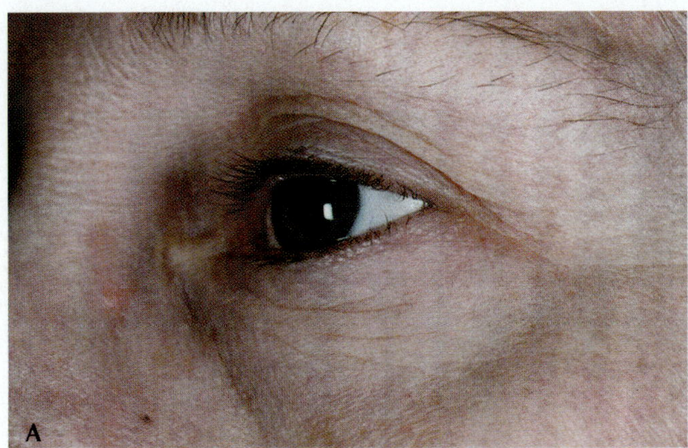

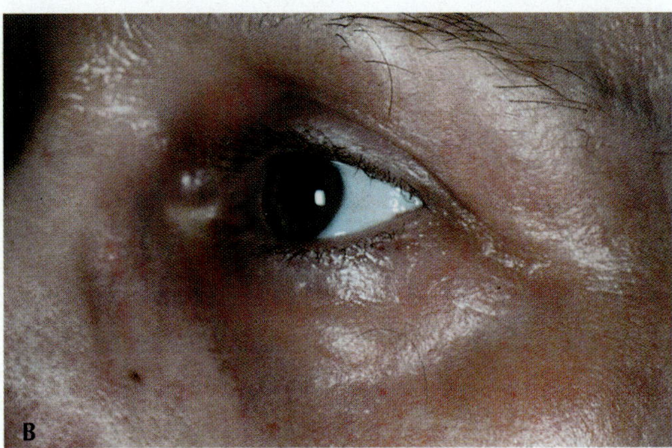

Figure 9–16. Moderate photoaging. (A) Before resurfacing. (B) Moderate erythema has developed 2 weeks after treatment. Settings for the two passes were 300 mJ with a density of 5 and 225 mJ with a density of 4, respectively.

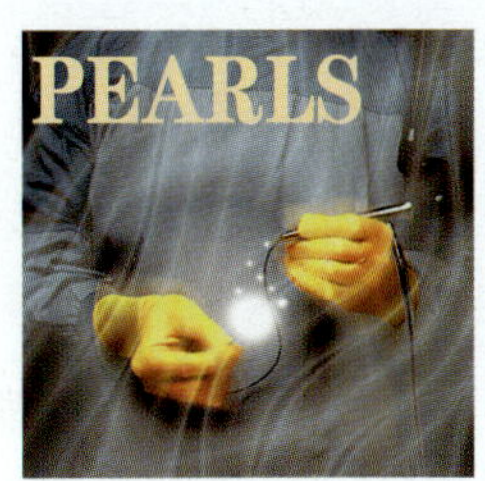

- The 3-mm collimated handpiece that is used with the UltraPulse laser allows precise delivery of consistent energy regardless of its distance from the skin.

- When used with a CPG, the UltraPulse laser permits faster (25% of the time needed without the scanner) and uniform resurfacing.

- CPG pattern 3 is preferred for most facial resurfacing with the UltraPulse laser, but other patterns may be used for the periorbital, perioral areas and for scars.

- Although wiping vaporized skin after each pass (except the last one) is standard procedure for most laser resurfacing, we do not wipe when resurfacing the neck because we use only a single pass in this very delicate area.

REFERENCES

1. David LM, Lask GP, Glassberg E, et al. CO_2 laser ablation for cosmetic and therapeutic treatment of facial actinic damage. *Cutis.* 1989;43:583–587.

2. Fitzpatrick RE, Ruiz-Exparaza J, Goldman MT. The depth of thermal necrosis using the CO_2 laser: a comparison of the superpulsed mode and the conventional mode. *J Dermatol Surg Oncol.* 1991;17:340–344.

3. Fitzpatrick RE, Goldman MP. Advances in carbon dioxide laser surgery. *Clin Dermatol.* 1995;13:35–47.

4. Lowe NJ, Lask G, Griffin ME, et al. Skin resurfacing with the ultrapulsed carbon dioxide laser: observation on 100 patients. *Dermatol Surg.* 1995;21:1025–1029.

5. Hruza GJ. Skin resurfacing with lasers. *J Clin Dermatol.* 1995;3:38–41.

6. Waldorf HA, Kauvar A, Geronemus RG. Skin resurfacing of fine to deep rhytides using a char-free carbon dioxide laser in 47 patients. *Dermatol Surg.* 1995;21:940–946.

7. Lask G, Keller G, Lowe N, et al. Laser skin resurfacing with the SilkTouch flashscanner for facial rhytides. *Dermatol Surg.* 1995;21:1021–1024.

8. Fitzpatrick RE, Tope WD, Goldman MP, et al. Pulsed carbon dioxide laser, tricholoroacetic acid, Baker-Gordon phenol, and dermabrasion: a comparative clinical and histological study in a porcine model. *Arch Dermatol.* 1996;132:469–471.

9. Cotton J, Hood AF, Gonin R, et al. Histologic evaluation of preauricular and postauricular human skin after high-energy short-pulsed carbon dioxide laser.

10. Lowe NJ, Lask G, Griffin ME. Laser skin resurfacing: pre- and posttreatment guidelines. *Dermatol Surg.* 1995;21:1017–1019.

CHAPTER 10

Single-Pass, High-Fluence, Carbon Dioxide Laser Skin Resurfacing

MAURICE M. KHOSH, WAYNE F. LARRABEE, AND BRUCE SMOLLER

This chapter discusses the effectiveness and safety of single-pass, high-fluence, carbon dioxide (CO_2) laser skin resurfacing. We propose that eliminating repeated laser passes by using a higher fluence helps minimize subsequent post-treatment erythema, and we present histologic and clinical data that support our proposed CO_2 laser parameters.

In the past decade, CO_2 laser resurfacing has gained prominence in our armamentarium for treating superficial facial rhytids. It is preferable to dermabrasion and chemical peeling for facial skin rejuvenation because of the lack of bleeding, precision in depth of ablation, and technical simplicity. Histologic studies on the long-term effects of laser resurfacing in skin demonstrate elimination of epidermal atrophy and atypia, development of new collagen in the dermis, proliferation of elastic fibers, homogenization of melanin distribution, and a reduction in the amount of glycosaminoglycans.[1] These histologic changes correlate with clinical findings of diminished fine wrinkles, enhanced color and texture, and overall skin rejuvenation.

To ablate skin without scarring, tissue vaporization and thermal damage must not extend to the deep reticular dermis. In human skin, char-free CO_2 laser vaporization requires a minimal energy density (fluence) of 5 J/cm². This critical amount of energy must be delivered within the thermal relaxation time of skin (0.695 msec) to minimize heat conduction and thermal injury to surrounding tissues. On average, each pass of the CO_2 laser vaporizes 20 to 30 μm of skin, leaving an additional

25 to 70 μm of sublethal thermal damage, which is proposed to contribute to postresurfacing erythema that lasts 2 to 6 months.

Although our knowledge of laser-skin interaction has increased and the technology in laser delivery and scanning devices has advanced, long-term postoperative erythema continues to be a significant problem with CO_2 laser resurfacing. In attempts to minimize posttreatment erythema, manufacturing companies have concentrated on developing laser devices with more rapid energy delivery capabilities and shallower ablation depths. Advances in scanning devices represented a significant development in this area.

Erbium:yttrium-aluminum-garnet (Er:YAG) lasers have gained popularity for skin resurfacing. They represent a class of lasers with much greater water absorption, shallower depth of skin ablation, and a thinner band of residual thermal damage in the skin. The major advantage of Er:YAG resurfacing has been the significantly shorter duration of posttreatment erythema, and the Er:YAG laser seemed poised to replace the CO_2 laser for all skin resurfacing indications. However, the long-term results of Er:YAG laser resurfacing have shown limited effectiveness in removing deeper facial rhytids. It has been postulated that effective collagen remodeling and deep rhytid effacement depend on laser-induced thermal damage in the deep dermal layer, such as that caused by the CO_2 laser. Therefore, proven long-term effectiveness, prevalence, and easy availability continue to power the popularity of CO_2 lasers for facial skin resurfacing.

In our practice, we use the Sharplan XJ150 laser (Sharplan, Inc., Allendale, NJ) with the FeatherTouch scanning device. In laser resurfacing, depth of skin ablation correlates with intensity of the laser pulse and the number of laser passes.[1,2] To achieve adequate depths of ablation with the FeatherTouch laser, many clinicians use multiple laser passes at 9 J/cm^2 or 36 W (the recommended power setting for the FeatherTouch system), especially in facial areas with more extensive rhytids such as the perioral region. Because of reduced water content in the dermis following the first laser pass, repeated laser passes cause progressively greater thermal injury in the dermis and less effective tissue vaporization.[3] Ideally, the desired depth of laser resurfacing should be achieved with one laser pass to minimize thermal conduction during repeated laser passes.

HISTOLOGIC STUDIES

In a histologic study with the UltraPulse CO_2 laser (Coherent Medical), Alster et al[3] showed that the first laser pass achieved epidermal removal and a 20- to 30-μm zone of damage to the dermis. The subsequent two or three passes yielded significantly greater depths of thermal damage. Tissue desiccation from each laser pass increases the capacity for heat transfer to adjacent tissues. Each laser pass delivered the same amount of energy, but because of the decreased water content in the dermis, secondary and tertiary laser passes caused less vaporization and more extensive heat damage. It can be deduced that the desired depth of skin ablation should be achieved with a single laser pass so that the effects of tissue desiccation can be circumvented.

To determine the histologic effects of CO_2 laser resurfacing, we spot-treated the preauricular skin of five patients prior to their undergoing rhytidectomy. All five patients were female and between 55 and 64 years old with Fitzpatrick skin types I or II. We used a 3-mm spot to treat the preauricular skin on six sites on either side of the face for a total of 60 sites. Resurfaced skin was wiped after each laser pass. A list of the laser parameters and number of passes appears in Table 10–1. After skin excision during rhytidectomy, punch biopsies were taken from the laser-treated areas and submitted for histologic evaluation. The hematoxylin-eosin stained biopsy specimens were evaluated for depth of skin ablation, depth of thermal damage in the residual skin, and evidence of thermal damage in the reticular dermis.

Table 10–1. Histologic Results of Resurfacing in the Preauricular Skin

No. of passes	Energy Fluence (J/cm^2)	Power (W)	Depth of Ablation or Thermal Injury (μm)		No. of Sites Tested
			Epidermis	Dermis	
1	7	32	20–60	0–20	2
1	8	34	20–60	0–40	3
1	9	36	20–60	0–40	3
1	12	50	FT*	20–80	3
2	12	50	FT	60–100	3
1	14	60	FT	40–100	3
2	14	60	FT	80–100	3
1	16	65	FT	40–60	3
1	17	70	FT	60–100	5
2	17	70	FT	60–140	5

*FT, full thickness.

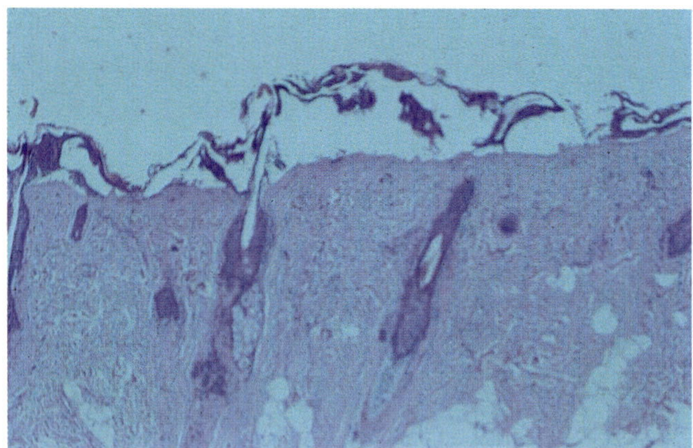

Figure 10–1. Histologic results of single-pass CO_2 laser resurfacing at 36 W (9 J/cm²).

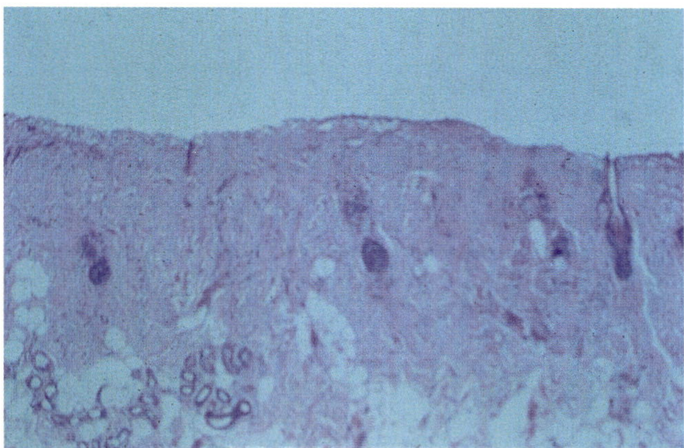

Figure 10–2. Histologic results of single-pass CO_2 laser resurfacing at 70 W (17 J/cm²).

Our study showed that laser passes with 7, 8, or 9 J/cm² (32, 34, or 36 W) ablated the epidermis but rarely penetrated the papillary dermis (Fig. 10–1). It was at fluences of 12 J/cm² (50 W) or greater that full epidermal ablation was achieved with a single pass. A single laser pass at 17 J/cm² (70 W) caused total ablation of the epidermis and partial ablation of the papillary dermis. At this power setting, the depth of thermal injury in the papillary dermis was 60 to 100 μm. There was no evidence of injury to the reticular dermis (Fig. 10–2). Absence of thermal injury in the reticular dermis indicated that laser resurfacing at 17 J/cm² (70 W) could be carried out without injuring the pilosebaceous apparatus and risking scarring (see Table 10–1 for results).

CLINICAL STUDIES

Clinical reports on the Coherent UltraPulse laser indicate posttreatment erythema extends from 8 to 16 weeks.[4–7] Studies with the SilkTouch laser report the duration of erythema to be 6 to 18 weeks.[8,9] Our experience with the

Sharplan XJ150 laser and FeatherTouch scanner is outlined below.

During a 6-month period, 30 patients underwent single-pass high-fluence CO_2 laser resurfacing. All patients were female and between 34 and 71 years old. Fitzpatrick and Glogau skin class distributions are listed in Tables 10–2 and 10–3. None of the patients had ever received radiation therapy or used isotretinoin (Accutane) in the preceding 2 years. All patients had adequate lower lid tone. The indication for skin resurfacing was fine facial rhytids or solar keratosis. The resurfaced regions included the entire face in 19 patients, the perioral area in 2 patients, and the periorbital plus the perioral area in 9 patients. Patients who had isolated periorbital resurfacing were not included because the periorbital region was always resurfaced at lower fluences (9 J/cm², or 36 W). Pretreatment protocol included glycolic acid, kojic acid, prophylactic antibiotics, and antiviral therapy. Concomitant cosmetic procedures (including rhytidectomy, blepharoplasty, and endoscopic forehead plastic surgery)

Table 10–2. Fitzpatrick Skin Class Distribution

	Number	Percentage
Type I	10	33%
Type II	16	54%
Type III	4	13%
Type IV–VI	0	0%

Table 10–3. Glogau Photoaging Distribution

	Number	Percentage
Type 1	0	0%
Type 2	14	47%
Type 3	12	40%
Type 4	4	13%

were performed in 60% of patients. In rhytidectomy patients, the undermined area was not resurfaced.

Resurfacing was accomplished with the Sharplan XJ150 laser and the FeatherTouch scanner. A 200-mm handpiece with a 3- to 11-mm spot size was used. Except for the periorbital area, all facial regions were treated with a single pass at 17 J/cm^2 (70 W). The periorbital area was treated with a single pass at 9 J/cm^2 (36 W) because epidermal and dermal width in the eyelids is significantly thinner than in the rest of the face.[10]

Postoperative wound care included Flexzan (Dow Hickams Pharmaceuticals, Inc., Sugarland, TX) or Silon-TSR (Bio Med Sciences, Inc., Bethlehem, PA) dressings and bovine collagen ointment. Steroid creams were not used. Patients had regular office follow-up visits for evaluation and photographic documentation that ranged from 6 to 12 months.

Skin reepithelialization was complete by day 10 in all patients. There were no major complications such as scarring, hypopigmentation, infection, or scleral show. In three patients, hyperpigmentation was noted at postoperative weeks 2 to 4. Treatment with topical bleaching agents resolved the hyperpigmentation by the third postoperative month. Results were judged as good to excellent by 90% of patients (Figs. 10–3 to 10–5). The effectiveness of rhytid effacement and skin rejuvenation was similar to that in 20 patients who had been treated previously with two or more passes of average fluence (9 J/cm^2, or 36 W). Posttreatment erythema in the single-pass group lasted 4 to 8 weeks (mean, 6 weeks)

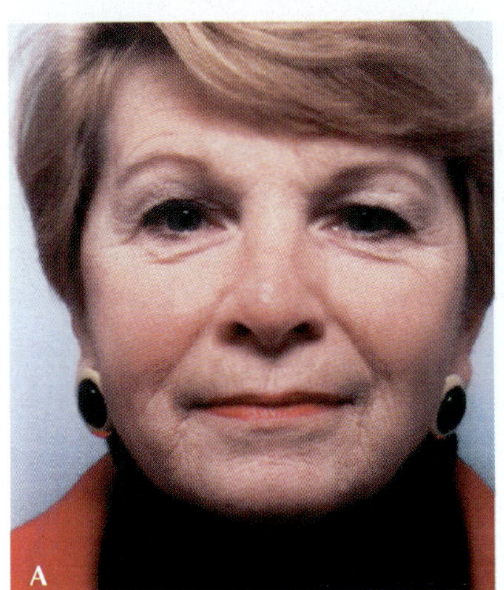
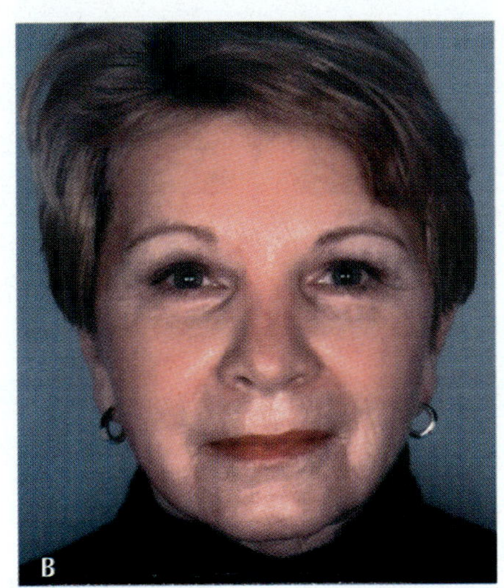

Figure 10–3. A 62-year-old woman before (A) and 6 months after (B) full-face laser resurfacing, endoscopic forehead lift, laser blepharoplasty of the upper lids, laser transconjunctival blepharoplasty of the lower lids, and neck lift.

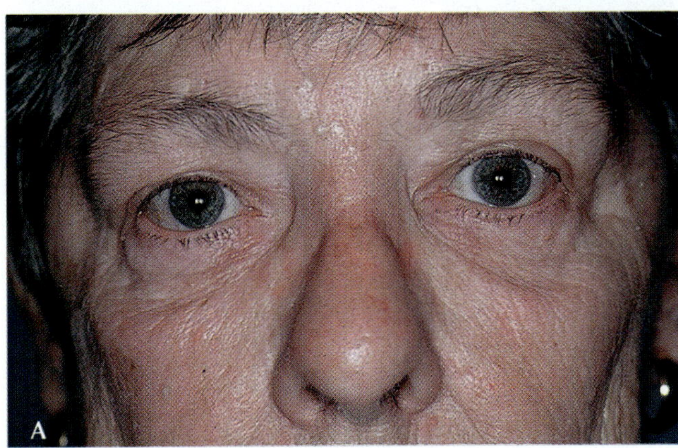
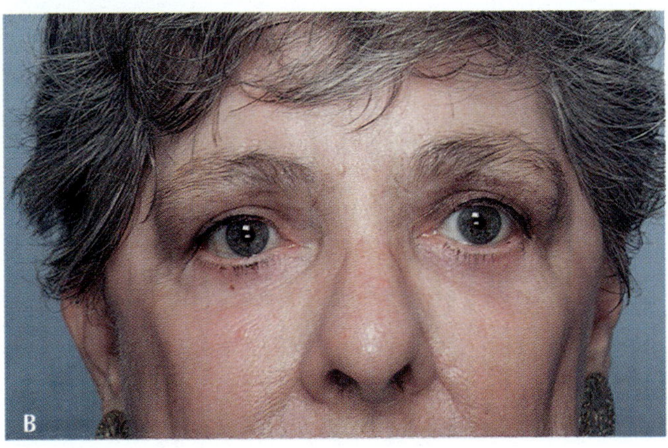

Figure 10–4. A 67-year-old woman before (A) and 6 months after (B) laser resurfacing and blepharoplasty.

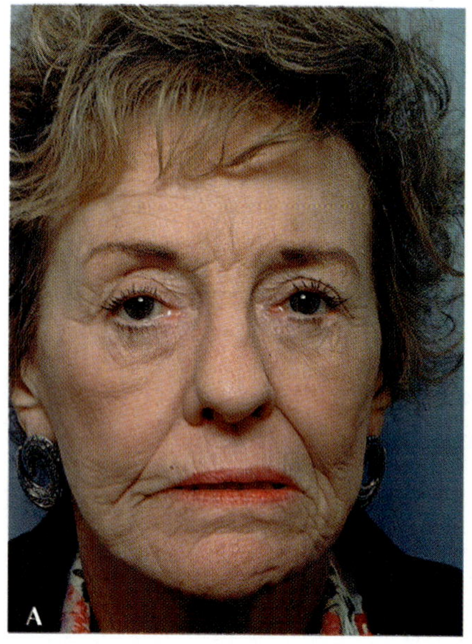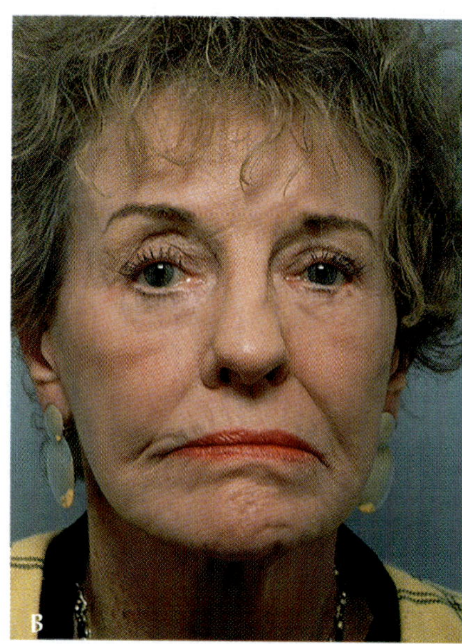

Figure 10–5. A 75-year-old woman before (A) and 1 month after (B) laser resurfacing and neck lift.

compared with 8 to 16 weeks in the multipass group. Therefore, our results indicate that high-fluence, single-pass, CO_2 laser resurfacing is as effective clinically as multipass laser resurfacing, while reducing the duration of posttreatment erythema.

CONCLUSIONS

Carbon dioxide laser resurfacing is a reliable and precise method of superficial skin rejuvenation, but post-treatment skin erythema invariably occurs despite avoidance of skin irritants, prophylaxis against infections, and use of topical steroids. The proposed mechanisms include thermal damage to the deep dermis, contact or irritant dermatitis, atopy, vasodilating medications, and superficial infection.[11] Because erythema after laser treatment is significantly less with the Er:YAG laser, it is believed that the depth of sublethal thermal damage contributes to the intensity and duration of posttreatment erythema.

Reducing the number of laser passes minimizes tissue desiccation and limits the extent of thermal damage in the adjacent dermis. For effective and safe CO_2 laser resurfacing, we recommend high-fluence laser resurfacing with a single pass, specifically the FeatherTouch laser at a

power setting of 17 J/cm² (70 W), based on our own experience. The recommended laser parameters have been tested in all facial regions except the periorbital region because prior studies have shown that the skin (or dermis) in this region is significantly thinner than in the rest of the face. In our group of patients, these laser parameters resulted in good to excellent clinical outcome while minimizing the duration and intensity of posttreatment erythema.

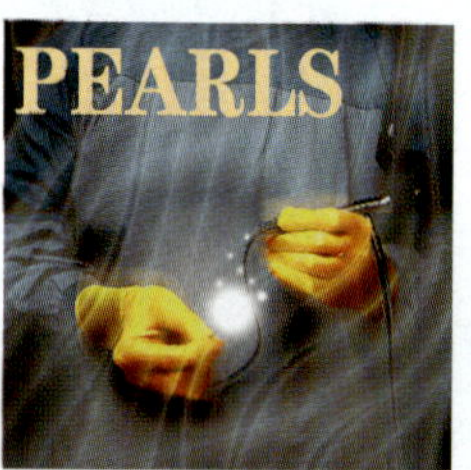

- The major advantage of Er:YAG resurfacing is significantly shorter duration of posttreatment erythema, but the long-term results of Er:YAG laser resurfacing have shown limited effectiveness in removing deeper facial rhytids. Therefore, the CO_2 laser's proven long-term effectiveness, prevalence, and easy availability continue to power its popularity.

- The periorbital area is treated with a single pass of the FeatherTouch laser at 9 J/cm² instead of 17 J/cm² because epidermal and dermal width in the eyelids is significantly thinner than in the rest of the face.

REFERENCES

1. Stuzin JM, Baker TJ, Baker TM, Klingman AM. Histologic effects of high energy pulsed CO2 laser on photoaged facial skin. *Plast Reconstr Surg.* 1997;99:2036–2055.
2. Cotton J, Hood AF, Gonin R, et al. Histologic evaluation of preauricular and postauricular human skin after high-energy short-pulse carbon dioxide laser. *Arch Dermatol.* 1996;132:425–428.
3. Alster TS, Kauvar AN, Geronemus RG. Histology of high-energy pulsed CO_2 resurfacing. *Semin Cutan Med Surg.* 1996;15:189–193.
4. Apfelberg DB. The UltraPulse carbon dioxide laser with computer pattern generator automatic scanner for facial cosmetic surgery and resurfacing. *Ann Plast Surg.* 1996;36:522–529.
5. Alster TS, Sanjay G. Treatment of facial rhytids with a high energy pulsed carbon dioxide laser. *Plast Reconstr Surg.* 1996;98:791–794.
6. Alster TS, West TB. Resurfacing of atrophic facial acne scars with a high energy pulsed carbon dioxide laser. *Dermatol Surg.* 1996;22:151–155.
7. Fitzpatrick RE, Goldman MP, Satur NM, Whitney DT. Pulsed carbon dioxide laser resurfacing of photoaged facial skin. *Arch Dermatol.* 1996;132:395–402.
8. Ho C, Nguyen Q, Nicholas JL, Griffin ME, Lask G. Laser resurfacing in pigmented skin. *Dermatol Surg.* 1995;21:1035–1037.
9. Bernstein LJ, Kauvar AN, Grossman MC, Geronemus RG. The short and long term side effects of carbon dioxide laser resurfacing. *Dermatol Surg.* 1997;23:529–525.
10. Gonzalez-Ulloa M, Castillo A, Stevens E, et al. Preliminary study of the total restoration of the facial skin. *Plast Reconstr Surg.* 1954;14:151.
11. Kilmer SL. Laser resurfacing complications. *Aesthetic Restorative Surg.* 1997;5:41–45.

CHAPTER 11

The Luxar Laser System

R. JAMES KOCH

The Luxar Laser System (Luxar Corp., Bothell, WA) consists of the Luxar LX-20SP NovaPulse carbon dioxide (CO_2) laser, the NovaScan 3-mm handpiece, and the SureScan computerized pattern-generator (CPG) handpiece (Fig. 11–1). Luxar's parent company, ESC Medical Systems (Yokneam, Israel), has recently released an improved CPG handpiece, the DermaScan, for use with this laser.

The NovaPulse is the base unit, and the NovaScan handpiece accepts tips up to 0.8 mm in size. The 8-mm tip is valuable for regional skin work, whereas the 0.4-mm tip (5 mm long) is used for blepharoplasty (upper eyelid) and the 0.3-mm tip (10 mm long) is used for transconjunctival blepharoplasty. The MG 125EC tip on the LXM-C microguide handpiece is used for endoscopic brow lift. Other handpieces are directly interchanged as desired for full-face laser skin resurfacing.

NOVAPULSE CO$_2$ LASER

The NovaPulse is a gated superpulsed CO_2 laser that also has continuous wave (CW) and gated continuous-wave (GCW) modes. Laser energy is delivered to the treatment site via a flexible hollow waveguide (fiber optic), which results in multimodal output beam geometry. The energy distribution of the multimodal beam eliminates the "hot spot" of Gaussian beam systems (cone-shaped delivery) and provides uniform fluence across the entire ablation region. The NovaPulse is a sealed radiofrequency-excited laser, so pulse energy is maintained well above the ablation threshold throughout the entire pulse duration.

With the NovaPulse laser the clinician sets the desired average power (watts), the pulse frequency (Hertz), and the delivery percentage (duty cycle). Pulse frequency and delivery percentage are set up as programs for ease of use and consistency: "A" for ablation and "C" for cutting. The operator selects the desired average power to control the depth of ablation and the program mode to determine the rate of tissue ablation. The system's microprocessor then sets the pulse duration and repetition frequency necessary to deliver the requested average power based on the actual measured peak power of the NovaPulse laser and delivery system.

As noted in earlier chapters, fluence (energy density) is more relevant to clinical tissue ablation than peak power because it is a measure of the energy in millijoules delivered to the treatment region based on spot size. Increasing the fluence increases the depth of ablation. A fluence above 5 J/cm^2 provides clean, efficient tissue ablation and dissipates much of the heat in the plume of vaporized tissue. The criteria for ablation with minimal thermal damage (i.e., superpulsed) are met in the Nova-Pulse mode.[1] In this mode, a fluence of up to 7 J/cm^2 per pulse is available using the standard 0.8-mm tip at a nominal peak power of 50 W.

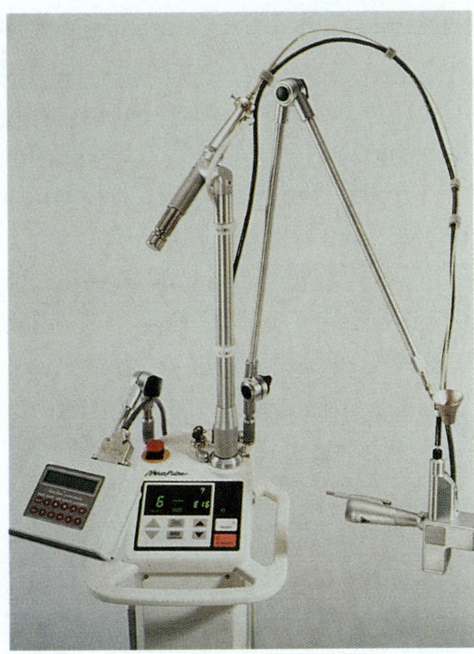

Figure 11–1. Luxar NovaPulse with SureScan CPG handpiece.

NOVASCAN HANDPIECE

The NovaScan handpiece is an accessory for the Nova-Pulse laser that creates a 3-mm-diameter spot size. To maintain the fluence necessary for superpulsed ablation, a small wedge-shaped tip spins inside of the handpiece. It covers an area 1/12 (30 degrees) of the total scanned area at any given time. Therefore, it delivers an arc of 12 superpulsed pulses to create the 3-mm-diameter spot size (Fig. 11–2). Because of the equal fluence delivered to

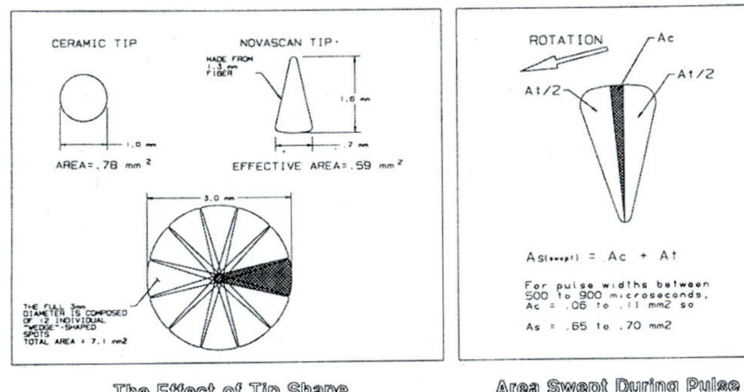

Figure 11–2. Generation of the NovaScan 3-mm-diameter spot size. Equal fluence is delivered to each of the 12 individual wedges without overlap.

each of the 12 "slices" (multimodal beam) and the wedge configuration, pulses do not overlap. Pulses occur every 5 milliseconds to ablate the full 3-mm-diameter spot uniformly in 60 milliseconds.

To control depth of ablation, the operator sets the average power, which is directly proportional to the energy delivered in each pulse. The microprocessor calculates a safe pulse duration for the 12 individual 50-W laser pulses on the basis of the average power set by the operator. Because the rotation time is fixed at 60 milliseconds per revolution, the energy delivered in each 3-mm spot is also controlled. For example, at a setting of 5 W, 300 mJ of energy are delivered per revolution (5 W $\times$ 60 milliseconds). A maximum of 540 mJ per 3-mm spot (7 J/cm^2) can be delivered with an average power setting of 9 W.

In addition to setting the average power for ablation depth, the operator can select the pulse frequency or repetition rate. These "E modes" are programs that vary repetitions from 2 to 16 pulses per second. This allows the clinician to select a handspeed that accommodates both the facial region being treated and the operator's technical expertise.

SURESCAN AND DERMASCAN COMPUTERIZED PATTERN GENERATOR HANDPIECES

The SureScan CPG (manufactured for Luxar by Clinicon, Inc., Carlsbad, CA) is an accessory for the NovaPulse laser that greatly facilitates full-face treatment and significantly reduces the resurfacing learning curve. Four patterns are available: square, parallelogram, triangle, and rectangle. Each pattern comes in three sizes, and density can be varied to allow overlap or underlap of the delivered pulses. The most frequently used pattern is the square, which has a maximum size of 11.7 $\times$ 11.0 mm. The SureScan CPG's "program mode" is always set to E-16 on the NovaPulse console.

As mentioned earlier, the DermaScan CPG for the NovaPulse laser recently became available in the United

States. This microprocessor-controlled scanning device will generate precisely defined, repeatable laser beam patterns. Scanning is performed by two rotating mirrors that deflect the laser beam in two perpendicular directions. This scanning process is synchronized with the laser pulses. The DermaScan has six programmable repeat-pattern scanning modes. Six patterns will be available in sizes 2 to 20 mm, continuously variable: square, rectangle, hexagon, parallelogram, line, and triangle. Repeat scans from 1 to 100 are available. Spot overlap can be varied from −50 to +50%. Other features include the capability to save parameter values in memory.

PREOPERATIVE PREPARATION

The Luxar superpulsed CO_2 laser is well-suited for treatment of perioral vertical furrows, periorbital dynamic lines (crow's feet), glabellar dynamic lines, actinic damage, generalized facial elastosis, shallow scars, and epidermal-dermal lesions. The patient's wrinkle severity is classified preoperatively. Regions are graded on a scale of 1 to 6, with 1 being essentially unwrinkled and 6 being profoundly wrinkled. The patient's sun-reactive skin type (Fitzpatrick scale) is also recorded preoperatively (see Table 6–3). Patients with Fitzpatrick type VI (black) skin are excluded. Patients with Fitzpatrick type IV or V skin (e.g., those of Asian or Hispanic descent, respectively) and those with potential hyperpigmentation problems are pretreated with a combination cream containing 5 to 8% hydroquinone, 1% hydrocortisone, and 0.05 to 0.1% retinoic acid (Retin-A) twice a day for 4 weeks. Absolute contraindications include active acne, deep acne pits or picks, and isotretinoin use in the past 2 years. A history of herpetic infection is only a relative contraindication because most patients do not know their true status.

TECHNIQUE

Two principles form the basis of treatment. The first is to always maintain a balance between results and morbidity (i.e., err on the conservative side). The second is never to set the wattage *below* that recommended for the handpiece being used. One must remember that sufficient energy is required to reach the fluence necessary for superpulsed ablation. Setting the wattage too low forces heat into the tissue instead of vaporizing tissue.

The most frequently used procedure-specific parameters for the Luxar laser are listed in Table 11–1. Remember, however, that the laser settings given in the table and discussed in this chapter are general guidelines only.

Table 11–1. Luxar System: Usual Parameters*

Treatment	Handpiece	Program	Watts
Full-face LSR	NovaScan	E-8 to E-10	5–6 W, 1–2 passes
	SureScan[†]	E-16	6–7 W, 1–2 passes
Perioral LSR	NovaScan	E-4 to E-6	5–6 W, 2–3 passes
	SureScan[†]	E-16	6–7 W, 2–3 passes
Periorbital LSR	0.8 mm	A-6	5–6 W, 2 passes maximum
Blepharoplasty	0.4 mm	C-1	6 W
Transconjunctival blepharoplasty	0.3 mm	C-2	6 W
Endoscopic brow lift[§]	MG 125EC	C-2	7 W

*LSR, laser skin resurfacing.

[†]Appropriate pattern shape and size at 0 density.

[§]Laser is used to vaporize edges of corrugator muscles.

All patients receive regional nerve blocks and subdermal local anesthetic. Single-pulse vaporization (i.e., no overlap of pulses) is always performed. Skin lesions and actinic regions are removed by sequential ablative passes. The endpoint is complete removal of the lesion base or a depth of penetration to the middle reticular dermis. Wrinkles are treated by direct yet gentle lasering into the furrows in an attempt to remodel the furrow base and take advantage of favorable dermal collagen heating. Next, the wrinkle shoulders are flattened using the laser as a planing tool. The region immediately adjacent to the wrinkle(s) is treated with ablative passes as indicated. In general, any subsequent passes are performed at a reduced wattage. Regions to be re-treated are wiped with sterile saline-soaked gauze prior to any additional passes.

POSTOPERATIVE CARE

A closed-wound care system is used to promote moist healing and prevent an exudative phase. Exudation causes crust formation, which impedes reepithelialization and can lead to infection and/or scarring. Complete facial coverage also decreases postoperative pain and provides camouflage.[2] I use RevitaDerm (PolyMedica Wound Care Co., Woburn, MA) a three-layer adhesive dressing with a membranous middle layer to absorb drainage and an outer vapor-permeable shell. The dressing is removed in 2 days, and Second Skin (Bionet Inc., Little Rock, AR) (hydrogel: 96% sterile H_2O plus 4% polyethelene mesh) is applied for an additional 2 days (changed twice daily by the patient). The RevitaDerm allows maximal wound coverage and prevents crust formation in the critical first 2 days, and the Second Skin serves as an optimal wound-healing environment. Acetic acid soaks are then initiated until reepithelialization occurs.

Routine postoperative medications include ciprofloxacin, 500 mg twice a day for 5 days, for *Pseudomonas* coverage. Herpes prophylaxis for all laser patients is valacyclovir, 500 mg twice a day, starting 2 days preoperatively and continuing until postoperative day 10. Valacyclovir is a prodrug for acyclovir that achieves higher plasma concentrations and is less expensive than acyclovir.[3] The need for narcotic analgesics has greatly diminished since I started using occlusive dressings. After reepithelialization, patients are instructed to use an ultraviolet sunscreen with a sun-protective factor (SPF) of more than 25 on treated areas for 1 year.

RESULTS

To date, more than 750 patients have undergone laser skin resurfacing at the Facial Plastic Surgery Clinic at Stanford University Medical Center. Based on a questionnaire survey, approximately 90% of patients subjectively rated their result as satisfactory at 6 months postoperatively. Most patients improve their wrinkle grade by 2 (range of 1 to 3) on the 6-point scale. Typical results are shown in Figures 11–3 and 11–4.

Complications have included 5 patients with postinflammatory hyperpigmentation, 10 patients with persistent hyperpigmentation (Fitzpatrick skin types IV and V), and 8 patients with outbreaks of herpes (Fig. 11–5). All cases of hyperpigmentation resolved with bleaching regimens by 6 months. All patients with herpetic outbreaks had no sequelae after medical management. One patient had scar formation secondary to *Candida* infection. This patient underwent a very superficial resurfacing (epidermal) and missed her routine day-2 and day-7 follow-up visits. On her own, she applied antibiotic ointment for 1 month, and a skin fungal infection resulted. This case alone demonstrates that screening for patient compliance cannot be overemphasized.

ADVANTAGES AND DISADVANTAGES

The Luxar Laser System offers several distinct advantages: ability to interchange several different handpiece

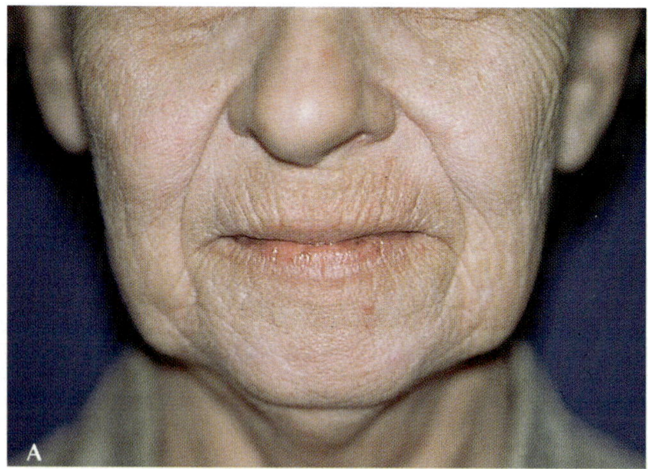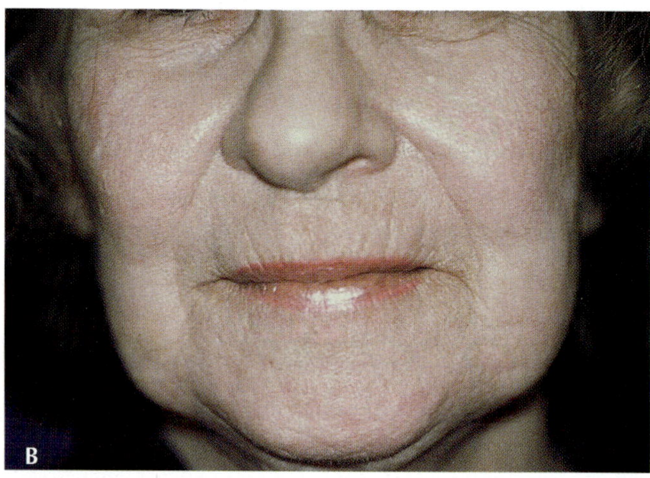

Figure 11–3. Typical result with full-face laser skin resurfacing. (A) Patient with severe facial elastosis, actinic damage, and perioral rhytids. (B) Postoperative view at 3 months.

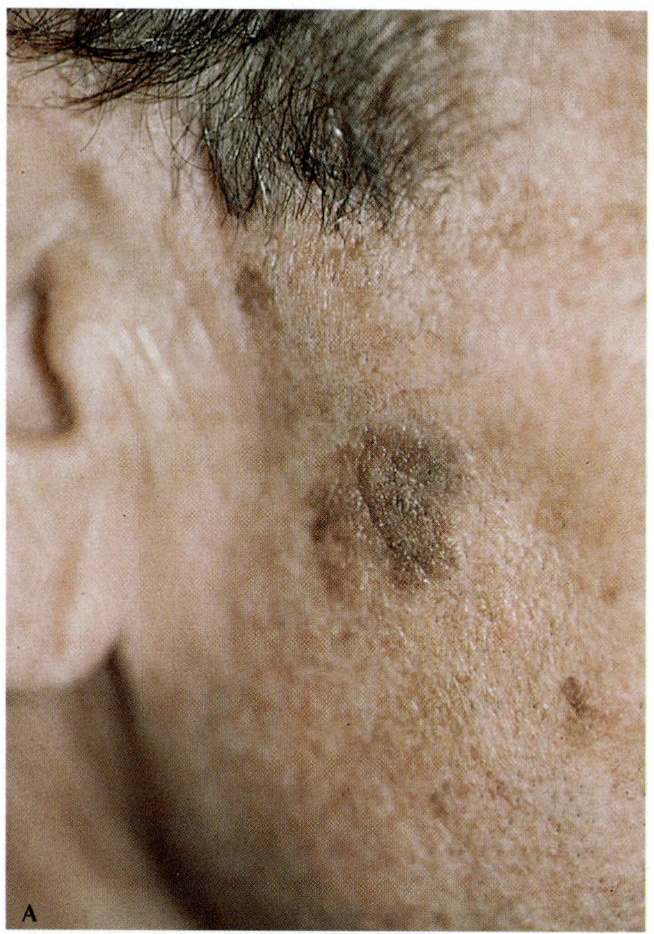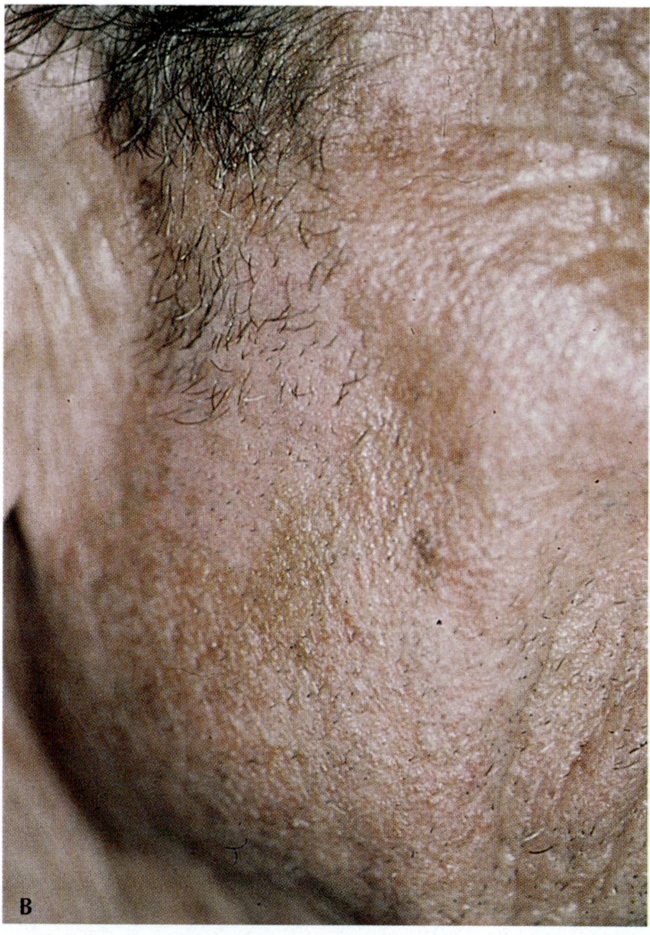

Figure 11–4. Typical early result of laser ablation of facial skin lesions. (A) Patient with a pigmented lateral cheek lesion (lentigines). (B) Postoperative view at 7 days.

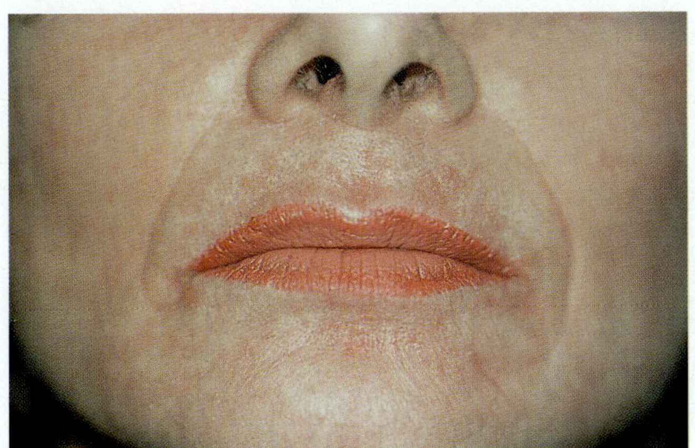

Figure 11–5. Minor herpetic outbreak 1 week postoperatively while the patient was on prophylaxis. There were no sequelae after increased dosing. Note regional hypopigmentation following prior phenol peel.

sizes for incisional and ablative procedures, portability, relatively low cost, and the flexible fiber optic delivery system that facilitates its use for other facial plastic surgical procedures (Fig. 11–6). Although some clinicians may consider the noncollimated beam a disadvantage, I believe that it adds an extra safety factor against unintentional lasing. Keeping the proper focal distance for a specific handpiece is not difficult, and the system permits defocusing for cauterization during cutting procedures.

ACKNOWLEDGMENTS

I wish to acknowledge Steven E. Wojcik, research and development manager, Luxar Corporation, for reviewing the technical description of the Luxar Laser System.

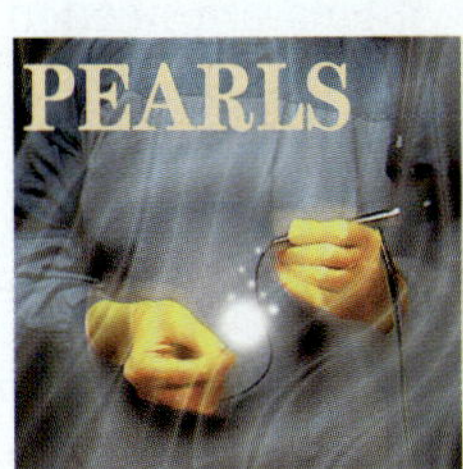

- Combining rhytidectomy with laser skin resurfacing is perfectly acceptable. Appropriate patients are those with severe facial elastosis, poor dermal recoil, and actinic damage. I prefer to do the face lift first, followed by laser resurfacing at 3 months. This allows laser resurfacing of the rhytidectomy scars. It is risky to resurface skin that has just been undermined because full-thickness skin loss may result.[4]
- Sequential treatments may yield the best results. Patients with severe rhytids should be managed in this way. Re-treatments generally are spaced 4 months apart.
- Full-face treatment is preferable to regional treatments to avoid lines of demarcation. Not only does this improve camouflage while healing, it also avoids obvious differences in skin quality and small step-offs between adjacent regions. If a regional procedure is performed, aesthetic units must be respected.

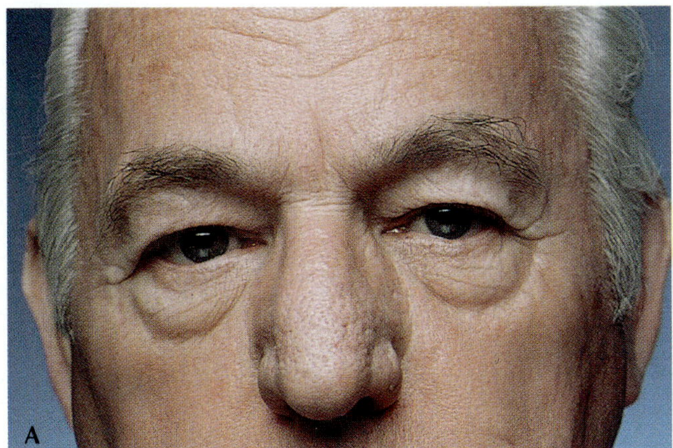
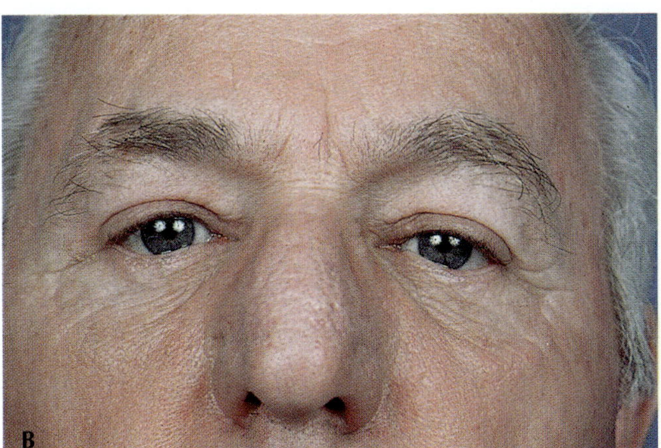

Figure 11–6. Laser blepharoplasty, periorbital laser skin resurfacing, and laser endoscopic brow lift. Lower eyelid skin resurfacing was performed immediately following retroseptal transconjunctival blepharoplasty. (A) Patient with brow ptosis, upper eyelid dermatochalasis, and lower eyelid pseudoherniated orbital fat. (B) Postoperative view at 1 year.

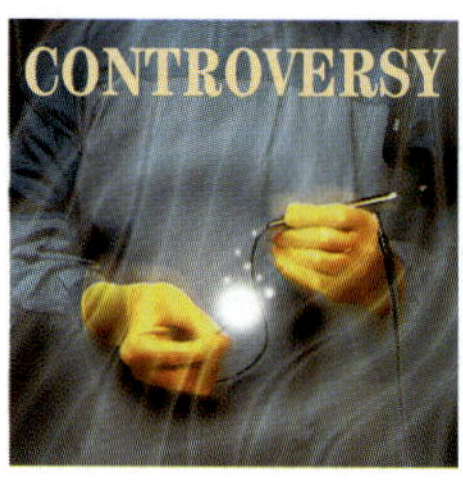

- Clinically, the superpulsed CO_2 laser appears to have a collagen-tightening effect. Some practitioners believe that a certain level of thermal damage and resulting erythema are needed for this effect. Others, including myself, believe that local mediators (growth factors) are involved. More basic science research is needed in this area.[5,6]

- The relatively low cost of the Luxar system opens this arena to many physicians. Although not required to by law, these physicians should attend a basic course on the use of their specific laser, attend a preceptorship to gain experience, and maintain a conservative approach until able to evaluate endpoints.

REFERENCES

1. Walsh JT, Flotte TJ, Anderson RR, et al. Pulsed CO_2 laser tissue ablation: effect of tissue type and pulse duration on thermal damage. *Lasers Surg Med.* 1988;8:108.
2. Newman JP, Koch RJ, Goode RL. Closed dressings after laser skin resurfacing. *Arch Otolaryngol Head Neck Surg.* 1998;124(7):751–757.
3. Jacobson MA. Valacyclovir (BW256U87): The L-valyl ester of acyclovir. *J Med Virol.* 1993;Suppl 1:150–153.
4. Hayes DK, Berkland ME, Stambaugh KI. Dermal healing after local skin flaps and chemical peel. *Arch Otolaryngol Head Neck Surg.* 1990;116:794–797.
5. Koch RJ, Goode RL, Simpson GT. Serum-free keloid fibroblast cell culture: an in vitro model for the study of aberrant wound healing. *Plast Reconstr Surg.* 1997;99: 1094–1098.
6. Nowak KC, McCormack MC, Koch RJ. The effect of superpulsed CO_2 laser energy on keloid and normal dermal fibroblast secretion of growth factors: a serum-free study. *Plast Reconstr Surg.* 2000 (May).

CHAPTER 12

Tru-Pulse Laser Resurfacing

BRIAN D. BUCALO AND RONALD L. MOY

The Tru-Pulse carbon dioxide (CO_2) laser delivers energy to the target tissue in a rapid series of pulses; this pulse rate may be adjusted from 1 to 12 Hz. Each pulse has a very short duration (60 microseconds) and a very high peak power (10,000 W), attributes which allow excellent control of ablation with minimal thermal damage.[1] The thermal cross section of the Tru-Pulse laser beam has a uniform energy density pattern, which differs from other lasers that have a Gaussian energy density pattern and result in a "hot spot" in the center of the laser beam.[2] Furthermore, the Tru-Pulse beam cross section is square shaped, allowing accurate placement of contiguous but nonoverlapping pulses across the surface of the skin.

The Tru-Pulse laser system, which weighs 165 lb and measures $20 \times 17 \times 52$ inches, is self-contained in a cabinet that easily rolls on wheels. A scanning pattern generator is available that provides many different shapes, including squares, rectangles, triangles, hexagons, lines, and rhombi, with up to four sizes for each shape. Laser energy is delivered via an articulating arm (Fig. 12–1), and there are several ergonomically designed handpieces: the standard handpiece, which delivers individual 3-mm² pulses, and the 1- and 2-mm handpieces. We generally use the standard handpiece with the 3-mm spot size, which features a helium–neon aiming beam that facilitates accurate placement of the ablation spot.

LASER–TISSUE INTERACTION

The Tru-Pulse laser produces less thermal damage per pass than continuous wave (CW) lasers and requires more passes to achieve an equivalent depth of ablation.[1] Because there is less tissue removed per pass, the physician exercises more accurate control over the resurfacing process. Decreased thermal damage by the Tru-Pulse laser correlates with shorter durations of posttreatment erythema, which is important because many patients, particularly males, object to prolonged periods of erythema. However, proponents of long-pulse-duration or long-dwell-time lasers have suggested that persistent erythema and inflammation are beneficial and necessary for rhytid improvement because they tighten the underlying collagen scaffold.[3]

In one contralateral study of six patients treated facially with the SilkTouch laser (mean passes, 1) and the Tru-Pulse laser (mean passes, 3.2), the average duration of erythema was judged by patients to be 4 weeks on the Tru-Pulse laser side and 9 weeks on the SilkTouch laser side. There were equal degrees of rhytid improvement with both lasers.[1] Table 12–1 summarizes the relative histologic effects of the Tru-Pulse and SilkTouch lasers.

Researchers investigating the effects of the Tru-Pulse laser have proposed that contraction of skin occurs not from an erythema-driven mechanism but rather as a result

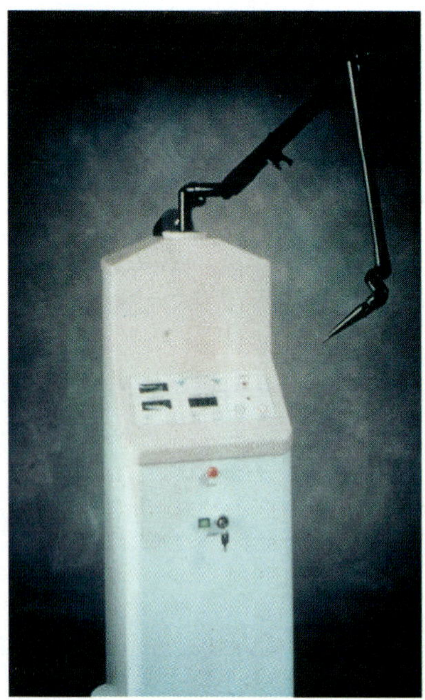

Figure 12–1. Tru-Pulse laser with articulating arm.

of the deposition of new stromal cells and concomitant actin filaments, which results in tightening of lax skin and improvement of creases.[4] Other researchers have suggested that a subepidermal repair zone of fibrosis accounts for clinical improvement after laser treatment.[5]

Dessication and collagen shrinkage have also been proposed as mechanisms for rhytid improvement.[6]

Recent data indicate that for an equal ablation depth, long-dwell-time lasers such as the SilkTouch initially produce 18% greater linear contraction than the Tru-Pulse laser immediately after treatment. This contraction effect tends to diminish with time so that 4 weeks after treatment there is only 10% more linear contraction with the SilkTouch when compared with the Tru-Pulse laser.[7] This observation is consistent with reports that contraction of laser-treated skin following resurfacing decreases after the treated skin has been rehydrated.[8]

LASER PROTOCOL

When performing laser resurfacing, it is important to remember that no single approach is appropriate for every patient. Safe resurfacing requires planning and forethought by the physician as well the patient. Physicians who are learning the art of facial resurfacing should first observe another physician perform the procedure; preceptorships for the Tru-Pulse laser can be arranged through the Polomar Corporation.

INDICATIONS AND CONTRAINDICATIONS

We have used the Tru-Pulse laser to treat a variety of conditions, including facial rhytids, acne scars, surgical

Table 12–1. Comparison of Histologic Findings Using Tru-Pulse and SilkTouch Lasers (N = 10)

Laser	Depth of Resurfacing (μm)	Depth of Thermal Damage (μm)
Tru-Pulse (500 mJ, 3 mm)		
1 pass	100	17 ± 3
2 passes	150	26 ± 6
3 passes	200	34 ± 3
4 passes	250	44 ± 6
5 passes	300	52 ± 4
6 passes	350	63 ± 7
SilkTouch (18 W, 0.2 s, 6 mm)		
1 pass	180	50 ± 8
2 passes	300	86 ± 6
3 passes	380	138 ± 15

scars, and actinic damage, but the patient's age, physical condition, and skin type must be considered. As with all resurfacing procedures, certain individuals should not receive treatment: pregnant or immunosuppressed people; people with diabetes; those with a history of keloid formation, poor wound healing, radiation treatment, collagen-vascular or autoimmune disease, photosensitivity due to medications or preexisting skin conditions, or postinflammatory hypo- or hyperpigmentation; those who require constant anticoagulants; those who have received Accutane (isotretinoin) therapy within the past 12 months; and those with seizures or active herpes simplex infections. People who have unrealistic expectations of the procedure and those who are unable to follow postoperative care instructions also should not be treated.

Several months should elapse after any facial surgery, such as a face lift or facial implants, before resurfacing. This allows the effects of surgery to settle down and will decrease the risk of scarring or delayed wound healing from a compromised vascular supply to the skin.

In those patients who are at significant risk for hypo-or hyperpigmentation, a small area, such as the posterior auricular sulcus of the ear, should be tested. People of Mediterranean or Asian heritage are at greater risk for postinflammatory hyperpigmentation, and these patients should be treated with caution. Those patients who are at risk for an extended period of erythema include patients with fair skin or rosacea and those of northern European or Celtic heritage. These patients must be told that postoperative erythema may last substantially longer than it does for the average patient. We do not recommend that black patients be treated because of the risk of significant dyschromia.

PREOPERATIVE PREPARATION

All patients undergoing skin resurfacing should complete an informed consent form during their initial consultation. Preoperative photographs are very important. One day before laser treatment, patients begin a 12-day course of oral antibiotics, typically Keflex (cephalexin 500 mg twice a day) or erythromycin (250 mg every 6 hours).

Valtrex (valacyclovir; 500 mg twice a day for 12 days) is also prescribed with or without any history of herpes. Darker-skinned individuals need topical hydroquinone for at least 1 month prior to laser resurfacing to avoid hyper- or hypopigmentation.

Using a mirror on the day of laser resurfacing, the patient points out specific areas that need special attention. These areas are then marked with a Gentian violet skin-marking pen. If complete full-face resurfacing is planned, the resurfacing border, just under the jawline, is also marked.

Anesthesia for laser resurfacing may be provided in the form of local infiltration of 1% lidocaine with or without nerve blocks. Tumescent anesthesia has also been used, whereas some patients prefer intravenous sedation or general anesthesia. It is essential that eye shields be used to avoid damage by the laser light.

PROCEDURE

It is important to remember that when treating rhytids, your goal is not complete erasure of every rhytid at the time of treatment, particularly the deeper lines. A mild improvement or softening of the rhytids should be expected at the end of the laser procedure, which emphasizes the importance of keeping the patient's preoperative photographs within view for reference during the procedure.

Treatment of facial rhytids may be accomplished by treating individual rhytids, small areas, whole cosmetic units such as the perioral area, or the entire face. If multiple rhytids in the same area are being treated, it is generally better to resurface the entire cosmetic unit or the entire face. By blending separately treated areas together, a more uniform overall cosmetic result is achieved. The guidelines for treating facial rhytids listed in Table 12–2 are only a rough guide. Each physician must use his or her judgment when performing laser resurfacing.

A patient can always return for a touch-up treatment of an area. Therefore, if there is any question in the physician's mind, additional laser passes must be avoided. Although we have never seen scarring with the Tru-Pulse laser, it is theoretically possible, and scarring is extremely difficult to

Table 12–2. Treatment Guide for Facial Rhytides with the Tru-Pulse Laser

Rhytid Location	No. of Passes
Forehead	3–6*
Crow's feet	2–5*
Eyelids	1–3†
Perioral	3–7*
Cheeks	3–7*
Neck	1–2

Note: Tru-Pulse laser parameters: 500 mJ energy, standard nonscanning handpiece, 3-mm spot size; pulse repetition rate: adjust from 1 to 12 Hz, based on proficiency.

*Final pass may be done directly on the rhytid in a linear fashion.

†Eyelid laxity should be assessed before treatment. If lids are tight, treatment should be avoided.

correct. One absolute endpoint to remember is the appearance of a faint chamois-yellow color of the skin. This color indicates that you have reached the level of the reticular dermis—further treatment will likely cause scarring.

Between each pass of the laser, charred debris may be wiped off with dry gauze or gauze moistened in sterile saline and the surface gently patted dry with sterile dry gauze. After the final resurfacing pass and subsequent wipe, the area is covered in an overlapping fashion with Flexan dressing that is left in place for 4 days. After 4 days, the patient moistens the Flexan with water-soaked gauze

and then gently removes the dressing. Petrolatum ointment is then applied four to five times a day for an additional 10 days. Patients should not apply the ointment with their bare fingers because this could lead to infection. The petrolatum should be applied copiously to sterile gauze and then gently patted, not rubbed, onto the skin surface.

Patients may return for follow-up visits 1 week and then again 2 weeks following resurfacing. If any change in skin appearance is noted by the patient or there is unusual discomfort or discharge from the skin, the patient should return immediately for follow-up evaluation. Sun avoidance should be stressed during this period of healing. The patient may start using sunscreen and go outdoors following the reepithelialization period, which is usually complete in 2 weeks. For darker-skinned patients, diligent sun avoidance during reepithelialization and rigorous application of sunscreen thereafter is important, and patients at risk for pigmentary problems must adhere to a regimen of hydroquinone for at least 1 month after resurfacing. Rhytids continue to improve for 3 to 4 months as collagen remodeling occurs. Patients must be informed of this fact so that they do not become anxious about their rate of improvement. Reevaluation of the patient at 5 months provides a good perspective on the result. Figure 12–2 provides preoperative and postoperative views of a patient treated with the Tru-Pulse laser.

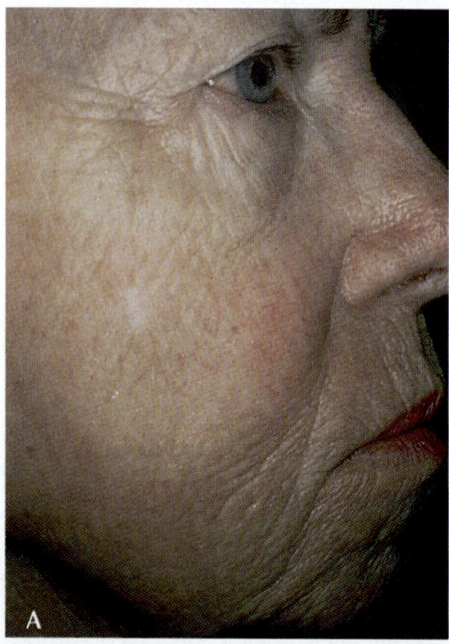

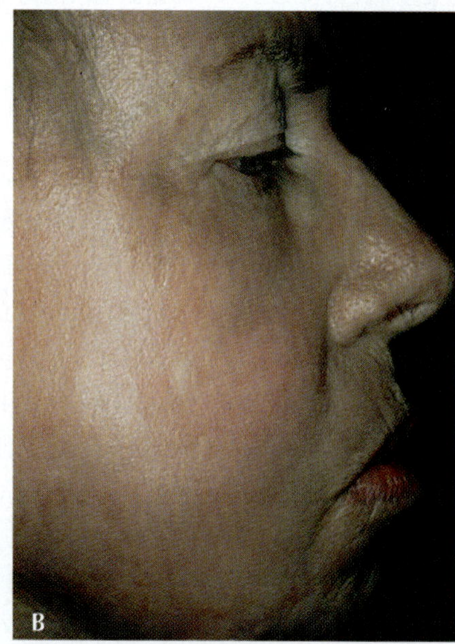

Figure 12–2. Patient (A) before and (B) after resurfacing with the Tru-Pulse laser.

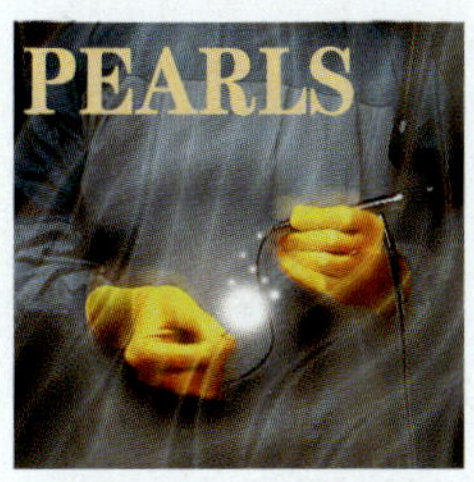

- The Tru-Pulse laser beam has a uniform energy density pattern, unlike other lasers, which have a Gaussian energy density pattern and resultant "hot spot" in the center of the laser beam.

- The authors prefer to use the standard handpiece with the 3-mm spot size, which features a helium-neon aiming beam that facilitates accurate placement of the ablation spot.

- Because there is less tissue removed per pass with the Tru-Pulse laser, there is a shorter duration of posttreatment erythema. However, certain patients are at risk for an extended period of erythema: those with fair skin or rosacea and those of northern European or Celtic heritage.

- Having the patient point out using a mirror which rhytids need special attention allows the physician to see which rhytids are of particular concern to the patient.

- Because rhytids continue to improve for 3 to 4 months, patients must be assured immediately after the procedure that over time the desired result will occur.

REFERENCES

1. Moy RL, Bucalo BD, Lee MH, Wieder JM, Chalet MD, Ostad A. Skin resurfacing of facial rhytids and scars with the 90 microsecond short pulse CO_2 laser: comparison to the 900 microsecond dwell time CO_2 laser and clinical experience. *Dermatol Surg.* 1998;24(12):1390–1396.
2. Harris DM, Bell T, From L, Schacter D. Facial skin resurfacing with a very short pulsed CO_2 laser: beam-characterization and initial histological results. *Lasers Dermatol Plast Surg.* 1996.
3. Fitzpatrick RL, Goldman MP. Reply to Smith et al. *Arch Dermatol.* 1997;133:107.
4. Smith KJ, Graham JS, Hamilton TA, Hackley BE, Skelton HG, Hurst CG. Additional observations using a pulsed carbon dioxide laser with a fixed pulse duration. *Arch Dermatol.* 1997;133:105–106.
5. Cotton JC, Hood AH, Gonin R, Beeson WH, Hanke W. Histologic evaluation of preauricular and postauricular human skin after high energy, short pulse carbon dioxide laser. *Arch Dermatol.* 1997;132:425–427.
6. Ross EV, Domankevits Y, Skrobal M, Anderson RR. Effects of CO_2 laser pulse duration in ablation and residual thermal damage: implications for skin resurfacing. *Lasers Surg Med.* 1996;19:123–129.
7. Moy RL, Bucalo BD. Quantitative comparison of inflammatory infiltrate and linear contraction in human skin treated with 90 microsecond pulsed and 900 microsecond dwell time carbon dioxide lasers. *Dermatol Surg.* 1998;24(12):1314–1316.
8. Gardiner ES, Reinisch L, Stricklin GP, Ellis DL. In vitro changes in non-facial human skin following CO_2 laser resurfacing: a comparison study. *Lasers Surg Med.* 1996;19:379–387.

CHAPTER 13

The Derma 20 Erbium:YAG Laser

R. JAMES KOCH

The Derma 20 Erbium:Yttrium-Aluminum-Garnet (Er:YAG) Laser (ESC Medical Systems, Yokneam, Israel) produces a wavelength of 2940 nm at a pulse length of 350 millisecond (Fig. 13–1). Pulse energy levels range from 0.1 to 1.7 J/pulse. The Derma 20 has a maximum average power of 20 W and a pulse repetition rate of 5 to 12 pulses per second. Interchangeable handpieces produce spot sizes ranging from 0.2 to 6.0 mm (noncollimated) for laser skin resurfacing (Fig. 13–2). In addition, a 6.0-mm collimated handpiece is available for rapid resurfacing.

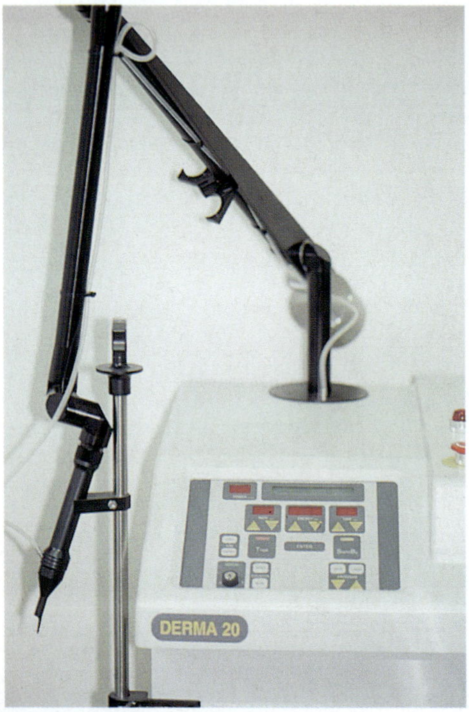

With the Derma 20 system the clinician sets the desired pulse energy (joules per single pulse) and the pulse repetition rate (pulses per second) (Fig. 13–3). The system's microprocessor calculates average power based on these values. The operator selects the desired pulse energy to control the fluence for depth of ablation. Then the operator sets the pulse repetition rate to accommodate the facial region being treated and his or her technical expertise.

The DermaScan computerized pattern generator (CPG) handpiece (ESC Medical Systems) is a microprocessor-controlled scanning device that generates

Figure 13–1. Derma 20 Er:YAG Laser System.

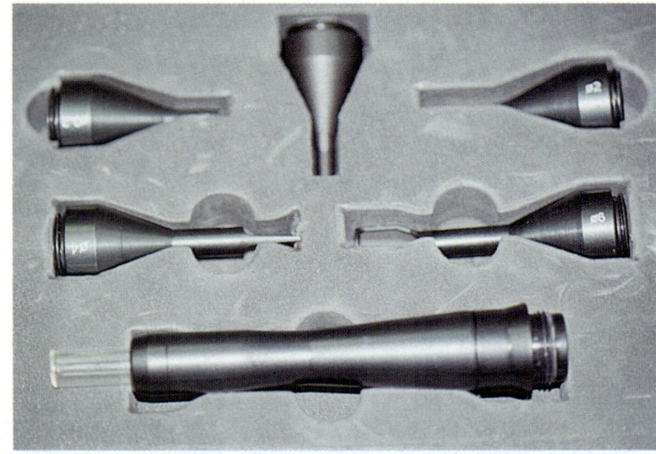

Figure 13–2. Handpieces with spot sizes ranging from 0.2 to 6.0 mm are directly interchangeable.

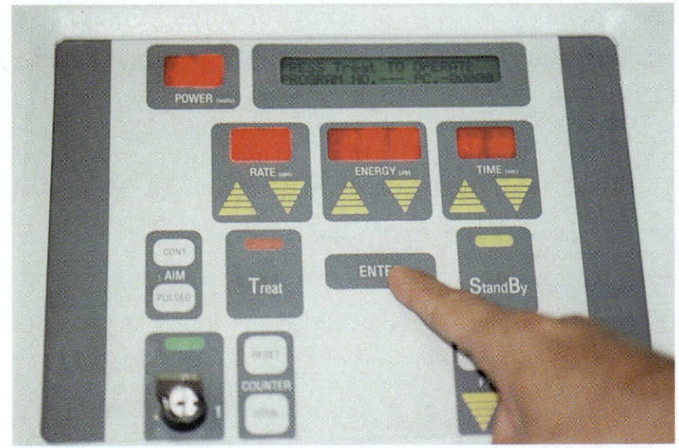

Figure 13–3. The pulse energy (joules per single pulse) and the pulse repetition rate (pulses per second) are selected by the operator.

repeatable laser beam patterns. Scanning is performed by two rotating mirrors that deflect the laser beam in two perpendicular directions. This scanning process is synchronized with the laser pulses. The DermaScan has six programmable repeat pattern scanning modes: square, rectangle, hexagon, parallelogram, line, and triangle. Pattern sizes can be varied continuously from 2 to 20 mm. Repeat scans are available from 1 to 100. Spot overlap can be set from −50 to +50%. Although full-face laser skin resurfacing is extremely rapid with the Derma 20 system and its accessory handpieces (using spot sizes greater than 4.0 mm), the availability of the DermaScan CPG handpiece is an attractive feature.

LASER PHYSICS AND TISSUE EFFECTS

The Derma 20 Er:YAG laser produces a beam in the infrared (IR) spectrum (2940 nm), and its absorption by water is approximately 10 to 12 times greater than that of the carbon dioxide (CO_2) laser (at 10,600 nm). The resulting tissue interaction provides true ablation with minimal thermal damage. Significantly, the optical penetration is approximately 1/20 that of the CO_2 laser.

The energy distribution of the Derma 20's multimodal output eliminates the "hot spot" of Gaussian beam systems (cone-shaped delivery) and provides uniform fluence (energy density) across the entire target tissue.

This ensures that the periphery of the pulse has the same energy as the center.

Each pulse removes only 25 to 30 μm of tissue, compared with the 50 to 100 μm of tissue removed by the superpulsed CO_2 laser. Because the thermal conduction is only approximately 5 μm with the Derma 20 Er:YAG laser, there is less collateral dermal energy (the superpulsed CO_2 laser produces 30 to 50 μm of thermal conduction). In the dermis, the Derma 20's output is selectively absorbed by collagen and dermal proteins, whereas the CO_2 laser continues to vaporize extracellular water. Thus, each pass of the Derma 20 generates the same amount of ablation as in the epidermis with a very small additive effect of increasing thermal damage, whereas the superpulsed CO_2 laser produces less vaporization depth and more thermal damage with each pass.

PATIENT SELECTION AND PREPARATION

Patients with actinic damage and/or superficial rhytids are excellent candidates for Er:YAG laser skin resurfacing. An equally important factor is patient request for early recovery; that is, patients may want laser treatment yet may request that they "not be red for months." Unlike the CO_2 laser, the Er:YAG laser appears safe for use on the skin of the neck, chest, and hands, which expands its role. The patient's sun-reactive skin type (Fitzpatrick scale) is recorded preoperatively, and there may be a decreased incidence of hyperpigmentation in patients with Fitzpatrick skin types IV and V with the Er:YAG laser (Figs. 13–4 and 13–5). However, it is the relative need for aggressive treatment that dictates which laser I use.

Patients with Fitzpatrick type VI (black) skin are excluded from treatment (see Table 6–3). Other absolute contraindications include active acne, deep acne pits or picks, and isotretinoin use in the past 2 years. A history of prior herpetic infection is only a relative contraindication.

Once accepted for treatment, the first step is to classify the patient's wrinkle severity. Regions are graded on a scale of 1 to 6, with 1 being essentially unwrinkled and

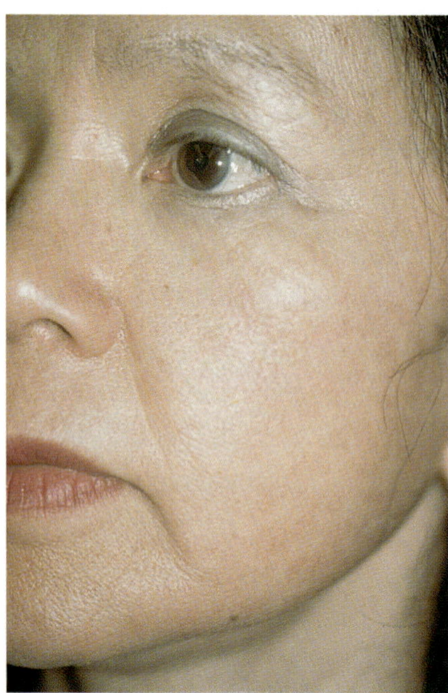

Figure 13–4. Typical residual hyperpigmentation 4 months following superpulsed CO_2 laser resurfacing in a patient with Fitzpatrick skin type V (Tahitian descent).

6 being profoundly wrinkled. Patients with Fitzpatrick type IV or V skin (such as those of Asian or Hispanic descent, respectively) and those with a potential for hyperpigmentation are pretreated with a combination cream containing 5 to 8% hydroquinone, 1% hydrocor-

tisone, and 0.05 to 0.1% retinoic acid twice daily for 4 weeks. Herpes prophylaxis for all laser patients includes valacyclovir, 500 mg twice daily, starting 2 days preoperatively.

All patients receive regional nerve blocks and topical anesthesia. Treatment with the Er:YAG laser is not painless, but it is significantly less painful than treatment with the CO_2 laser. A eutectic mixture of local anesthetics (EMLA cream, Astra Pharmaceuticals; a topical lidocaine) applied 2 hours prior to procedure provides sufficient topical anesthesia.

TECHNIQUE

The most frequently used procedure-specific parameters for the Derma 20 Er:YAG Laser are shown in Table 13–1. It should be noted that the laser settings given in the table and in this chapter are general guidelines only.

Single-pulse vaporization (i.e., no overlap of pulses) is attempted first. It is not as critical from a tissue interaction standpoint to avoid overlap as with the superpulsed CO_2 laser because virtually no tissue debris is produced by the Er:YAG laser. However, it is still possible to burn a hole in the skin if the laser is fired repeatedly at

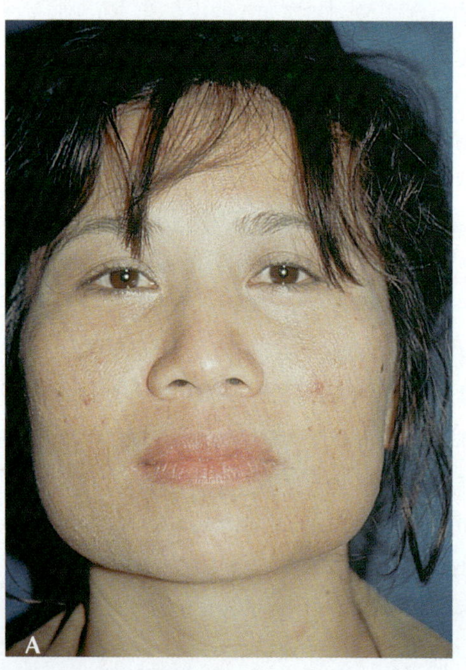

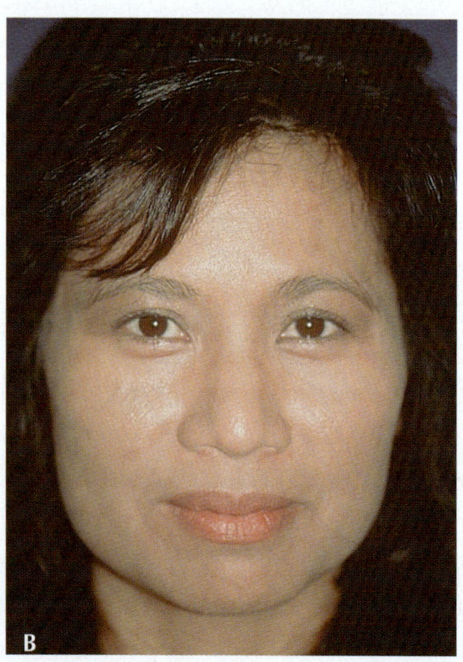

Figure 13–5. Results of Er:YAG laser skin resurfacing of a patient with Fitzpatrick skin type V (Hawaiian descent).
(A) Preoperative view.
(B) Postoperative view at 1 month. Note relatively slight hyperpigmentation.

Table 13–1. Usual Parameters for the Derma 20 Er:YAG Laser

Area and Depth	Pulse Energy	Pulse Rate	Spot Size	Passes
Full face				
Superficial	1.5 J/pulse	8–10 pulses/s	4 mm	2–3
Medium	1.7 J/pulse	8–10 pulses/s	4 mm	4–5
Deep	1.7 J/pulse	10–12 pulses/s	6 mm	6
Other sites				
Periorbital	0.8 J/pulse	5–6 pulses/s	2.5 mm	2–3
Neck and chest	1.5 J/pulse	10–12 pulses/s	6 mm	2–3
Hands	1.5 J/pulse	8 pulses/s	4 mm	2–3

the same spot. Skin lesions and actinic regions are removed by sequential ablative passes. Wrinkles are treated with direct yet light lasering into the furrows. Then the wrinkle shoulders are flattened using the laser as a planing tool. There is no need to mechanically abrade these areas with a sponge.

Because the Er:YAG laser does not produce coagulation necrosis, one does not see the characteristic skin-depth color changes evident with the superpulsed CO_2 laser. One useful depth indicator is the pinpoint bleeding that occurs in the papillary dermis. If the papillary dermis continues to ooze, hold a lidocaine-epinephrine–soaked sponge over the region for 15 to 30 seconds.

Use of a smoke evacuator is mandatory because this high-powered laser turns the superficial skin layer into airborne particulate matter. In addition to eye protection suitable for 2940 nm, personnel should wear laser masks that filter 0.1-μm particles.

POSTOPERATIVE CARE

After superficial Er:YAG laser resurfacing, mupirocin is applied to keep the face moist for 2 days. Patients undergoing medium and deep Er:YAG laser peels receive the same wound care as that for CO_2 laser patients (closed-wound care for 2 days; see Chapter 10). A closed-wound care system is used to promote moist healing while preventing exudation (Fig. 13–6).

Exudation causes crust formation, which impedes reepithelialization and can lead to infection and/or scarring. In addition, complete facial coverage decreases postoperative pain and provides camouflage.[1] The closed-wound dressing is removed after 2 days.

After 2 days, patients are instructed to wash their face two to three times a day with Cetaphil soap (Galderma

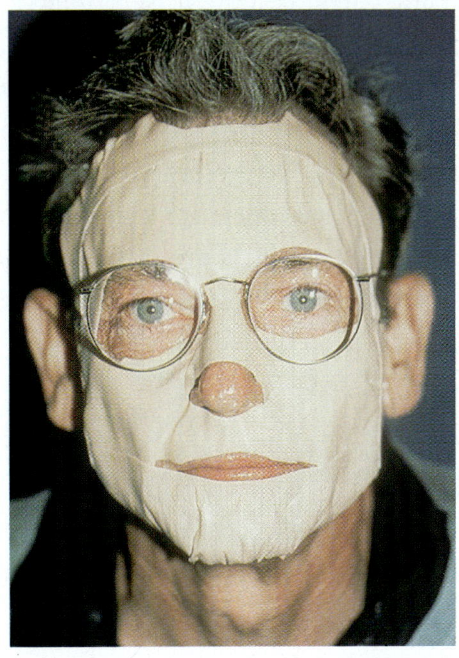

Figure 13–6. RevitaDerm (PolyMedica Wound Care Co., Woburn, MA) is a three-layer adhesive dressing with a membranous middle layer to absorb drainage and an outer vapor-permeable shell. A closed-wound care system is used to promote moist healing while preventing exudation.

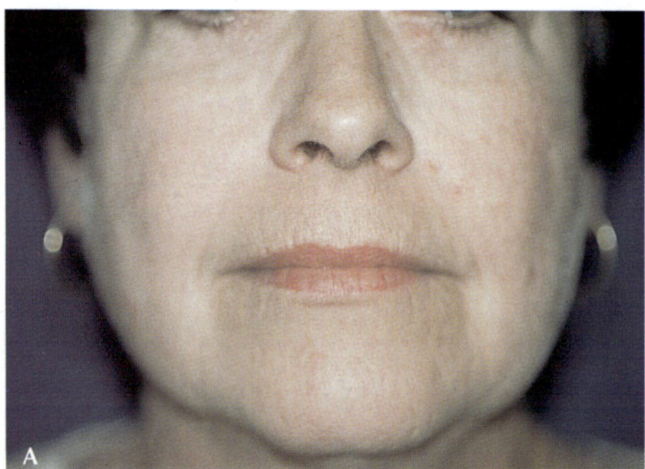

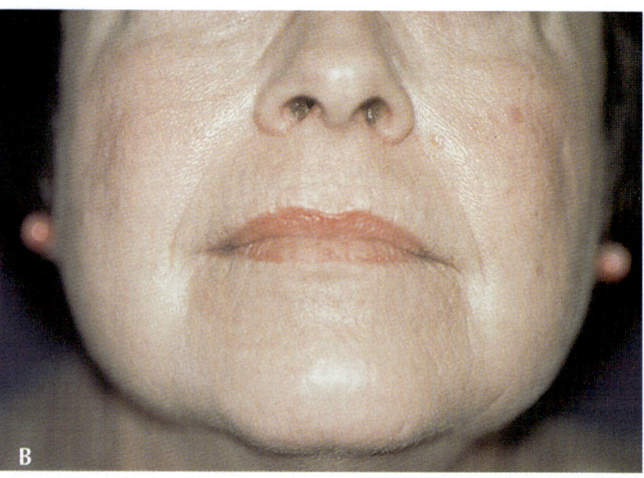

Figure 13–7. Typical result of Er:YAG laser skin resurfacing. (A) Preoperative view of a patient with actinic damage and perioral rhytids. (B) Postoperative view at 1 month. Early result shown to illustrate lack of erythema.

Laboratories Inc., Fort Worth, TX). They are told to not rub their skin but to gently pat it dry. Patients also are instructed to soak the treated region(s) with dilute acetic acid soaks (1 tablespoon of white vinegar per pint of tap-water) for at least 15 minutes three to four times a day. After soaking, a light coating of petrolatum is applied until the skin is reepithelialized.

Routine postoperative medications include ciprofloxacin, 500 mg twice a day for 5 days, for *Pseudomonas* coverage. Herpes prophylaxis for all laser patients continues postoperatively for 10 days. After reepithelialization, patients are instructed to use an ultraviolet sunscreen with a sun-protective factor (SPF) of greater than 25 on treated areas for 1 year.

RESULTS

To date, more than 340 patients have undergone Er:YAG laser skin resurfacing at the Facial Plastic Surgery Clinic at Stanford University Medical Center. Compared with the superpulsed CO_2 laser, findings indicate less perioperative discomfort, reepithelialization in 4 to 5 days, no erythema for more than 4 weeks, fewer lines of demarcation with spot treatments, and a much less exudative wound with the Er:YAG laser. My colleagues and I are in the process of formally evaluating subjective patient satisfaction, so no definitive data are available, but patients seem pleased primarily with their rapid healing and lack of erythema. There have been no complications. Typical results are shown in Fig. 13–7.

ER:YAG AND CO_2 LASER COMBINATION TREATMENT

Recently, my colleagues and I examined the histologic effects of combining CO_2 and Er:YAG laser modalities during a single treatment session.[2] Using preauricular skin that was lasered 7 days prior to rhytidectomy, we found that limiting CO_2 laser passes and finishing up with the Er:YAG laser produces less collagen injury, less thermal necrosis, and more robust epithelial and dermal fibrous tissue regeneration. Treating with the CO_2 laser followed by the Er:YAG laser produces similar thermal necrosis and collagen injury as the Er:YAG laser alone. It is our belief that this results from Er:YAG laser removal of areas of thermal injury produced by the CO_2 laser. In

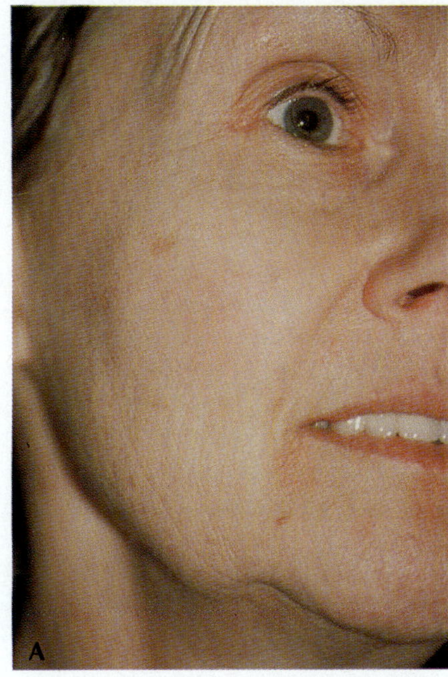 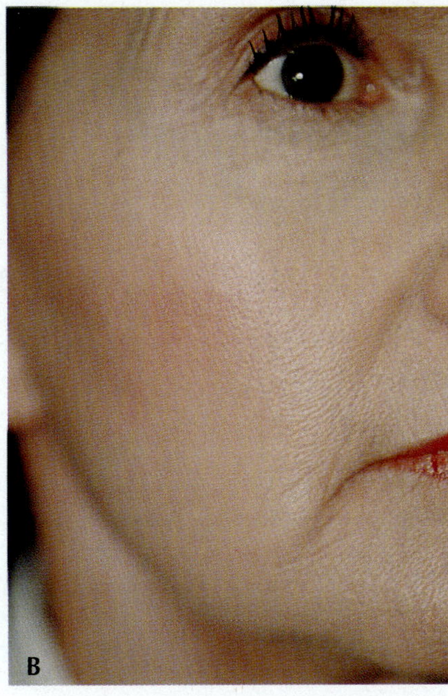

Figure 13–8. Typical result with combined superpulsed CO_2 and Er:YAG laser skin resurfacing. (A) Preoperative view of a patient with facial elastosis and actinic damage. (B) Postoperative view at 3 months.

other words, following CO_2 laser passes with the Er:YAG laser removes the zone of thermal necrosis and promotes prompt healing.

Our clinical experience supports the histologic findings of this study. Our patients who undergo superpulsed CO_2 resurfacing require 7 or more days to heal completely and may have erythema for up to 4 months. Despite these apparent disadvantages, CO_2 laser patients show very satisfying results in terms of skin tightening, skin rejuvenation, and rhytid removal. The thermal injury produced by the CO_2 laser may be the cause of both the prolonged healing and the improved results.[3,4] The Er:YAG laser patients, on the other hand, tend to heal in 3 to 4 days and have less erythema and fewer wound complications. Their results, however, may be somewhat less satisfying in terms of rhytid resolution and skin tightening.

The results of our preliminary study have prompted us to begin treating patients with combination laser therapy (e.g., two passes with the CO_2 laser followed by two to four passes with the Er:YAG laser) to exploit the specific advantages of each laser. Wound healing

with this combination treatment is expedient, usually within 4 days (as with the Er:YAG laser alone), and patient satisfaction with the skin rejuvenation, rhytid removal, and skin tightening is high (as with the CO_2 laser alone; Fig. 13–8).

ACKNOWLEDGMENTS

I would like to thank Mr. Mitch DeShon of ESC Medical Systems, without whom testing of the Derma 20 would not have been possible.

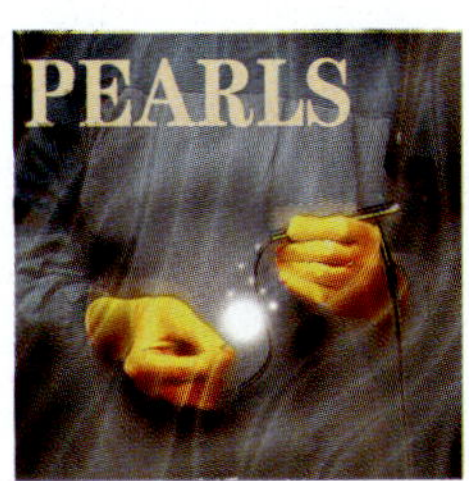

- When in doubt about which resurfacing laser to use, use the Er:YAG laser.
- A purely cosmetic practice should have both the Er:YAG and the CO_2 lasers, but if you are purchasing only one laser for use in facial plastic surgery, buy the more versatile superpulsed CO_2 laser. It has the added benefit of incisional capabilities.

- Following CO_2 laser passes with Er:YAG laser passes may produce the perfect balance of results and recovery. Combination modalities give you "the best of both worlds."
- Healing after Er:YAG laser treatment is significantly quicker than after CO_2 laser treatment because of minimal thermal damage and inflammation, as compared with the surrounding thermal damage and the resulting rim of thermal necrosis that are produced by a CO_2 laser.
- The Er:YAG laser may allow a return to regional treatments because of its lack of lines of demarcation and posthealing step-offs.
- Although concurrent subcutaneous rhytidectomy and CO_2 laser skin resurfacing is not recommended, the lack of thermal necrosis may allow use of the Er:YAG laser in this capacity.

REFERENCES

1. Newman JP, Koch RJ, Goode RL. Closed dressings after laser skin resurfacing. *Arch Otolaryngol Head Neck Surg* 1998;124(7):751–757.
2. Utley DS, Koch RJ, Egbert BM. Histologic analysis of the thermal effect on epidermal and dermal structures following treatment with the superpulsed CO_2 and the Erbium:YAG lasers: an in vivo study. *Lasers Surg Med* 1999;24:93–102.
3. Trelles MA, Mordon S, Svaasand LO, Mellor TK, Rigau I, Garcia L. The origin and role of erythema after carbon dioxide laser resurfacing: a clinical and histological study. *Dermatol Surg.* 1998;24:25–29.
4. Ruiz-Esparza J, Barba-Gomez JM, Gomez de la Torre OL, David L. Erythema after laser skin resurfacing. *Dermatol Surg.* 1998;24:113–117.

CHAPTER 14

The Erbium:YAG Laser versus the Carbon Dioxide Laser

WILLIAM K. BOSS, JR., MICHAEL A. FIORILLO, AND HAKAN USAL

The term *laser* is an acronym for *light amplification by stimulated emission of radiation*. In 1917, Einstein suggested the concept of stimulated emission, whereby a photon of light is emitted as an atom or a molecule returns to the ground state from an excited state and collides with a similarly excited atom. In 1959, Dr. Theodore Maiman at Hughs Aircraft Research Laboratory in California developed the first laser.[1] In 1963, Dr. Leon Goldman did the first tests on this ruby laser.[2]

LASER PRINCIPLES

Light emitted from a laser has three distinct properties: monochromaticity, coherence, and collimation. *Monochromaticity* refers to the fact that laser light is of a single wavelength. Laser light travels in phase with respect to time and space; this is *coherence*. *Collimation* means that laser light is emitted in a parallel fashion through a narrow, intense beam, which permits propagation without divergence or loss of intensity along an optical fiber and allows focus on a small spot size. Lasers are characterized by wavelength, or the color of light emitted. Most lasers are within the visible region of the electromagnetic spectrum, from 400 nm (blue range) to 700 nm (red range). Some lasers fall into the infrared (>700 nm) and ultraviolet (<400 nm) regions of the electromagnetic spectrum.

Laser light produces energy when it is absorbed. Different molecules absorb laser light differently. Tissue is not homogeneous, and there is competition by various chromophores—substances that absorb specific wavelengths—for absorbing laser light; therefore, the goal of laser treatment is to maximize absorption in the intended tissue and minimize absorption in the competing chromophores.

In 1983, an important concept known as *selective photothermolysis* was described (see Chapter 4).[3] Selective thermolysis involves the specific absorption of laser energy to achieve temperature-mediated localized injury in a target. The amount of selective tissue ablation depends on the laser's wavelength and the target tissue's *thermal relaxation time*, which is the time it takes for a tissue to cool following laser irradiation. Using this concept, many lasers have been developed that treat specific cutaneous conditions.

COSMETIC APPLICATIONS

The cosmetic applications of lasers, specifically to skin resurfacing, have been one of the fastest growing areas of laser use. The advantage of laser-induced tissue ablation over chemical peeling and dermabrasion lies in the laser's precise ability to remove thin layers of skin. The aim of laser skin resurfacing is to remove abnormal skin with minimal collateral damage to normal skin. The carbon dioxide (CO_2) laser emits light in the infrared region of the electromagnetic spectrum (10,600 nm) that is largely absorbed by water, so it readily ablates skin, which is made up largely (90%) of water. Carbon dioxide lasers have been used in dermatology since the 1970s, but their use in cosmetic surgery has been relatively recent.[4] The first-generation of CO_2 lasers were continuous wave (CW) lasers that were associated with nonspecific heat diffusion in surrounding skin, resulting in unwanted thermal necrosis and unacceptable rates of hypertrophied scarring and pigmentary changes.[5,6]

Over the past few years, technologic advances have led to the development of CO_2 laser systems that are pulsed (as opposed to CW).[7–9] Pulsed lasers minimize thermal damage when they are applied to the skin because the pulse duration is less than the thermal relaxation time of the target tissue, namely, skin, which is less than 1 millisecond. This advance has led to the development of a number of pulsed, char-free CO_2 laser systems.[10,11] Skin resurfacing with the CO_2 laser causes rapid epidermal ablation on the first pass and partial papillary dermal ablation on subsequent passes.[12] Dermal repair then occurs via replacement of coagulated dermis with new collagen production by fibroblasts from the underlying reticular dermis that continues for many months.[13]

Despite these recent improvements in CO_2 lasers, complications and undesirable skin effects still occur. The most common complications include, in decreasing order, prolonged erythema, bacterial infections, hyperpigmentation, hypopigmentation, allergic reactions, herpes/viral infections, hypertrophic scars, excessive telangiectasia, and ectropion.[14]

ERBIUM:YTTRIUM-ALUMINUM-GARNET LASER SYSTEM

The erbium:yttrium-aluminum-garnet (Er:YAG) laser is the newest generation of infrared lasers used for the treatment of photoaged skin, wrinkles, scars, and skin lesions. It was developed as an effective skin resurfacing tool with a significantly diminished incidence of complications. Prior to this, the CO_2 laser (with a wavelength of 10,600 nm) had the best water absorption characteristics available. In 1984, it was shown that laser light at the water absorption peak of 2940 nm in the infrared spectrum could cut tissue with a minimal (<1 μm) zone of thermal damage adjacent to the targeted tissue.[15] The Er:YAG laser produces energy with a wavelength of 2940 nm (the peak of water absorption) and targets the chromophore water, so its ability to be absorbed by water is 10 to 15 times that of CO_2 lasers.[16] This wavelength penetrates superficially, is readily absorbed by water, and exhibits minimal thermal scatter. Therefore, the Er:YAG laser efficiently ablates tissue while producing minimal thermal damage.[16–18]

LASER–TISSUE INTERACTIONS

Because the Er:YAG laser produces wavelengths at the peak of water absorption, the laser energy penetrates only about 15 to 25 μm into the skin per laser pass, compared with about 100 μm with a CO_2 laser used at similar energies.[19–21] The thermal damage produced by the Er:YAG laser is therefore much less than with the CO_2 laser, that is, about 5 to 20 μm versus about 75 to 100 μm for the CO_2 per pass. Because of this, the average healing time with the Er:YAG laser is 5 to 10 days, compared with 10 to 14 days for the CO_2 laser.[22] In addition, postinflammatory pigmentary changes and prolonged erythema have been reported to be less severe with the Er:YAG laser when compared with the CO_2 laser.[22] Therefore, the Er:YAG laser may be the treatment of choice in patients with higher Fitzpatrick skin types (see Table 6–3).

Proponents of the CO_2 laser point to the positive effects of the noticeable skin contraction following CO_2 laser skin resurfacing, but skin contraction is also seen following Er:YAG laser resurfacing.[23] Another benefit of the Er:YAG laser is that treatment is less painful than with the CO_2 lasers and can be performed under local anesthesia. Moreover, the infection rate has been reported to be lower than with CO_2 laser treatment, probably due to faster reepithelialization and less thermal damage with the Er:YAG laser.[24,25]

CLINICAL EFFICACY

Early reports indicated that two to three passes with the Er:YAG laser could be very effective in skin resurfacing with rapid healing and minimal prolonged erythema. We found this to be true, but rhytid improvements lasted only 3 to 4 months, and patients became dissatisfied (Fig. 14–1). We then increased the number of passes as described in Box 14–1 and obtained results comparable with CO_2 laser results. However, postoperative erythema was also prolonged significantly.

More recent studies have supported the clinical effectiveness of the Er:YAG laser for skin resurfacing of the face and neck, as well as scar revisions.[26,27] Most such studies have demonstrated good to excellent results. The same complications are seen as with the CO_2 laser (e.g., erythema, infection, hyperpigmentation, hypopigmentation, allergic reactions, scars, telangiectasia, and ectropion), but they appear less frequently.

Combination Therapy

In an effort to minimize the disadvantages of the CO_2 laser system and lessen the prolonged erythema seen with the Er:YAG protocol, we tried combination therapy with the Er:YAG laser and the CO_2 laser (Sharplan XJ150 laser set on "feather touch" mode; Sharplan, Inc., Allendale, NJ) on one side of the face and the CO_2 laser and the Er:YAG laser on the other side with fewer passes

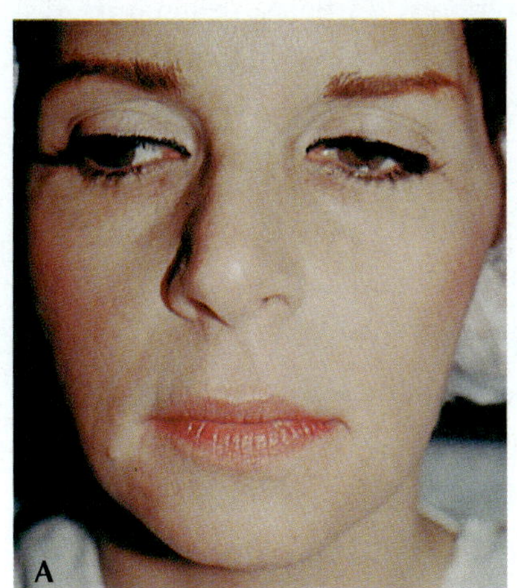
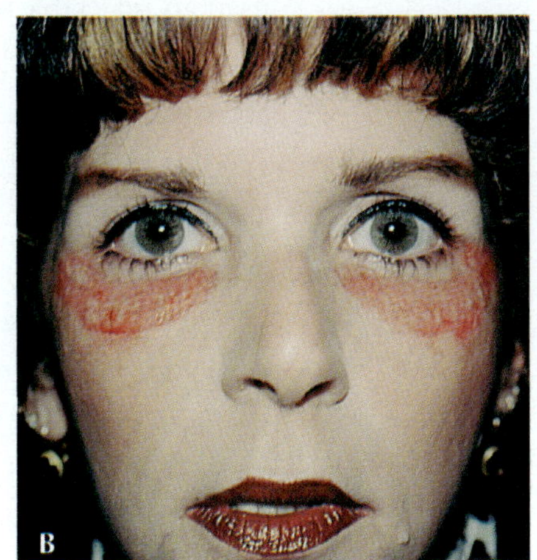
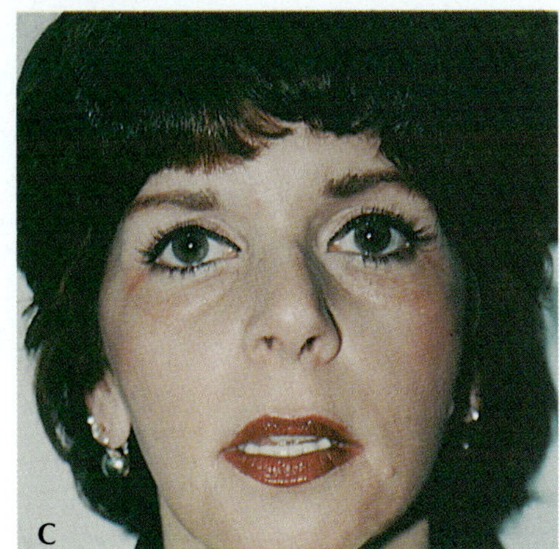
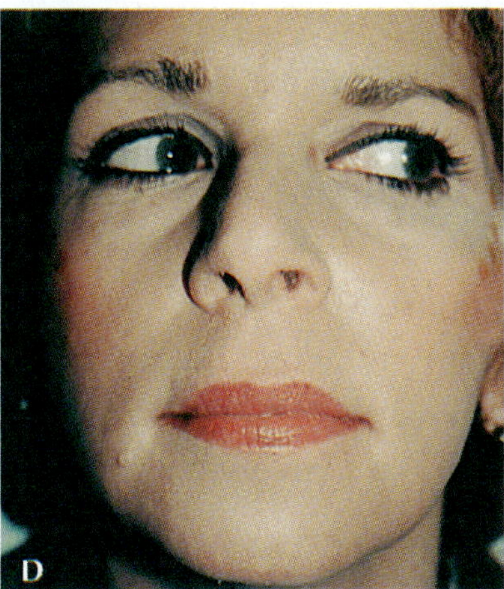

Figure 14–1. (A) Preoperative view. (B) Two days postoperatively (2–3 passes, Er:YAG laser). (C) Ten days postoperatively (note minimal erythema). (D) Appearance at 4 months (note the lack of change in rhytids from preoperative view).

Box 14–1. Erbium:YAG Laser Skin Resurfacing Protocol

Preoperative Skin Treatment (2–6 weeks)

1. Retin-A—retinoic acid

2. Hydroquinone

3. Antistaphylococcal antibiotics

4. Antivirals (2 days preoperatively)

5. Sunscreens/sun avoidance

Surgery

1. Topical anesthesia—eutectic mixture of local anesthetics

2. Nerve block or local infiltration (lidocaine with epinephrine)

3. Face wash with soap and water, Betadine wash, alcohol wipe

4. Eye shields, tooth protection, safety check

5. 3-mm spot size, 800 mJ to 1.0 J

6. Six to eight passes on cheeks, nose, chin, forehead, and perioral area; three to four passes in periocular area

7. Endpoint is rhytid ablation and elimination of the shoulders of rhytids

Postoperative Treatment

1. Open or closed dressing system

2. Patients should wash face six times per day for 2 days using bacitracin and then apply Vaseline until reepithelialization

3. Sunscreens/sun avoidance

4. Resume preoperative skin treatment—glycolic micropeel system with daily glycolic acid creams

---

(one CO_2 laser pass and three Er:YAG laser passes). (See Chapter 7 for a discussion of the Sharplan system.) We did not notice any differences between the two sides, nor did we see a significant lessening of erythema (Fig. 14–2).

Comparative Study

To better evaluate the purported advantages of the Er:YAG laser and to try to find a technique to minimize the disadvantages of the CO_2 laser, we did a comparative study on the same patient. The Er:YAG laser set at 15 J/cm^2 with a 3-mm spot size was used with an effective number of passes (four to six) on half the face, and a single pass with the high-power CO_2 laser (Sharplan XJ150 FeatherTouch, 80–100 W on the face, 40–50 W in the periocular area) was used on the contralateral side (Fig. 14–3). Interestingly, we found no difference in efficacy, postoperative erythema, or complications.

Isolagen Injections

In another attempt to maximize the results of Er:YAG laser treatment and minimize postoperative erythema, we used an injectable autologous fibroblast cell culture system [Isolagen (Technologies Inc., Paramus, NJ)]. Certain areas were pretreated with Isolagen injections, and Isolagen was then injected in the same areas following Er:YAG laser treatment. We found a significant improvement in long-term results and minimal postoperative erythema with only three laser passes (Figs. 14–4 and 14–5). Histologically, Isolagen results in increased collagen production at 4 months after injection, which continues up to 24 months. Increased collagen deposition for about 1 year after laser treatment has also been documented.[27]

Disadvantages

With so many theoretical and reported advantages, the Er:YAG laser has become the first choice of many surgeons who perform skin resurfacing. Nevertheless, there are several disadvantages to Er:YAG laser treatment, including the smaller spot size and the need for multiple passes, which prolong the procedure. However, new computerized pattern generators allow this pulsed system to ablate thin layers of skin safely and quickly. They

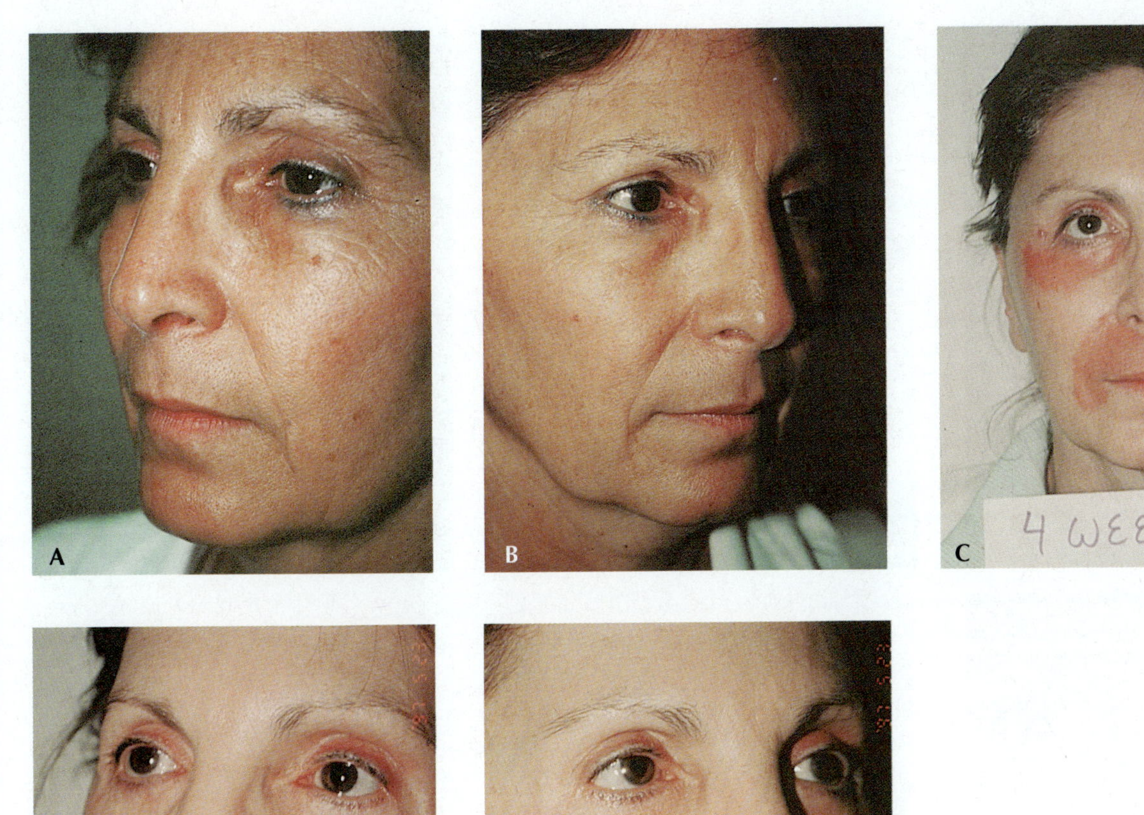

Figure 14–2. Preoperative left (A) and right (B) views. (C) Er:YAG laser only on lids. Er:YAG laser followed by CO_2 laser on left and CO_2 laser followed by Er:YAG laser on right (note that there is no difference in erythema). (D,E) Appearance 8 months postoperatively showing good results on both sides and a good Er:YAG-only result on the lids.

also permit larger spot sizes, which increases the speed of the procedure. Other drawbacks of the erbium include the difficulty in determining the proper endpoint and the occurrence of bleeding, which is not an issue with the CO_2 laser.

CONCLUSIONS

In conclusion, the Er:YAG laser is the newest advance for resurfacing aged and sun-damaged skin. It is effective in reducing facial wrinkles and superficial skin lesions, as well as in treating scars from surgery, accidents, or acne. It can also be used in conjunction with various surgical procedures. The Er:YAG laser produces minimal thermal damage and minimizes postoperative erythema, leading to quicker healing time than many conventional lasers. Postoperative complications and morbidity have been minimal. In addition, the Er:YAG laser is less expensive than the CO_2 laser, although less powerful, less expensive CO_2 laser systems are now available (the less

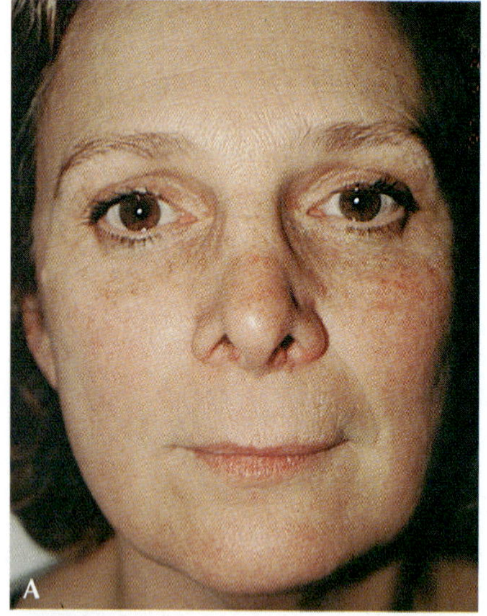
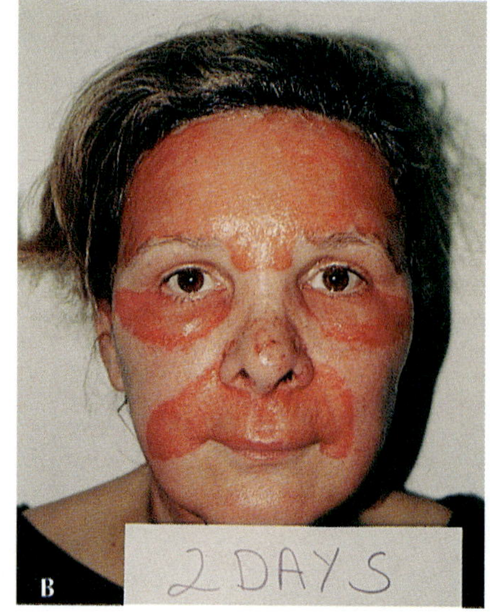

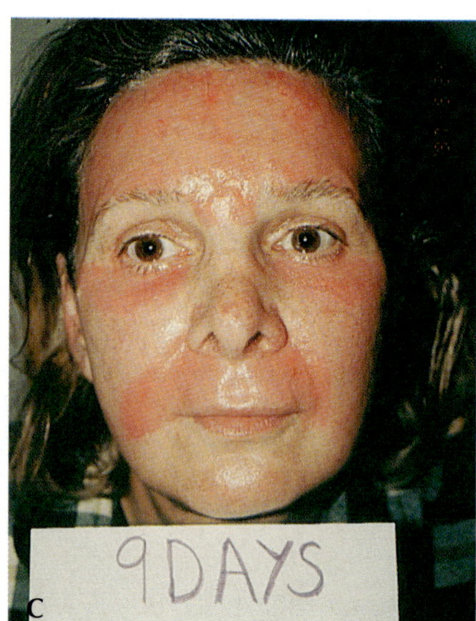

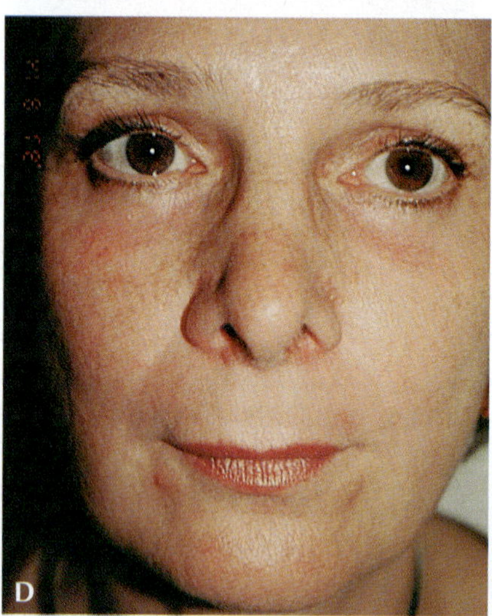

Figure 14–3. (A) Preoperative view. (B) Two days postoperatively (Er:YAG laser on the right and CO_2 laser on the left). (C) Nine days postoperatively. (D) Appearance 9 months postoperatively, with good overall improvement and no difference between the CO_2- and Er:YAG-treated sides.

expensive CO_2 lasers require a greater number of passes and greater erythema for equivalent results).

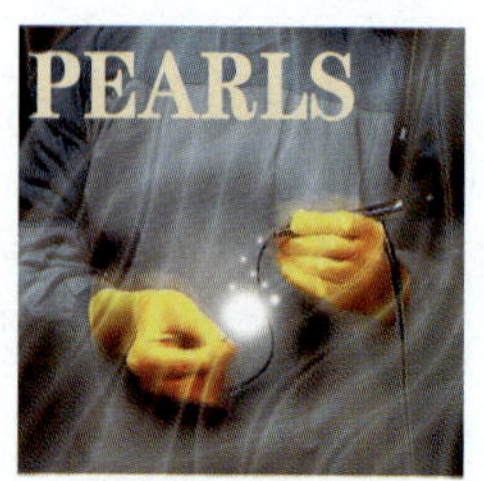

PEARLS

- The Er:YAG laser has a significantly diminished incidence of complications when compared with the CO_2 laser because its energy is readily absorbed by water. Because it penetrates superficially and exhibits minimal thermal scatter, the Er:YAG laser efficiently ablates tissue while producing minimal thermal damage.
- Average healing time with the Er:YAG laser is 5 to 10 days, compared with 10 to 14 days for the CO_2 laser.

- Because there are less severe postinflammatory pigmentary changes with the Er:YAG laser than with the CO_2 laser, the Er:YAG laser may be the treatment of choice in patients with higher Fitzpatrick skin types.

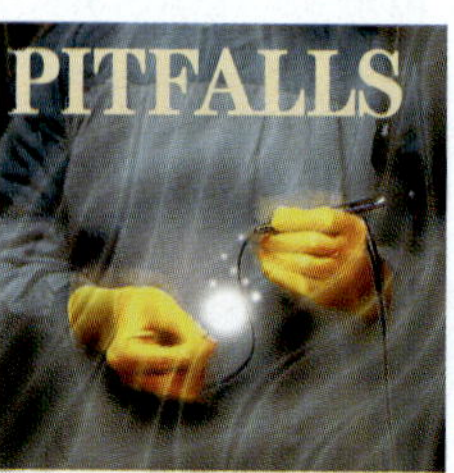

PITFALLS

- Two to three passes with the Er:YAG laser effectively resurfaces skin with rapid healing and minimal prolonged erythema, but rhytid improvements last only 3 to 4 months, which leads to patient dissatisfaction.
- The smaller spot size and the need for multiple passes with the Er:YAG laser prolong the procedure, although

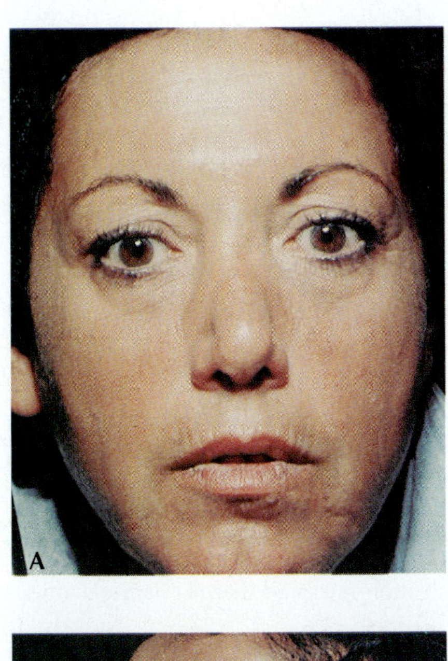
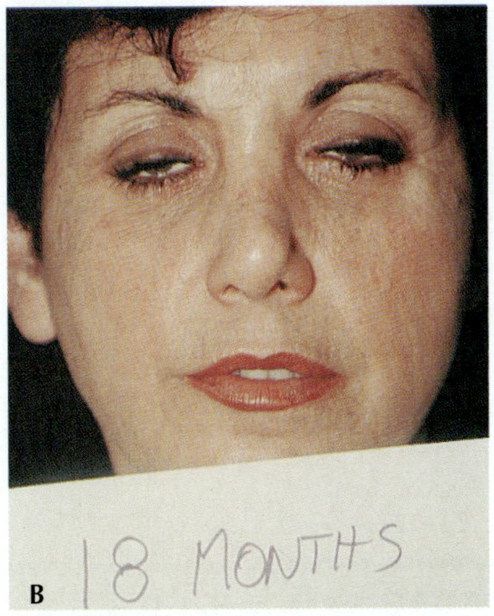

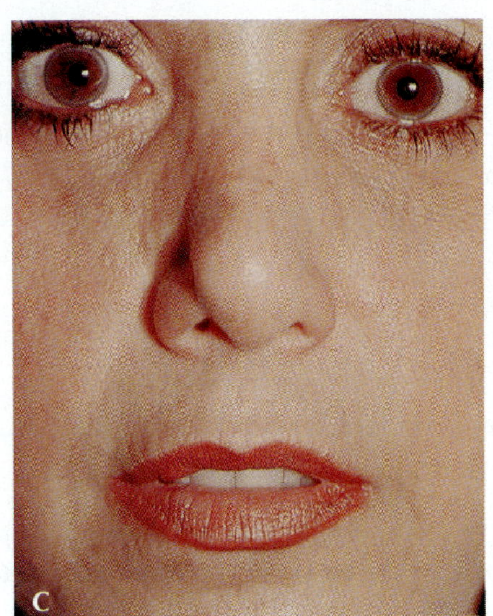
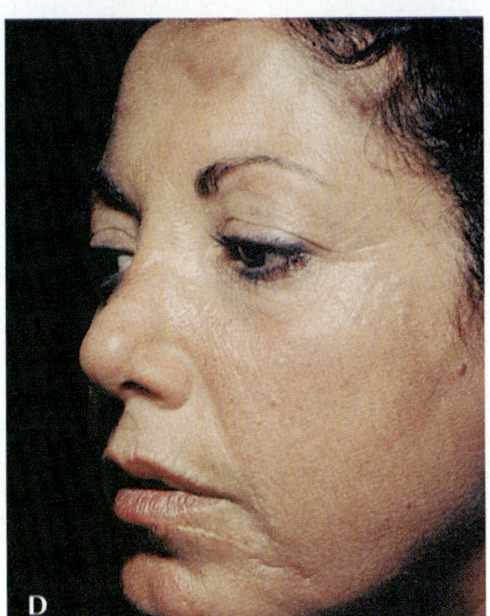
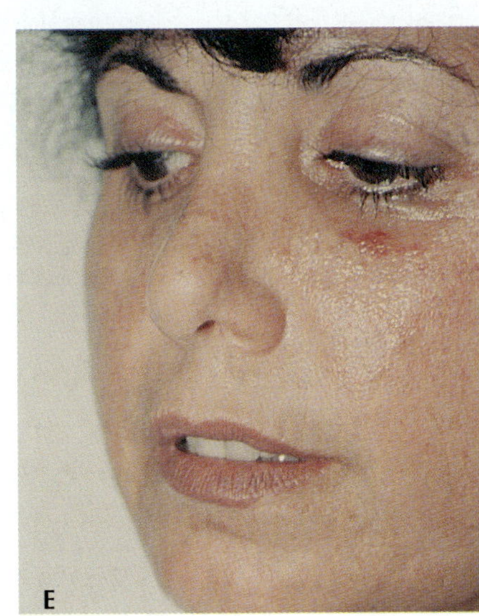

Figure 14–4. (A) Preoperative view (note depressed left nasal bone, upper lip rhytids, and left lower lip and chin scar). (B) Appearance 18 months after Isolagen injections to the left side of the nose, upper lip, and chin scar and Er:YAG laser treatment of the upper lip and chin scar. Preoperative front (C) and side (D) views. (E) Side view 24 months postoperatively.

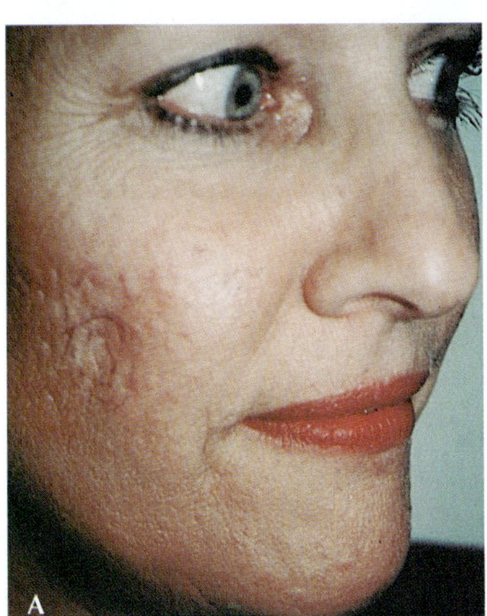
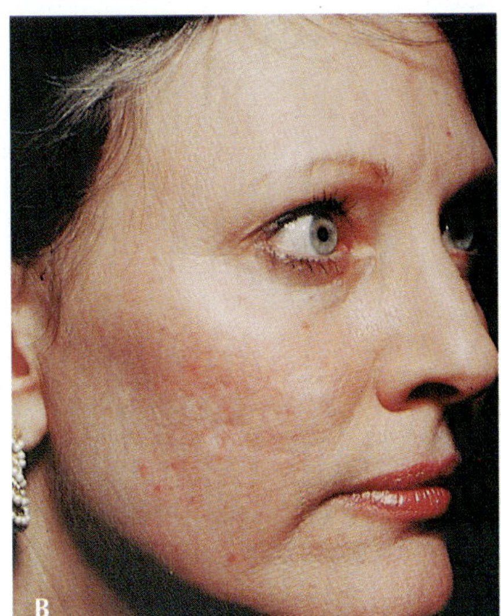
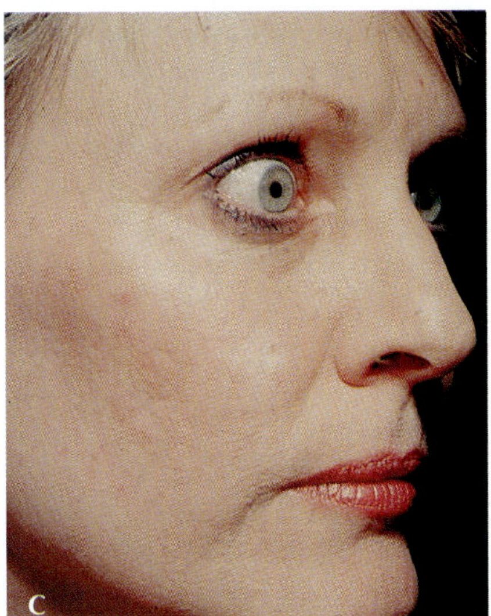

Figure 14–5. (A) Preoperative view (before acne scar treatment). (B) Appearance 8 months after three Isolagen injections. (C) Appearance 6 months after Er:YAG laser treatment.

new computerized pattern generators allow quick ablation of thin layers of skin and larger spot sizes. The occurrence of bleeding and the difficulty of determining an appropriate endpoint are additional pitfalls with the Er:YAG laser.

REFERENCES

1. Maiman TH. Stimulated optical radiation in ruby. *Nature.* 1960;187:483–494.
2. Goldman L, Blaney DJ, Kindel DJ, et al. Effect of the laser beam on the skin. *J Invest Dermatol.* 1963;40:121–122.
3. Anderson RR, Parish JA. Selective photothermolysis: precise microsurgery by selective absorption of pulsed radiation. *Science.* 1983;22:524–527.
4. Baker SS, Muenzler WS, Small RG, et al. CO_2 laser blepharoplasty. *Ophthalmology.* 1984;91:238–243.
5. Friedman M, Gal D. Keloid scars as a result of CO_2 laser for molluscum contagiosum. *Obstet Gynecol.* 1987;70:394.
6. Olbricht SM. Complications of cutaneous laser surgery. *Arch Dermatol.* 1987;123:345–349.
7. Hobbs ER, Bailin PL, Wheeland RG, Ratz JL. Superpulsed lasers: minimizing thermal damage with short duration, high pulses. *J Dermatol Surg Oncol.* 1987;13:955–964.
8. Fitzpatrick RE, Ruiz-Esparza J, Goldman MP. The depth of thermal necrosis using the CO_2 laser: a comparison of the superpulsed mode and conventional mode. *J Dermatol Surg Oncol.* 1991;17:340–344.
9. Zweigh AD, Meierhofer B, Muller OM, et al. Lateral thermal damage along pulsed laser incisions. *Lasers Surg Med.* 1990;10:262–274.
10. Apfelberg DB. The ultrapulse carbon dioxide laser with computer pattern generator automatic scanner for facial cosmetic surgery and resurfacing. *Ann Plast Surg.* 1996;36:522.
11. Fitzpatrick RE, Goldman MP. Advances in carbon dioxide laser surgery. *Clin Dermatol.* 1995;13:35.
12. Walsh JJ, Flott TJ, Anderson RR, Deutsch TF. Pulsed CO_2 laser tissue ablation effect of tissue type and pulse duration on thermal damage. *Lasers Surg Med.* 1988;8:108–118.
13. Clarke RF. Cutaneous tissue repair: basic biological considerations. *J Am Acad Dermatol.* 1985;13:701.
14. Apfelberg DB. Summary of the 1997 ASAPS/ASPRS laser task force on laser resurfacing and laser blepharoplasty. *Plast Reconstr Surg.* 1998;101:511.
15. Wolbarsht ML. Laser surgery: CO_2 or HF. *J Quant Elect* 1984;Qe20:1426–1432.
16. Kaufmann R, Hibst R. Pulsed erbium:YAG laser ablation in cutaneous surgery. *Lasers Surg Med.* 1996;19:324–330.
17. Walsh JT, Deutsch TF. Er:YAG laser ablation of tissue: measurement of ablation rates. *Lasers Surg Med.* 1989;9:327–337.
18. Hibst R, Kaufmann R. Effects of laser parameters on pulsed Erbium:YAG laser skin ablation. *Lasers Med Sci.* 1991;6:391–397.
19. Hohenleutner U, Hohenleutner S, Baumier W, Landthaler M. Fast and effective skin ablation with an Er:YAG laser: determination of ablation rates and thermal damage zones. *Lasers Surg Med.* 1997;20:242–247.
20. Kaufmann R, Hartmann A, Hibst R. Cutting and skin-ablative properties of pulsed mid-infrared laser surgery. *J Dermatol Surg Oncol.* 1994;20:112–118.
21. Kaufmann R, Hibst R. Pulsed 2.94-micron erbium:YAG laser skin ablation–experimental results and first clinical application. *Clin Exp Dermatol.* 1990;15:389–393.
22. Hughes PS. Skin contraction following erbium:YAG laser resurfacing. *Dermatol Surg.* 1998;24:109–111.
23. Ando Y, Aoki A, Watanabe H, Ishikawa I. Bactericidal effect of erbium:YAG laser on periodontopathic bacteria. *Lasers Surg Med.* 1996;19:190–200.
24. Spiprachya-Anunt S, Fitzpatrick RE, Goldman MP, Smith SR. Infections complicating pulsed-carbon dioxide laser resurfacing for photoaged facial skin. *Dermatol Surg.* 1997;23:527–536.
25. Teikemeier G, Goldberg DJ. Skin resurfacing with the Er:YAG laser. *Dermatol Surg.* 1997;23:685–687.
26. Weinstein C. Computerized scanning erbium:YAG laser for skin resurfacing. *Dermatol Surg.* 1998;24:83–89.
27. Weinstein C, Alster TS. Skin resurfacing with high energy, pulsed carbon dioxide lasers. In: Alster TS, Apfelberg DB, eds. *Cosmetic Laser Surgery.* New York: John Wiley and Sons; 1996:9–27.

CHAPTER 15

Nonexfoliating Laser Rejuvenation of Facial Rhytids

W. GREGORY CHERNOFF

Since 1994, there has been a rapid evolution in the treatment of facial rhytids. Currently, 20,000 people per day turn age 50 in North America; well over half the U.S. population will be 45 years of age or older by the year 2000. In addition, most aesthetic surgical practices have seen an increase in the number of men seeking aesthetic improvement. All these factors have led to a monumental increase in the number of patients seeking aesthetic plastic surgery. The most appealing scenario to many of these patients is one of minimal risk, pain, and healing time—but with maximal results. This combination has placed pressure on physicians to develop new, less invasive procedures, such as nonexfoliating laser rejuvenation, to offer this ever more demanding patient population.

The list of modalities available to patients for the purposes of counteracting the effects of photoaging and chronologic aging is continually growing. As health care providers, aesthetic surgeons have a responsibility to be familiar with both old and new technologies, as well as the fads that Internet-savvy clients may ask about. With general wellness in mind, more practitioners are promoting the benefits of "skin care from within," advocating various oral supplements that have been proven scientifically to maximize collagen structure. Preventive maintenance has also entered the limelight with "photo protection education." Increasing evidence of the negative effects of free radicals on aging skin, coupled with reports on the benefits of antioxidant therapies, is opening new pathways to youthful skin. The use of retinoic acid, with its positive effects on collagen stimulation, is rapidly growing.[1] Tissue-culturing techniques have enabled us to implement autologous fibroblast injections for the purposes of filling expression lines and deeper folds. Many scientists and clinicians are struggling to explain to their patients the facts versus fiction regarding the multitude of skin care products available. It is widely recognized that using some form of general exfoliant coupled with a moisturizer has long-term benefits to patients.[2,3]

When preventive maintenance and skin care fail to stave off the inexorable effects of time and sun damage, a growing number of patients seek surgical intervention. The armamentarium available to aesthetic plastic surgeons for the treatment of facial rhytids is extensive. Historically, chemical peels and dermabrasion were the first lines of therapeutic intervention. The carbon dioxide (CO_2) laser, with its extremely accurate depth control, has overtaken these modalities in popularity. The modern CO_2 laser has proven to be a very effective and predictable instrument for the purposes of softening fine, static rhytids on the face.[4] The complication rate is similar to that of deeper trichloroacetic acid (TCA) or phenol peels once the operator is familiar with the procedure. More recently, erbium:yttrium-aluminum-garnet (Er:YAG) laser systems have proven to be somewhat safer than the

CO_2 laser on a per pass basis because less ablation is coupled with less thermal deposition into the residual tissue.[5]

All the aforementioned modalities provoke a strong wound-healing response that, in theory, leads to a reduction in static rhytids.[6] A major pitfall of these procedures, however, is the fact that they require exfoliation of the epidermis to effect the desired changes. This exfoliation and the subsequent controlled healing reaction may be accompanied by complications such as persistent erythema, scarring, infection, and pigmentary changes, including hyper- and hypopigmentation. Edema, serous drainage, and discomfort may persist for a week, which requires patients to alter their schedule of regular activities.

The mechanism of action of laser exfoliation has been the subject of much study. Ablation of the epidermis and a portion of the dermis with a subsequent thermal reaction leads to long-term wound healing and dermal collagen remodeling. As new collagen and extracellular matrix materials are synthesized, a softening of the rhytids is noticed. This healing phase typically extends over a period of months. The exact amount of collagen shrinkage proportional to laser energy delivered to the dermis also has been the subject of tremendous study.[4-7]

Although many patients present with epidermal lentigines that necessitate epidermal ablation, new research reveals that epidermal and dermal ablation may not be a prerequisite for collagen remodeling. While dermal collagen shrinkage induced by the exfoliating/rejuvenating instruments has been studied in vitro in human skin healing experiments and in vivo in pig skin experiments, the process may only be incidental to long-term rhytid reduction. Long-term wound healing and dermal remodeling are probably the major mechanisms of action responsible for long-term facial rhytid reduction.[8,9]

NONABLATIVE (NONEXFOLIATIVE) COLLAGEN REMODELING

Topical application of substances such as retinoic acid (Retin-A) and alpha-hydroxy acids has been shown to increase papillary type-I dermal collagen production and subsequently yield a softening of rhytids. With this in mind, several studies have been undertaken to examine methods designed to provoke a dermal wound-healing response. Most of this research has been performed using the 1320-nm neodymium:yttrium-aluminum-garnet (Nd:YAG) laser. Some research has also been performed using the 980-nm diode laser. Currently, nonablative laser therapy is designed to produce selective papillary dermal injury, yielding fibroblast activation and the synthesis of new collagen and extracellular matrix while avoiding significant epidermal injury.[10,11] To produce this result at the collagen level, two goals must be achieved:

1. The laser wavelength, pulse width, and appropriate fluences capable of reaching and damaging the papillary dermis adequately to induce a long-term wound healing response must be determined.
2. The epidermis must be protected prior to and during laser exposure with methods that provide superficial cooling.

The ultimate challenge of this form of therapy is to choose a wavelength that will penetrate the dermis to at least 100 to 200 μm, cause significant thermal reaction within the dermis, and yet cause no exfoliation of the skin, which would result in an open wound. The ability to deliver a coolant to the epidermis must not, on the other hand, impede sufficient heating of the dermis, or no results will be achieved.

COOL TOUCH NEODYMIUM: YTTRIUM-ALUMINUM-GARNET LASER

I have done an extensive study using the New Star 130 Cool Touch Nd:YAG system. This laser produces a beam of infrared (IR) radiation at a wavelength of 1320 nm. The laser emission is a pulsed waveform of three symmetrical 300-microsecond pulses at 100 Hz forming a 20-millisecond duration macropulse. The system incorporates dynamic cooling technology that allows a metered dose of cryogen spray (a form of tetrafluoroethylene) to be delivered to the treatment surface a fraction of a second prior to delivery of the laser energy. A thermal sensor in the handpiece measures the changes in skin surface temperature produced by the nonablative laser. Appropriate fluences, dwell times, and cooling have been determined by examining known models of laser–tissue interaction.[12–17]

At 1320 nm, the primary tissue chromophore is water, which has an absorption coefficient of 1.82 cm^{-1}.[18,19] Ablative lasers such as the CO_2 and Er:YAG lasers produce wavelengths of light that are almost entirely absorbed within the upper 10 to 50 μm of skin. The 1320-nm wavelength produces heating necessary to create thermal damage to the papillary and superficial reticular dermis at a depth of 100 μm. This damage is sufficient to induce a wound-healing response with each treatment.

CONTROLLING VARIABLES OF NONABLATIVE LASER THERAPY

A great deal of work has been performed on relative light distributions and subsurface scattering. Light absorption and temperature increases are proportional to the light distribution function. Thermal damage in the epidermis is nearly the same as that in the papillary dermis if conventional Nd:YAG laser treatment is performed. By using dynamic cryogen cooling, selective protection of the epidermis through the stratum corneum can be achieved immediately before laser treatment.[20–24] Studies have shown that temperature increases between 30 and 40°C above physiologic temperature applied over a period of several milliseconds cause a phase transition of type-I collagen within the papillary dermis and superficial reticular dermis. This thermal modification of collagen is sufficient to activate fibroblasts to produce a long-term wound-healing response. Therefore, the controlling variables of nonablative laser therapy include the following:

1. Dynamic cooling (cryogen type and application time)
2. Temporal delay (between the cryogen cooling pulse and the laser heating pulse)

3. Laser heating (radiate exposure, as well as wavelength and waveform in other lasers)

Further "fine tuning" is being studied to examine the benefits of a "precryogen warming pulse" to gradually warm the skin in situations where large temperature fluctuations exist. This illustrates one of the tremendous benefits of the surface temperature thermal sensor.

HISTOLOGIC STUDIES

Histologic analyses of the dynamic cooling methodology coupled with the "thermescent" technique have been completed. Human blepharoplasty and rhytidectomy skin specimens were used to first determine the cryogen duration and then the delay between cryogen bursts and laser firing. A cooling duration of 20 milliseconds with a subsequent delay of 30 milliseconds from the end of cooling to onset of laser firing has been found to be most efficacious in terms of yielding a consistent, safe response.

These dynamic cooling parameters, coupled with fluences in the range of 28 to 32 J/cm^2, yield sufficient energy to cause a wound-healing response. Using a radiant exposure distribution calculated by Monte Carlo modeling indicates that achieving surface temperatures in the range of 40 to 45°C correlates with heating of the dermis to 80°C to a depth of 100 μm.[25–27] This creates sufficient thermal damage to activate fibroblasts and stimulate a long-term wound-healing response, including new collagen synthesis.[28] A side effect of this process is subsequent reduction in fine rhytids.

Figure 15–1 shows a 4-mm punch biopsy of preauricular skin immediately after treatment with the thermescent technique. The epidermis at the left of the specimen shows the results of not using cryogen with a fluence of 28 J/cm^2. There is significant blistering of the epidermis with coagulative damage to the epidermis. Clinically, this would equate with a prolonged healing response. The right side of the specimen reveals the effect of using a cryogen spray with a duration of 20 milliseconds and a delay of 30 milliseconds before firing 28 J/cm^2 of laser energy into the tissue. Note the

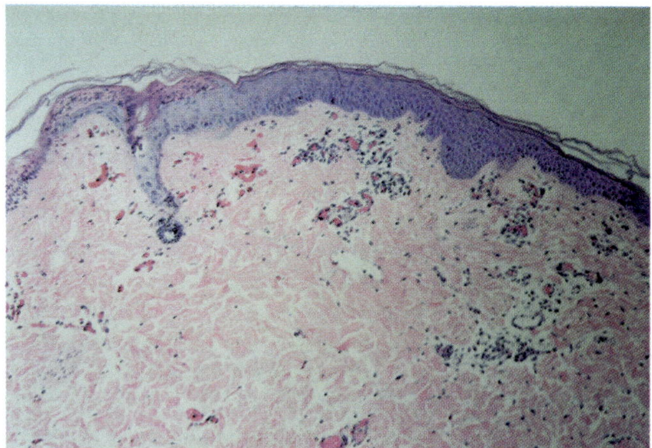

Figure 15–1. Histologic specimen treated with the Cool Touch laser at 28 J/cm² showing an intense fibroblast response. On the left side of the specimen, no cryogen cooling was used, and epidermolysis is evident. On the right, the epidermis was treated with cryogen cooling for 20 milliseconds with a 30-millisecond delay prior to laser firing. Note preservation of the epidermis.

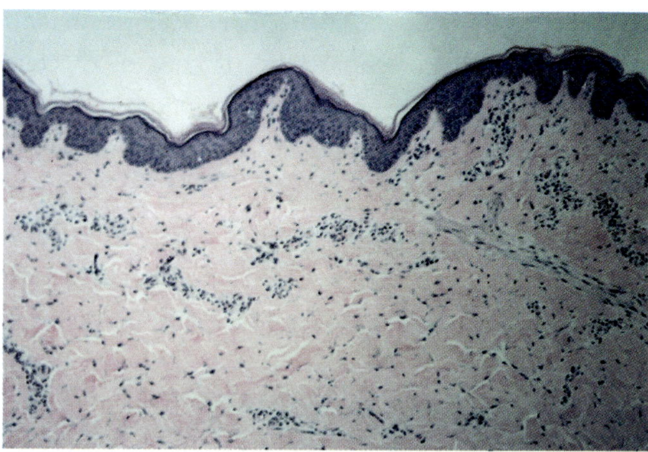

Figure 15–2. Histologic specimen 1 week following one pass with the Cool Touch laser at 28 J/cm². Continued fibroblast stimulation is seen.

preservation of the epidermis and the fibroblast response. Figure 15–2 shows a biopsy from the same patient taken 1 week after treatment. A continued fibroblast response is noted. Figure 15–3 shows a biopsy from the same patient 1 week after treatment. The production of neocollagen is observed. This sequence can be observed histologically with each subsequent treatment. Figure 15–4A is a control biopsy, and Figure 15–4B is a 1-year biopsy after three treat-

ments at 28 J/cm² spaced 6 weeks apart. A new band of collagen is noted in the papillary dermis along with compaction. A grading scale has been implemented for patients to subjectively score their degree of rhytid improvement (Box 15–1). Most patients report a grade 1 to 2 improvement in rhytids subsequent to this therapeutic regimen.

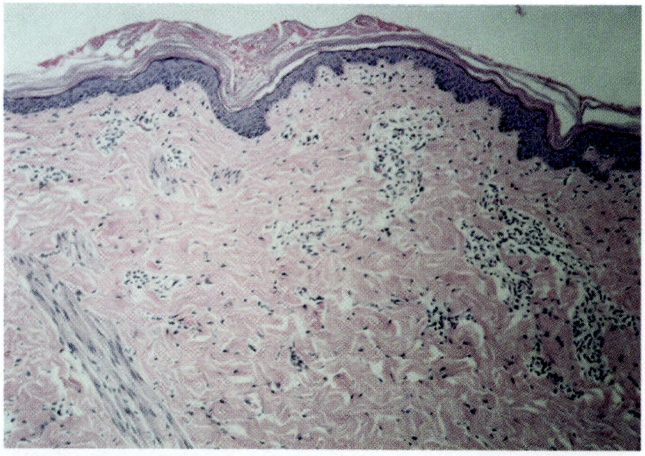

Box 15–1. Grading Scale of Rhytid Improvement		
Grade 1	0 to 25%	improvement
Grade 2	25 to 50%	improvement
Grade 3	50 to 75%	improvement
Grade 4	75 to 100%	improvement

TREATMENT

Static Rhytids

Success has been achieved in treating fine static rhytids with the Cool Touch laser in the infraorbital and perioral regions, but patients should know the difference between *static rhytids* and *dynamic folds* such as glabellar folds, crow's feet, and perioral expression lines. Patients are frequently concerned about dynamic folds, but the efficacy of the

Figure 15–3. Neocollagen formation 1 week following one pass with the Cool Touch laser at 28 J/cm².

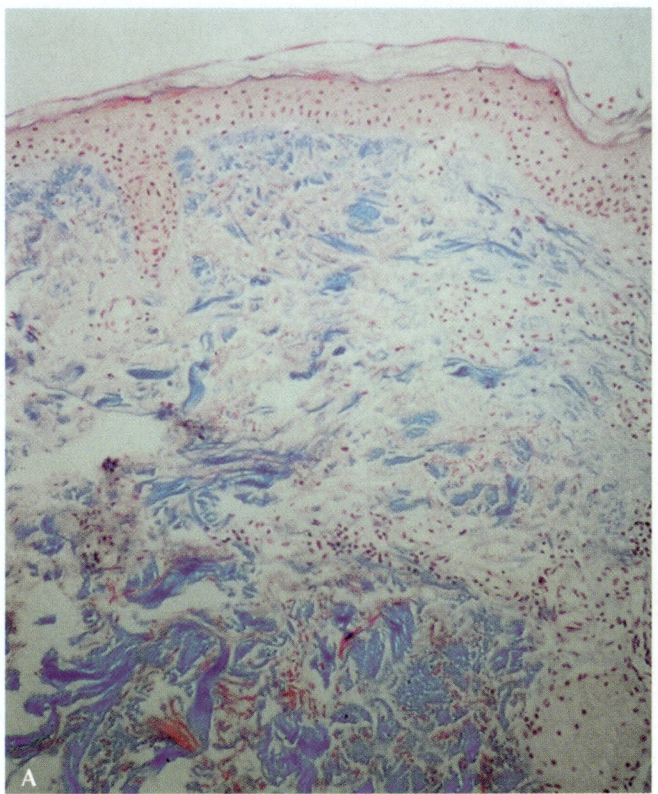 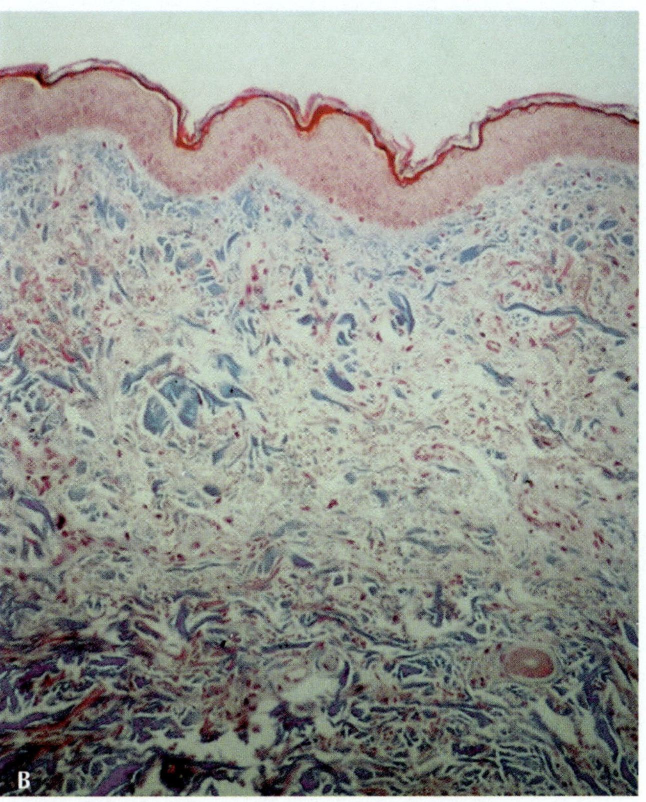

Figure 15–4. (A) Control. (B) One-year after Cool Touch laser treatment at 28 J/cm^2 with cryogen cooling of 20-millisecond duration with a 30-millisecond delay. Note collagen contraction and maintenance of neocollagen.

nonablative laser should not be substituted for filling materials such as Gore-Tex, Isologen, and collagen.

Patients must also be educated about the fact that the laser is stimulating their own fibroblasts to produce new collagen. Because each additional treatment brings added benefits, patients must understand that this is not a "one-time" treatment. As patients appreciate the softening of the fine lines and improvement in the quality, tone, and texture of their skin, they seek further treatments. In addition, the practitioner should encourage these patients to begin an antiaging skin care program.

Contraindications to treatment include general poor health, active herpetic lesions, and unrealistic patient expectations. Patients should be prescribed prophylactic antiviral medication to prevent any potential outbreak of herpetic lesions.

After obtaining proper photographic documentation of the regions to be treated, the skin is cleansed of oils with alcohol. A topical eutectic mixture of local anesthetics (EMLA cream/Astra Pharmaceuticals) is applied for a period of 10 to 15 minutes in the treatment areas.[29] After observing a blanching of the skin, a test pulse beginning at 28 J/cm^2 is initiated. Once the peak temperature is observed ($>40°C$ to $\leq 45°C$), the fluence is adjusted until this temperature peak is obtained. The laser pulses are overlapped by approximately one third with each application. A common combination therapy in the periorbital region is coupling the Cool Touch laser with botulinum toxin (Botox) administration. This yields a meticulous softening of both the expression lines and the static infraorbital rhytids. One clinical endpoint is the appearance of even erythema without epidermal lysis or blistering.

Treatment of the fine rhytids in the perioral area has also been successful. When coupled with injection of Isologen or autologous fibroblasts, increased bulk in the lip has been noted. The injected fibroblasts are given a

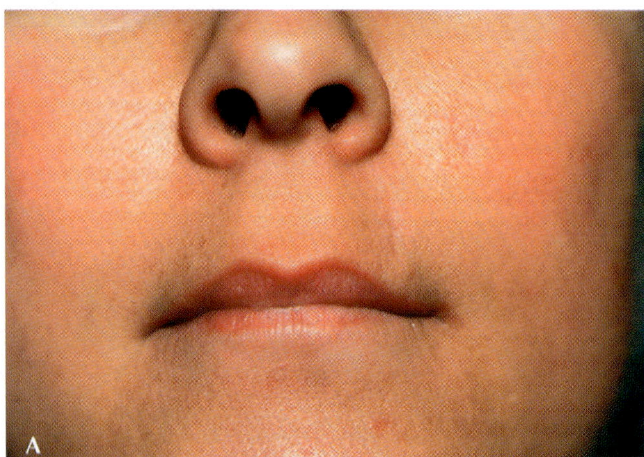

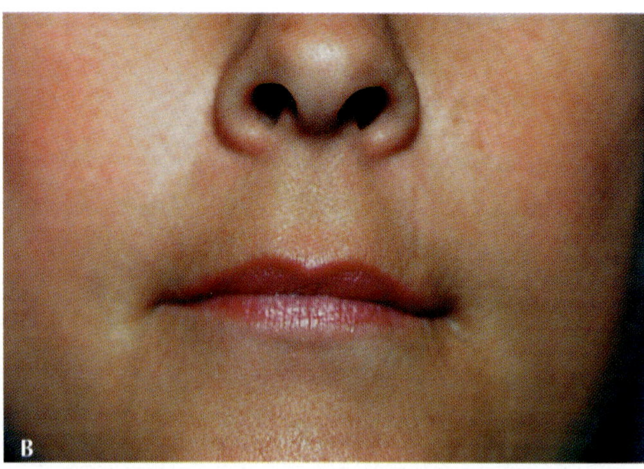

Figure 15–5. (A) Preoperative view of a 42-year-old woman. (B) Same patient 1 year later after three Isologen injections and three Cool Touch laser treatments at 32 J/cm^2 1 month after each Isologen injection.

period of 4 to 6 weeks to develop their blood supply and are subsequently stimulated with the Cool Touch laser at intervals of 2 weeks for three applications. After 6 months, an increase in bulk along the vermilion border is routinely noted (Fig. 15–5).

Another subset of patients who have received benefit from the Cool Touch laser consists of those who have previously undergone Er:YAG or CO$_2$ laser resurfacing. Patients who had already undergone laser resurfacing and who went on to have Cool Touch therapy were noted to have further softening of perioral rhytids. These patients were pleased that their treatment involved no additional time away from normal activities. Figure 15–6A shows a 51-year-old patient with severe photo damage who previously had undergone CO$_2$ exfoliation with minimal results. Figure 15–6B shows the same patient 1 year after four Cool Touch treatments spaced 6 weeks apart. She was pleased with the additional softening achieved.

After the procedure, patients are asked to grade their pain sensation with therapy. A linear pain scale is used,

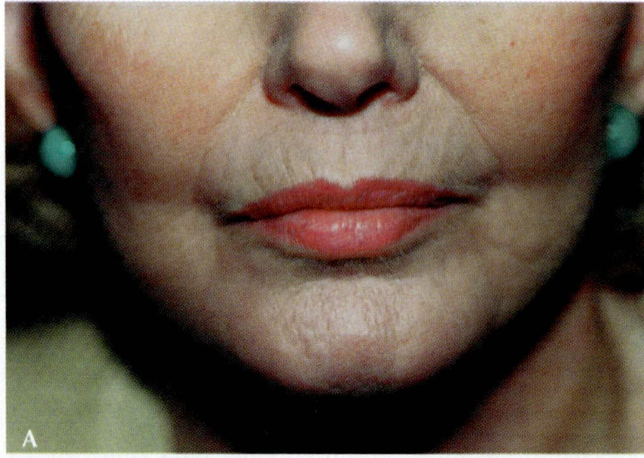

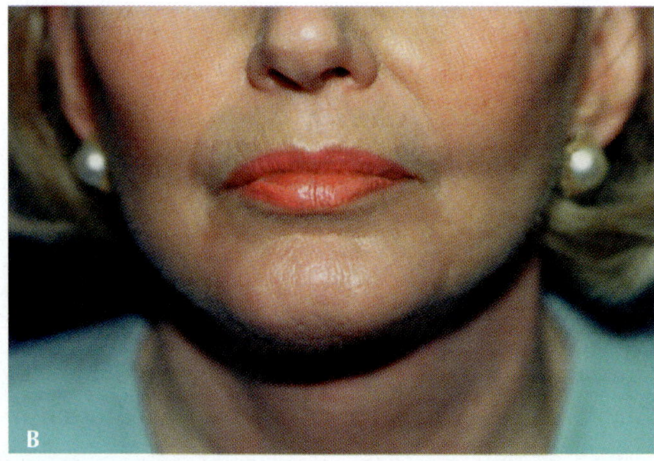

Figure 15–6. (A) Preoperative view of a 51-year-old woman. (B) Same patient 1 year later after four treatments at 32 J/cm^2 each 1 month apart.

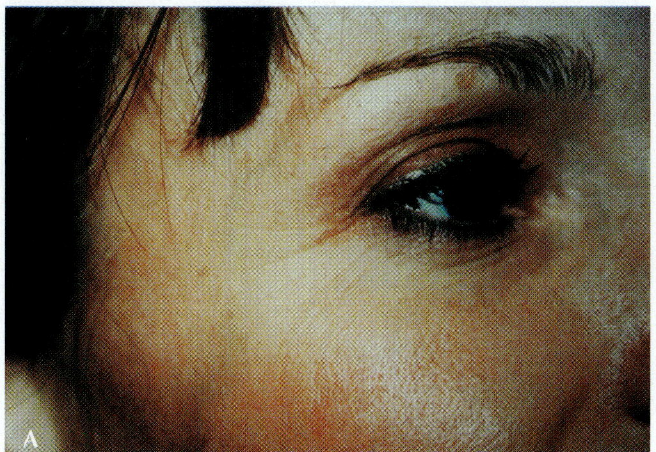
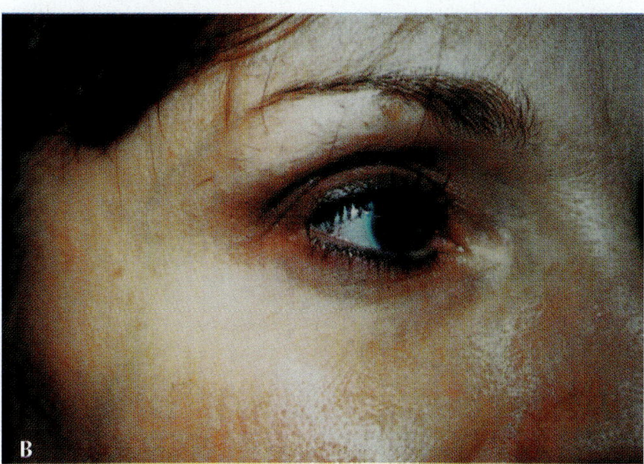

Figure 15–7. (A) Preoperative view of a 36-year-old woman. (B) Same patient 1 year after three treatments at 28 J/cm² each 1 month apart.

with 0 representing no pain and 10 representing the worst pain the patient could imagine. Most patients undergoing thermescent therapy relate pain levels of 3 or 4. After completion of therapy, a 4% aloe-based lidocaine gel is applied to the treatment area. This gel is often kept in a refrigerator and provides a very soothing postoperative experience for the patient. The lidocaine gel is left on for 5 minutes and then removed. Makeup is then applied before the patient leaves the office.

Photographic documentation at each sitting is absolutely essential because the results per treatment are more subtle than with ablative or exfoliating lasers. Most patients return for one to three treatments spaced 2 to 6 weeks apart, with one maintenance treatment recommended every 6 to 12 months. Figures 15–7 and 15–8 show examples of nonablative resurfacing with the thermescent technique at 1 year follow up.

If epidermolysis or blistering occurs, the area should be treated with moist occlusive dressings such as Vigilon or Second Skin. This response usually lasts for 24 to 48 hours and has no bearing on the final result. Such problems can occur if surface temperatures repeatedly exceed 45°C, so decreasing the fluence can prevent this complication.

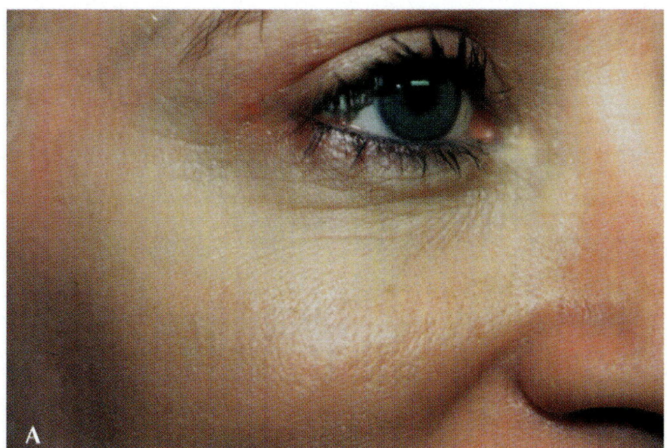
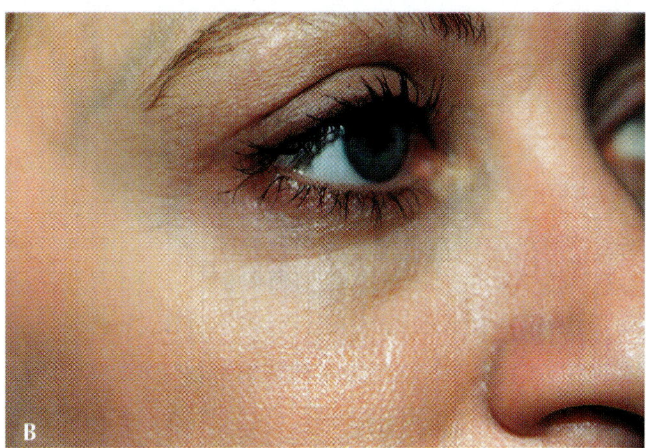

Figure 15–8. (A) Preoperative view of a 45-year-old woman. (B) Same patient 1 year later after three treatments at 32 J/cm² each 1 month apart.

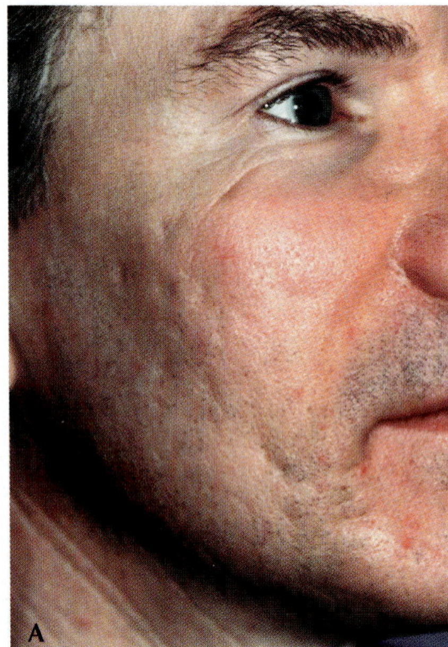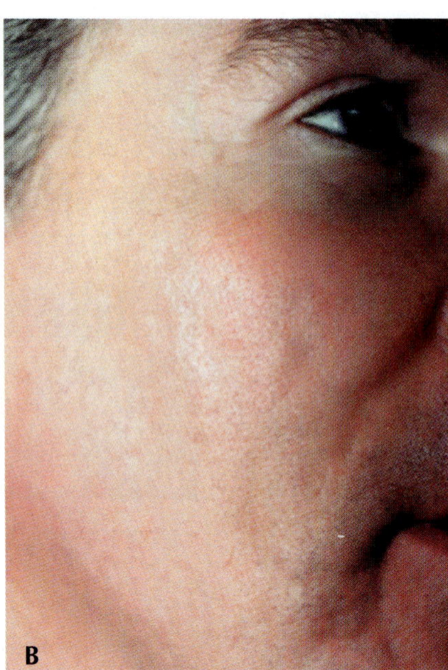

Figure 15–9. (A) Preoperative view of a 47-year-old man. (B) Same patient 1 year later after three Isologen injections and three Cool Touch laser treatments at 32 J/cm^2 1 month after each Isologen injection.

Acne Scars and Chickenpox Scars

Softening of acne scars and chickenpox scars also has been achieved with the thermescent technique, both with and without Isolagen injections. The protocol for treating the base of an acne scar is a double pulse at 28 to 32 J/cm^2. Patients should be aware that a minimum of three treatment sessions is required to achieve a degree of softening that will be noticeable. A greater degree of softening was noted when the Cool Touch laser was combined with injectable fibroblasts or Isolagen therapy. Figure 15–9A shows a 47-year-old patient before Cool Touch laser treatment for acne scarring. Figure 15–9B shows the same patient 1 year after three Isologen injections and three Cool Touch laser treatments.

Atrophic Scars

The treatment of atrophic scars has been successful with use of the Cool Touch laser. Caution must be exercised because the epidermis is much thinner in this region, and epidermolysis with subsequent blistering can occur easily. Starting at 26 J/cm^2 is recommended in the treatment of atrophic scars. Once again, if blistering is noted, these wounds should be treated with topical occlusive dressings such as Vigilon.

Stretch Marks

Early results show softening of stretch marks with each treatment with the Cool Touch laser (Fig. 15–10). Because these areas are also atrophic in nature, care must be taken to avoid epidermolysis in the same manner as in treating atrophic scars.

FUTURE DEVELOPMENTS

The field of nonablative (nonexfoliating) rejuvenation is growing rapidly. In the future it is likely that larger spot sizes will be employed with computer-generated facial patterns to treat larger areas in a shorter period of time. There has been a tremendous acceptance of this method of treatment by patients because no injectable anesthetic is required, no time off from regular daily activities is necessary, and yet softening of facial rhytids and photodamaged skin is achieved.

The search for a more effective method of treating facial wrinkles in photodamaged skin has led to tremendous advancements in the fields of laser physics and tissue biophysical applications. The ability to cause a controlled thermal response at a specific dermal level while preserving the epidermis is a tremendous advancement. Regu-

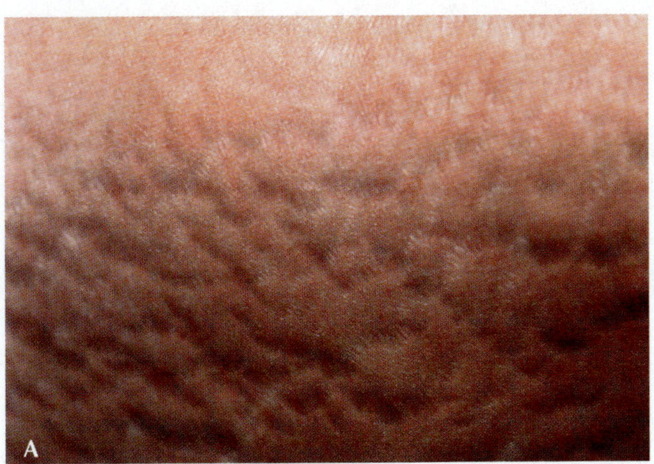

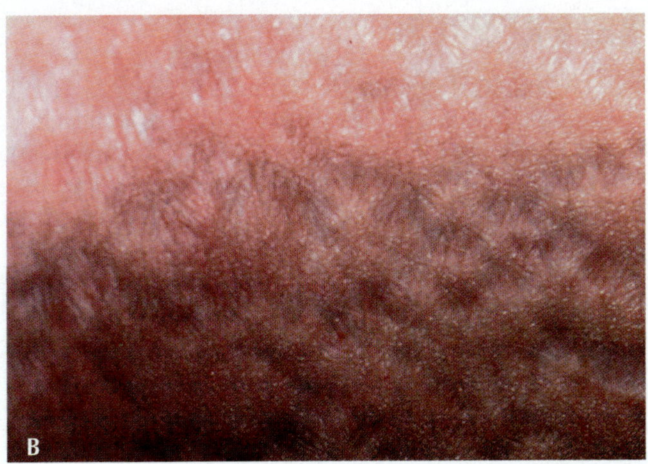

Figure 15–10. (A) Preoperative view of a 42-year-old woman with striae. (B) Same patient 1 year later after six Cool Touch laser treatments at 32 J/cm^2 each 1 month apart.

lating the depth where the thermal injury starts can yield a fibroblast response in the production of new collagen. Further studies examining collagen contracture with this modality are under way. The clinical correlates to what have been found histologically demonstrate a general improvement in skin tone and texture.

The persistent erythema present with the CO$_2$ laser treatment and to a lesser extent with Er:YAG laser treatments is not an issue. To date there have been no problems with hypopigmentation or hyperpigmentation. Hopefully, this will open laser technology to a larger population, including Asian, Hispanic, and African-American patients, who currently experience unacceptable levels of pigmentary complications from resurfacing lasers. The field of nonablative, nonexfoliating laser rejuvenation provides a welcome addition to the armamentarium of aesthetic surgeons.

- which may be accompanied by complications such as persistent erythema, scarring, infection, and pigmentary changes, including hyper- and hypopigmentation.
- New research reveals that epidermal and dermal ablation may not be a prerequisite for collagen remodeling. Long-term wound healing and dermal remodeling are probably the major mechanisms of action responsible for long-term facial rhytid reduction.
- A 4% aloe-based lidocaine gel that has been kept in the refrigerator provides a very soothing postoperative experience for the patient.
- Because each additional nonexfoliating laser treatment brings further softening of fine lines and improvement in the quality, tone, and texture of skin, patients must understand that this is not a "one-time" treatment. Each treatment seems to act as a positive reinforcement for patients.

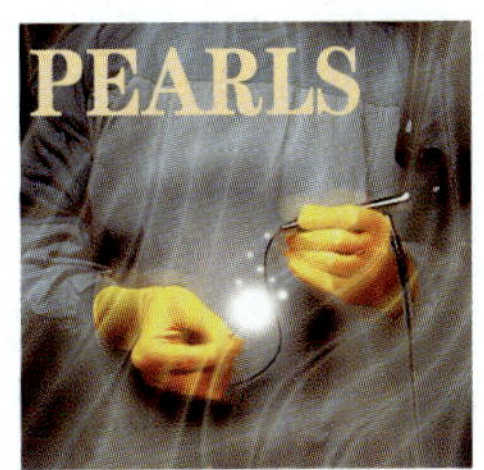

- Nonablative laser techniques soften rhytids without significantly injuring the epidermis. Other laser procedures require exfoliation of the epidermis to soften the appearance of rhytids,

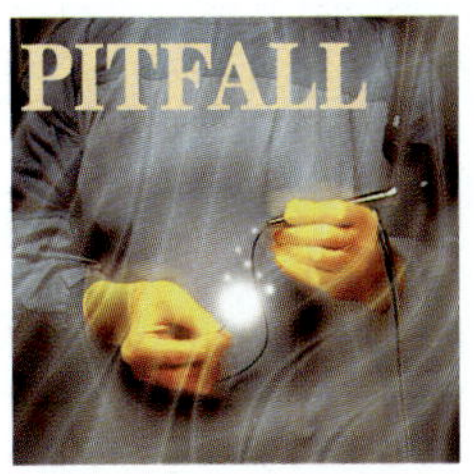

- Patients are frequently concerned about dynamic folds, but the efficacy of the nonablative laser should not be substituted for filling materials such as Gore-Tex, Isologen, and collagen.

REFERENCES

1. Griffiths CEM, Russman AN, Majmudar G, Singer RS, Hamilton TA, Voorhees JJ. Restoration of collagen formation in photodamaged human skin by tretinoin (retinoic acid). *N Engl J Med.* 1993;329:530–535.

2. Ditre CM, Griffin TD, Murphy GF, et al. Effects of α-hydroxy acids on photoaged skin: a pilot clinical, histologic, and ultrastructural study. *J Am Acad Dermatol.* 1996;34:187–195.

3. Grove GL, Grove MJ, Leyden JJ, et al. Skin replica analysis of photodamaged skin after therapy with tretinoin emollient cream. *J Am Acad Dermatol.* 1991;25:231–237.

4. Cotton J, Hood AF, Gonin R, Beeson WH, Hanke W. Histologic evaluation of preauricular and postauricular human skin after high energy short-pulse carbon dioxide laser. *Arch Dermatol.* 1996;132:425–428.

5. Fitzpatrick RE, Tope WD, Goldman MP, Satur NM. Pulsed carbon dioxide laser, trichloroacetic acid, Baker–Gordon phenol, and dermabrasion: a comparative clinical and histologic study of cutaneous resurfacing in a porcine model. *Arch Dermatol.* 1996;132:469–471.

6. Ashcroft GS, Horan MA, Ferguson MWJ. The effects of cutaneous wound healing in mammals. *J Anat.* 1995;187:1–26.

7. Stringer H, Parr J. Shrinkage temperature of eye collagen. *Nature.* 1964;204:1307.

8. Milner TE, Anvari B, Smithies DJ, et al. Analysis of nonablative skin resurfacing. *SPIE Proc.* 1997;2970.

9. Wheeland RG. Lasers for the stimulation or inhibition of wound healing. *J Dermatol Surg Oncol.* 1993;19:747–752.

10. Lask G, Lee PK, Seyfzadeh M, et al. Nonablative laser treatment of facial rhytides. *SPIE,* 1998.

11. Goldberg DJ. Evaluation of the Q-switched Nd:YAG laser for skin resurfacing. *Lasers Surg Med.* 1996; (suppl 8):35.

12. Pearce J, Thomsen S. Rate process analysis of thermal damage. In: Welch AJ, van Gemert MJC, eds. *Optical-Thermal Response of Laser-Irradiated Tissue.* New York: Plenum Press; 1995.

13. Milner TE, Smithies DJ, Goodman DM, Lau A, Nelson JS. Depth determination of chromophores in human skin by pulsed photothermal radiometry. *Appl Opt.* 1996;35:3379–3385.

14. Weaver JA, Stoll AM. Mathematical model of skin exposed to thermal radiation. *Aerospace Med.* 1969;40:24.

15. Milner TE, Goodman DM, Tanenbaum BS, Nelson JS. Depth profiling of laser-heated chromophores in biological tissues by pulsed photothermal radiometry. *J Opt Soc Am A.* 1995;12:1479–1488.

16. Duck FA. *Physical Properties of Tissue: A Comprehensive Reference Book.* London: Academic Press; 1990.

17. Valderrama GL, Fredin LG, Berry MJ, Dempsey BP, Harpole GM. Temperature distributions in laser-irradiated tissues. *SPIE Proc.* 1991;1427:200–213.

18. Kou L, Labrie D, Chylek P. Refractive indices of water and ice in the 0.65- to 2.5-μm spectral range. *Appl Opt.* 1993;32:3531–3540.

19. von Zglinicki T, Lindberg M, Roomans GM, Forslind B. Water and ion distribution profiles in human skin. *Acta Derm Venereol.* 1993;73:340–343.

20. Anvari B, Milner TE, Tanenbaum GBS, Kimel S, Svaassand LO, Nelson JS. Selective cooling of biological tissues: application for thermal mediated therapeutic procedures. *Phys Med Biol.* 1995;40:241–252.

21. Anvari B, Milner TE, Tanenbaum BS, Kimel S, Svaasand LO, Nelson JS. Selective cooling of biological tissues: application for thermally mediated therapeutic procedures. *Phys Med Biol.* 1995;40:241–252.

22. Nelson JS, Milner TE, Anvari B, Tanenbaum BS, Kimel S, Svaasand LO. Dynamic epidermal cooling during pulsed laser treatment of port wine stain—a new methodology with preliminary clinical evaluation. *Arch Dermatol.* 1995;131:695–700.

23. Anvari B, Tanenbaum BS, Milner TE, Kimel S, Svaasand LO, Nelson JS. A theoretical study of the thermal response of skin to cryogen spray cooling and pulsed laser irradiation: implications for the treatment of port wine stain birthmarks. *Phys Med Biol.* 1995;40:1451–1465.

24. Nelson JS, Milner TE, Anvari B, Tanenbaum BS, Svaasand LO, Kimel S. Dynamic epidermal cooling in conjunction with laser-induced photothermolysis of port wine stain blood vessels. *Lasers Surg Med.* 1996;19:224–229.

25. Jacques SL, Wang L. Monte Carlo modeling of light transport in tissues. In: Welch AJ, van Gemert MJC, eds. *Optical-Thermal Response of Laser-Irradiated Tissue.* New York: Plenum Press; 1995:73–100.

26. Anderson RR, Parrish JA. Optical properties of human skin. In: Regan JD, Parris JA, eds. *The Science of Photomedicine.* New York: Plenum Press; 1982:147–194.

27. Welch AJ, van Gemert MJC, Star WM, Wilson BC. Definitions and overview of tissue optics. In: Welch AJ, van Gemert MJC, eds. *Optical-Thermal Response of Laser-Irradiated Tissue.* New York: Plenum Press; 1995:15–46.

28. Thomsen S, Pearce JA, Cheong W-F. Changes in birefringence as markers for thermal damage in tissues. *IEEE Trans Biomed Eng.* 1989;36:1174–1179.

29. Gupta AK, Sibbald RG. Eutectic lidocaine/prilocaine 5% cream and patch may provide satisfactory analgesia for excisional biopsy or curettage with electrosurgery of cutaneous lesions. *J Am Acad Dermatol.* 1996;35:419–423.

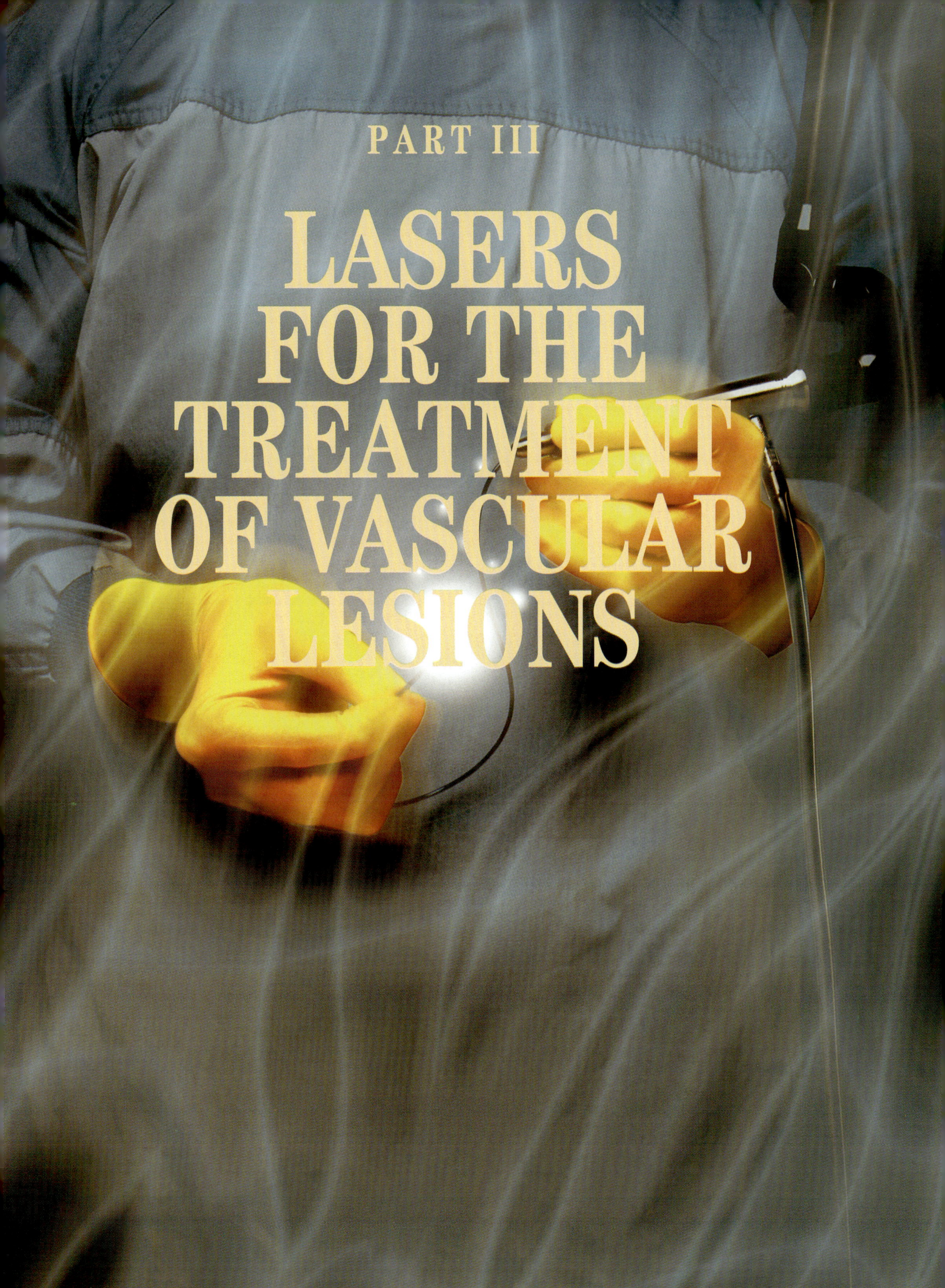

PART III

LASERS
FOR THE
TREATMENT
OF VASCULAR
LESIONS

CHAPTER 16

Vascular Laser Systems

PATRICK K. LEE

Laser therapy of vascular lesions was first developed in the mid-1960s, but it quickly reached a plateau in terms of clinical efficacy. However, within the past 15 years, great strides in laser theory have resulted in technological advancements and created a renaissance in laser therapy of vascular lesions. This chapter discusses the significant progress made in laser technology and cutaneous laser systems.

As discussed previously (see Chapter 1), the first working laser was the ruby laser developed by Maiman in 1960.[1] In 1964, the continuous wave (CW) argon and carbon dioxide (CO_2) lasers were developed and soon became the most frequently used lasers in dermatology.[2] They were used to treat a variety of vascular lesions such as port-wine stains and congenital hemangiomas. However, the treatment applications of these lasers were limited by the risks of unwanted scarring and texture changes[3,4] resulting from the nonspecific thermal injury seen with CW technology, and for many years there were few advances in the state of the art of laser treatment of cutaneous vascular lesions.

In 1983, however, Anderson and Parrish introduced the concept of *selective photothermolysis*,[5] a theory that revolutionized and expanded the applications of cutaneous laser surgery (see Chapter 4). This theory stated that selective tissue absorption of laser light could lead to selective destruction of only that tissue. First, this princi-ple examined the role of chromophores in laser use; chromophores absorb most of incidental laser light that contact the skin. Therefore, if laser light energy were directed at a specific chromophore and at the wavelength specific for that chromophore, then theoretically that chromophore could be selectively targeted and destroyed by the energy. Skin lesions could be treated with a laser that emits a wavelength corresponding to the absorption profile of the chromophore within the lesion. The main chromophores of the skin are hemoglobin, oxyhemoglobin, and melanin. Vascular lesions contain hemoglobin and oxyhemoglobin, which become the targets for wavelength-specific laser light energy.

However, selective photothermolysis involves more than wavelength specificity. In addition, the distribution of laser heating of a particular tissue is determined not only by the depth of light penetration and the particular wavelength used but also by the time over which the light energy is delivered (i.e., the pulse duration or pulse width). This aspect of laser theory is built on the concept of *thermal relaxation time*, which is the time it takes for a tissue irradiated by laser light to lose 50% of its incident heat.[6] If heat is produced in a tissue more slowly than the tissue can cool, that is, longer than its thermal relaxation time, then both the tissue and its surroundings will be heated, leading to greater collateral damage. However, if heat is produced in a tissue more quickly than the tissue can cool, the tissue will become very hot compared with its surroundings with little or no effect on those surroundings. It became apparent that by selective photothermolysis, specific tissues could be subjected to certain types of laser light that produced selective destruction of only that tissue if the light energy was delivered quickly enough (i.e., within the thermal relaxation time).

These principles helped to make clear why many CW lasers can produce widespread thermal damage and resulting scarring. For example, argon laser tissue exposure for photocoagulation of skin lesions is in the range of tens to hundreds of milliseconds. During this time, heat diffuses about 100 μm or more, which is greater than the distance between most blood vessels. Thus, even though the argon laser wavelength (488 nm) is strongly and selectively absorbed by hemoglobin, the entire superficial dermis is heated by thermal conduction during argon laser exposure, which can lead to scarring.[7]

Early experiments with selective photothermolysis on vascular lesions demonstrated how sensitive tissue was to the thermal relaxation time–pulse duration relationship. The first experiments were conducted with *submicrosecond* 577-nm pulses that caused extensive hemorrhage and yielded poor results in the treatment of port-wine stains.[8–11] However, pulses in the *submillisecond* range produced less hemorrhage and greater vessel wall injury, and higher energy fluences were necessary to effect tissue change at the longer pulse durations.[12] Finally, a pulse duration of several hundred *microseconds* was tested, proved to be effective clinically,[13] and soon was in widespread use with the flashlamp-pumped pulsed dye laser. Histologic studies[10–13] demonstrated controlled, selective destruction of treated blood vessels with no infarction of the skin and thus no scarring or textural changes. Development of the concept of selective photothermolysis and its successful clinical application in the flashlamp-pumped pulsed dye laser opened the doors for advances in cutaneous laser treatment of vascular lesions.

LASER TREATMENT OF VASCULAR LESIONS

PORT-WINE STAINS

Port-wine stains are benign proliferations composed of ectatic venules in the papillary dermis that occur in 0.3% of newborns.[14] The ectasia can be progressive, with the lesions becoming hypertrophic and/or nodular in 65% of patients by the fifth decade of life.[15] In addition to their social and psychological impact,[16] 5% of port-wine stains have been associated with Sturge-Weber and Klippel-Trenaunay-Weber syndromes.[14] Previously used treatment approaches include cryosurgery, excision, grafting, irradiation, and the tattooing of flesh-colored ink into affected areas.[17,18] With the advent of selective photothermolysis and advanced laser systems, laser treatment of port-wine stains has become the mainstay of treatment.

Yellow-light lasers, such as the krypton, flashlamp-pumped pulsed dye, and copper lasers, often equipped with a scanning device, are usually the first choice in laser treatment of port-wine stains. These lasers emit wavelengths of 568, 585, and 578 nm, respectively—ranges that are very appropriate for the oxyhemoglobin-deoxyhemoglobin absorbance spectra. In general, the earlier, pinker-appearing grade-I and -II port-wine stains respond very well to the flashlamp-pumped pulsed dye laser, whereas more advanced, nodular grade-IV and -V port-wine stains respond better to the krypton and copper lasers. There is considerable overlap between these lasers as well as the port-wine stain grades, so individual response to a certain laser may vary. Use of these yellow-light lasers yields a low incidence of scarring. Disadvantages include patient discomfort during treatment and posttreatment purpura with the flashlamp-pumped pulsed dye laser. In addition, multiple treatments are needed for significant clearing. Recently, a longer-pulse pulsed dye laser has been developed with wavelengths of 590, 595, and 600 nm, as well as the usual 585 nm. These additional wavelengths and longer pulse duration (1.5 millisecond) may increase the effectiveness of laser treatment for port-wine stains, as well as other lesions.

HEMANGIOMAS

Hemangiomas have been well classified.[19] They are usually present on the head and neck region either at birth or shortly thereafter.[20] Rapid proliferation of endothelial cells and thus immense growth characterize hemangiomas in the first year of life, often followed by complete or partial involution by age 12.[21,22] Smaller hemangiomas usually involute spontaneously without treatment with satisfactory cosmetic and functional results. However, as many as 10 to 20% of hemangiomas require surgical intervention,[23] often because of functional restriction or impingement on vital structures of the face, orbit, or airway. Rarely, the Kasabach-Merritt syndrome (platelet trapping in larger hemangiomas) can occur, causing thrombocytopenia and afibrinogenemia.[24] Early treatment of hemangiomas is preferred because of the psychological trauma of young patients having disfiguring facial lesions, sometimes even after involution.

Treatment in the past included electrocautery, radiation, sclerotherapy, and cryotherapy, which sometimes leave significant scarring. Systemic steroids, which inhibit angiogenesis, work in only 30% of patients during the proliferative phase.[25] The flashlamp-pumped pulsed dye laser and the copper laser can be used to target the superficial blood vessels, destroying them with little or no scarring. The flashlamp-pumped pulsed dye laser can be effective on superficial hemangiomas even if they are ulcerated;[23,26] however, further proliferation of the deeper component of the hemangioma may still occur.[27] Copper lasers have a deeper effect, possibly because of vasoconstriction.[28] Combination treatment with a yellow-light laser followed by surgical excision with a contact neodymium:YAG (Nd:YAG) laser has been used to eradicate deeper (cavernous) and mixed hemangiomas.[28,29]

FACIAL TELANGIECTASIAS

Facial telangiectasias can occur as essential telangiectasias or secondary to chronic sun exposure or chronic dermatologic conditions such as rosacea. Treatment options in the past have included electrocautery, cryotherapy, and sclerotherapy, with scarring and skin textural changes being major limitations. Numerous laser systems can be used to treat these lesions adequately. However, the flashlamp-pumped pulsed dye laser can be very effective, often in only one treatment. The posttreatment purpura, which can last 7 to 10 days, may be objectionable[30] to some patients. Copper lasers can be used to treat larger vessels, leaving only minimal or no erythema[31] and no purpura. The frequency-doubled Nd:YAG, or potassium-titanyl-phosphate (KTP) laser and the krypton laser also give very acceptable results. The long-pulse pulsed dye laser with multiple wavelengths also holds promise for treatment of larger facial vessels.

Also available to treat facial telangiectasias is the PhotoDerm system. It is not a laser but is a noncoherent, intense pulsed light source developed to treat a variety of benign cutaneous lesions, including facial and leg telangiectasias. The device uses a flashlamp as a light (i.e., thermal) source to generate energy and was developed with a great range of parameters. Because it is not a laser, it does not emit light at a specific wavelength; rather, it uses a series of cutoff filters. These filters cut out the spectrum of light emitted by the flashlamp below that of the particular wavelength; for example, a 550-nm cutoff filter allows transmission of light from 550 to approximately 900 nm.[32] This energy is directed into the skin and used to heat the vessels to coagulate them. By its inherent design for energy application, the PhotoDerm system is reportedly able to transfer heat such that the heat will dissipate within the vessels' thermal relaxation time, thus conforming to the principle of selective photothermolysis. The PhotoDerm system can treat facial vessels with little or no postoperative erythema or purpura.

LEG TELANGIECTASIAS

Abnormal leg veins occur in 29 to 41% of women and 6 to 15% of men in the United States.[33] Genetic predisposition, hyperestrogenic states, standing vocations, localized trauma, and obesity are all major predisposing factors.[34,35] Leg veins can be divided into two categories: *varicosities* of the greater and lesser saphenous veins, which are connected to the deep venous system, and *superficial telangiectasias*, with negligible deeper connections. For the former, conventional treatments have included support hose, surgery, aggressive sclerotherapy,[36] and more recently, ambulatory phlebectomy.[37] Superficial telangiectasias of the leg are primarily a cosmetic concern, but cosmesis is the most common reason patients seek treatment.[38]

The most common method for treating leg telangiectasias is sclerotherapy.[38] Its effectiveness is well documented; for more than two decades, the procedure has been shown to be reliable and predictable.[37] However, the most frequent side effects of sclerotherapy in general are postsclerosis pigmentation ($\geq 30\%$)[39] and telangiectatic matting (5 to 40%).[40] These side effects can be very difficult to treat.

Because of these side effects, there has been a search for alternative therapies for superficial telangiectasias of the leg, such as laser therapy. In the past, CW laser systems, such as the CO_2 and argon lasers, were tested for their effect on leg veins.[41] However, scarring, hypo- and hyperpigmentation, pain, and recurrence of treated vessels limited their use. These complications far outweighed the side effects of sclerotherapy.[38]

When the flashlamp-pumped pulsed dye laser proved effective for cutaneous vascular lesions, its use in the treatment of leg veins seemed to be a natural extension. However, treatment results were disappointing because of inconsistent response and persistent postinflammatory hyperpigmentation.[42] These poor results may have been due to the deeper location of leg telangiectasias, their larger diameter, and/or the presence of connections with the deep venous system, resulting in rapid recanalization of the coagulated vessel.[43] Moreover, pulsed dye laser treatment of leg veins combined with sclerotherapy offered no greater resolution than treatment by sclerotherapy alone.[38]

Specific laser systems for the treatment of leg telangiectasias are discussed in detail in subsequent chapters. The consensus appears to be that laser surgery

for leg telangiectasias should not be a first-line treatment but should be complementary to either prior or simultaneous injection sclerotherapy. The unpredictability of response of leg telangiectasias to either laser or PhotoDerm treatment cannot compete with the efficacy and cost-effectiveness of sclerotherapy as a first-line treatment.

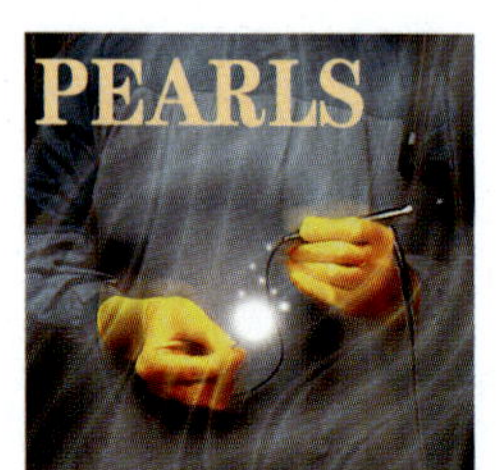

- Vascular lesions contain the chromophores hemoglobin and oxyhemoglobin, which become the targets for wavelength-specific laser light energy.
- Development of the concept of selective photothermolysis and its successful clinical application in the flashlamp-pumped pulsed dye laser opened the doors for advances in cutaneous laser treatment of vascular lesions.
- The flashlamp-pumped pulsed dye laser can be effective on superficial hemangiomas even if they are ulcerated; however, further proliferation of the deeper component of the hemangioma may still occur.
- The PhotoDerm system is not a laser so it does not emit light at a specific wavelength but uses a series of cutoff filters to cut out the spectrum of light emitted by the flashlamp below that of the particular wavelength. The PhotoDerm system can treat facial vessels with little or no postoperative erythema or purpura.

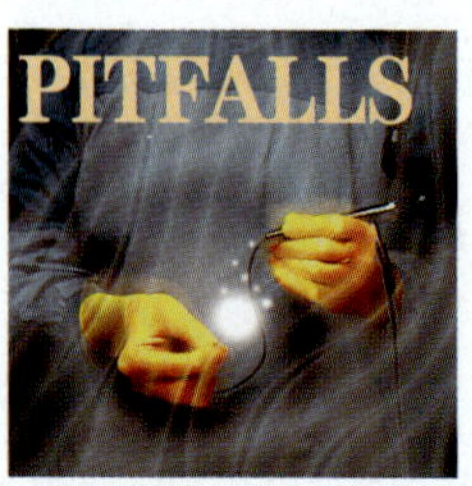

- Although the argon laser wavelength is strongly and selectively absorbed by hemoglobin, the entire superficial dermis is heated by thermal conduction during argon laser exposure, which can lead to scarring, thus making the argon laser unsuitable for treating vascular lesions.

- Disadvantages with the flashlamp-pumped pulsed dye laser for the treatment of port-wine stains include patient discomfort during treatment and posttreatment purpura. In addition, multiple treatments are needed for significant clearing.

REFERENCES

1. Maiman T. Stimulated optical radiation in ruby. *Nature.* 1960;187:493–494.
2. Arndt KA, Noe JM. Lasers in dermatology. *Arch Dermatol.* 1982;118:293–295.
3. van Gemert MJC, Welch AJ, Tan OT, et al. Limitations of carbon dioxide lasers for treatment of port-wine stains. *Arch Dermatol.* 1987;123:71–73.
4. Noe JM, Barsky SH, Geer DE, et al. Port wine stains and the response to argon laser therapy: successful treatment and the predictive role of color, age, and biopsy. *Plast Reconstr Surg.* 1980;65:130–139.
5. Anderson RR, Parrish JA. Selective photothermolysis: precise microsurgery by selective absorption of pulsed radiation. *Science.* 1983;220:524–527.
6. Tan OT, Sherwood K, Gilchrest BA. Treatment of children with port-wine stains using the flashlamp-pulsed tunable dye laser. *N Engl J Med.* 1989;320:416–421.
7. Anderson RR, Levins PC, Grevelink JM. Lasers in dermatology. In: Fitzpatrick TB, Eisen AZ, Wolff K, et al, eds. *Dermatology in General Medicine.* 4th ed. New York: McGraw-Hill, Inc.; 1993:1755–1766.
8. Anderson RR, Parrish JA. Microvasculature can be selectively damaged using dye lasers: a basic theory and experimental evidence in human skin. *Lasers Surg Med.* 1981; 1:263–276.
9. Greenwald J, Rosen S, Anderson RR, et al. Comparative histologic studies of the tunable dye (at 577 nm) laser and argon laser: the specific vascular effects of the dye laser. *J Invest Dermatol.* 1981;77:305–310.
10. Anderson RR, Jaenicke KF, Parrish JA. Mechanisms of selective vascular changes caused by dye lasers. *Lasers Surg Med.* 1983;3:211–215.
11. Hulsbergen-Henning JP, van Gemert MJ, Lahaye CT. Clinical and histological evaluation of port-wine stains with a microsecond pulsed dye laser at 577 nm. *Lasers Surg Med.* 1984;4:375–380.
12. Garden JM, Tan OT, Kerschmann R, et al. Effect of dye laser pulse duration on selective cutaneous vascular injury. *J Invest Dermatol.* 1986;87:653–657.
13. Morelli JG, Tan OT, Garden JM, et al. Tunable dye laser (577 nm) treatment of port-wine stains. *Lasers Surg Med.* 1986:6:94–99.
14. Jacob AH, Walton RG. The incidence of birthmarks in the neonate. *Pediatrics.* 1976;58:218–222.
15. Geronemus RG, Ashinoff R. The medical necessity of evaluation and treatment of port-wine stains. *J Dermatol Surg Oncol.* 1991;17:76–79.
16. Kalick SM. Toward an interdisciplinary psychology of appearance. *Psychiatry.* 1978;41:243–253.
17. Hidano A, Ogihara Y. Cryotherapy with solid carbon dioxide in the treatment of nevus flammeus. *J Dermatol Surg Oncol.* 1977;3:213–216.
18. Conway H, Montry RE. Permanent camouflage of capillary hemangiomas of face by intradermal injection of insoluble pigments (tattooing): indications for surgery. *N Y State J Med* 1965;65:876–885.
19. Mulliken JB, Glowacki J. Hemangiomas and vascular malformations in infants and children: a classification based on endothelial characteristics. *Plast Reconstr Surg.* 1982;69: 412–422.
20. Simpson JR. Natural history of cavernous hemangiomata. *Lancet.* 1959;2:1057–1059.
21. Lister WA. The natural history of strawberry nevi. *Lancet.* 1938;253:1429–1434.
22. Bowers RE, Graham EA, Tomlinson KM. The natural history of the strawberry nevus. *Arch Dermatol.* 1960; 82:667–680.
23. Sherwood KA, Tan OT. Treatment of a capillary hemangioma with the flashlamp-pumped-dye laser. *J Am Acad Dermatol.* 1990;22:136–137.
24. Kasabach HH, Merritt KK. Capillary hemangioma with extensive purpura. *Am J Dis Child.* 1940;59:1063–1070.
25. Enjolras O, Riche MC, Merland JJ, et al. Management of alarming hemangiomas in infancy: a review of 25 cases. *Pediatrics.* 1990;85:491–498.
26. Ashinoff R, Geronemus RG. Capillary hemangioma and treatment with the flash lamp-pumped pulsed dye laser. *Arch Dermatol.* 1991;127:202–205.
27. Ashinoff R, Geronemus RG. Failure of the flashlamp-pumped pulsed dye laser to prevent progression of the deep component of hemangiomas. *Pediatr Dermatol.* 1993; 10:77–80.
28. Waner M, Suen JY, Dinehardt S. Treatment of hemangiomas of the head and neck. *Laryngoscope.* 1992;102:1123–1132.
29. Waner M, Key JM. Vascular lesions of the lips [abstract]. *Lasers Surg Med.* 1994;13(suppl 6):48.
30. Gonzalez E, Gange RW, Momtaz KT. Treatment of telangiectases and other benign vascular lesions with the 577 nm pulsed dye laser. *J Am Acad Dermatol.* 1992; 27:220–226.

31. Dinehart SM, Waner M, Flock S. The copper vapor laser for treatment of cutaneous vascular and pigmented lesions. *J Dermatol Surg Oncol.* 1993;19:370–375.

32. Goldman MP, Eckhouse S. Photothermal sclerosis of leg veins. *Dermatol Surg.* 1996;22:323–330.

33. Engel A, Johnson ML, Haynes SG. Health effects of sunlight exposure in the United States: Results from the first national health and nutrition examination survey: 1971–1974. *Arch Dermatol.* 1988;124:72–79.

34. Sadick NS. Predisposing factors of varicose and telangiectatic leg veins. *J Dermatol Surg Oncol.* 1992;18:883–836.

35. Lofgren KA. Varicose veins: their symptoms, complications, and management. *Postgrad Med.* 1979;65:131–139.

36. Fitzpatrick TB, Eisen AZ, Wolff K, et al, eds. *Dermatology in General Medicine*, 4th ed. New York: McGraw-Hill; 1993: 2095–2096.

37. Weiss MA, Weiss RA. Sclerotherapy in the U.S. *Dermatol Surg.* 1995;21:393–396.

38. Goldman MP, Fitzpatrick RE. Pulsed-dye laser treatment of leg telangiectasia: with and without simultaneous sclerotherapy. *J Dermatol Surg Oncol.* 1990;16:338–344.

39. Goldman MP, Kaplan RP, Duffy DM. Postsclerotherapy hyperpigmentation: a histologic evaluation. *J Dermatol Surg Oncol.* 1987;13:547–550.

40. Duffy DM. Understanding sclerotherapy. In: Lask GP, Moy RL, eds. *Principles and Techniques of Cutaneous Surgery.* New York: McGraw-Hill; 1996:411–412.

41. Apfelberg DB, Maser MR, Lash H, et al. Use of the argon and carbon dioxide lasers for treatment of superficial venous varicosities of the lower extremity. *Lasers Surg Med.* 1984; 4:221–231.

42. Lask GP, Glassberg E. 585–nm pulsed dye laser for the treatment of cutaneous lesions. *Clin Dermatol* 1995;13:63–67.

43. Polla LL, Tan OT, Garden JM, et al. Tunable pulsed dye laser for the treatment of benign cutaneous vascular ectasia. *Dermatol* 1987;174:11–17.

CHAPTER 17

Management of Vascular Lesions of the Head and Neck

MILTON WANER

Lasers have revolutionized the treatment of vascular lesions and have become indispensable. We are now able to ablate subcutaneous vessels of certain dimensions through intact skin and destroy very little but the targeted vessels. However, there are still limitations. Lasers currently in use destroy only the most superficial of vessels, and there is no single laser that can successfully treat all vascular lesions. Lesions consisting of large or deep vessels are still not amenable to laser treatment and should be treated with other modalities. There exists, however, an unfortunate tendency among physicians to treat all lesions with the same modality, which accounts for much of the confusion about which modality is best for which lesion. The major objective of this chapter is to describe a logical approach to the treatment of vascular lesions using different lasers in different situations.

BASIC LASER PRINCIPLES

Two requirements are necessary to selectively destroy a given population of blood vessels with a laser. The laser should emit the correct wavelength of light, and the length of time the vessels are exposed to this light should be sufficient to destroy only the vessels and not the surrounding tissue. There is, thus, a finite exposure time that is related to the thermal relaxation time of the skin.

WAVELENGTH

The wavelength of the laser light is important for two reasons: (1) the light should penetrate a sufficient depth to reach the affected vessels, and (2) the wavelength of light used should be selectively absorbed by these vessels. Unfortunately, there is no ideal wavelength that fulfills both these requirements. However, within the visible spectrum, a longer wavelength of light has a smaller degree of scatter and, thus, deeper penetration. Therefore, I prefer to use the longest possible wavelength that is absorbed by the target. Because the depth of the vessels can vary from a few hundred microns to several centimeters, the limited depth of penetration of light within tissue restricts one's ability to effectively treat all but the most superficial of vascular lesions.

The abundance of hemoglobin (both the oxygenated and the deoxygenated forms) makes it a convenient intravascular target. The absorption spectrum of oxyhemoglobin dictates the use of yellow or green light because there is ample absorption at these wavelengths (Fig. 17–1). The absorption coefficient drops off sharply after 600 nm, but melanin still absorbs strongly throughout the visible spectrum. As a result, these wavelengths (532 and 585 to 600 nm) have been exploited.[1–3] Because there is strong absorption at both 532 and 585 nm, most published data concern these two wavelengths. Unfortunately, light at these wavelengths will only penetrate the first 2 to 3 mm of tissue.

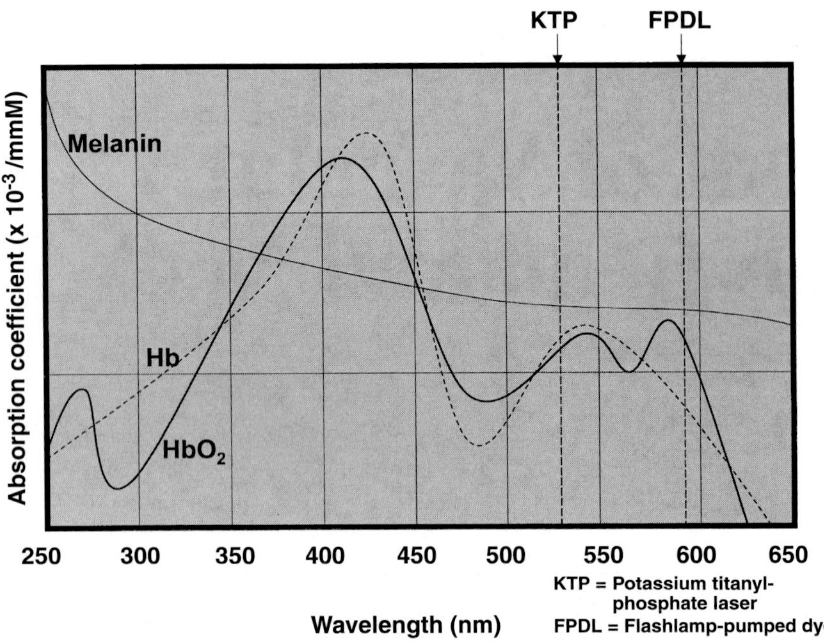

Figure 17–1. The absorption spectrum of hemoglobin (Hb), oxyhemoglobin (HbO_2), and melanin.

Recent studies have shown that a longer wavelength (1064 nm) can destroy deeper and larger vessels.[4,5] Because there is no selective absorption by hemoglobin at this wavelength, it is important to limit exposure time to prevent damage to the overlying mucosa or skin.[6]

EXPOSURE TIME

Once the light is absorbed by hemoglobin, it is converted to thermal energy and heats up the vessel. After the vessel is saturated with thermal energy, the energy is conducted to the surrounding tissue. To confine the damage to the vessels and spare the surrounding tissue, exposure time is crucial. The time it takes to fully saturate the target vessel with thermal energy is known as the *thermal loading time*, which is roughly equivalent to the *thermal relaxation time*, or the time it takes for 50% of the heat in a tissue to dissipate.[7]

The thermal loading time is related to the size of the vessel; a larger vessel has a longer thermal loading time (i.e., it takes more time to heat the vessel to thermally saturate it). It is important to consider the average vessel diameter of the lesion being treated to determine the appropriate exposure time (see Table 17–1). Because vascular lesions vary so widely in terms of vessel diameters,

Table 17–1. The Relationship between Vessel Diameter and Thermal Relaxation Time

Vessel Diameter	Thermal Relaxation Time
30 μm	0.86 ms
40 μm	1.54 ms
50 μm	2.40 ms
100 μm	9.60 ms

the ideal vascular lesion laser needs to vary its pulse width or exposure time in the range of microseconds to seconds. Unfortunately, no such laser exists. Therefore, it is necessary to subclassify vascular malformations according to vessel diameter and then use the most appropriate laser.

Small vessel disorders consist of vessels 100 μm or less in diameter. These include early port-wine stains and proliferating hemangiomas (Figs. 17–2 and 17–3). Because the thermal loading time is in the microsecond range, a flashlamp-pumped dye laser is used (exposure time 500 to 1500 microseconds).

Medium-sized vessel disorders have vessels 100 to 400 μm wide. Intermediate and advanced port-wine stains, as well as some involuting hemangiomas, are in this category (Figs. 17–4 and 17–5). Exposure times for vessels this size

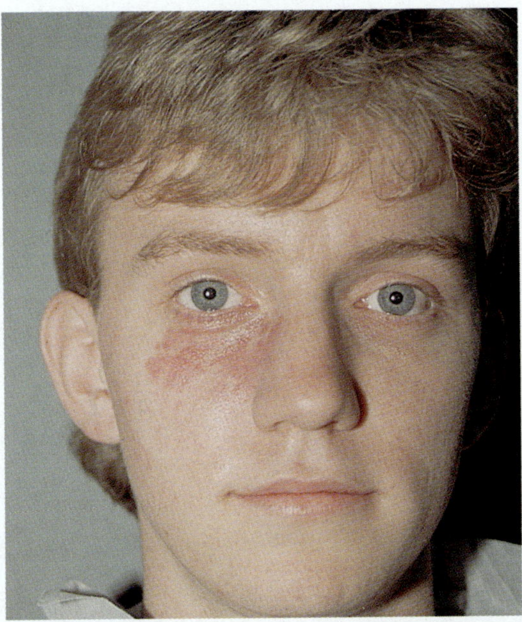

Figure 17–2. A teenager with a grade-I port-wine stain involving his right cheek.

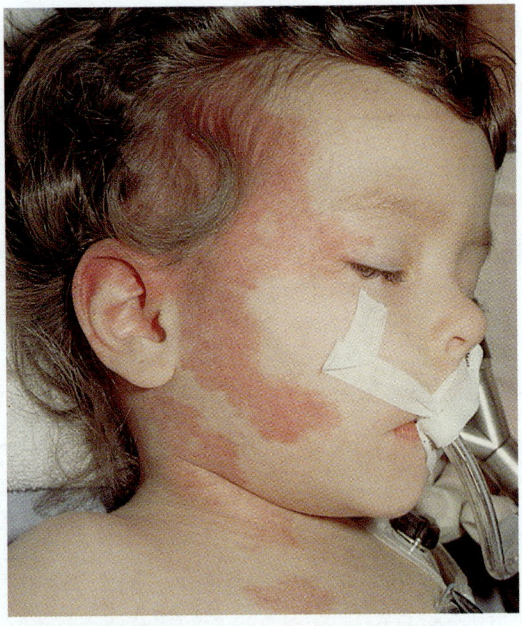

Figure 17–3. A child with a grade-II port-wine stain.

vary between 10 and 100 milliseconds, and a potassium-titanyl-phosphate (KTP) laser is an appropriate choice.

Large vessel disorders consist of vessels larger than 400 μm. Advanced port-wine stains and venous malformations make up this category and are best treated with a long-pulsed or continuous-wave neodymium:yttrium-aluminum-garnet (Nd:YAG) laser (Figs. 17–6 and 17–7). These lasers are capable of exposure times in the range of 1 second, and I typically use exposure times of between 0.1 and 0.5 second.

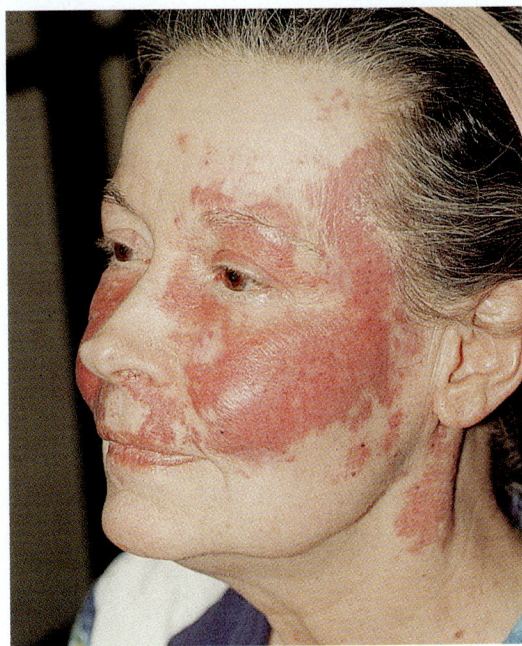

Figure 17–4. An adult with a grade-III port-wine stain.

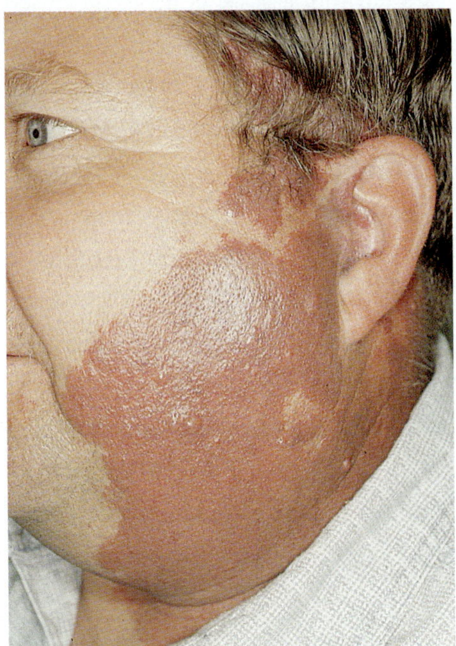

Figure 17–5. An adult with a grade-IV port-wine stain. Note the presence of early cobblestone formation.

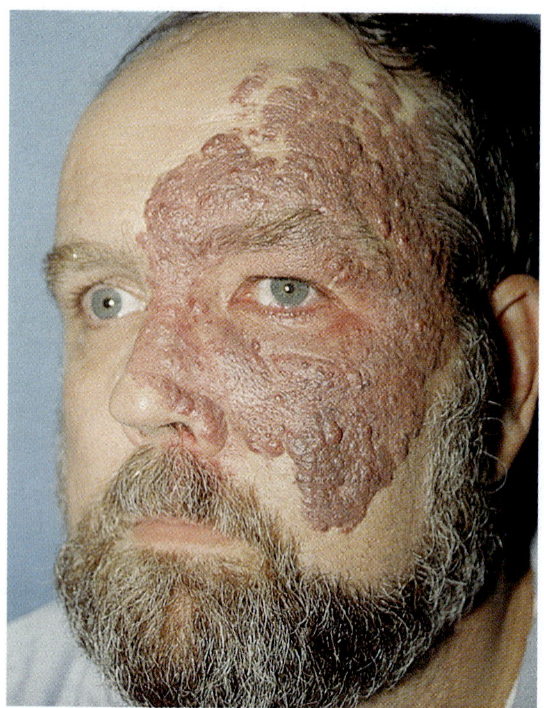

Figure 17–6. An adult with an advanced port-wine stain showing cobblestone formation. These vessels are greater than 400 μm in diameter.

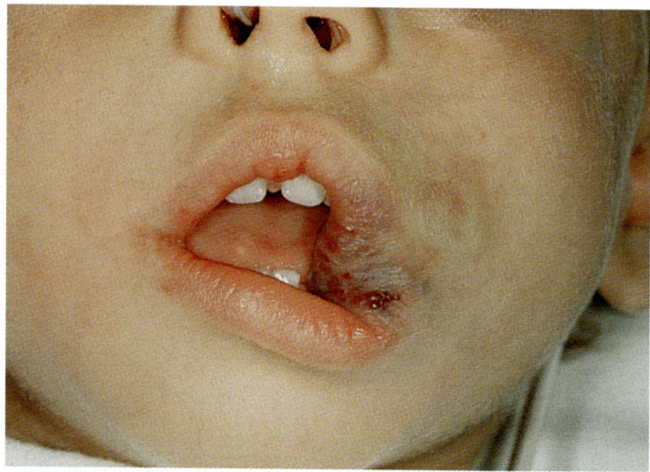

Figure 17–7. An infant with a venous malformation involving the vermilion of the upper lip and buccal mucosa. These vessels are much larger than 400 μm in diameter.

CLASSIFICATION OF VASCULAR LESIONS

The reclassification of congenital vascular lesions was the next major advance in the management of vascular lesions.[8] The term *hemangioma* is no longer used generically to describe all vascular lesions. Recent work has shown that there are two main groups of vascular lesions: hemangiomas and vascular malformations.[8] Hemangiomas are pediatric tumors that usually are not present at birth, proliferate during the first year of life, and then involute. These tumors are the most common tumors in infants and are found in 1 of every 10 infants.[9] *Vascular malformations*, on the other hand, are always present at birth, never proliferate, and never involute. This latter group is further subdivided according to vascular content: venous, venular, arteriovenous, lymphatic, or mixed.[10] Vascular malformations are much less common and are seen in about one of every 1000 live births.[11]

HEMANGIOMAS

Hemangiomas are usually not present at birth, although the incidence at birth is about 30%. Their course is con-

sistent in that they invariably proliferate during the first year of life and then ultimately involute over the next 5 to 10 years. Although 10% of infants are affected, a smaller percentage require some form of intervention, perhaps a further 1 in 10 of this 10%. Hemangiomas are much more common in females, and the male-to-female ratio is believed to be 1:6.[12] Hemangiomas may be superficial or deep with respect to skin or mucosa. Superficial lesions present as the classic *strawberry birthmark*, whereas deep hemangiomas were previously known as *cavernous hemangiomas* (Figs. 17–8 and 17–9). These terms are confusing because the pathology of these lesions is identical; the only difference is their depth. Therefore, I refer to them as superficial and deep (or compound) hemangiomas.

Toward the end of the first year of life, hemangiomas cease to proliferate and begin their inevitable, although sometimes protracted, course of involution. Involution may or may not be complete (Fig. 17–10), probably depending on the speed of the process. In general, lesions that complete the process of involution before 6 years of age are much less likely to require corrective surgery than lesions that take much longer to involute.[13]

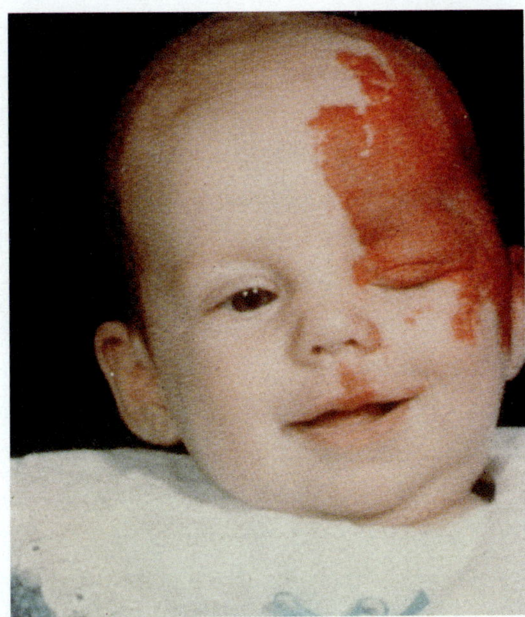

Figure 17–8. An infant with a superficial hemangioma. This type of lesion was known previously as a *strawberry birthmark*.

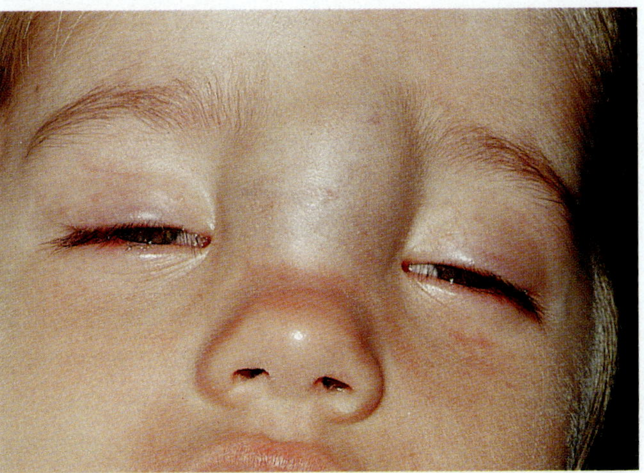

Figure 17–9. A child with a deep glabellar hemangioma. This type of lesion was known previously as a *cavernous hemangioma*.

VASCULAR MALFORMATIONS

In contrast with hemangiomas, vascular malformations are always present at birth (although they may not be readily apparent), never proliferate, and never involute.[8] Their natural history is characterized by slow, steady expansion with advancing age. This is due to progressive ectasia of the existing vessels that make up the lesion. Vascular malformations are further subdivided according to the vessel type that makes up the lesion (Box 17–1).[8,12] Vascular malformations are much less common than hemangiomas and affect males and females equally. Although there are no published data regarding their overall incidence, it is known that the incidence of venular malformations is around 3 per 1000 live births.[11]

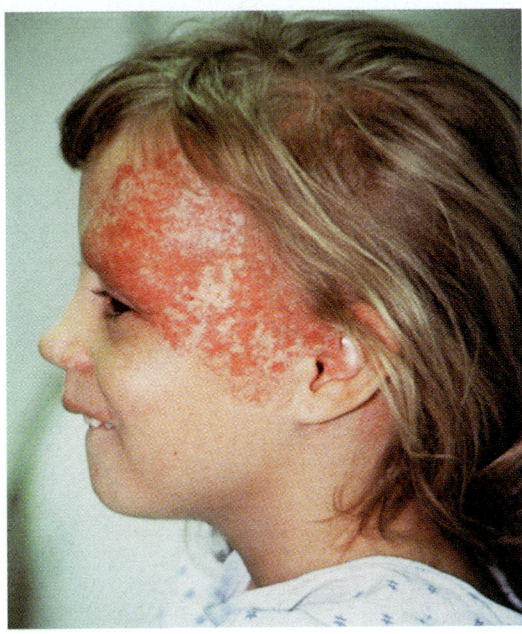

Figure 17–10. A child with a hemangioma that has not completely involuted. The child still has residual telangiectasia as well as some epidermal atrophy and a small amount of residual deep hemangioma overlying her eyebrow. This is the same child as was shown in Figure 17–8.

Box 17–1. Vascular Malformations Categorized by Vessel Type

Venous malformations

Venular malformations (port-wine stains)

Arteriovenous malformations

Lymphatic malformations

Mixed malformations (e.g., mixed venous lymphatic malformations, mixed venous venular malformations, mixed venous lymphatic capillary malformations)

Venular Malformations (Port-Wine Stains)

These are the best known vascular malformations and appear to be the most common. Venular malformations conform to the dermatomal distribution of cutaneous sensory innovation, and recent evidence suggests that their etiology is related to a relative or absolute deficiency of autonomic vascular innovation within the papillary plexus.[14,15] This deficiency results in a loss of venomotor tone, which in turn leads to vasodilatation; the number of vessels does not increase, but vessel diameter does increase. This lack of innervation has two important clinical implications: (1) the lack of venomotor tone results in progressive ectasia. Therefore, lesions progress from flat, light macules to dark, thick papules with a "cobblestoned" appearance (the result of coalescence of the vessels). (2) The rate of this progression is inversely related to degree of innervation. An absolute lack of innervation results in a complete loss of venomotor tone, which speeds the rate of progress.[10]

Venular malformations can be subclassified according to the degree of ectasia of the component vessels.[16] Although this classification is somewhat arbitrary, it does have clinical relevance in that the type of laser used to treat the lesion is determined by vessel diameter. The response to treatment, however, appears to be related to the depth of the vessels rather than to their diameter. Early lesions (i.e., grade-I and -II lesions) consist of vessels less than 100 μm in diameter. Vessels of this size have a thermal relaxation time in the microsecond range and are best treated with a pulsed dye laser. Although the vessel diameter of grade-III lesions is 100 to 400 μm, treatment response is seen with both the pulsed dye laser and the KTP laser. The vessel size of the more advanced grade-IV lesions ($>$400 μm) precludes treatment with a pulsed dye laser. The KTP laser has exposure times of up to 100 milliseconds and is thus more suitable for these lesions.

Venous Malformations

Venous malformations are made up of the many larger, deeper vessels that populate the subcutaneous, submucosal, and intramuscular venous plexi. They commonly involve the buccal fat space, tongue, and upper or lower lips[10] (Figs. 17–11 and 17–12). They are frequently multifocal

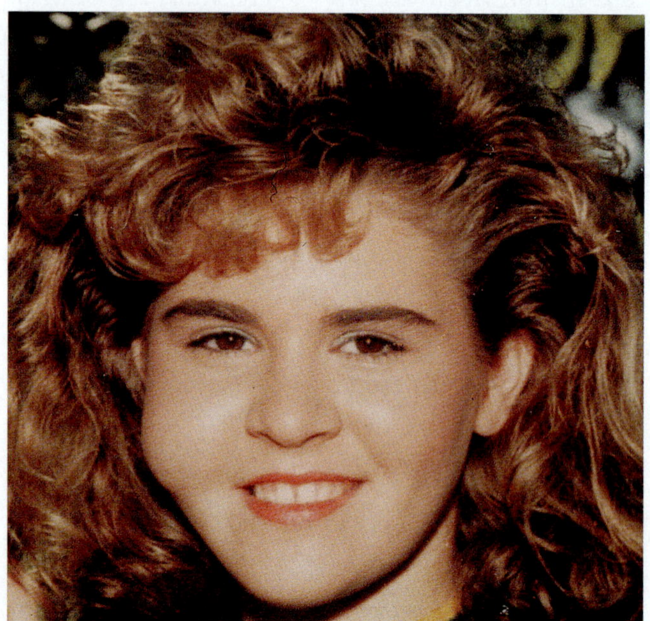

Figure 17–11. A teenager with a venous malformation involving her buccal fat space, which is a common site for these lesions. Although no vascular lesion was evident on clinical inspection, an MRI and surgical histology confirmed the presence of a venous malformation.

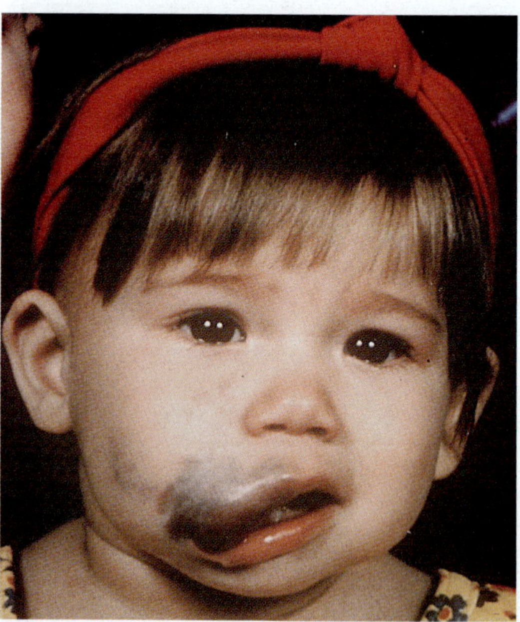

Figure 17–12. An 18-month-old with a venous malformation of the upper lip as well as some involvement of the buccal fat space. These are common sites for venous malformations.

and often intramuscular. This latter group was known previously as *intramuscular hemangiomas*. Lesions close to the surface have a bluish discoloration, whereas deeper lesions have no discoloration.[10] All venous malformations of the head and neck are soft and compressible and empty easily with pressure. They also fill and distend with raised intravascular pressure. Phleboliths are pathognomonic of the diagnosis and sometimes can be felt clinically. Their natural history is similar to that of venular malformations in that they tend to hypertrophy (enlarge) with advancing age.[10]

Arteriovenous Malformations

Arteriovenous malformations (AVMs) are congenital vascular malformations, whereas their counterpart, the arteriovenous fistula, is an acquired lesion usually made up of a single fistula tract.[8] The components of an AVM are the nidus, the afferent hypertrophied arterial supply, and the efferent dilated venous drainage (Fig. 17–13). As with other vascular lesions, AVMs enlarge with advancing age, and the three components become less distinct.[17] Recent evidence suggests that the underlying abnormality appears to be deficient control at the precapillary sphincter.[17] This allows unimpeded flow into the capillary bed, which expands to form the nidus. With time, and as a consequence of increased flow across the capillary bed, the afferent arteries hypertrophy and the efferent venous system dilates.

Arteriovenous malformations appear as a firm mass that does not compress easily, and, occasionally, an arterial pulsation may be palpable, although this is surprisingly infrequent. The skin overlying the mass occasionally is discolored, which should be an indication of skin involvement.

Lymphatic Malformations

Previously used terms such as *lymphangiomas* and *lymphangiohemangiomas* are all synonymous with the term *lymphatic malformation*. Lymphatic malformations are congenital lesions (always present at birth), although they may not be readily apparent until later. These lesions represent an area of poor lymphatic drainage[10,18] and appear histologically as an area of dilated cyst-like lymph-filled spaces.[19] The lesion may be macrocystic, microcystic, or mixed. Macrocystic lesions usually are found in the neck and tend to be localized, whereas microcystic lesions usually are facial and tend to be poorly localized (Fig. 17–14).

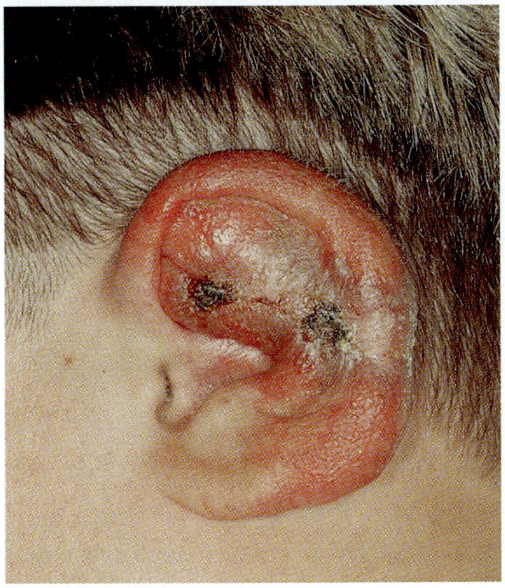

Figure 17–13. An arteriovenous malformation involving a child's pinna. The lesion parasitized a blood supply from the superficial temporal vessels as well as from the postauricular vessels. These vessels were, consequently, dilated and hypertrophied.

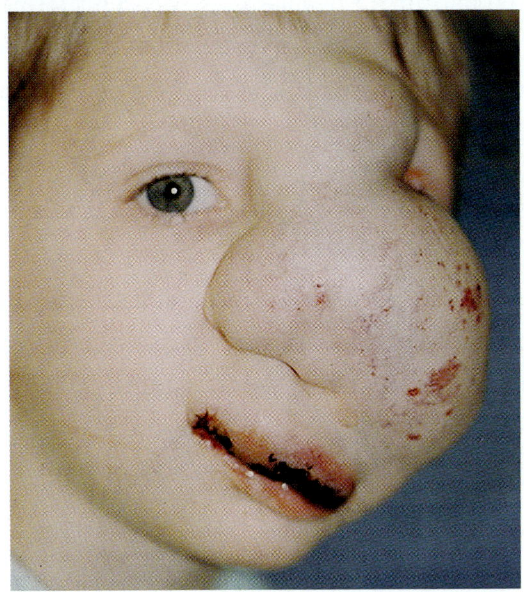

Figure 17–14. A 6-year-old with an extensive lymphatic malformation involving his midface. This lesion was microcystic and poorly localized.

Lymphatic malformations may be superficial or deep. Superficial lesions usually present with small cutaneous or mucosal lymph-filled vesicles. The natural history of lymphatic malformations is punctuated with periods of fluctuation in the size of the lesion.[20] These episodes are associated with periods of increased lymph production, such as during an infection or after trauma. The lesion usually diminishes in size after these events, giving a false sense of security to the patient and his or her physician, only to reexpand at some later stage. Lymphatic malformations usually are firm on palpation, and the overlying skin often exhibits a brawny edema. Lesions involving skin or a mucosal surface will exhibit small vesicles measuring about 1 to 2 mm in diameter.

Mixed Malformations

Mixed malformations are less common in the head and neck. The one most frequently encountered is the mixed venous venular malformation. Mixed arteriovenous capillary malformations are cited as an example of a mixed malformation, but I believe that these merely reflect cutaneous involvement. Another often-cited example is the mixed venous lymphatic malformation, which I think merely reflects hemorrhage or the presence of altered blood products in the lymph spaces. Mixed malformations display the characteristics of their various components.

DIAGNOSIS OF A CONGENITAL VASCULAR LESION

The beauty of Mulliken's classification lies in its simplicity. In the vast majority of patients, a diagnosis can be reached by history and physical examination alone. To establish a diagnosis, further investigation is rarely necessary but is needed to plan the management of a more complex lesion.

HISTORY AND EXAMINATION

Most hemangiomas are not present at birth, but 30% are. This is especially true for premature infants, in whom the incidence is much higher. Hemangiomas are also much more common in females. The typical profile of a child with a hemangioma is a premature female with a vascular lesion that was noticed at birth or very soon thereafter. The lack of a history of proliferation during the early neonatal period mitigates against the diagnosis of a hemangioma.

Vascular malformations, however, are always present at birth, although they may not be immediately apparent; in the case of arteriovenous malformations, several years may elapse before they become evident. These lesions always hypertrophy with advancing age. The rate of expansion varies between individuals and helps to distinguish high-grade lesions from low-grade lesions; high-grade lesions expand rapidly, whereas low-grade lesions expand more slowly.

The physical features of all the lesions assist in diagnosis, which is usually obvious. However, when confronted with a child with a subcutaneous blue mass, the diagnosis may not seem that obvious. The lesion may be a deep hemangioma, a lymphatic malformation, a venous malformation, or an arteriovenous malformation. A hemangioma usually declares itself by virtue of its behavior, by proliferating or showing some sign of involution. A lymphatic malformation is more likely to fluctuate in size, especially in relation to upper respiratory infections. A venous malformation is softer and more compressible. Furthermore, venous malformations often enlarge when in a dependent position, and in the case of a head and neck lesion, when the patient is recumbent.

SPECIAL INVESTIGATIONS

Magnetic resonance imaging (MRI) is used when the diagnosis is in question or when planning surgical strategy preoperatively. From a diagnostic standpoint, the features of an MRI scan interpreted together with the history and physical examination usually finalize the diagnosis. If an arteriovenous malformation is suspected, an arteriogram is indicated to confirm the diagnosis and determine whether it is possible to embolize the lesion. The features of the various lesions detected by MRI are summarized in Box 17–2.[21]

> **Box 17–2. Features of Congenital Vascular Lesions Seen on MRI**
>
> *Hemangiomas.* These are high-flow lesions in which there is an obvious parenchymal component. Tubular flow voids are obvious on T1- and T2-weighted images, and there is a moderate signal intensity increase on T2-weighted images. These lesions enhance with gadolinium.
>
> *Arteriovenous malformations.* These are also high-flow lesions, but there is no appreciable parenchymal component, and there is no enhancement with gadolinium. Tubular flow voids are evident on T1- and T2-weighted images, and there is minimal signal intensity increase on T2-weighted images.
>
> *Venous malformations.* Venous malformations are low-flow lesions. There is a uniform increase in signal intensity on T2-weighted images and a signal intensity equal to muscle on T1-weighted images. There is moderate enhancement with gadolinium.
>
> *Lymphatic malformations.* These are low-flow lesions with a similar signal intensity to muscle on T1-weighted images and an increased signal intensity on T2-weighted images. There may be some enhancement with gadolinium. Macrocystic lesions usually exhibit fluid-fluid levels.

Histologic confirmation of the diagnosis is only rarely required but must be considered when the diagnosis of a vascular lesion is in question. This is especially important if one or more of the features of the lesion are atypical. A sarcoma is always a possibility, especially if the features are atypical.

MANAGEMENT OF HEMANGIOMAS

The management of hemangiomas has undergone dramatic changes over the past few years. Although there is still some degree of controversy, the consensus is shifting away from a policy of benign neglect toward a more expectant policy of management. Several modalities are useful in the management of hemangiomas: pharmacotherapy (e.g., steroids, interferon), laser photocoagulation, and surgical resection.

Hemangiomas pass through two physically and physiologically distinct stages during their life cycle. The mechanism of action of each of these modalities is different, and, therefore, no single modality is good for all stages of the condition. The focus must shift away from the modality and toward the stage of the lesion.

The majority of hemangiomas are small, benign, and inconsequential. A small percentage of lesions, however, do warrant treatment. These may either be large or facial or may present with a complication, such as visual obstruction, airway obstruction, or ulceration or cardiac failure. In general, during proliferation, my mainstay of treatment is the use of steroids to retard or inhibit the process. Interferon is reserved for life- or sight-threatening hemangiomas that fail to respond to steroids in patients in whom surgery is contraindicated. Surgery is also a viable option during proliferation, provided the entire lesion can be resected. Any residuum remaining during this stage invariably results in recurrence.

Once the lesion has entered the phase of involution, it is advisable to wait until the child is 3 to 3.5 years old. By this stage it is usually possible to determine whether a good outcome is likely if the lesion is left untreated. A hemangioma that is involuting rapidly is likely to have very little residuum and is probably best left untreated. A lesion that appears to be involuting slowly is extremely likely to require some form of intervention, and it is best to do so before the child enters preschool.

PHARMACOTHERAPY

In general, steroids are only effective during proliferation, and a dose of up to 5 mg/kg may be necessary to obtain the desired effect.[22] This is usually continued for up to 2 weeks and then tapered. The speed of the taper varies with the age of the patient and the circumstances of the lesion. A long, slow taper may be chosen in a younger child because the lesion has a potentially longer period of proliferation. On the other hand, a shorter taper may be prescribed under the same circumstances for patients treated for the first time and the long, slow taper reserved for rebound growth. All children on systemic steroids should be given an appropriate dose of Zantac (rantidine hydrochloride) to prevent gastritis. Intralesion steroids are preferred by some who feel that this route of administration diminishes the likelihood of systemic adverse effects.[23,24] The recommended combination of drugs is triamcinolone (3 to 5 mg/kg of body weight) and betamethasone (0.5 to 1.0 mg/kg of body weight). These agents should be injected separately and with separate syringes. The rationale for this combination is that the short-acting betamethasone begins its effect fairly soon after administration, whereas the effect of triamcinolone takes several days to commence. Unfortunately, the effect of a single dose appears to be short-lived, and the dose may need to be repeated.

Interferon has been confirmed by several investigators to be extremely useful.[25,26] Unfortunately, a large percentage of patients develop neurologic deficits as a consequence of its use. The incidence of this complication appears to be as high as 25%, and a significant proportion of the deficits appear to be permanent.[27] For this reason, interferon has been abandoned as a routine agent and is reserved for life-threatening complications of hemangiomas. A daily dose of 1 million units given as a subcutaneous injection is usually initiated, and once the effect is confirmed, the dose is cut back to alternate days. The child should be examined by a neurologist at the start of treatment and monthly thereafter. At the first sign of a neurologic deficit, one should seriously consider stopping treatment with interferon.

LASER PHOTOCOAGULATION

The limitations of laser treatment must be emphasized. Because of the limited depth of penetration of light in the visible spectrum, lasers only benefit the most superficial lesions.[28,29] Furthermore, treating the superficial component of a compound lesion fails to affect the deeper component at all.

The current laser of choice is the flashlamp-pumped dye laser (pulsed dye laser), and most published experience concerns the conventional pulsed dye laser (pulse width 450 microseconds, wavelength 585 nm). Recently, two major modifications to this laser have been made. The first concerns the wavelength and pulse width. To improve the response rate, a longer wavelength was chosen to increase the depth of penetration, and the pulse width was lengthened to allow photocoagulation of some of the larger vessels. Wavelengths up to 600 nm are available, and exposure times up to 1500 microseconds are used commonly. These are relatively recent modifications, however, and only limited data are available. The second and perhaps most interesting modification is the addition of surface cooling, which can be accomplished in several ways to cool the surface sufficiently so that higher fluences can be used without destroying the epidermis. The impact of this is a deeper effect (due to the higher fluence) and more efficient photocoagulation of some of the larger vessels. Lasers have been found to be helpful in several circumstances.

Proliferation

In the presence of a superficial proliferating lesion, photocoagulation with a pulsed dye laser retards proliferation and in some cases even completely resolves the lesion (Fig. 17–15). A larger spot size is chosen (the larger the spot size—up to 1 cm—the deeper the penetration), and an appropriate fluence is set (see Table 17–2). The endpoint of bluish gray discoloration indicates sufficient vascular damage, and it may be necessary to double or even triple pulse each area until this endpoint is evident. It may be necessary to re-treat every 4 to 5 weeks for up to six sessions for an optimal effect.[29] If a

Table 17–2. Fluences (J/cm²) Commonly Used for Port-Wine Stains with the Flashlamp-Pumped Dye Laser (450-μm pulse width and 585 nm)

Spot Size	Face	Neck	Limb
5 mm	6–7.5	5–6.5	5–6.5
7 mm	5–6.5	4–5.5	4–5.5
10 mm	4–5.5	3–4.5	3–4.5

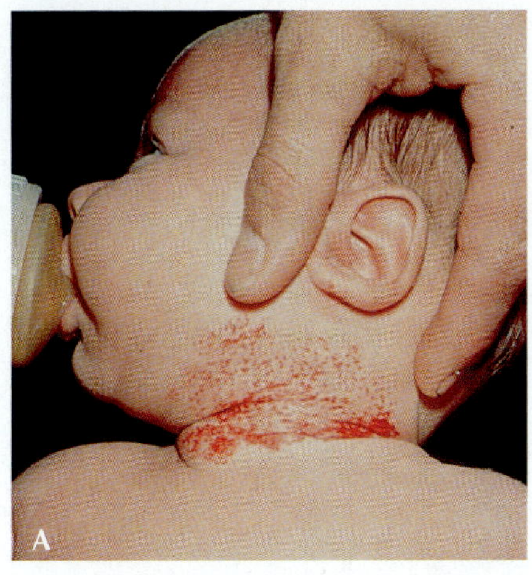
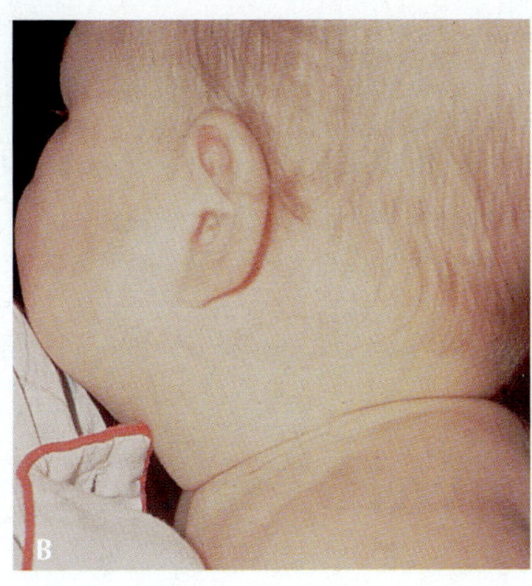

Figure 17–15. (A) Preoperative and (B) postoperative views of an infant with an extensive superficial proliferating hemangioma of his neck. This lesion responded dramatically to laser photocoagulation with a pulsed dye laser.

compound lesion is treated, the laser only affects the most superficial aspect of the lesion and leaves the deeper portion undisturbed.

Involution

Residual telangiectasia usually responds well to treatment with a pulsed dye laser; however, some of these vessels may be much larger and require treatment with a longer pulse width (Fig. 17–16), such as that of a KTP laser.

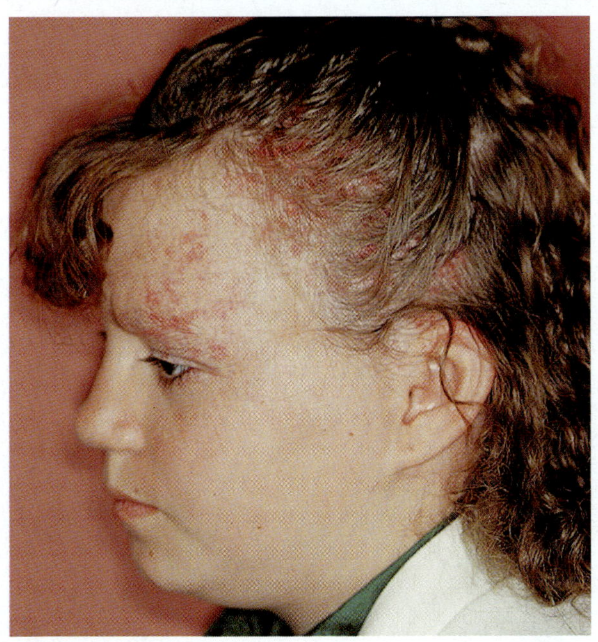

Figure 17–16. The same child as shown in Figures 17–8 and 17–10. At the end of proliferation, the child was left with a significant degree of telangiectasia (Fig. 17–10). She is now shown after several treatments with a pulsed dye laser. Most of the smaller vessels have responded to treatment. A few residual, larger vessels remain and these will be treated with a KTP laser.

The parameters are the standard power settings used to treat telangiectasia (see Table 17–3). Vasoconstriction without blanching the overlying skin is the goal. If this is not possible, some blanching is acceptable.

Skin Changes

Atrophic and hypertrophic skin changes that often remain after completion of involution can be remedied with skin resurfacing.[30] The standard power settings and parameters of a carbon dioxide (CO_2) laser used in skin resurfacing are appropriate. Postoperative care options are similar. Although I prefer a closed method of wound management, this can be challenging for children, so one may need to revert to an open technique with petrolatum. This process is also useful for hypertrophic scarring if surgery is impractical.

Surgical Resection

Once again, surgical remedies should not replace any of the other modalities simply because one has a higher level of comfort using this modality. Surgical resection can be accomplished at any stage of a lesion (Fig. 17–17). However, one principle is of paramount importance: When resecting a proliferating lesion, any residuum left at the end of surgery invariably continues proliferating. If it is the intention of the surgeon to debulk the lesion, this concern is less relevant. On the other hand, if the intention is to remove the entire lesion, no vestige should

Table 17–3. Parameters Commonly Used with the Aura KTP Laser

Spot Size	Fluence	Exposure Time	Pulses per Second
Telangiectasia (endpoint: vasoconstriction with little or no blanching of the overlying skin. Always use lowest parameters to achieve endpoint)			
1 mm	10–20 J/cm^2	10–30 ms	5
Port-wine stain (use scanner whenever possible. Endpoint: slight graying of the lesion without blanching of the overlying skin)			
Scanner	2–4 J/cm^2	2–4 ms	Scanner

remain at the end of surgery. If this is not possible, the timing of surgery is important. One might consider delaying surgery until proliferation has commenced; in the presence of an involuting lesion it is less important to remove the entire lesion because any residual lesion left at the end of surgery will merely continue to involute.

A surgical technique that I have developed has overcome previous concerns about blood loss. Using either a thermoscalpel (a thermally heated scalpel; Shaw Scalpel, Xomed, Memphis, TN) or a contact laser instrument (a laser fiber used in direct contact with the tissue as a scalpel) simplifies the task of hemostasis. The application of heat at subablative thresholds ($<100°C$) coagulates some of the smaller vessels. The critical size of vessel affected by this technique is not known, but it is probably restricted to small vessels and, therefore, should be supplemented with conventional electrocautery. In addition to achieving hemostasis, finding the correct surgical plane is also extremely important. Rapidly expanding hemangiomas condense a soft tissue plane around their advancing margin and do not invade adjacent structures. This plane is relatively avascular, and excessive bleeding can be avoided if the surgeon stays within this plane and does not stray into the actual hemangioma.

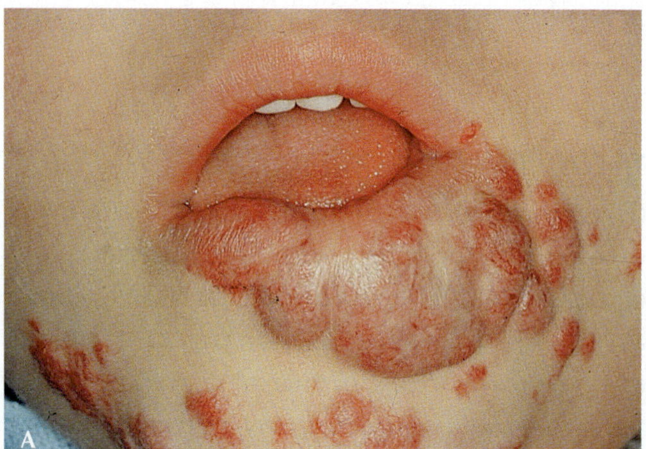
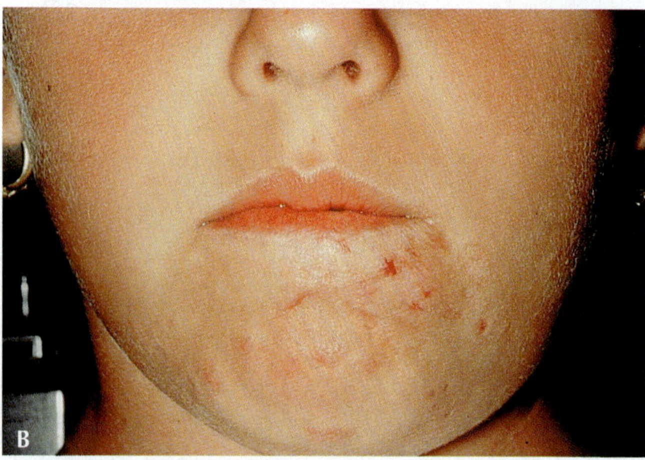

Figure 17–17. (A) Preoperative and (B) postoperative view of a 3-year-old with an extensive hemangioma involving her lower lip. The lesion had ulcerated and left significant atrophic scarring. The residual hemangioma was excised through a wedge lip excision. The residuum was then treated with a pulsed dye laser as well as skin resurfacing. Three or four small areas of telangiectasia have remained. These are made up of vessels with a much wider diameter and are, therefore, best treated with a KTP Nd:YAG laser.

MANAGEMENT OF VASCULAR MALFORMATIONS

The natural history of vascular malformations is progressive enlargement or expansion of the lesion. High-grade lesions expand more rapidly, and low-grade lesions tend to do so at a much slower rate. Because vascular malformations never involute, they almost always warrant treatment. The type of treatment depends on several factors, including the type of lesion, its degree of aggression (grade), and its anatomic location. Three forms of management are available, and, as with hemangiomas, all are valuable, but no single modality should not be used to the exclusion of the others (Box 17–3).

Box 17–3. Modalities for Treating Vascular Malformations

Laser photocoagulation

Surgery

Interventional radiology

   Sclerotherapy

   Embolization

LASER PHOTOCOAGULATION

Lasers are the treatment of choice for venular malformation (port-wine stains).[1] As mentioned earlier, the type of laser used depends on the stage of the lesion and, therefore, the size of the vessel.[6] Early port-wine stains are made up of smaller vessels and are best treated with a flashlamp-pumped pulsed dye laser. As the vessels become more ectatic, their diameters approach the upper limits of the capability of pulsed dye laser, and eventually, with advanced lesions, a much longer exposure time is necessary. The KTP and copper bromide lasers, with their millisecond exposure times, are, therefore, important tools.

As with the treatment of hemangiomas, much of the published data concern the earlier model (pulse width, 450 microseconds; wavelength, 585 nm).[1,31] An appro-priate endpoint is a uniform gray discoloration of the lesion. The fluences necessary to achieve this are shown in Table 17–2. With the KTP or copper bromide lasers, the endpoint is similar, and the parameters necessary are shown in Table 17–3. See Chapter 18 for a discussion of copper bromide lasers.

The treatment of "cobblestones" can be difficult without the right laser. The vessels that make up a cobblestone are sometimes several millimeters in diameter and, therefore, are best treated with an Nd:YAG laser. The endpoint is vasoconstriction with a small blanched spot seen at the surface,[32] which clearly indicates cutaneous destruction (a scar ≤ 1 mm in diameter may appear). With careful use of these lasers, such scars usually are avoided. A series of treatment spots is delivered via the optical quartz fiber in the free-beam mode. The laser fiber is held perpendicular to the skin about 2 mm from the surface of the skin, and each spot is separated from its adjacent spot by 1 to 2 mm.[6]

Venous malformations are made up of ectatic subcutaneous veins. The size and depth of the vessels preclude use of the pulsed dye laser. The Nd:YAG laser, however, is effective and can be used to treat submucosal and subcutaneous lesions.[32] By minimizing exposure time, subcutaneous lesions can be treated with little risk of scarring. The endpoint should be vasoconstriction with very little or no blanching of the overlying skin. On the other hand, when treating mucosal lesions, a small amount of blanching is acceptable. In general, two or three treatments are necessary, and the lesion may need to be re-treated every few years.[32]

Lasers are not effective in treating arteriovenous malformations but do have a role in the treatment of lymphatic malformations. The mucosal vesicles seen in superficial lesions can be vaporized with a CO_2 laser to provide temporary relief, which, in low-grade lesions, may be longstanding. Many of the superficial vesicles are connected with a much larger submucosal reservoir, and, therefore, when treating mucosal vesicles, especially on the tongue, vaporization should extend to the depth of these vesicles.

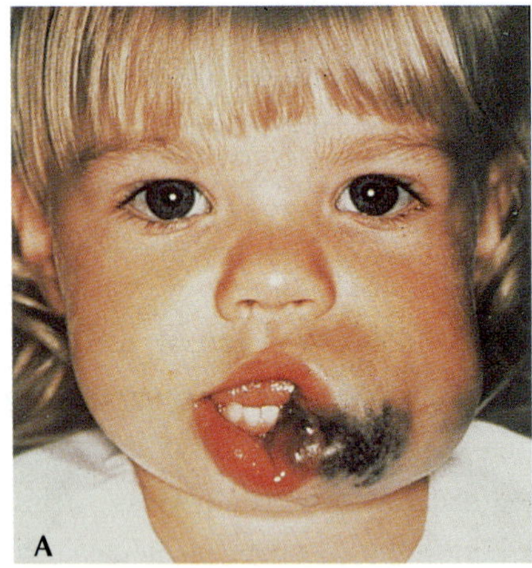
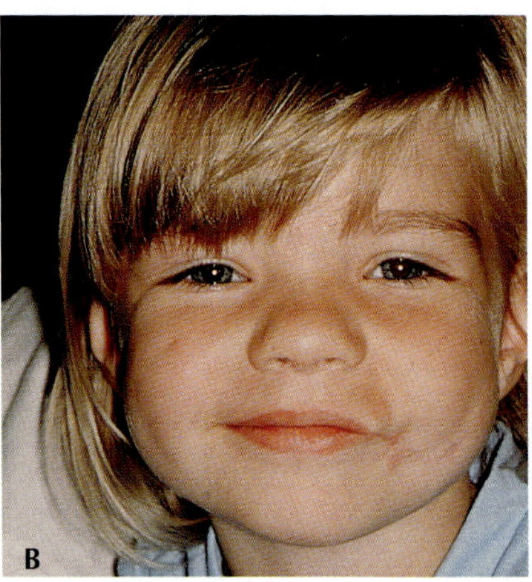

Figure 17–18. (A) Preoperative and (B) postoperative view of a 3-year-old with an extensive buccal fat space and commisural venous malformation. The child was treated with an Nd:YAG laser followed with surgical resection. This picture was taken just prior to her final procedure, during which a scar revision and a dermal implant were performed.

SURGERY

Surgical problems and techniques are almost identical to those described for proliferating hemangiomas. Any residuum remaining after surgery invariably leads to recurrence. This is especially true of arteriovenous malformations, where the entire nidus should be excised to prevent recurrence. Unfortunately, vascular malformations do not expand rapidly and, therefore, are not surrounded by a condensed soft tissue capsule. Moreover, vascular malformations, especially venous malformations, infiltrate tissue planes and are, therefore, much more difficult to excise (Fig. 17–18). With regard to lymphatic malformations, there are no easily recognizable margins, and the need for re-treatment at a later stage to complete what was thought to be a complete excision is very common. For this reason, many physicians have explored the possibility of sclerosing agents for the treatment of these lesions.

INTERVENTIONAL RADIOLOGY

Interventional radiology is an important modality for the management of vascular malformations and hemangiomas. Two procedures, sclerotherapy and embolization, are indispensable in this regard. Percutaneous sclerotherapy is accomplished using a variety of alcohol derivatives, as well as OK432.[33,34] Alcohol derivatives have been used for some time as a percutaneous agent in the sclerosis of venous malformations.[33] This can be done as a preoperative strategy to minimize blood loss during surgery or, alternatively, as a sole method of treatment. Sclerotherapy needs to be performed several times to maximize its effect. One of the risks concerns the accidental entry of the sclerosing agent into the cavernous sinus circulation. The veins of the face lack valves, and the infraorbital veins drain directly into the cavernous sinus. For this reason, one should exercise extreme caution, especially when performing sclerotherapy in the middle third of the face. The risk of cavernous sinus thrombosis can be avoided by performing the procedure with direct screening at all times.

Sclerotherapy using OK432 has become extremely useful for the management of lymphatic malformations.[34] Macrocycstic lesions appear to respond best, but the technique is also useful for the large cervicofacial mixed lesions.[34,35]

Embolization is extremely useful in the management of both arteriovenous malformations and hemangiomas.[36] It is occasionally advocated for the treatment of venous malformations but is usually best avoided. With regard to arteriovenous malformation, embolization can be used as a preoperative strategy to reduce blood loss during surgery or, alternatively, as a therapeutic modality in difficult lesions that cannot be resected. It must be understood that the effects of embolization are, at best, temporary and that the arteriovenous malformation almost invariably recurs. Preoperative embolization of hemangiomas is also a useful strategy if significant blood loss can be avoided.

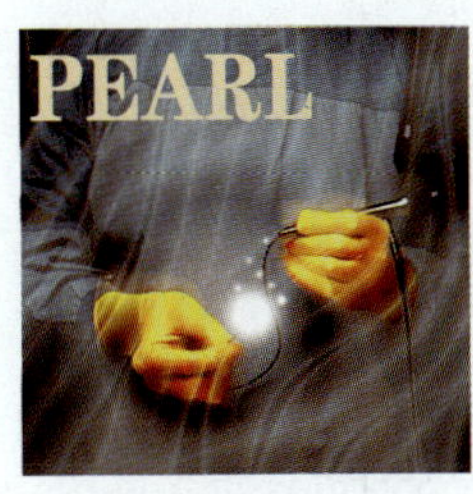

PEARL

- Histologic confirmation is rarely necessary but must be considered when the diagnosis of a vascular lesion is in question, especially if one or more of the features of the lesion are atypial. If the features are atypical, sarcoma is a possibility.

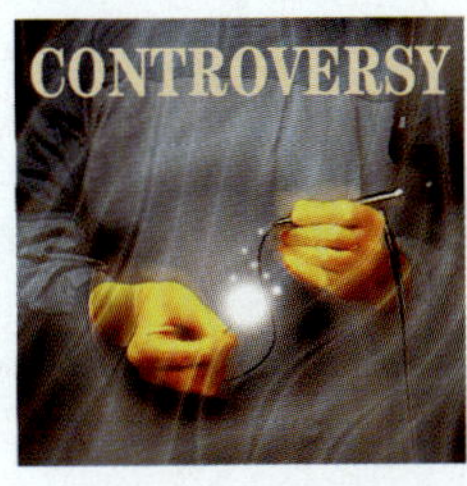

CONTROVERSY

- The management of hemangiomas has undergone dramatic changes over the past few years, and the consensus is shifting away from a policy of benign neglect toward a more expectant policy of management, including pharmacotherapy, laser photocoagulation, and surgical resection.

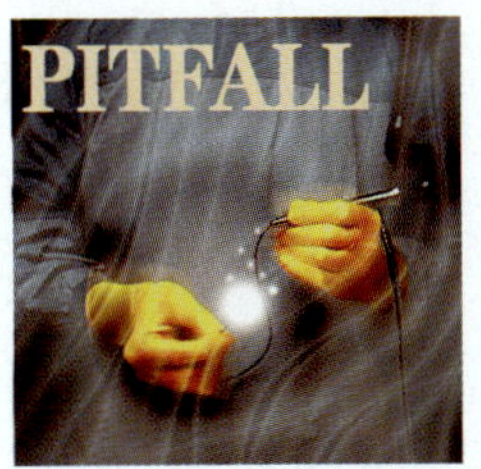

PITFALL

- Because the incidence of neurological deficit may be as high as 25% and a significant proportion of the deficits appear to be permanent, interferon has been abandoned as a routine agent and is reserved for life-threatening complications of hemangiomas. At the first sign of a neurologic deficit, one should seriously consider stopping treatment with interferon.

REFERENCES

1. Orten S, Waner M, Flock S, Roberson P, Kincannon J. Port-wine stains: an assessment of 5 years of treatment. *Arch Otolaryngol Head Neck Surg.* 1996;122:1174.
2. Hsia J, Lowery JA, Zelickson B. Treatment of leg telangiectasia using a long-pulse dye laser at 595 nm. *Lasers Surg Med.* 1997;20:1–5.
3. Adrian RM. Treatment of leg telangiectasias using a long-pulse frequency-doubled neodymium:YAG laser at 532 nm. *Dermatology.* 1998;4:19–23.
4. Suen J, Waner M. Treatment of oral cavity vascular malformations using the neodymium:YAG laser. *Arch Otolaryngology Head Neck Surg.* 1989;115:1329–1333.
5. Landthaler M, Haina D, Brunncr R, Waidelich W, Braun-Falco O. Neodymium-YAG laser therapy for vascular lesions. *J Am Acad Dermatol.* 1986;14:107–117.
6. Waner M, Suen J. Treatment options for the management of vascular malformations. In: Waner M, Suen JY, eds. *Hemangiomas and Vascular Malformations of the Head and Neck.* New York: John Wiley & Sons; 1999:315–350.
7. Anderson R, Parrish J. Selective photothermolysis: precise microsurgery by selective absorption of pulsed radiation. *Science.* 1983;220:521–527.
8. Mulliken JB, Glowacki J. Hemangiomas and vascular malformations in infants and children: a classification based on endothelial characteristics. *Plast Reconstr Surg.* 1982;69:412.
9. Hollinger L, Toriumi D, Anandappa L. Subglottic cysts and asymmetrical subglottic narrowing on neck radiograph. *Pediatr Radiol.* 1988;18:306.
10. Waner M, Suen JY. A classification of congenital vascular lesions. In: Waner M, Suen JY, eds. *Hemangiomas and Vascular Malformations of the Head and Neck.* New York: John Wiley & Sons; 1999:1–12.
11. Jacobs AH, Walton RG. The incidence of birthmarks in the neonate. *Pediatrics.* 1976;58:218.
12. Waner M, Suen JY. The natural history of vascular malformations. In: Waner M, Suen JY, eds. *Hemangiomas and Vascular Malformations of the Head and Neck.* New York: John Wiley & Sons; 1999:47–82.
13. Finn MC, Glowacki J, Mulliken JB. Congenital vascular lesions: Clinical applications of a new classification. *J Pediatr Surg.* 1983;18:894.
14. Rydy M, Malm M, Jernbeck J, Dalsgaard C. Ectatic blood vessels in port-wine stains lack innervation: possible role in pathogenesis. *Plast Reconstr Surg.* 1991;87:419.
15. Smoller BR, Rosen S. Port-wine stains: a disease of altered neural modulation of blood vessels. *Arch Dermatol.* 1986;122:177.
16. Waner M. Classification of port-wine stains. *Facial Plast Surg.* 1989;6:162–166.
17. Baker LL, Waner M, Thomas JR, Suen JY, Bussard D. Extracranial arteriovenous malformations of the head and neck. *Arch Otolaryngol Head Neck Surg.* 1999. (In press).
18. Levine C. Primary disorders of the lymphatic vessels—a unified concept. *J Pediatr Surg.* 1989;24:233.
19. North P, Mihm M. The surgical pathology approach to pediatric vascular tumors and anomalies. In: Waner M, Suen JY, eds. *Hemangiomas and Vascular Malformations of the Head and Neck.* New York: John Wiley & Sons; 1999:93–170.
20. Broomhead IW. Cystic hygroma of the neck. *Br J Plast Surg.* 1964;17:225.
21. Green CJ. Diagnostic imaging of congenital vascular lesions. In: Waner M, Suen JY, eds. *Hemangiomas and Vascular Malformations of the Head and Neck.* New York: John Wiley & Sons; 1999:171–216.
22. Sadan N, Woloch B. Treatment of hemangiomas with high doses of prednisone. *J Pediatr.* 1996;128:141–146.

23. Azzolini A, Nouvenne R. Nuove prospettive nella terapia degli angiomi immaturi dell'infanzia. 115 lesioni trattate con infiltrazioni intralesionali di triamcinnolone acetonide. *Ateneo Parmense.* 1970;41(suppl):51.

24. Kushner B. Local steroid therapy in adnexal hemangioma. *Ann Ophthamol.* 1979;11:1005–1009.

25. Ezekowitz R, Phil D, Mulliken J, Folkman J. Interferon ALFA-2a therapy for life-threatening hemangioma of infancy. *N Engl J Med.* 1992;326:1456.

26. Ohlms L, McGill T, Jones D, Healy G. Interferon alpha-2A therapy for airway hemangioma. *Ann Otol Rhinol Laryngol.* 1994;103:1.

27. Barlow CF, Priebe CJ, Mulliken JB, et al. Spastic diplegia as a complication of interferon alpha-2 treatment of hemangiomas in infancy. *J Pediatr.* 1998;132:527–530.

28. Waner M, Suen JY, Dinehart S, Mallory SB. Laser photocoagulation of superficial proliferating hemangiomas. *J Dermatol Surg Oncol.* 1994;20:43.

29. Garden JM, Bakus AD, Paller AS. Treatment of cutaneous hemangiomas by the flashlamp-pumped pulsed dye laser: prospective analysis. *J Pediatr.* 1992;120:555–560.

30. Waner M. Laser resurfacing and the treatment of involuting hemangiomas. *Lasers Surg Med Suppl.* 1996; Abstract 219, 40.

31. Waner M, Suen J. The treatment of vascular malformations. In: Waner M, Suen JY, eds. *Hemangiomas and Vascular Malformations of the Head and Neck.* New York: John Wiley & Sons; 1999;351–390.

32. Tan O, Carney M, Margolis R, et al. Histologic response of port-wine stains treated by argon, carbon dioxide and tunable dye lasers. *Arch Dermatol.* 1986;122:1016–1022.

33. de Lorimier A. Sclerotherapy of venous malformations. *J Pediatr Surg.* 1995;30:188–194.

34. Ogita S, Tsuto T, Deguchi E, Tokiwa K, Nagashima N, Iwai N. OK432 therapy for resectable lymphangiomas in children. *J Pediatr Surg.* 1991;26:263–270.

35. Smith RJ, Burke DK, Sato Y, Poust RJ, Kimura K, Bauman NM. OK432 therapy for lymphangiomas. *Arch Otolaryngol Head Neck Surg.* 1996;122:1195–1199.

36. Yakes W, Haas D, Parker S, et al. Symptomatic vascular malformations: Ethanol embolotherapy. *Radiology.* 1989;170:1059–1066.

CHAPTER 18

Copper Vapor and Copper Bromide Lasers

SUE E. McCOY

The copper vapor laser (CVL) and copper bromide laser (CBL) each use copper atoms as the lasing medium, so both emit identical wavelengths of laser light, at 511 (green) and 578 (yellow) nm. The CVL tube is composed of zirconia alloy, and the elemental copper contained within is heated to a vapor at around 1600°C. Electrical "pumping" induces lasing. The CBL tube is composed of a silica, and its reservoirs contain the compound copper bromide. At 600°C, copper bromide becomes gaseous, and electrical pumping again induces lasing. The essential difference between these lasers, therefore, is the temperature at which they operate, their efficiency, their overall size, and their power output. (Efficiency = percent conversion of total energy input to light energy emission. For CVLs, efficiency is about 0.5%, and for CBLs, it is about 1%.) The CBLs are considerably smaller than the CVLs but emit light at a higher power (a few watts) than most CVLs (a few hundred milliwatts), although large, high-powered CVLs do exist in some specialized clinics.[1]

Both lasers emit light as a train of extremely short pulses of high peak power but low energy, at frequencies of 11 to 16 kHz. The width of these pulses is on the order of tens of nanoseconds, with pulse intervals ranging from 63 to 91 microseconds. Such pulse intervals are shorter than the thermal relaxation time of the targeted tissue, and hence these lasers are considered quasi-continuous wave (quasi-CW) for physiologic purposes. The power output is measured as an average of the train of pulses rather than as the peak of individual nanosecond pulses. This quasi-CW light is then either mechanically "chopped" to produce exposures of tens to hundreds of milliseconds or used in continuous mode.

The green and yellow laser light is transmitted by a flexible quartz fiber to either a lensed handpiece or directly to the skin. Spot sizes can be varied with both laser systems, but because of the limited power of these systems, spot sizes are kept small to maximize power density. Either laser can be coupled to a computer-controlled scanning system for more uniform coverage of large skin areas, as is often desirable when treating port-wine stains. The primary chromophores of the wavelengths emitted by copper lasers are hemoglobin (578-nm yellow light) and melanin (511-nm green light).

TREATMENT OF VASCULAR LESIONS

When the component vessels of a vascular lesion are between about 75 and 300 μm in diameter and located in the papillary or upper reticular dermis (to a depth of around 500 μm from the dermal–epidermal junction), copper lasers are highly effective. Although parameters that allow selective photothermolysis can be employed if the spot size and exposure duration are manipulated within the limits of the available power, these "ideal" parameters are rarely used in clinical practice. The CBL is able to approximate theoretical ideals more closely than

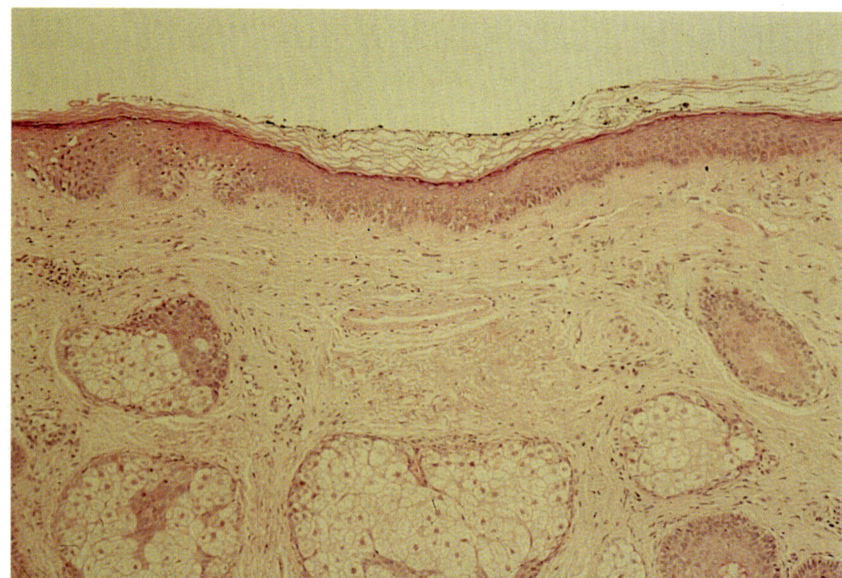

Figure 18–1. Photomicrograph of facial skin containing a single telangiectatic vessel that was laser irradiated 3 hours previously with a CBL using yellow light at 2.6 W and 15-millisecond exposures in an 0.8-mm spot (10.3 J/cm^2). The vessel is empty of red cells, and the endothelium and vessel wall are clearly damaged. There is minimal perivascular injury, and the overlying epidermis is intact. This degree of selective vessel damage is unlikely to result in permanent sclerosis.

most CVLs because of its higher power output in the yellow wavelength. With CVLs, a smaller spot size (100 to 150 μm) to increase power density and/or a longer exposure time (50 to 200 milliseconds) to increase the total energy delivered are used to compensate for the limited available power. The higher-powered CBL, in contrast, can be used with spot sizes up to 1 mm and exposure times of 15 to 40 milliseconds.

Nonetheless, although histologic responses consistent with selective vessel necrosis are seen using short exposures, satisfactory clinical results appear to require longer exposures.[2] It may be that a moderate degree of perivascular damage is necessary to achieve permanent vessel sclerosis. If the photothermolysis is too selective and only the vessel wall is damaged, recanalization may occur. This certainly seems to be the case when larger (>150 μm) vessels are targeted with yellow light. If the exposure duration is within the thermal relaxation time of the vessel, absorption by hemoglobin is so complete in the upper portion of the vessel that a superficial crescent of blood is coagulated, leaving the deeper portion of the vessel shielded from further injury. This has been demonstrated using flashlamp-pumped pulsed dye lasers.[3,4]

However, lasers employing longer exposure times at lower power seem to operate by a different mechanism.

During copper laser irradiation, vessels are emptied of blood, perhaps because of a comparatively slower coagulation process that allows shrinkage of a small portion of vessel wall, thus squeezing out the red cells as the laser is moved along the vessel. This proposed mechanism is theoretical, although this emptying of vessels can be seen clearly during laser treatment, and histologic examination of vascular skin immediately after treatment reveals few red cells within the vessel lumen[5] (Fig.18–1).

There is no doubt that at commonly employed exposure times copper lasers produce a predictable and inevitable degree of epidermal injury. However, most studies suggest that this injury heals rapidly with few late adverse effects. Generally, such injury is less severe with CBLs than with most CVLs, as evidenced by the extent and duration of posttreatment sequelae (see below).

TELANGIECTASIAS

Copper lasers are arguably the most effective method of treating facial telangiectasias with a minimum of adverse short- and long-term sequelae and a high level of patient satisfaction. These common cosmetic blemishes are dilatations of the most superficial dermal venules that measure from 50 to over 400 μm in diameter in vivo. Vessels smaller than about 50 μm present as a generalized

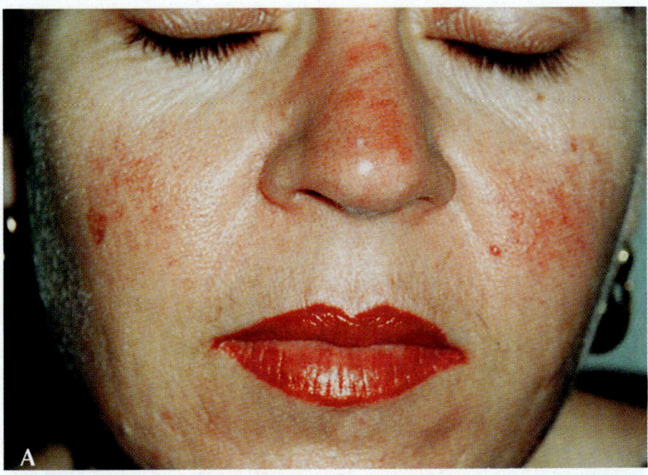
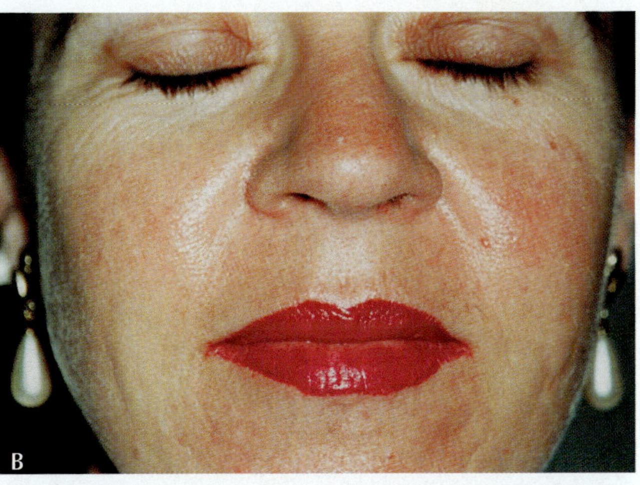

Figure 18–2. (A) Moderate essential telangiectasia on the cheeks and nose of a 41-year-old woman. A lentigo is evident on the left cheek. (B) Four months after one CBL treatment lasting about one half hour and using 2.2 W and 30- to 40- millisecond exposures for the telangiectasia. The lentigo was treated with green light, 4.2 W and 15-millisecond exposures until the denatured hypermelanotic epidermis easily wiped away.

blush rather than as individual telangiectasias and are more suited to treatment with shorter-pulsed lasers.

Although scanners have been used for telangiectasias, the most common treatment method is manual vessel tracing. A CVL with a 100- to 300-μm spot size is used in either CW or pulsed mode, the vessel being irradiated until a minimal whitening of the skin overlying the vessel is seen. The CBL is used only in pulsed mode with a 750- to 900-μm spot size depending on whether a naked fiber tip or a lensed handpiece is used. Exposure lengths are increased in 5-millisecond increments, commencing at 15 to 20 milliseconds and increasing to 40 milliseconds or occasionally longer for very large vessels. The endpoint for effective treatment with this laser is immediate disappearance of the vessel but no residual whitening of the skin.

Within minutes of treatment, the lased area becomes erythematous and slightly edematous. It is nonetheless still possible to assess the region for missed vessels by digital stretching of the skin. With this maneuver, untreated vessels are discernible.

The degree and duration of edema following treatment vary depending on the size, number, and density of vessels in an area. Because CVLs are used with nonselective parameters, posttreatment reactions tend to be more severe, commonly with some blistering and subsequent crusting. These sequelae are rare with CBL treatments, but edema may persist for 3 to 5 days.

Patients presenting with essential telangiectasias of the cheeks, preauricular areas, nasal bridge, or forehead may expect 75 to 90% reduction of the size and number of visible vessels within 6 to 8 weeks of one treatment (Fig. 18–2). Ectatic vessels at the bases of the nasal alae and those in the sebaceous skin of the nasal bulb or the chin are more often resistant to treatment or recur within weeks despite thorough blanching at the time of laser therapy. Because a similar outcome is seen when virtually any laser is used on these types of vessels, it is surmised that the cause of these less-than-optimal results is the pathology itself rather than the efficacy of a particular laser system. I prefer to microsclerose such vessels immediately prior to laser treatment. The visible narrowing of the vessels that ensues (whether caused by spasm or endothelial edema) presents a smaller-diameter target for the laser. When a sclerosed vessel is laser irradiated within minutes, the vessel does not blanch but instead turns purple. Inspection of such vessels under magnification suggests trapped intravascular coagulum. This may be a result of laser irradiation of slowed blood flow. Vessels that demonstrate this

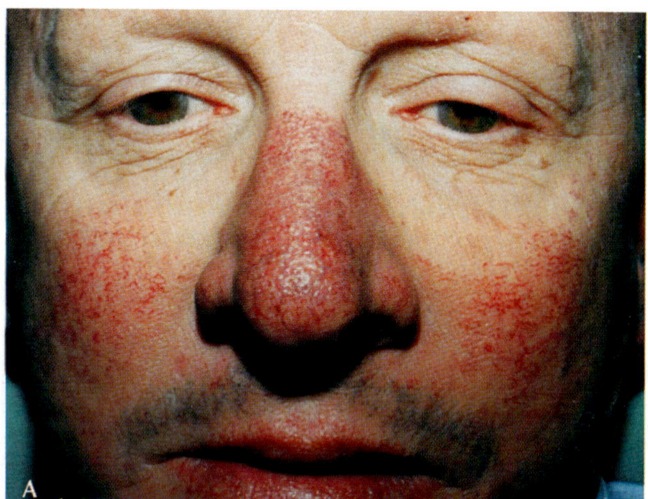

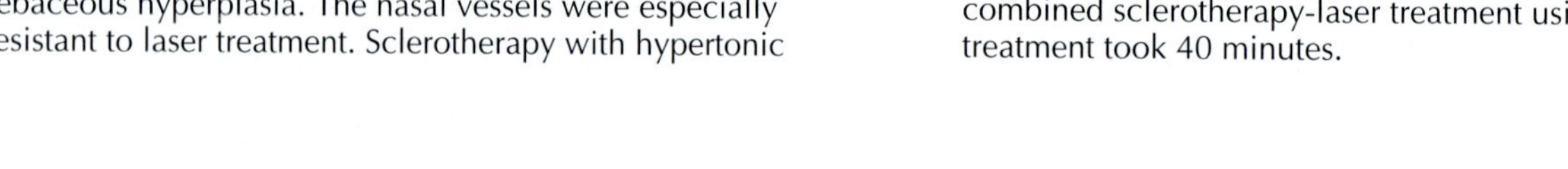

Figure 18–3. (A) This 60-year-old man had telangiectasia and sebaceous hyperplasia. The nasal vessels were especially resistant to laser treatment. Sclerotherapy with hypertonic saline had proved unsuccessful. (B) Appearance after one combined sclerotherapy-laser treatment using the CBL. The treatment took 40 minutes.

response inevitably respond much better to laser treatment (Fig.18–3).

While laser treatment of telangiectasias secondary to systemic or topical corticosteroid use or to diseases such as lupus erythematosus and acne rosacea is frequently very successful, patients must be warned that recurrence of the vessels with time is likely. Patients should be advised that there is no contraindication to subsequent treatments to maintain cosmetic improvement, even if the disease itself remains active.

Long-term adverse effects of CVL or CBL treatment of telangiectasia are uncommon. Transient hyperpigmentation has been described after CVL use, though not with the CBL, presumably due to lesser thermal injury with the latter laser. Hypopigmentation may occur with either laser along the track of treated vessels. It is more likely if the clinical endpoint of treatment was definite skin whitening than if vessel blanching without residual skin whitening was seen. In my opinion, hyperpigmentation occurs early and is transient, whereas hypopigmentation occurs late and is permanent. While minor skin atrophy in areas where large vessels have been treated has been noted after CBL treatment, macroscopic scarring after treatment of telangiectasias with copper lasers has not been described.

Angiomas

Spider Angiomas

Spider angiomas (nevus araneus) arise from an ascending artery that ends in a thin-walled subepidermal ampulla and then branches into numerous capillaries. Their etiology is unclear, but they may have some hormone dependence. In prepubescent children, I prefer to counsel the patient and family to leave the lesion untreated, because most resolve spontaneously, without visible residue, whereas laser treatment can result in a small hypopigmented pit. In adults, sclerotherapy is the preferred initial treatment option because it is successful in over 90% of patients and leaves no mark if extravasation is avoided. Both copper lasers can be used for resistant lesions, although the recurrence rate is relatively high. This may be due to the fact that the feeding arteriole of the spider angioma is oriented perpendicular to the skin and may extend from the deep dermis, thus being unreachable with yellow laser light. Treatment using increased energy (longer exposures) generally only results in pinpoint scarring.

Cherry Angiomas

Cherry angiomas (De Morgan spots, senile angiomas) are extremely common benign papules composed of numerous dilated capillaries that arise in the dermal papillae.

They respond dramatically to copper laser irradiation. The CW or pulsed mode can be used with equal efficacy, although pulsed mode may be better tolerated with regard to pain. The immediate response is graying and shrinkage of the lesion. Within a week it is difficult to identify the site of the original lesion.

Pyogenic Granulomas

Pyogenic granulomas (proliferative angiomas) are lobular capillary hemangiomas that occasionally arise following trauma but most often occur without a predisposing event. These lesions can be up to 2 cm in diameter and are usually papular or pedunculated, presenting the problem of lack of penetration of laser light through the full thickness of the lesion. They are treated successfully using relatively high energies. Very thick lesions can be treated initially with combined wavelength light using an ablation method. Once the lesion is reduced to a level flush with the skin following sequential laser ablations and wiping with saline-soaked gauze, the base can be irradiated with yellow light. It is important to wipe the lesions gently, because active bleeding prohibits further immediate laser treatment. Since laser treatment can destroy the vascular nodule with minimal coincidental damage to surrounding skin, the inevitable scar is minimized compared with other tissue-destructive methods.

Angiofibromas

Angiofibromas are composed of numerous fibroblasts and dilated blood vessels arranged around follicles and present macroscopically as red papules. Treatment with a copper laser is as effective as treatment with the carbon dioxide laser, if not more so. The endpoint of treatment with the copper laser, using long exposure times, is complete blanching of the lesion. This implies protein denaturing and is desirable to photocoagulate the dense collagen of these lesions. Healing by secondary intention over a mildly injured underlying dermis may leave minor hypopigmentation, but the result is cosmetically preferable to the scar that results from excision and suture or other thermal methods of tissue destruction (Fig.18–4).

Adenoma Sebaceum

Adenoma sebaceum, the pathognomonic skin manifestation of tuberous sclerosis, is, in fact, numerous angiofibromas. Treatment is similar to that for angiofibromas. Some crusting and scab formation are to be expected for 7 to 10 days.

Port-Wine Stains

Argon, argon-pumped dye, and CVLs were used to treat port-wine stains long before the theory of selective photothermolysis spurred the development of a laser with a pulse width shorter than the thermal relaxation time of

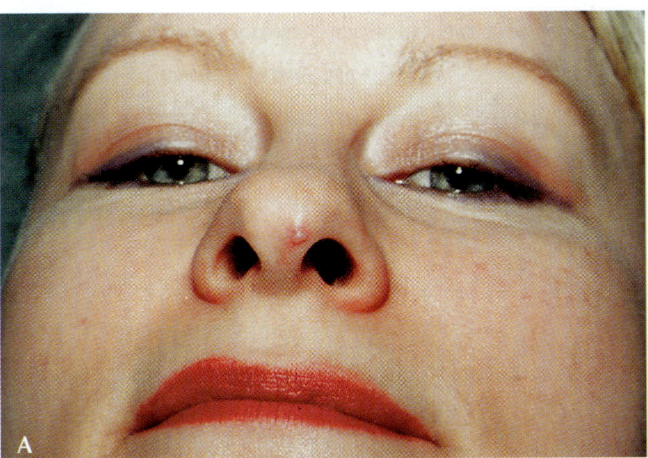

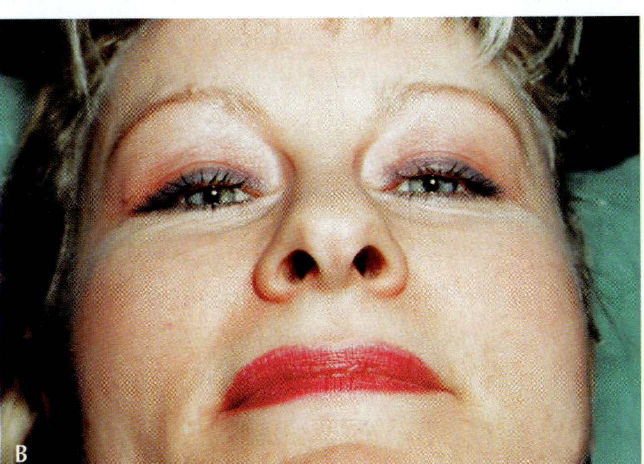

Figure 18–4. (A) An isolated angiofibroma on the nasal tip of a 31-year-old woman. (B) Appearance after one CBL treatment using yellow light at 1.8 W with 100-millisecond exposures until the lesion was completely blanched. The follow-up period is 3 months.

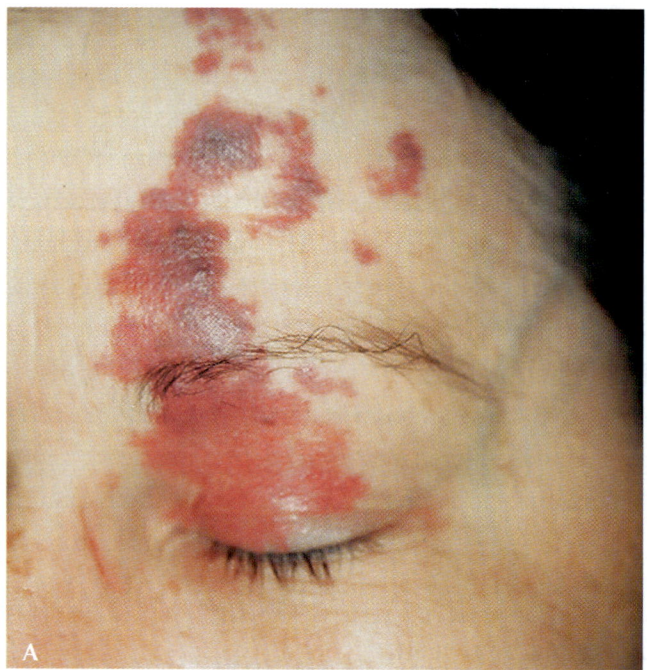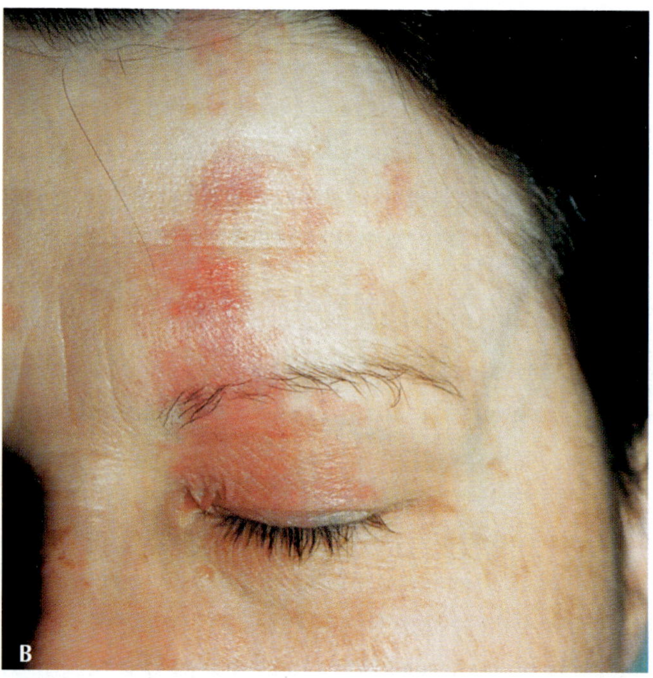

Figure 18–5. (A) Grade-IVa port-wine stain in the ophthalmic nerve area of a 48-year-old woman having had no previous treatment. (B) Appearance 3 months after two treatments with a CBL using 2 W with 30 and 35-millisecond exposures and a supraorbital nerve local anesthetic block. The lesion is now ready for treatment with a shorter-pulsed laser such as a pulsed dye system.

vascular lesion microvessels (see Chapters 16 and 17). The thermal effects of these lasers were largely nonspecific, and a degree of epidermal necrosis with the subsequent healing of what amounted to a superficial burn was usual.

The addition of automated scanners that placed controlled exposures evenly on the skin in orderly, nonadjacent patterns improved the performance of CVLs in the treatment of port-wine stains on test areas and histologic specimens, but published clinical results of large studies are lacking. The CBL, with its higher average power in the yellow wavelength and the capacity to employ shorter exposure times, has proved useful for the treatment of grades III, IV, and IVa port-wine stains. Blistering, crusting, and scabbing are uncommon after CBL treatment, although swelling for several days is usual. Results such as those shown in Figure 18–5 can be achieved with relatively few treatments.

Copper lasers are contraindicated for port-wine–stain treatment in children and in anyone with grade-I or -II lesions. An exposure sufficiently short to confine damage to the targeted vessels with the limited available power from these lasers does not equate to adequate energy density for vessel necrosis.

Methods of treatment rely on the same clinical endpoint described for telangiectasias. Point-by-point coverage of the lesional skin as quickly as is mechanically feasible is desirable, because the triple response that rapidly ensues may reduce the effectiveness of the laser in areas adjacent to those already treated (Fig.18–6). To this end, automated scanners are useful, although most port-wine stains are not uniform in color (vessel size) so care must be taken with these geometric pattern systems not to over- or undertreat regions within one scanner pattern.

Rapid treatment is painful. Most treatments can be performed with regional nerve blocks, especially of the head and neck, where port-wine stains frequently and conveniently follow the distribution of one or more dermatomes of the trigeminal nerve. Topical anesthesia can be used but has the disadvantage of causing vasoconstriction and has a limited duration of effectiveness in hypervascular port-wine–stain skin. Since copper lasers are used

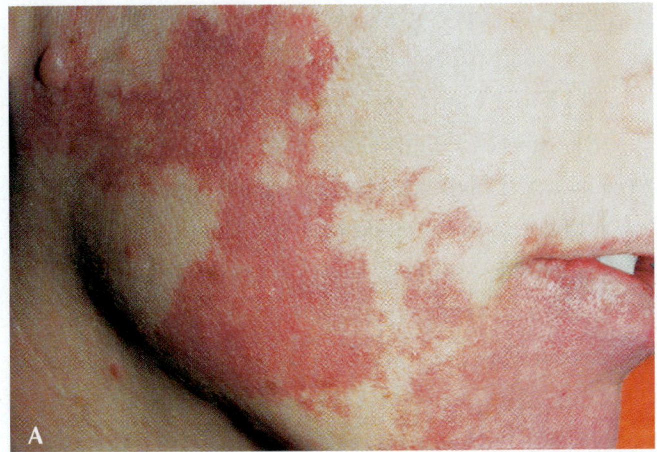

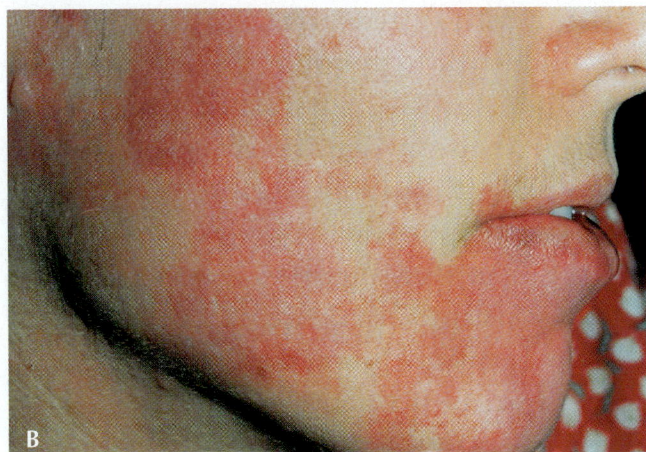

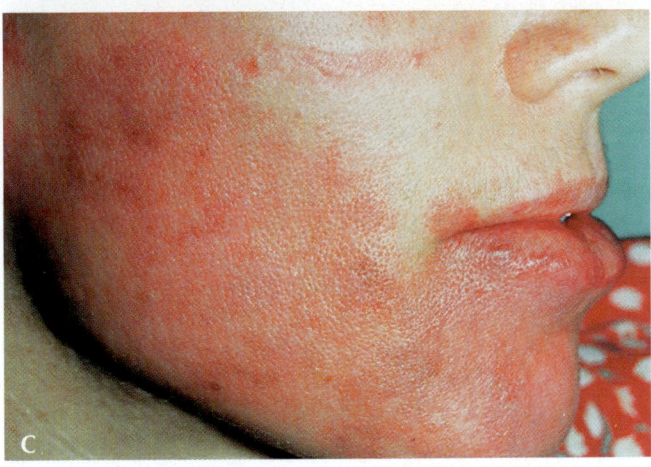

Figure 18–6. (A) Grade-III to -IV port-wine stain in the mandibular nerve territory of a 34-year-old woman. (B) Appearance nearly 12 months after one treatment with a CBL using a manual "coloring in" technique. (C) The entire area was treated again with the CBL under local mandibular nerve block. This is the appearance immediately after treatment. It is anticipated that any further treatment would require a shorter-pulsed laser.

rarely in the pediatric age group, the need for general anesthesia is infrequent.

Treatment of large skin areas is less forgiving with respect to complications than treatment of discrete, small areas. Thus hypopigmentation and/or minor atrophy may occur more readily or be more noticeable than after treatment of discrete lesions such as telangiectasia, especially if multiple treatments are performed. It is worth recognizing the point at which repeated treatment with a copper laser is likely to result in a diminishing response, and the patient should be referred for further therapy with a shorter-pulsed laser.

ACTINIC KERATOSES

If the keratin is scraped or curetted from an actinic (solar) keratosis, the underlying lesion is frequently hyperemic.

After malignancy is excluded by careful examination, dermatoscopy, or biopsy where appropriate, most of these lesions are suitable for treatment with a copper laser.

The absorbing chromophore is generally hemoglobin, although melanin contributes to the light absorption in many instances. Copper laser ablation of these lesions is nonspecific. Either wavelength or both can be used, although combined light yields higher power and shorter exposures, thereby reducing perilesional thermal damage. The abnormal epidermis is irradiated to gray-white denaturing and is then easily wiped off, akin to treatment with the CO_2 laser. This process can be repeated until the lesional area is flat and flush with surrounding skin. Larger spot sizes and considerably longer exposures (50 to 80 milliseconds with the CBL and several hundreds of milliseconds with the CVL) can be used because tissue destruction is the goal.

Anecdotally, keratoses thermolysed with a copper laser heal as rapidly as those treated with CO_2 lasers and more rapidly than those treated with cryosurgery, electrocautery, or surgical curettage. Accordingly, the cosmetic result is more acceptable, with less noticeable hypopigmentation and atrophy.

Despite the fact that keratoses generally are limited to the epidermis, careful follow-up of all treated patients should be encouraged because the presence of keratoses denotes significant sun damage. Laser treatment in these patients should be part of a more comprehensive management plan for their skin.

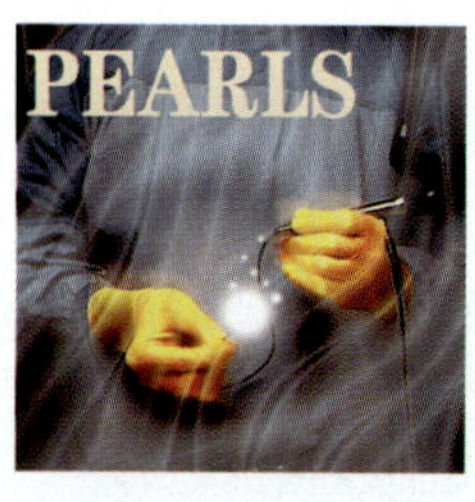

- Good results with copper lasers depend on good technique. The laser practitioner inevitably finds that results improve as more patients are treated. Conveying the subtle details of treatment methods to a newcomer to copper laser therapy is difficult. The best advice is to follow the basic guidelines and then modify technique based on experience.
- Copper lasers consume the copper lasing medium the entire time they are lasing, regardless of whether they are being used to treat a patient. To maximize laser lifespan, it is best to treat one patient after another without interruption. If there is a gap of more than 5 minutes between treatments, the laser should be put into standby mode to preserve the copper lasing medium. This is particularly true of the CBL, which has a warm-up time of 12 to 15 minutes from a cold start but reactivates from stand-by in just a few minutes.
- Like most high-powered air-cooled laser systems, significant heat is generated while copper lasers are in operation. Although it is desirable to have a patient warm when treating vascular lesions, the room temperature will become uncomfortably hot after a couple of hours. This problem is easily overcome by installing additional cooling systems or hot-air extraction fans, but new laser purchasers should be aware of it.

REFERENCES

1. Walker EP, Butler PH, Pickering JW, et al. Histology of port wine stains after copper vapor laser treatment. *Br J Dermatol.* 1989;121:217–223.
2. Neumann RA, Leonhartsberger H, Bohler-Sommeregger K, et al. Results and tissue healing after copper-vapour laser (at 578 nm) treatment of port-wine stains and facial telangiectasias. *Br J Dermatol.* 1993;128:306–312.
3. Hohenleutner U, Hilbert M, Wlotzke U, Landthaler M. Epidermal damage and limited coagulation depth with flash-lamp-pumped pulsed dye laser: a histochemical study. *J Invest Dermatol.* 1995;104:798–802.
4. Kimel S, Svaasand LO, Hammer-Wilson M, et al. Differential vascular response to laser photothermolysis. *J Invest Dermatol.* 1994;103:693–700.
5. Tan OT, Stafford TJ, Murray S, Kurban AK. Histologic comparison of the pulsed dye laser and copper vapor laser on pig skin. *Lasers Surg Med.* 1990;10:551–558.

CHAPTER 19

Flashlamp-Pumped Pulsed Dye Laser

WILLIAM RUSSELL RIES AND PATRICK K. LEE

The flashlamp-pumped pulsed dye laser (FPDL) is unique in that it is one of the first medical lasers developed for a specific function (i.e., the treatment of benign vascular cutaneous lesions). Before the development of medical yellow-dye lasers, lasers with other wavelengths (primarily the argon laser) were used in treating vascular skin lesions. Many laser surgeons have had great success using carbon dioxide (CO_2),[1,2] potassium-titanyl-phosphate (KTP),[3] neodymium:yttrium-aluminum-garnet (Nd:YAG),[4] and argon[5,6] lasers for ablation of vascular malformations, but their results very often depend on the expertise of the laser surgeon.

The FPDL is not a panacea for these lesions, but it is one of the easiest lasers to use, and consistently good results are less dependent on an individual's expertise if the operator is properly trained in use of the FPDL.[7–9] Recently, the next generation of the FPDL was devel-oped—the long-pulse flashlamp-pumped pulsed dye laser (LP-FPDL), which gives laser surgeons a greater range of treatment wavelengths as well as a longer tissue exposure time (i.e., pulse duration).

The FPDL works on the principle of selective photothermolysis. As set forth by Anderson and Parrish,[10,11] this principle states that selective damage to a target vessel is a function of the wavelength of the laser light and exposure time (Fig. 19–1). The FPDL's wavelength is 585 nm, which is visible yellow light. This wavelength closely matches the third absorption peak of the target chromophore oxyhemoglobin (577 nm) (Fig. 19–2).[12]

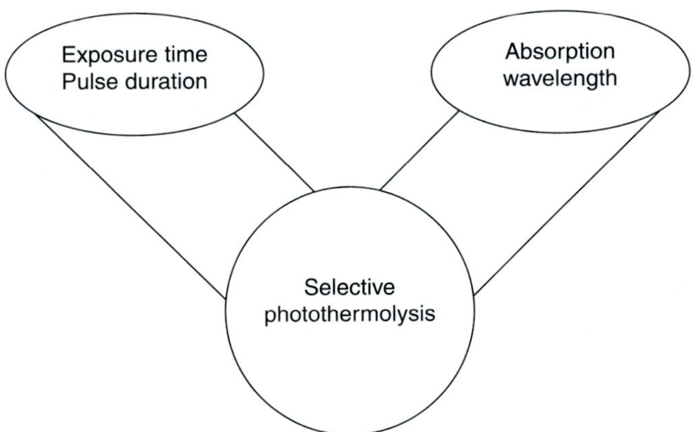

Figure 19–1. Principle of selective photothermolysis.

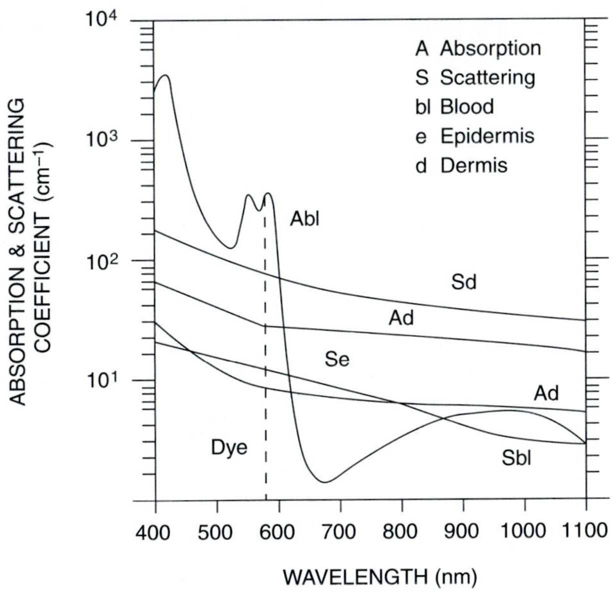

Figure 19–2. Absorption spectrum of oxyhemoglobin with superimposed absorption and scattering graphs for epidermis and dermis.

Earlier lasers used the 577-nm wavelength, but increasing the wavelength to 585 nm cleared the lesion more effectively without a loss in vascular selectivity;[13] chromophores such as melanin absorb less light in the wavelength range of 577 to 585 nm.[14] For the LP-FPDL, the available wavelengths are 585, 590, 595, and 600 nm, which translate into deeper penetration and even less absorption by other chromophores.

The exposure time, or pulse duration, is critical because the blood within the vessel must be coagulated; then the heat is allowed to conduct to the vessel wall to cause ablation and fibrosis, which manifests clinically as lightening of the lesion.[15] If the exposure time is too short, the blood may be coagulated, but the vessel wall may not be heated sufficiently. If the exposure time is too long, then the heat is conducted to surrounding dermis and overlying epidermis, resulting in scarring or pigmentation changes or both. The FPDL has a set exposure time of 450 microseconds, which was determined by calculating the thermal relaxation time of an average-sized vessel found within a vascular lesion[10] using the equation

$$T = G\frac{D^2 PC}{K}$$

where G = geometry factor, D = size of object, P = density, C = specific heat, and K = thermal conductivity. It is important to note that thermal relaxation is directly proportional to the square of the object's diameter D. The pulse duration of the LP-FPDL (1.5 milliseconds) is three times that of the FPDL and closer to the thermal relaxation time of many adult port-wine stains and leg telangiectasias, which can result in more efficient selective photothermolysis of these lesions.

TREATMENT CONSIDERATIONS
SAFETY

It is essential that the laser surgeon and all ancillary personnel be thoroughly trained in the proper operation, use, and safety features of dye lasers before they use the lasers clinically. It is the responsibility of the medical facility and its laser safety officer to ensure that personnel receive the necessary didactic and hands-on instruction. Training in the use of another visible-light laser such as the argon laser should not be accepted as adequate training for the FPDL or the LP-FPDL.

The FPDL and LP-FPDL's wavelengths of 585 to 600 nm require that all individuals in the laser suite wear protective eyewear specifically for that range of wavelengths. Eyewear designed for other visible-light lasers (e.g., KTP and argon lasers) is not adequate protection from these wavelengths. It is best if the patient wears opaque eye shields to block completely any errant radiation. If the patient has a vascular lesion involving the eyelids, then a metal scleral shield should be inserted after the eye has been anesthetized with topical anesthetic. An extra set of protective eyewear should be placed outside each entrance to the laser suite (which should have the proper warning signs clearly posted) so that someone entering the room has the appropriate eye protection.

Since dye lasers require a high-voltage power supply, it is imperative that no attempt be made to circumvent the interlock switches that prevent operation of the laser if any of the outer covers or panels are open. The capacitors within the laser can maintain potentially fatal high-voltage charges even with the laser turned off, so any maintenance or servicing of the high-voltage components should be done by an authorized laser technician.

The dye used within the lasers also represents a potential danger, and it should be handled and disposed of in a manner suitable for this type of hazardous material.

Dye lasers achieve their clinical effect by heating the intraluminal blood to at least 75°C. Therefore, it is important to remember that they will heat other material that could ignite combustible substances if precautions are not taken. The skin should not be prepared with any flammable material, such as alcohol, ether, or acetone. Drapes are usually not required, but if used, they should be moistened with saline or water. Lesions that extend into the hairline or the eyebrows require that the laser surgeon keep the patient's hair wet and inform the patient of the possibility that some hair may be singed.

INDICATIONS

Box 19–1 lists some of the benign vascular cutaneous lesions that are amenable to treatment with the FPDL and LP-FPDL. Effective primary treatment of cavernous hemangiomas has not been shown due to the thickness of the lesion, larger blood vessel diameters, and high flow rate of blood. However, small residual lesions that may persist after using other modalities may be treated with the FPDL or LP-FPDL.

Box 19–1. Benign Cutaneous Vascular Lesions Treatable with FPDL

Port-wine stains (vascular malformation)

Strawberry hemangioma

Blue rubber bleb syndrome

Facial telangiectasias

Rosacea

CREST (calcinosis, Raynaud's disease, esophageal dysmotility, sclerodactyly, telangiectasia)

Angioma

   Spider

   Campbell De Morgan (cherry)

Angiofibroma (tuberous sclerosis)

Venous lakes

Patients with port-wine stains treated with other modalities, such as the argon, CO_2, or KTP laser, electrocautery, radiation, or tattooing, may experience less lightening and improvement in the port-wine stains. Scarring that results from other laser therapies, electrocautery, or radiation may be made more apparent after the surrounding port-wine stain is lightened using the dye laser. All patients who have received previous treatment with other modalities should be cautioned about this possibility as well as the fact that their response to the dye laser may be reduced by the presence of scar tissue.

The pigments in tattoos used to camouflage port-wine stains may act as competing chromophores to oxyhemoglobin, and the repeated needle injections used during the tattoo process cause a certain amount of der-

mal fibrosis that can result in increased scattering and decreased absorption of the laser light energy.

Patients with Fitzpatrick skin types IV and V may not derive as much benefit from the dye laser or any other visible-light laser because of the increased amounts of competing chromophores (i.e., melanin) present in their skin. A test spot is recommended for many patients, but it has added importance in these patients.

PATIENT PREPARATION AND PRETREATMENT

During the patient's first office visit, the initial step is a detailed history and physical examination. It is important to address the following questions: How long has the lesion been present? Has it changed in size? Has there been any bleeding from the lesion or any associated ophthalmologic, neurologic, or upper airway symptoms? Are there any other family members with similar lesions? If the history and physical examination indicate an isolated benign vascular cutaneous lesion, the consultation continues with careful photographic documentation of the present state of the lesion. This is important for medicolegal reasons and also because some patients and family members have a tendency to forget the severity of the condition once they have begun to see improvement in a particular lesion.

Expectations

It should be emphasized that the goal of this therapy is improvement and not perfection. Pretreatment discussions should be forthright. The patient and family should understand that multiple treatments may be necessary; one study demonstrated an average of 6.5 treatments per lesional area for children with port-wine stains.[16] Risks and complications such as skin texture changes, hypopigmentation, and scarring exist but are extremely rare. Nevertheless, these risks must be addressed. If the patient agrees to treatment, depending on the lesion and the patient's skin type, a test spot may be recommended.

Spot Testing

Port-wine stains usually are tested at various energy levels ranging from 5.5 to 7.5 J/cm^2 using a 5-mm spot size for the FPDL; because of the longer pulse duration and penetration of the LP-FPDL, test energy levels are lower. Children's lesions, macular pink lesions, and lesions of the eyelids and neck are also usually treated at lower energy levels; darker lesions and elevated lesions may require higher energy levels with the FPDL.[16] Treatment doses should vary with color, location, and type of lesion and skin type. A test spot usually consists of eight to ten contiguously placed spots, and it should be done in an inconspicuous but representative area of the lesion. Before performing a test spot, the patient should be informed that the area will appear bruised and/or blue-gray for 7 to 10 days, and then it should start to lighten. The patient is asked to return about 6 weeks after treatment to assess the test spot and adjust the energy density, if necessary, before further treatment is undertaken.

TECHNIQUES AND PARAMETERS

Treatment techniques and parameters vary according to the lesion. For port-wine stains, the energy density is adjusted based on the location of the lesion. A hemifacial port-wine stain around the eyes, lips, or cervical region requires a decrease in energy density. The size of the facial or cervical area to be treated depends on the patient's tolerance of the treatment. Local anesthesia is not used, and patients describe the sensation as "like being popped with a rubber band." Most often large facial port-wine stains in adults are divided and treated by aesthetic facial units. This allows for treatment sessions of 15 to 30 minutes, which often can be tolerated even by patients with extremely low pain thresholds. Very young children (less than 2 years of age) usually require some type of restraint during the procedure and often need to be treated under general anesthesia. In children older than 2 years, a mild sedative or even general anesthesia may be considered to reduce anxiety. Large lesions can be treated rapidly under general anesthesia. Eyelid

lesions in children of any age require administration of general anesthesia because scleral shields must be used for eye protection.

COMPLICATIONS

Complications with the dye lasers are rare. Hyperpigmentation is the most common complication, occurring in approximately 10 to 15% of patients treated with the FPDL.[17] Hyperpigmentation occurs more often in darkly pigmented individuals and when higher energy levels are used; it usually resolves within 2 to 3 months. Hypopigmentation occurs less frequently (<5% of patients) and usually resolves within a couple of months. Transient hyperpigmentation and hypopigmentation were seen in the treatment of leg telangiectasias with the LP-FPDL, but these resolved within a few months with no textural changes or other sequelae.[18] Scarring occurs in less than 1% of patients[17] and is generally atrophic in nature.[19] Infections are extremely rare, usually resulting from trauma to treated areas. Retinal damage is totally avoidable with proper use of eye protection. Superficial burns have occurred with ignition of hair. Proper care must be taken with general anesthesia, when high concentrations of oxygen are present.

PORT-WINE STAINS

A port-wine stain is approached with the dye laser by placing contiguous treatment spots within the area to be treated. A small amount of overlap at the periphery of the spots is acceptable, because the lens system in the handpiece causes a slight dissipation of the laser energy at the edges (5–10%). Large overlaps of the spots or repeated pulses to the same area may result in complications (Fig. 19–3).

After a treatment session, cold compresses are applied to the area. Patients undergoing treatment for facial port-wine stains are instructed not to wear makeup for the next 5 to 7 days because of the fragility of the epidermis

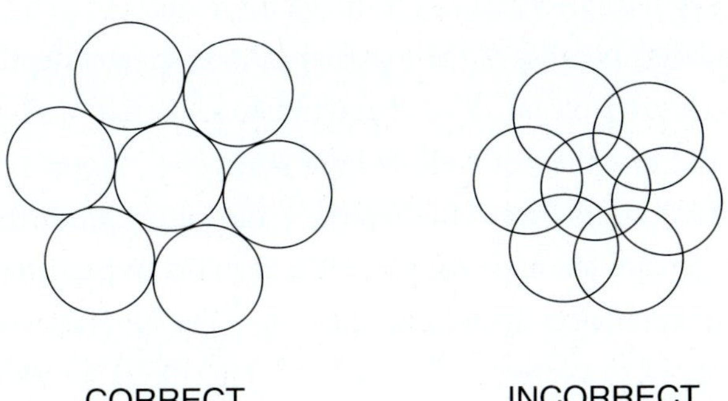

Figure 19–3. Correct and incorrect placement of laser pulses.

during the immediate posttreatment period; makeup could increase the risk of infection and result in scarring. If the area feels dry and tight or if any crusting appears, patients are asked to lightly coat the area with bacitracin ointment two to three times a day. For about 2 weeks after treatment, patients are asked to refrain from any activity in which there may be a chance of traumatizing the treated area (e.g., contact sports). Furthermore, they are instructed to avoid excessive exposure to sunlight and, if they must be outside, to wear a broad-brimmed hat and use sunscreen. Patients who work in dirty or dusty environments should cover the treated area with a light nonstick dressing until the blue-gray discoloration fades, usually in 7 to 10 days.

The same area may be re-treated safely 6 to 8 weeks after the first visit if the desired effect has not been achieved; most port-wine stains require several treatment sessions, but this depends on the color, size, and location of the lesion, as mentioned earlier. Facial port-wine stains appear to respond best to treatment (Fig. 19–4), those of the neck less well, and those of the trunk and extremities least favorably.[20] Age of the patient also plays a role; although younger patients have appeared to respond more favorably, recent results show that port-wine stains treated in early childhood or at a later age led to similar results.[21] Complete eradication of the port-wine stain is the ideal goal, but some patients may reach a point where further treatments fail to produce any additional improvement. Other patients have stopped treatments because they were satisfied with the improvement in their appearance, even if further lightening of the lesion were possible. The decision to end treatment is usually made by the physician and patient.

If a patient desires further improvement and has been treated with the FPDL or the LP-FPDL at 585 nm with no further improvement, then treatment test spots with the longer wavelengths (590–600 nm) available on the LP-FPDL may be indicated. As mentioned earlier, because longer wavelengths have greater penetration, they may reach deeper components of the port-wine stain. In addition, the longer pulse duration (1.5 milliseconds) of the LP-FPDL enables a greater delivery of energy to these deeper components, further improving the chances for increased lightening.

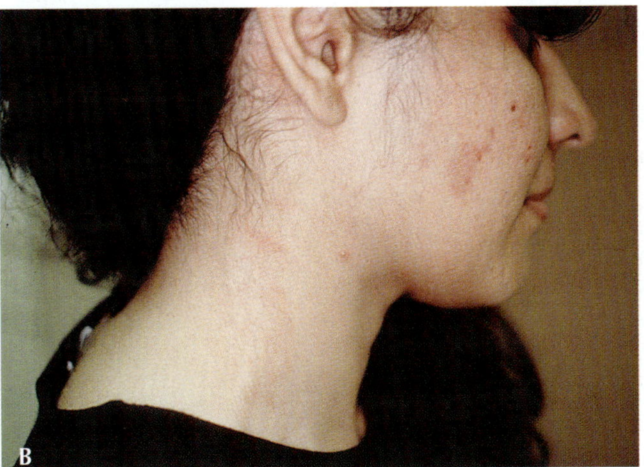

Figure 19–4. Facial port-wine stain before (A) and after (B) FPDL treatment.

TELANGIECTASIAS

Telangiectasias can be divided into two types: facial and leg telangiectasias. Treatment techniques for facial telangiectasias are similar to those described for port-wine stains in terms of test spots, treatment intervals, and post-treatment care. Treatment differences between port-wine stains and telangiectasias may be the energy densities used and the way in which the laser energy is applied. As a general rule, energy densities for telangiectasias are approximately 0.5 J/cm^2 less than those used for port-wine stains, and often individual facial telangiectasias require only one treatment. For larger facial vessels or for those for which the FPDL was ineffective, the LP-FPDL can be employed (Figs. 19–5 and 19–6).

Leg telangiectasias can be much more difficult to treat with lasers because of their greater caliber, greater depth, and varying blood flow characteristics. Earlier studies showed that the non-yellow-light lasers (i.e., argon and Nd:YAG lasers) were ineffective[22] and often produced scarring and textural changes; FPDL resulted in persistent postinflammatory hyperpigmentation.[23] The LP-FPDL was developed to address these problems (Fig. 19–7). In addition to standard treatment handpieces, it is equipped with a 2 × 7-mm elliptical spot handpiece designed to allow leg telangiectasias to be traced out. Moreover, the longer wavelengths and pulse durations allow higher energy delivery to these larger-caliber vessels, similar to the approach to resistant port-wine stains. Although results from some studies are encouraging,[24] the response of leg

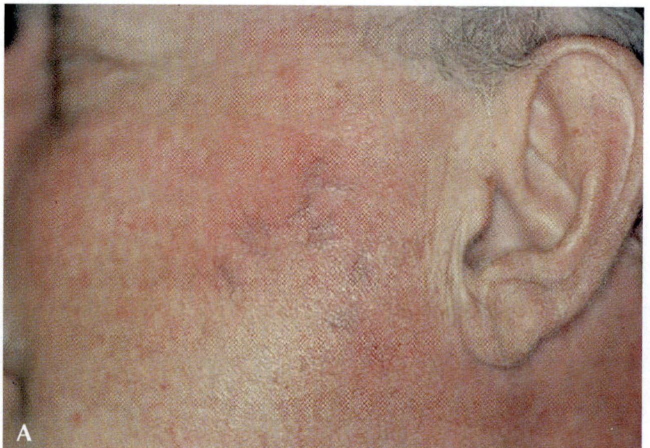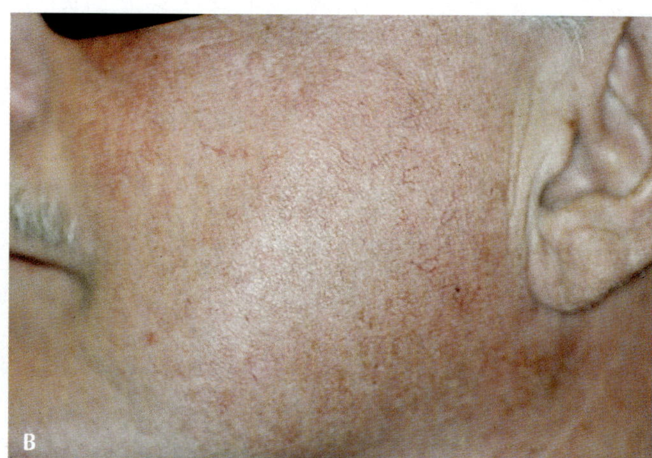

Figure 19–5. Facial telangiectasias before (A) and after (B) LP-FPDL treatment.

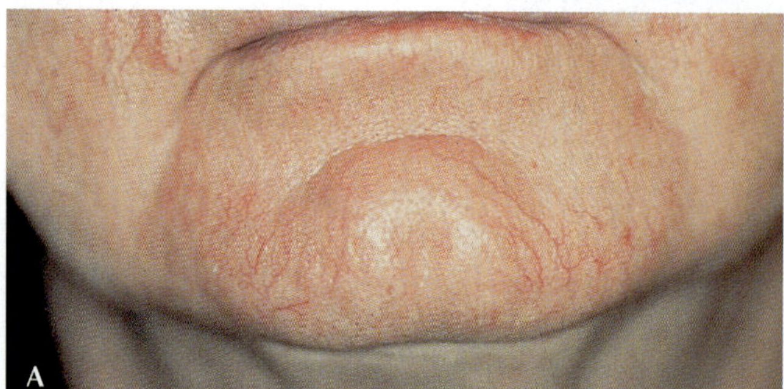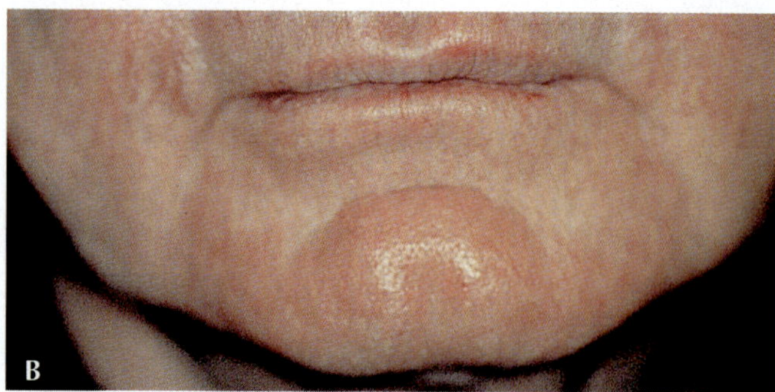

Figure 19–6. Facial telangiectasias before (A) and after (B) LP-FPDL treatment.

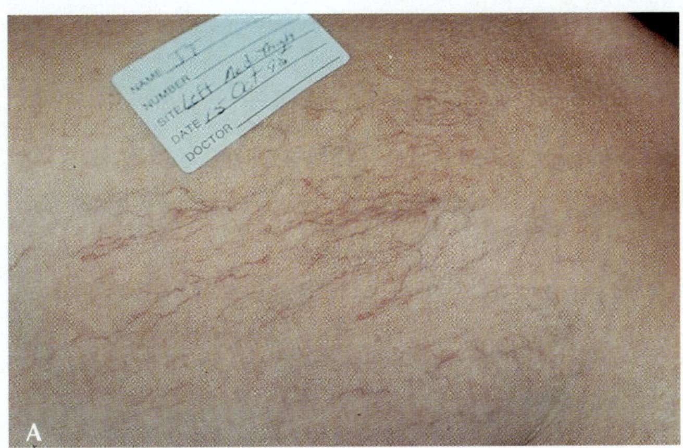 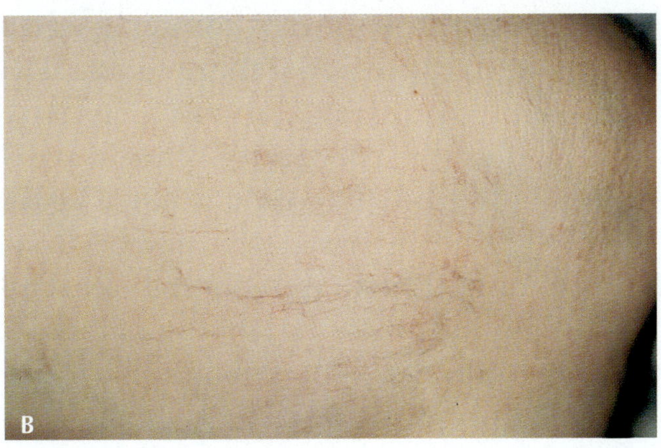

Figure 19–7. Leg telangiectasias before (A) and after (B) LP-FPDL treatment.

telangiectasias has been inconsistent and unpredictable, again most likely because of varying calibers and flow characteristics, such that LP-FPDL treatment is probably best employed as adjunctive therapy to other techniques such as sclerotherapy.

HEMANGIOMAS

Early reports of treatment of capillary hemangiomas with the FPDL are very encouraging, with complete resolution or impedance of growth of the lesions.[25–28] Treatment energy levels are about the same as for port-wine stains, and treatment can be repeated in 2 to 4 weeks to impede further growth. The endpoint of treatment is complete resolution of the lesion or no anticipation of further growth.[19]

The FPDL can be very effective in early treatment of hemangiomas near vital structures such as the eye. Cavernous hemangiomas are not responsive to the FPDL, as was discussed earlier. Capillary hemangiomas are best treated in the first few weeks of life when the lesions are small and macular. Once the lesion has matured and thickened, the response is much less dramatic.[19]

SCARS AND STRIAE

Erythematous and hypertrophic scars have been shown to improve with FPDL treatment.[29,30] The laser can significantly reduce the overlying erythema and may flatten the scar by decreasing collagen synthesis. Multiple treat-

ments are necessary, especially with thick scars, and often adjunctive treatment, such as intralesional steroid injection, hastens improvement.

Low-energy FPDL treatment can improve the appearance of erythematous and silvery striae.[31] The mechanism of action is unknown but may be related to an increase in elastin content; visible-light lasers at low fluences stimulate fibroblast proliferation, which can increase collagen and elastin production.

WARTS

The FPDL has been used for flat warts as well as recalcitrant common warts. One study of exclusively recalcitrant warts found that 72% of the patients were cleared of their warts after an average of 1.68 treatments, and overall response rates were in the range of 83 to 99%.[32] The mechanism of action again is unclear, but the technique of double or triple pulsing the FPDL light may cause thermal destruction of the wart primarily. Multiple treatments 2 to 6 weeks apart are often necessary.

CONCLUSIONS

The FPDL and LP-FPDL have been proven to be safe, effective, and very valuable tools for the treatment of a variety of cutaneous vascular lesions. Future studies should delineate their effectiveness and their role in the treatment of many other cutaneous lesions and disorders.

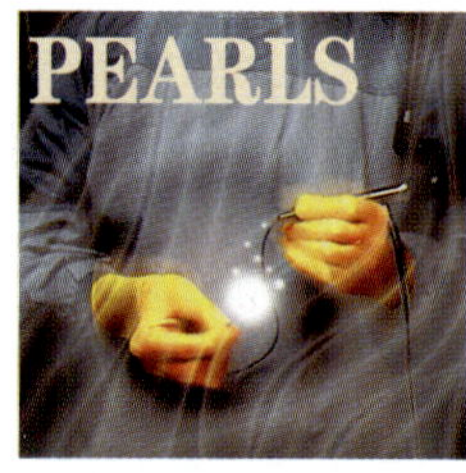

- The FPDL is one of the easiest lasers to use, relying more on an individual's training than his or her expertise. Despite its ease of use, didactic and hands-on instruction are imperative. Training in the use of another visible-light laser such as the argon laser should not be accepted as adequate training for the FPDL or the LP-FPDL.

- It is important that all individuals in the laser suite wear protective eyewear specifically for the range of wavelengths of the FPDL and LP-FPDL. Eyewear designed for other visible-light lasers is not adequate protection from these wavelengths.

- Adult patients describe the sensation of FPDL treatment as "like being popped with a rubber band." Older children may need a mild sedative, but children less than 2 years of age usually require some type of restraint and often need to be treated under general anesthesia.

- Capillary hemangiomas are best treated with FPDL in the first few weeks of life when the lesions are small and macular. Port-wine stains are also more effectively treated in younger patients.

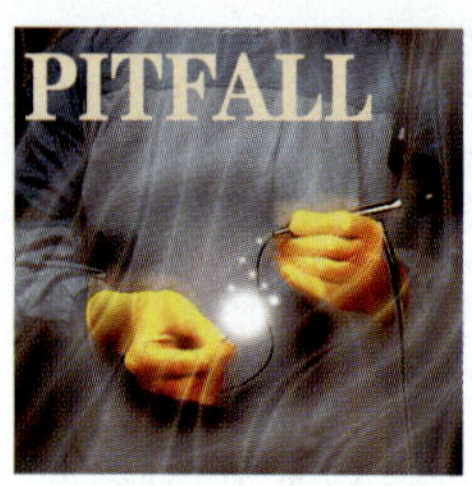

- If a port-wine stain has been treated with another modality, such as the argon, CO_2, or KTP laser, electrocautery, radiation, or tattooing, FPDL treatment may provide less lightening and improvement. Scarring from other laser therapies, electrocautery, or radiation may be made more apparent after treatment with the FPDL.

REFERENCES

1. Ratz JL. Current concepts of CO_2 laser therapy of port-wine stains. *Lasers Surg Med.* 1984;3:335.
2. Bailin PL. Treatment of port-wine stain with the CO_2 laser: early results. In: Arndt KA, Noe JM, Rosen S, eds. *Cutaneous Laser Therapy: Principles and Methods.* New York: John Wiley and Sons, 1983:129–136.
3. Apfelberg DB, Bailin P, Rosenberg H. Preliminary investigation of KTP/532 laser light in the treatment of hemangiomas and tattoos. *Lasers Surg Med.* 1986;6:38–42.
4. Rosenfeld H, Sherman R. Treatment of cutaneous and deep vascular lesions with the Nd:YAG laser. *Lasers Surg Med.* 1986;6:20–23.
5. Noe JM, Barsky SH, Geer DE. Port wine stains and the response to argon laser therapy: successful treatment and predictive role of color, age, and biopsy. *Plast Reconstr Surg.* 1980;65:130–136.
6. Silver L. Argon laser photocoagulation of port wine stain hemangiomas. *Lasers Surg Med.* 1986;6:24–28.
7. Glassberg E, Lask GP, Tan EML, Uitto J. The flashlamp-pumped 577–nm pulsed tunable dye laser: clinical efficacy and in vitro studies. *J Dermatol Surg Oncol.* 1988;14:1200–1208.
8. Garden JM, Polla LL, Tan OT. The treatment of portwine stains by the pulsed dye laser: analysis of pulse duration and long-term therapy. Arch Dermatol 1988;124:889–896.
9. Tan OT, Carney JM, Margolis R, et al. Histologic responses of port-wine stains treated by argon, carbon dioxide, and tunable dye lasers. *Arch Dermatol.* 1986;122:1016–1022.
10. Anderson RR, Parrish JA. Microvasculature can be selectively damaged using dye lasers: a basic theory and experimental evidence in human skin. *Lasers Surg Med.* 1983;1:263–276.
11. Anderson RR, Parrish JA. Selective photothermolysis: precise microsurgery by selective absorption of pulsed radiation. *Science.* 1983;22:524–527.
12. Anderson RR, Hu J, Parrish JA. Optical radiation transfer in the human and applications in in vivo remittance spectroscopy. In: Marks R, Payne PA, eds. *Bioengineering and the Skin.* London: MPT Press, 1980:253–265.
13. Tan OT, Murray S, Kurban AK. Action spectrum of vascular specific injury using pulsed irradiation. J Invest Dermatol. 1989;92:868–871.
14. VonGemert MJC, Welch AJ, Amin AP. Is there an optimal laser treatment for port wine stains? *Lasers Surg Med.* 1986;6:76–83.
15. Garden J, Tan OT, Kerschmann R, Boll J, Parrish JA. Effect of pulsewidth on vessel specific changes induced by a pulsed laser radiation. J Invest Dermatol. 1986;87:653–657.
16. Tan OT, Sherwood K, Gilchrest BA. Treatment of children with port-wine stains using the flashlamp-pulsed tunable dye laser. N Engl J Med. 1989;320:416–421.
17. Glassberg E, Lask GP, Tan EML, Uitto J. The flashlamp pumped 577 nm tunable dye laser: clinical efficacy and in vitro studies. J Dermatol Surg Oncol. 1988;14:1200–1208.
18. Lee PK, Lask GP. Treatment of leg veins by long pulse dye laser (Sclerolaser). *Lasers Surg Med.* 1997;suppl 9:40.
19. Lask GP, Glassberg E. 585 nm pulsed dye laser for the treatment of cutaneous lesions. Clin Dermatol. 1995;13:63–67.

20. Renfro L, Geronemus RG. Anatomical differences of port-wine stains in response to treatment with the pulsed dye laser. *Arch Dermatol.* 1993;129:182–188.

21. van der Horst CM, Koster PH, de Borgie CA, Bossuyt PM, van Gemert MJ. Effect of the timing of treatment of port-wine stains with the flash-lamp-pumped pulsed dye laser. *N Engl J Med.* 1998;338:1028–1033.

22. Apfelberg DB, Smith T, Maser MR, Lash H, White DN. Study of three laser systems for treatment of superficial varicosities of the lower extremity. *Lasers Surg Med.* 1987;7:219–223.

23. Goldman MP, Fitzpatrick RE. Pulsed dye laser treatment of leg telangiectasia: with and without simultaneous sclerotherapy. *J Dermatol Surg Oncol.* 1990;16:338–344.

24. Hsia J, Lowery JA, Zelickson B. Treatment of leg telangiectasia using a long-pulse dye laser at 595 nm. *Lasers Surg Med.* 1997;20:1–5.

25. Glassberg E, Lask GP, Rabinowitz LG, Tunnessen WW. Capillary hemangiomas: case study of a novel laser treatment and a review of therapeutic options. *J Dermatol Surg Oncol.* 1989;15:1214–1223.

26. Ashinoff R, Geronemus RG. Capillary hemangiomas and treatment with flashlamp-pumped dye laser. *Arch Dermatol.* 1991;127:202–205.

27. Garden JM, Bakus AD, Paller AS. Treatment of cutaneous hemangiomas by the flashlamp-pumped pulsed dye laser: prospective analysis. *J Pediatr.* 1992;120:555–560.

28. Geronemus RG. Pulsed dye laser treatment of vascular lesions in children. *J Dermatol Surg Oncol.* 1994;19:303.

29. Alster TS, Kurban AK, Grove GL, et al. Alteration of argon laser-induced scars by the pulse dye laser. *Lasers Surg Med.* 1993;13:368–373.

30. Alster TS, Williams CM. Improvements of hypertrophic and keloidal median sternotomy scars by the 585 nm flashlamp-pumped pulse dye laser: a controlled study. *Lancet.* 1995;345:1198–1200.

31. McDaniel DH, Ash K, Zukowski M. Treatment of stretch marks with the 585 nm flashlamp-pumped pulse dye laser. *Dermatol Surg.* 1996;22;332–337.

32. Tan OT, Hurwitz RM, Stafford TJ. Pulsed dye laser treatment of recalcitrant verrucae: a preliminary report. *Lasers Surg Med.* 1993;13:127–137.

CHAPTER 20

The VersaPulse Laser

EMIL A. TANGHETTI

The VersaPulse laser has become an important asset to the cosmetic laser surgeon for the treatment of vascular lesions because it heats blood vessels more slowly than other lasers, resulting in vessel ablation, not rupture. Conversely, the pulsed-dye laser at 585 nm with a 0.45- to 1.5-millisecond pulse duration heats vessels very rapidly, which leads to rupturing of the targeted blood vessels and purpura.

The importance of the millisecond pulse duration was suggested by the work of van Gemert et al[1] and Dierickx et al.[2] Based on their theoretical foundation, the VersaPulse laser was designed with pulse durations ranging from 1 to 10 milliseconds. This was later expanded with the HELP G, which permits pulse durations of up to 50 milliseconds.

BASIC PRINCIPLES AND PROCEDURES

The 532-nm laser light generated by the VersaPulse is well absorbed by hemoglobin (Fig. 20–1). However, melanin also selectively absorbs this wavelength. With use of a contact "chill tip" and a relatively long pulse duration, the heat generated in the epidermis by the VersaPulse can be wicked away, allowing continued penetration of the laser beam through the epidermis and into the targeted areas of the papillary and reticular dermis. The epidermis is not frosted or significantly damaged by

the laser pulse and can be lased repeatedly. Rather than destroying the targeted blood vessels in one pass, repeated passes can accomplish this task with little damage to surrounding tissues.

With these principles in mind, the VersaPulse laser generally is used with pulse durations ranging from 10 to 50 milliseconds, fluences of 9 to 24 J/cm^2, and a chiller set at 4 to 5°C. Spot sizes generally range from 3 to 6 mm. The larger spot size should be used whenever possible to allow for deeper penetration of the laser light into the dermis. Blood vessels generally are treated from the distal to the proximal end, thus preventing proximal spasm and premature disappearance of the entire target. Blood vessels are traced with consecutive passes rather than double or triple pulses to prevent unwanted heat accumulation. It is important to develop a smooth, flowing hand movement. Initially repetition rates of 1 to 2 Hz are used. As one becomes more experienced, repetition rates of 3 to 6 Hz are useful.

Ultrasound gel has become an important agent in VersaPulse laser treatments because it permits rapid and smooth movement by the operator and allows remarkably tight contact between the chill tip and skin surface, facilitating heat transfer away from the epidermis. The refractive index is also better matched when using the gel. When treating tight spaces such as nasolabial folds, this gel fills in gaps where the chill tip does not have direct contact with the skin and allows the entire area to be cooled.

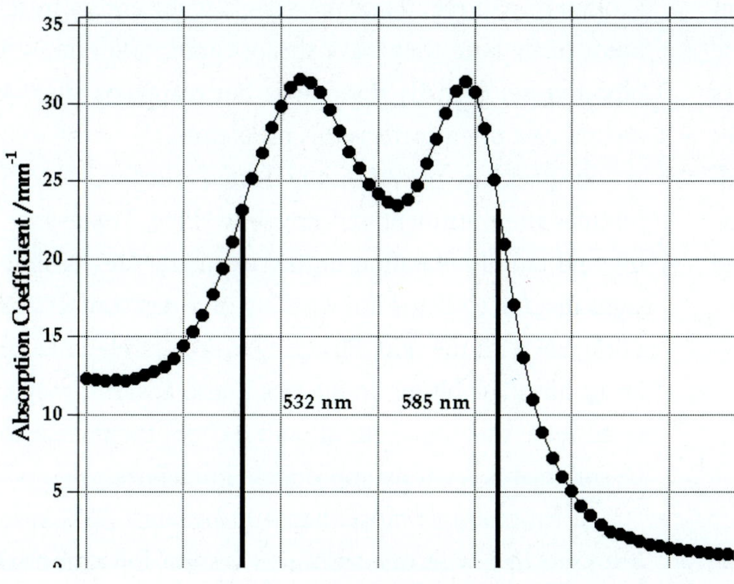

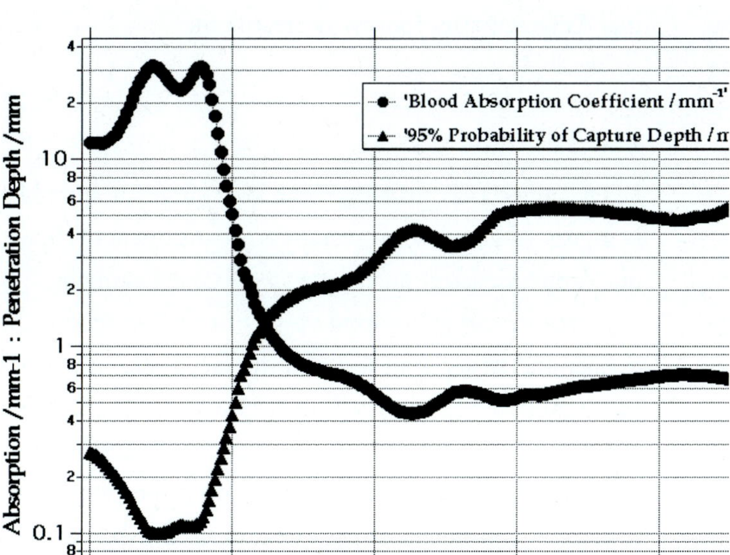

Figure 20–1. (A) Absorption of light generated by VersaPulse by hemoglobin. (B) Comparison of blood absorption and penetration of VersaPulse.

GENERAL CONTRAINDICATIONS AND ADVERSE EFFECTS

Treating patients with darker skin types (Fitzpatrick skin types V and VI) or deep tans can be a problem, but patients with Fitzpatrick skin types I to III are excellent candidates. When the epidermis is heavily melanized, the laser light is significantly absorbed and can damage the epidermis and papillary dermis. It is best to allow deep tans to fade for 30 days and to supplement this process with hydroquinones and sunscreens. During this time, the patient should avoid sun exposure. In patients with darker skin types, it is best to treat a few test spots before contemplating a more extensive procedure.

Immediate graying or blistering during test treatment can signify a problem, and the surgeon should cease treatments. It is important to evaluate whether there was proper contact of the chill tip with the skin or whether the fluence was too high. It is also wise to check the chill tip to be sure that it is cool and to check the output setting on the chiller to be certain that it is at the desired temperature.

TREATMENT OF SPECIFIC LESIONS

FACIAL TELANGIECTASIAS

Unwanted facial blood vessels are a problem seen frequently in most cosmetic dermatology practices. The VersaPulse laser can be particularly useful when treating patients with 0.1- to 1.5-mm-wide vessels because of the low rate of morbidity and the need for little or no time away from normal daily activities on the day of treatment. In contrast, pulsed-dye lasers result in purpura that can last from 7 to 14 days.

Blood vessels smaller than 0.3 mm in diameter are treated with fluences of 9 to 13 J/cm^2, a 4- to 5-mm spot size, the chiller set at 4 to 5°C, and pulse durations ranging from 10 to 30 milliseconds. I favor a 5-mm spot, 20-millisecond pulse durations, and fluences of 9.5 to 10 J/cm^2. If vessels are slow to respond, I often change to a 4-mm spot, 10-millisecond pulse duration, and 9 to 9.5 J/cm^2. Generally, one to three passes are required. If after repeated passes I do not see an adequate response, I often proceed to other areas. After several minutes, I retreat the first area with another pass. The partially damaged blood vessels seem to be much more vulnerable after 10 to 30 minutes and often respond favorably to another pass.

Blood vessels larger than 0.4 mm in diameter are treated with fluences of 10 to 14 J/cm^2, a 50-millisecond pulse duration, the chiller set at 4°C, and a spot size of 5 to 6 mm. Again, one to three passes are necessary. It is often best to reevaluate the vessels at the end of treatment to be sure they have disappeared. Sometimes a blood vessel partially disappears but reappears later. A second pass often corrects this problem.

Ice packs are placed on the treated area for 10 to 15 minutes after treatment to decrease swelling. Tissue graying and tan discoloration during treatment are warning signs that the chiller is not working or direct contact was not made with the skin. Blistering is seen rarely in facial areas, but a late blister on the face is also a warning sign. In all these situations, one should recheck the fluence to be sure that it is within appropriate guidelines.

In treatment of more than 400 patients, 85% have been satisfied with one treatment session for abnormal facial telangiectasias.[3,4] Another 15% required a second treatment session to achieve an acceptable result. This was accomplished with no purpura and a rapid return to normal daily activities following treatment.

LEG TELANGIECTASIAS

Leg telangiectasias challenge both laser surgeons and phlebologists. Although sclerotherapy is the treatment of choice, the VersaPulse laser can also be an effective treatment.

Because targeted blood vessels in the leg tend to be deeper and larger than those in the face, pulse durations of 50 milliseconds with a 5-mm spot size, the chiller set at 4°C, and fluences of 17 to 20 J/cm^2 are generally used. One to three passes are adequate. If no response is noted or if the vessels reappear after treatment, the spot size can be reduced to 4 mm and the fluence raised to 20 to 24 J. If the blood vessels are small, that is, less than 0.2 mm in diameter, and do not respond, a 3-mm spot size, 10-millisecond pulse duration, and fluences of 13 to 14 J/cm^2 may be necessary.

Graying and immediate blistering of the tissues indicate that it is necessary to reevaluate cooling and fluence settings. However, unlike on the face, delayed blistering with these fluences is not uncommon. As long as the areas of laser damage are superficial and treated appropriately postoperatively, low (if any) morbidity is experienced, and generally no scarring is seen. Small blisters can be treated with showering and Aquaphor healing ointment.

The favorable response to treatment of leg veins with the VersaPulse laser is approximately 60% for appropriately targeted blood vessels measuring 0.3 to 1 mm in diameter. A second treatment increases this response to approximately 80%.[5]

PORT-WINE STAINS

Port-wine stains remain a therapeutic challenge. The pulsed-dye laser has long been recognized as the "gold standard" of treatment for this problem. However, this device has its limitations and is often plagued with mechanical problems. Van Gemert et al[1] and Dierickx et al[2] have suggested that a longer pulse duration of 1 to 10 milliseconds is ideal to treat this vascular abnormality.

Recent work with the VersaPulse laser for the eradication of port-wine stains has been encouraging. Mature port-wine stains, which are often a dark purple color and slightly raised above the skin surface,[6] are difficult to treat with pulsed-dye lasers but have shown a remarkably positive response with the VersaPulse laser system. Using a 4-mm spot size, a fluence of 9 to 12 J/cm^2, and a 10 to 40-millisecond pulse duration, I have used the VersaPulse on pulsed-dye laser patients with excellent results after just one or two treatments.

When treating infants with port-wine stains, who generally are not treated with the pulsed-dye laser, it is especially important to do test spots to determine the proper fluence. I have seen successful eradications with pulse durations of 20, 30, and 40 milliseconds, which appears to contradict current scientific knowledge. However, this response is not unexpected if one understands the nature of the pulse duration of the VersaPulse unit. A 10-millisecond pulse with the VersaPulse laser is a true 10-millisecond square-wave pulse. However, all pulses of 15 to 50 milliseconds are composed of blocks of pulses that are on for 3 milliseconds then off for 3 milliseconds (Fig. 20–2). Therefore, these longer pulses actually allow

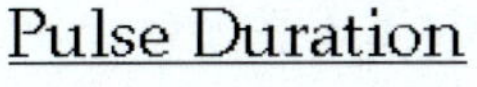
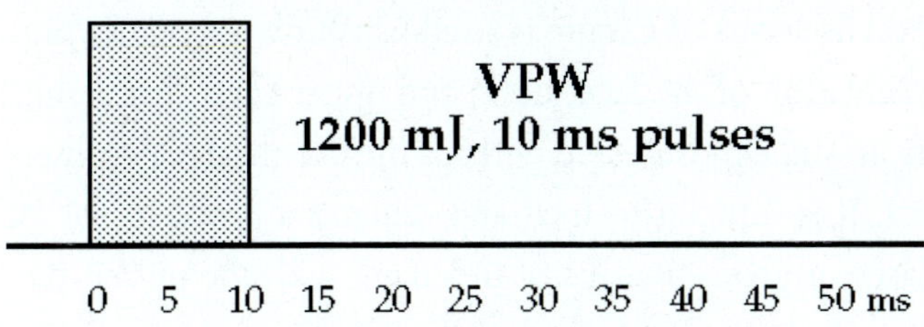

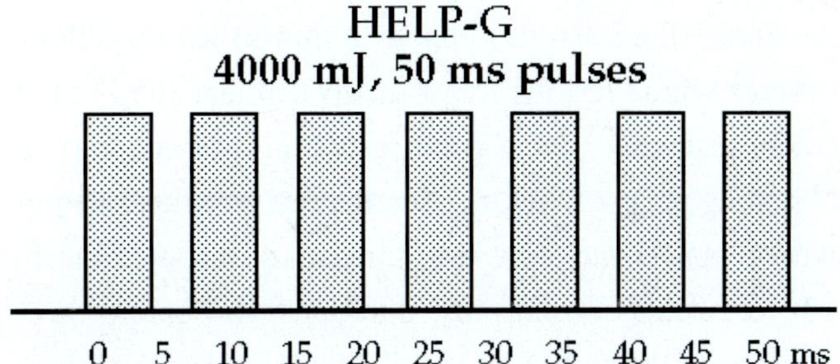

Figure 20–2. Pulse duration of VersaPulse (VPW) versus HELP-G lasers.

true multiple-pulse photocoagulation of the abnormal blood vessels in a port-wine stain. This concept was suggested by Dierickx et al[7] and actually appears to be an important part of the response seen with the VersaPulse laser. I generally perform one to three passes using ultrasound gel and look for disappearance of the abnormal red or maroon pigmentation. If there is graying or tan discoloration, it is best to check cooling and decrease the fluence.

These results are very preliminary, and there is much more to be learned about the use of the VersaPulse laser in treating port-wine stains. However, the VersaPulse has been remarkably helpful in eradicating larger, more mature port-wine stains. that previously were unresponsive to therapy.

HEMANGIOMAS

Hemangiomas, especially facial lesions, can appear unsightly. I often treat these lesions initially with a 50-millisecond pulse duration at 10 to 13 J/cm^2 and later follow them with a 10- to 20-millisecond pulse duration at 9.5 J/cm^2. Gradually the lesions respond, sometimes in one treatment session. At other times, however, two to three treatments are necessary.

POIKILODERMA OF CIVATTE

Poikiloderma of Civatte is a reddish-brown reticular pigmentation of the face, neck, and upper chest that results from sun exposure and perhaps the chemicals in cosmetics. It is difficult to treat and remains a problem for all laser surgeons. Results of treatment with the pulsed-dye laser have not been good, and generally, patient satisfaction is low. However, my preliminary results suggest that the VersaPulse laser may help treat this difficult problem. Patients whose lesions are primarily vascular (i.e., red in color) generally have a good response. After a 1-month bleaching program before laser therapy, treatment begins with a 4- to 5-mm spot size, fluences of 9 to 9.5 J/cm^2, 10- to 20-millisecond pulse durations, and one to three passes with the chiller set at 4°C. Results with one to three treatment sessions have been gratifying. Textural changes, hypopigmentation, and scarring have not been seen.

CONCLUSIONS

The VersaPulse laser has become an essential part of my laser practice. It is truly the treatment of choice for facial telangiectasias and certainly has a place in the treatment of hemangiomas, poikiloderma of Civatte, and port-wine stains. While no therapy is perfect for leg telangiectasias, it is my belief that the VersaPulse laser is the best choice for treating this difficult problem.

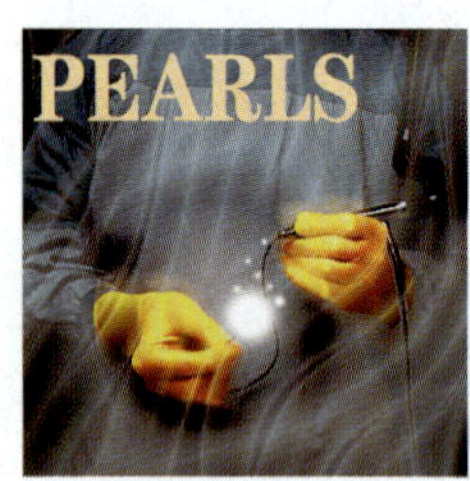

- Ultrasound gel permits rapid and smooth movement by the VersaPulse operator and allows remarkably tight contact between the chill tip and skin surface, facilitating heat transfer away from the epidermis. The refractive index is also better matched when using the gel. The gel fills in gaps in tight spaces where the chill tip does not have direct contact with the skin and allows the entire area to be cooled.

- A larger spot size should be used whenever possible to allow for deeper penetration of the laser light into the dermis.

- Blood vessels generally are treated from the distal to the proximal end, thus preventing proximal spasm and premature disappearance of the entire target. Blood vessels are traced with consecutive passes rather than double or triple pulses to prevent unwanted heat accumulation.

- When the epidermis is heavily melanized, the laser light can damage the epidermis and papillary dermis, so it is best to allow deep tans to fade for 30 days. Do a few test spots before contemplating a more extensive procedure.

- If after repeated passes for facial telangiectasias I do not see an adequate response, I often proceed to other parts of the face and then return to the area. The partially damaged blood vessels seem to be much more vulnerable after 5 to 10 minutes and often respond favorably to another pass.

- Reevaluate blood vessels at the end of treatment to be sure they have disappeared. Sometimes a blood vessel partially disappears but reappears later.

REFERENCES

1. van Gemert MJC, Welch AJ, Amin AP. Is there an optimal treatment for port-wine stains? *Lasers Surg Med.* 1986;6:76–83.
2. Dierickx CC, Casparian JM, Venugopalan V, et al. Thermal relaxation of port-wine stain vessels probed in vivo: the need for a 1–10 millisecond laser pulse treatment. *J Invest Dermatol.* 1995;105:709–714.
3. Tanghetti ET, Adrian RM. Long pulse 532–nm laser treatment of facial telangiectasia. *Dermatol Surg.* 1997;24:71–74.
4. Tanghetti ET, Adrian RM. Long-pulsed 532-nm laser treatment of facial telangiectasias. *Lasers Surg Med.* 1998;10:45.
5. Adrian RM, Tanghetti ET. Long pulse 532-nm laser treatment of lower extremity telangiectasias: a clinical and histologic study. *Lasers Surg Med.* 1998;10:31.
6. Tanghetti ET, Adrian RM. Long-pulsed 532-nm laser treatment of port wine stains. *Lasers Surg Med.* 1998;10:36.
7. Dierickx CC, Farinelli WA, Anderson RR, et al. Multiple pulse photocoagulation of port-wine stain blood vessels with a 585 nm pulsed dye laser. *Lasers Surg Med.* 1995;7:56.

CHAPTER 21

Noncoherent Filtered Flashlamp Intense Pulsed Light Device (PhotoDerm VL)

ROBERT A. WEISS AND MARGARET A. WEISS

One of the most frequently requested cosmetic procedures is elimination of facial and leg telangiectasias. Telangiectasias of the face are relatively uniform in size and depth, but ultrastructural studies show that the blood vessels of the leg vary in size and exist at different depths.[1,2] Leg veins are also under hydrostatic pressure and differ widely in the degree of oxygenation. Therefore, treatment of leg veins using laser light is much more difficult than treatment of facial veins.

One of the newest light-based methods applied to this cosmetic problem is the noncoherent filtered flashlamp intense pulsed light (IPL) device (PhotoDerm VL, MultiLight, ESC/Sharplan Inc., Boston, MA). The goal is to achieve selective photothermolysis of the blood vessel using light energy. The absorption coefficient of blood within blood vessels is higher than that of the bloodless dermis for a very broad range of wavelengths. When filtered, the IPL device is capable of emitting a bandwidth of light from 515 to approximately 1200 nm. This bandwidth is then modified by application of filters that exclude the lower wavelengths. Presently, applied filters are 515, 550, 570, and 590 nm, and longer filters, such as 615 and 645 nm, may soon be available.

THEORETICAL AND PRACTICAL IMPLICATIONS

Theoretically, selectivity for deoxyhemoglobin is obtained at 600 to 750 nm. Whereas oxyhemoglobin is characterized by very high absorption coefficients of up to 630 nm, absorption drops at longer wavelengths but rises again to a broad peak in the near-infrared region in the 800- to 900-nm range (Fig. 21–1). Deoxyhemoglobin has similar absorption characteristics to oxyhemoglobin up to 600 nm, but at 600 to 750 nm, absorption does not drop as fast as for oxyhemoglobin. Therefore, because the purple telangiectasias of the leg contain less oxygen than red telangiectasias,[3] wavelengths in the 600- to 750-nm range are preferable for treating these relatively deoxygenated violaceous leg telangiectasias.

An additional advantage of working at higher wavelengths is that longer wavelengths are absorbed less by melanin. Melanin absorption is greatest in the ultraviolet

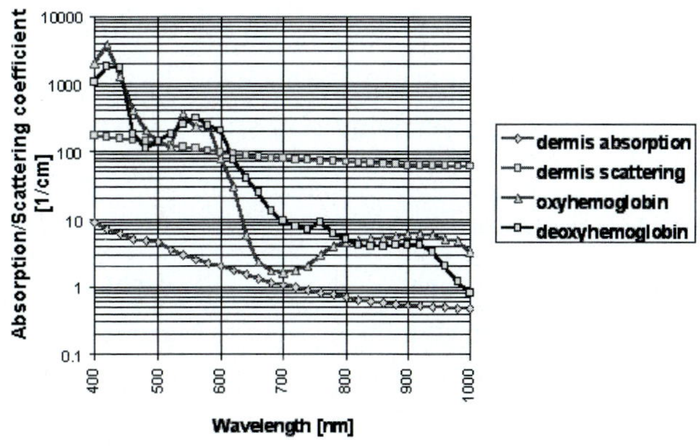

Figure 21–1. Absorption curve of hemoglobin in different states of oxygenation. Because collagen absorbs very little light on its own, the primary components absorbing light are hemoglobin and melanin (melanin not shown). There is a zone from 600 to 750 nm in which deoxyhemoglobin has preferential absorption.

range (240–360 nm) and decreases steadily as a function of increasing wavelength. Because absorption of light by skin is determined primarily by the skin's melanin content, not only do longer wavelengths penetrate more deeply, reaching relatively deeper blood vessels, but, in addition, more nonspecific melanin absorption with accompanying epidermal damage is avoided.

In treatment of blood vessels of the legs by a laser or IPL source, spot size plays a very important role because it, along with wavelength, has a direct effect on depth of penetration. Small spot size leads to rapid scatter and rapid decay of fluence by depth.[4] Penetration is therefore more efficient with a large spot size. A depth of 4 mm can be attained with the 8 × 35 mm rectangular spot size of the IPL device, considering an average wavelength of 800 nm (Table 21–1).

The large planar front of light emitted by the large-footprint IPL device must be directed using a water-based interface between the crystal and the skin. This water-based gel enhances optical coupling, minimizes reflections, and maintains continuity of the index of refraction of the skin–air interface. Clinical experience has emphasized the role of the gel as a heat sink. The heat generated by near-infrared wavelengths in the epidermis during the 2 to 8 milliseconds of the flashlamp pulse is very efficiently absorbed by the water-based gel. The gel may serve an additional function in that water absorbs some wavelengths beyond 1000 nm, thus filtering some of the higher near-infrared wavelengths. In the treatment of deeper, larger vessels, one may increase the fluence safely while protecting the overlying skin with chilled gel. A

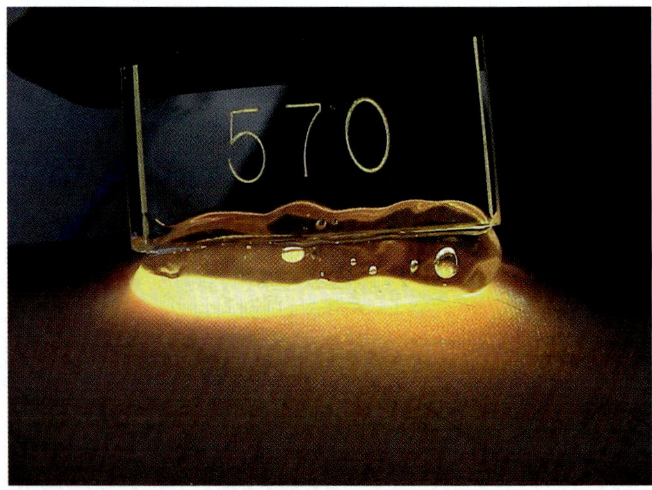

Figure 21–2. Proper spacing of the crystal from the skin with a 2-mm layer of gel. When the crystal is pressed onto the skin, the gel is directed to the sides of the crystal, leaving very little gel as a heat sink.

general rule is that when working with the large footprint of an IPL device, a 1- to 2-mm layer of gel between the crystal and the skin is highly desirable (Fig. 21–2).

Allowing a proper thermal relaxation time between pulses theoretically prevents elevation of epidermal temperatures above 70°C and is an inherent advantage of the multiple sequential pulsing of the IPL device. The epidermis generally is 100 μm thick, and its thermal relaxation time therefore is approximately 10 milliseconds. A typical blood vessel is 100 μm (0.1 mm) thick, and its thermal relaxation time is approximately 4 milliseconds. A telangiectatic blood vessel may be as large as 300 μm (0.3 mm), with a thermal relaxation time of about 10 milliseconds. Therefore, vessels larger than 0.3 mm cool more slowly than the epidermis when subjected to a single pulse. For larger vessels, however, multiple pulses with delay times of 10 milliseconds or more between pulses may be advantageous for epidermal cooling. This delay time must be increased with larger vessels because thermal diffusion across larger vessels increases the thermal relaxation time. Multiple sequential pulsing with delay times permits successive heating of targeted vessel(s) with adequate cooling time for the epidermis and surrounding structures.

The practical implications of these theoretical points are (1) vessels smaller than 0.3 mm should be treated

Table 21–1. Spot Size versus Wavelength

Spot Size	Light Penetration Depth (595 nm)	Light Penetration Depth (800 nm)*
1 mm	0.8 mm	1.5 mm
2 mm	1.1 mm	2.0 mm
5 mm	1.25 mm	2.5 mm

*For 800 nm the penetration appears to be half the diameter of the spot size. Therefore, an 8-mm-wide crystal should permit penetration as deep as 4 mm.

with a single pulse, (2) double or triple pulses should be spaced 10 milliseconds or more, (3) bright red lesions (containing oxyhemoglobin) are better treated with 515- or 550-nm filters, (4) violaceous lesions (containing deoxyhemoglobin) should be treated with 570- or 590-nm filters, and (5) darker skin (containing more melanin) should always be treated with 570- or 590-nm filters.

The newest theoretical advancement incorporated into the IPL device is elongation of pulse duration for larger vessels and the combination of short and long pulse widths. For many lasers used in the treatment of leg veins, a longer pulse duration (up to 50 milliseconds) has led to better clinical results.[5] Heat distribution for small vessels (0.3 mm) is assumed to be instantaneously Gaussian, but for larger vessels a Gaussian distribution cannot be assumed because more time is required for the heat to pass all the way to the core. Additional cooling time is required for the heat conduction from the core to the vessel surface. These principles were demonstrated using double-pulse experiments with the 585-nm yellow-dye laser in which larger vessels of port-wine stains (>0.1 mm) absorbed higher fluences after double pulses spaced 3 to 10 milliseconds apart before producing purpura.[6]

In another recent study using pulsed laser irradiation at 585 nm, short (0.45-millisecond) and long (10-millisecond) pulses were compared.[7] Results demonstrated that long-duration pulses caused coagulation of the larger-diameter vessels, whereas small-caliber vessels and capillaries showed resistance to photothermolysis at these parameters. Similarly, increasing pulse duration for the IPL device up to 12 milliseconds produces effective clinical photothermal coagulation of larger vessels (0.5 mm or greater) while sparing the epidermis.[8] Based on the principles of thermokinetic selectivity, we believe that the smaller overlying vessels in the papillary dermis do not absorb efficiently at longer pulse durations, causing less epidermal heating. Longer thermal diffusion times for larger vessels are best served with longer pulse durations with the IPL device.

TREATMENT OF LEG TELANGIECTASIAS

Over the past 2 years we have treated several hundred patients with the IPL device employing multiple parameters in an attempt to obtain the most consistent results. Typically, our patients have been screened for the absence of major reverse flow or reflux using a digital photoplethysmograph, Doppler flowmeter, and/or duplex ultrasound. If major reflux from the saphenous or lateral venous system is present, ligation with or without stripping, ambulatory phlebectomy, or sclerotherapy is the first treatment. Many telangiectatic webs are often seen in association with reticular veins in the lateral leg. These reticular veins show reverse flow in the direction of the telangiectatic veins. An unpredictable response occurs when telangiectasias are obliterated and associated reticular veins remain connected, regardless of the technique used to treat the telangiectatic veins.

For testing efficacy of the IPL device on telangiectasias, multiple pulse durations, pulse intervals, and spectrum parameters are used. Treatment results are evaluated at 4-week intervals. Clearance rates are estimated by comparison photographs. The most successful initial parameters for leg telangiectasias (50% improvement with three treatments) included a "double-pass technique" employing a triple pulse at 50-millisecond intervals (20-millisecond delay between pulses) with a 590-nm cutoff filter for a total fluence of 45 J/cm^2 for deeper, larger vessels, followed by a second pass with a single 5-millisecond pulse at 30 to 35 J/cm^2 (550-nm cutoff filter) for superficial, smaller vessels (Fig. 21–3).

Based on the theoretical points discussed earlier, we have devised a progressive series of new parameters for more effective treatment of leg telangiectasias. We use both a short and a long pulse of 2.4 and 6 milliseconds at a fluence of 40 J/cm^2 with a 570-nm cutoff filter, and the pulses are separated by a 10-millisecond delay (thermal relaxation interval). Visual endpoints include complete darkening of the targeted vessel(s) with a 2-mm or greater urticarial flare

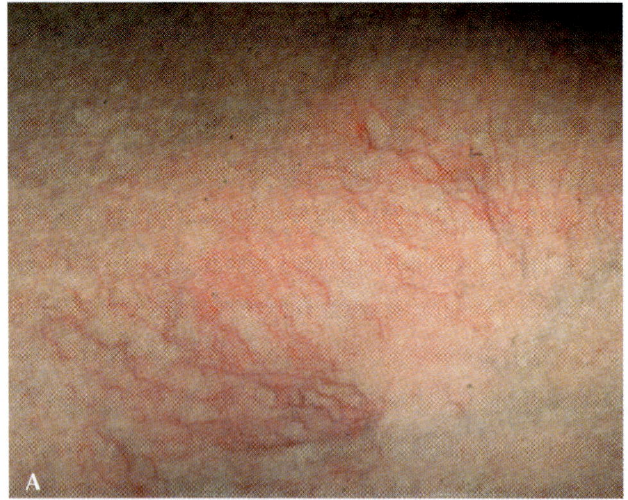

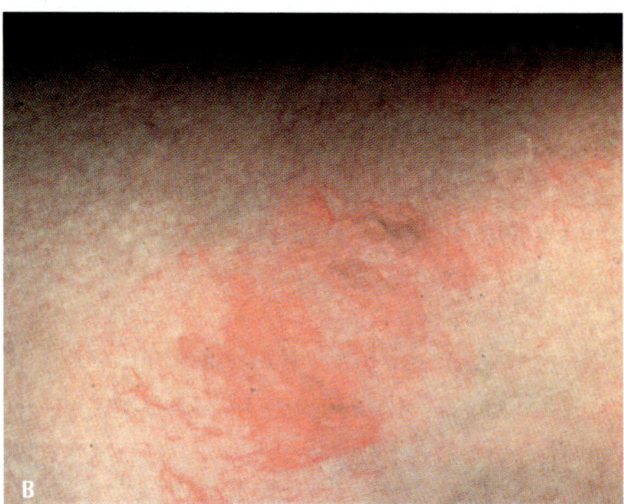

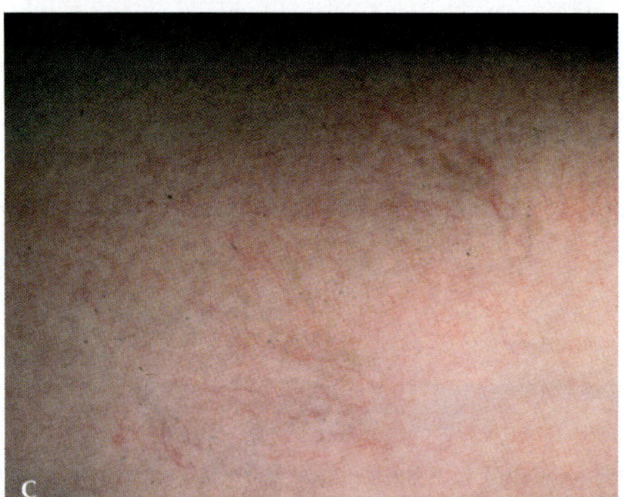

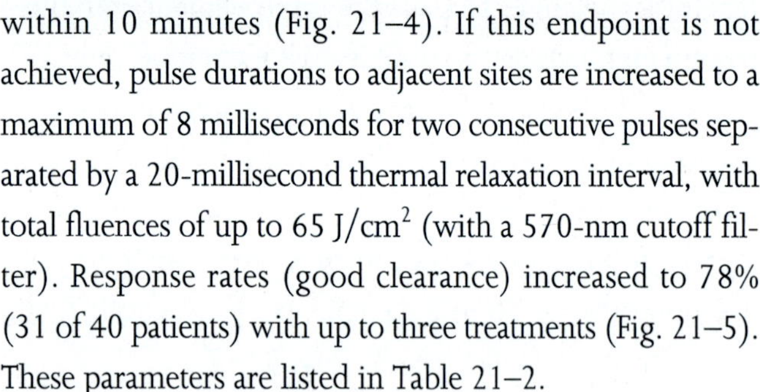

Figure 21–3. Double-pass technique. (A) Deeper vessels are targeted initially with a triple pulse using a 590-nm filter. (B) A second pass for more superficial vessels is then undertaken using a 550-nm filter. (C) This region on the lateral thigh was unresponsive to sclerotherapy but cleared following three IPL treatments spaced 1 month apart.

within 10 minutes (Fig. 21–4). If this endpoint is not achieved, pulse durations to adjacent sites are increased to a maximum of 8 milliseconds for two consecutive pulses separated by a 20-millisecond thermal relaxation interval, with total fluences of up to 65 J/cm^2 (with a 570-nm cutoff filter). Response rates (good clearance) increased to 78% (31 of 40 patients) with up to three treatments (Fig. 21–5). These parameters are listed in Table 21–2.

TREATMENT OF FACIAL TELANGIECTASIAS

The treatment of facial telangiectasia is more rewarding with any light-based device, including the IPL device. Facial telangiectasias generally are more uniform in size and depth and have a thinner overlying epidermis than

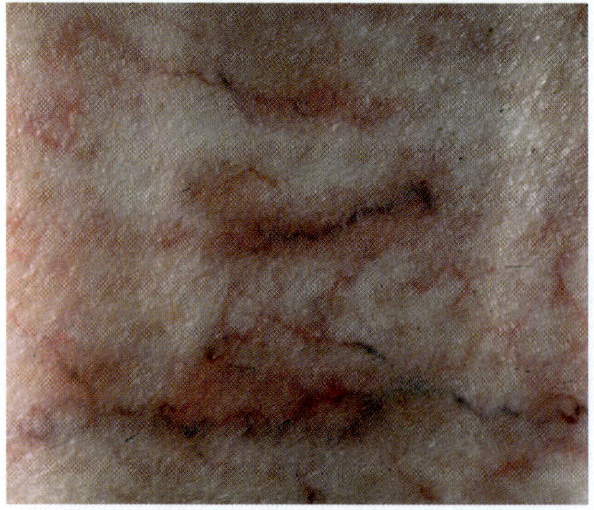

Figure 21–4. Endpoints of photothermal coagulation. Vessel is dark with surrounding urticarial edema.

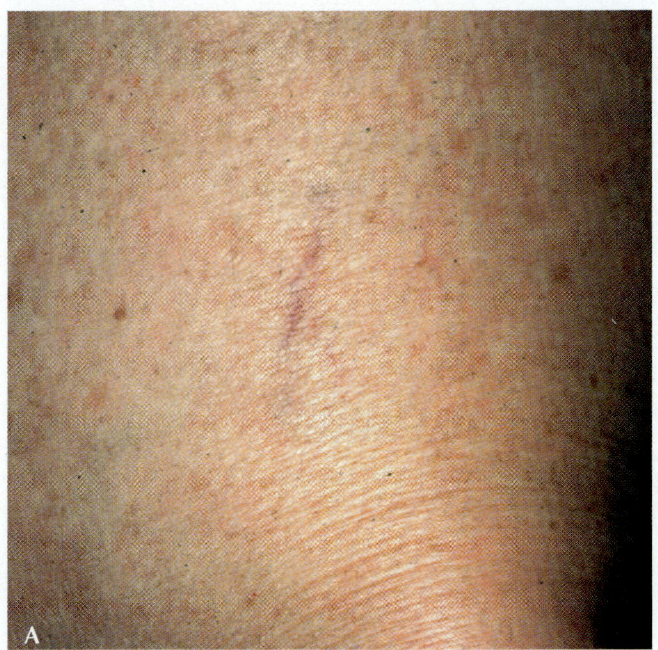
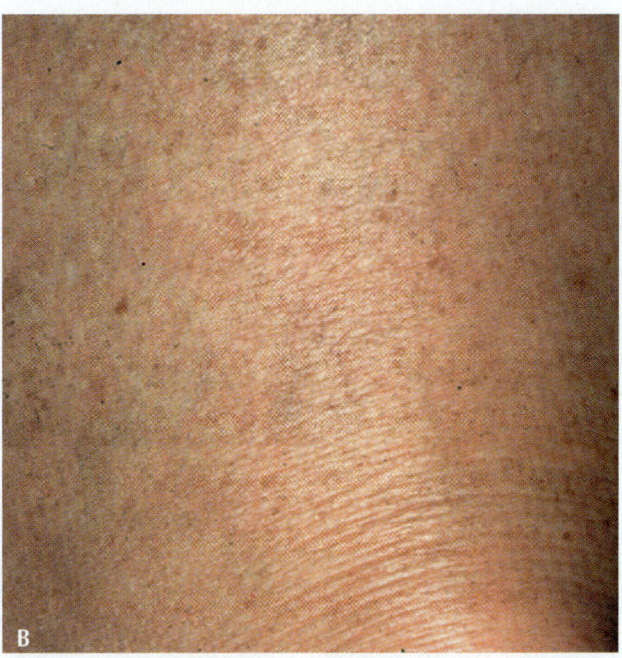

Figure 21–5. (A) Isolated area of telangiectasia on tanned thigh. (B) Treated with a short pulse followed by a long pulse. Parameters were 2.4 milliseconds, 10-millisecond delay, 7-millisecond pulse, 570-nm filter, 44 J/cm². Two treatments were required to clear this vascular lesion.

Table 21–2. Suggested IPL and 1064-nm Laser Parameters for Leg Veins

Vein Size (mm)	Filters (nm)	First Pulse (ms)	Delay Time (ms)	Second Pulse (ms)	Fluence (J/cm²)
Less than 0.5	550	3	10	3	30–35
0.5–1.0 mm	570	2.4	10	6	36–40
1.0–1.5 mm	570	2.4	10–20	7–8	40–45
1.5–2.0 mm	570	8	20–30	8	45–60
Unresponsive to ≥ 2.0 mm	590	Long pulse mode, 12	30–40	Long pulse mode, 12	60–70
0.4–0.7 mm	1064-nm laser	10	—	—	110–120
0.7–2.0 mm	1064-nm laser	16	—	—	120–140
>2.0 mm	1064-nm laser	16	500	16	130–140

leg telangiectasias; they are thus more susceptible to penetration by photons. Response is more predictable, with our clinical results approaching an 85% resolution rate of facial telangiectasias after one to three treatments.

The IPL device parameters for treatment of facial telangiectasias include a single or double pulse of approximately 3 milliseconds duration with a 550-nm filter typical, using delay times of 10 milliseconds between pulses. Fluences are much lower than for leg veins, typically in the range of 25 to 35 J/cm². The advantage of the IPL device is that with its large spot size an entire cheek of telangiectatic matting can be treated with fewer than a

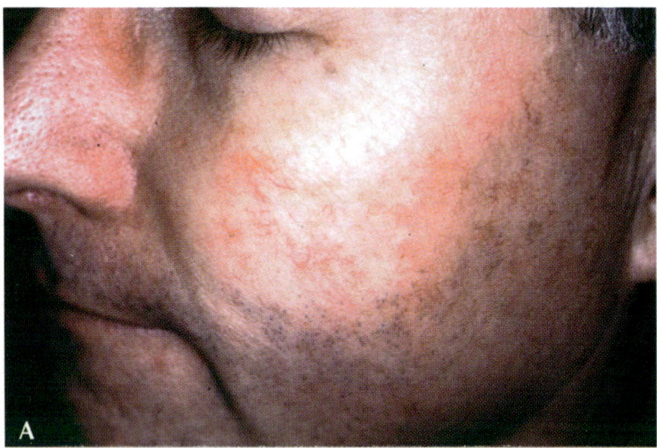 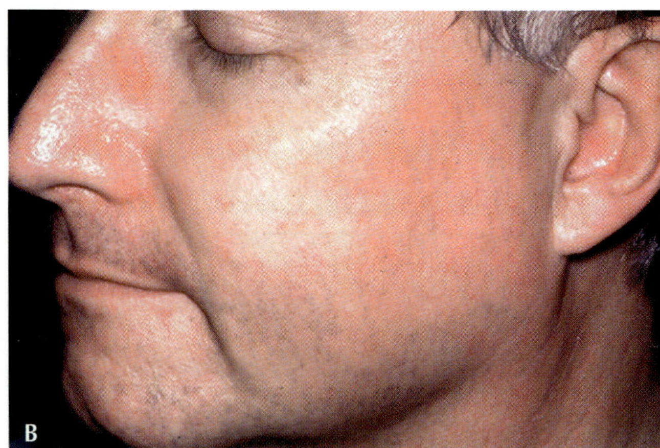

Figure 21–6. (A) Entire cheek treated with 12 pulses. (B) Results after three treatments spaced 1 month apart.

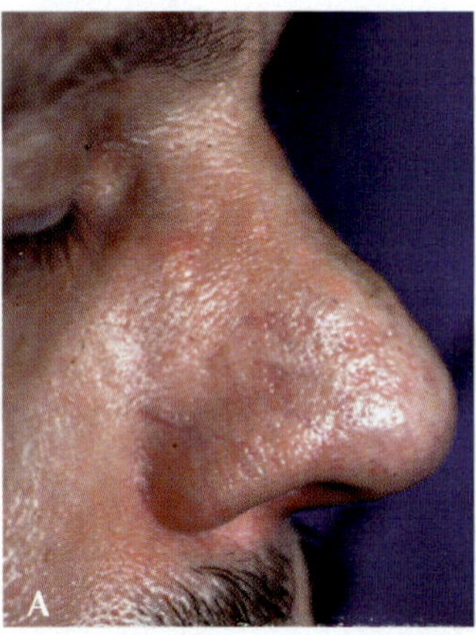 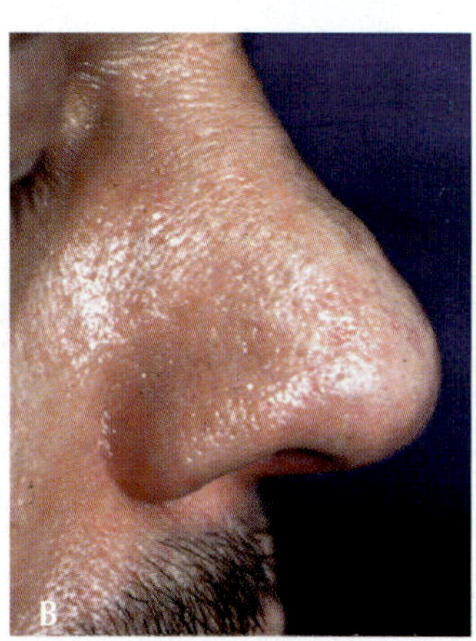

Figure 21–7. (A) Nasal alae telangiectasias. Treatment parameters were 2.4-millisecond pulse, 10-millisecond delay, 7-millisecond pulse, 570-nm filter, 40 J/cm^2. (B) Results after one treatment at 1 month. Slight skin smoothing is also seen.

dozen pulses in less than 10 minutes (Fig. 21–6). For larger, more purple telangiectasias (typically seen on the nasal alae) or for venous lakes or adult port-wine stains, the same settings may be employed as for small vessels of leg, that is, a short pulse followed by a long pulse (Fig. 21–7). For areas of poikiloderma on the neck and lower cheeks consisting of pigmentation and capillary matting, the IPL device with a 515-nm filter is ideal because the light energy is absorbed by melanin (Fig. 21–8). Parameters for various types of facial vascular lesions are listed in Table 21–3.

ADVERSE REACTIONS

During our initial inexperience with the IPL device, two tanned legs developed immediate desquamation of the epidermis, resulting in hypopigmentation (2.5%) lasting

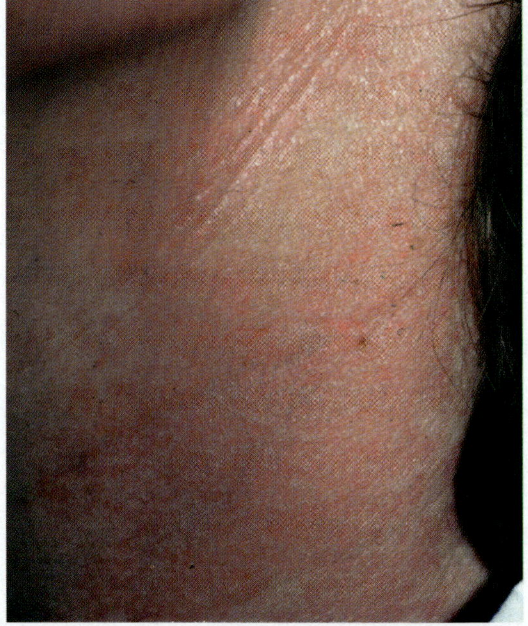

Figure 21–8. Treatment of poikiloderma of neck. Initial treatment with a single 3-millisecond pulse at 25 J/cm^2 with a 515-nm filter shows clearance in area of two test pulses.

Table 21–3. Suggested IPL Parameters for Facial Vascular Lesions

Vascular Lesion	Filters (nm)	First Pulse (ms)	Delay Time (ms)	Second Pulse (ms)	Fluence (J/cm²)	Number of Sequential Pulses
Telangiectatic matting	550	2.4–3.0	10	2.4–3.0	22–30	Single or double
Nasal alae telangiectasia	570	2.4	10	7	38–44	Double
Hemangioma	570	2.4	10	7	38–44	Double
Poikiloderma	515, 550	2.4–3.0	10	2.4–3.0	22–30	Single or double

4 to 6 months but no permanent pigment changes. This occurred at 40 J/cm² with a single pulse of 3 milliseconds. No such reaction has been observed on the face. No long-term sequelae were seen. Some crusting may be seen several days after treatment but no sequelae have been observed (Fig. 21–9).

The new parameters that we developed have markedly reduced the incidence of adverse reactions. Side effects include a mild burning sensation noted by 45% of patients that lasts less than 10 minutes and erythema that typically lasts from several hours to 3 days. The incidence of purpura is less than 5% and occurs typically when the fluence is too high for the size of the treated vessel. Most importantly, no epidermal injuries have been seen with the new parameters. Short-term hyper- or hypopigmentation (<2 months) has been noted in approximately 8 to 15% of the sites treated. Use of long pulses with the IPL device allows more effective treatment of 1- to 2-mm leg telangiectasias with a marked reduction in cutaneous side effects.

Most patients tolerate IPL treatments easily without requiring local anesthetic. Patients describe the pulse as feeling like a "brief grease splatter, electric shock, or rubber band snapping" on the skin. We are presently conducting multicenter trials on the use of active epidermal cooling to achieve more patient comfort and to allow the application of higher fluences for even better clinical results.

VASCULIGHT

A recent development has been the use of IPL source electronics in conjunction with a hand-held laser device (Vasculight) that outputs a high-energy 1064-nm wavelength with a maximum 16-millisecond pulse duration. Initial studies on 50 patients have shown that

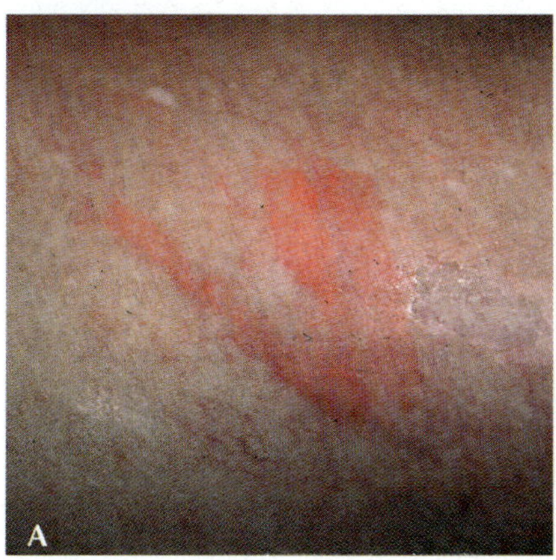
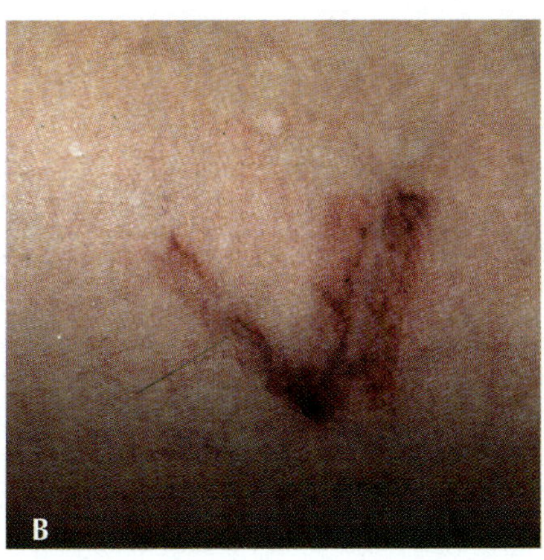

Figure 21–9. (A) A rectangular footprint leads to a small amount of crusting and temporary hypopigmentation. With the new parameters, this is no longer observed. (B) This only occurs when an erythematous rectangular footprint is observed immediately after treatment.

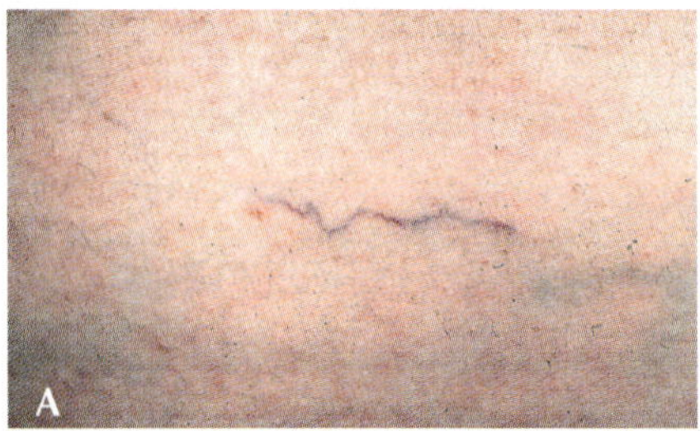
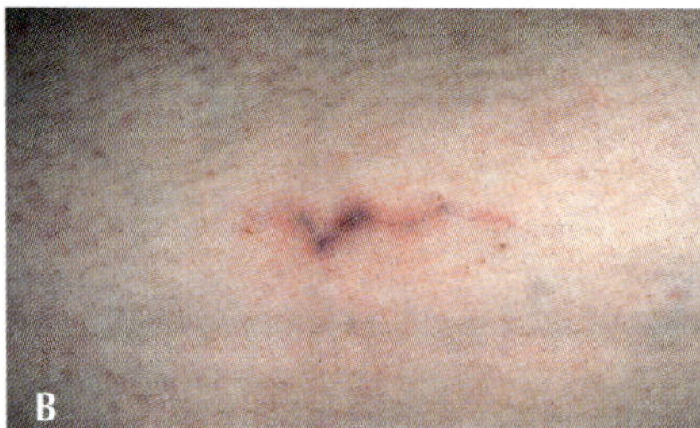
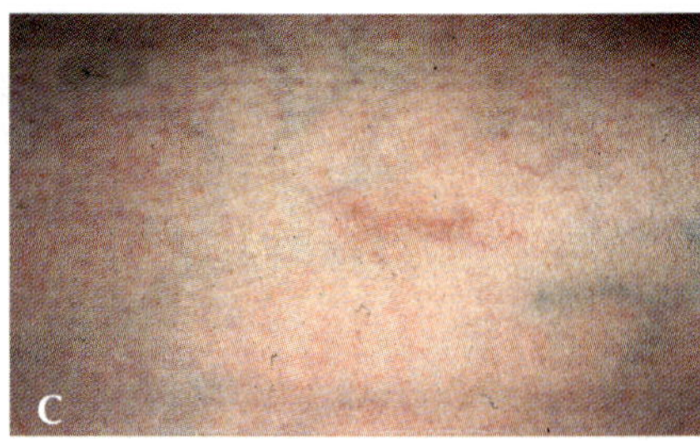

Figure 21–10. (A) Thigh telangiectasia of a 43-year-old woman prior to treatment with the 1064-nm laser (Vasculight). (B) Result at 1 month shows complete closure but some residual hyperpigmentation. Parameters used include a 14-millisecond pulse, 120 J/cm², 6-mm spot, with a 1064-nm laser. (C) Pigmentation cleared at 3 months.

immediate closure of violaceous leg telangiectasias is possible. Three-month follow-up has shown closure and resolution of approximately 75%, with an initial incidence of hyperpigmentation of approximately 50%. Results are preliminary but very encouraging, as shown in Fig. 21–10.

CONCLUSIONS

The PhotoDerm VL and Vasculight are potentially valuable treatment modalities for leg and facial veins. All regions of the leg may be treated, but significant reflux must be absent or poor response and increased side effects may be seen. Because the leg contains vessels of various sizes and depths, it is reasonable to begin with a short pulse combined with a long pulse. Excellent clinical results have been achieved through the use of longer pulses and a progressive increase in pulse duration and fluence based on vessel size. Safety is greatly enhanced. Many patients resistant to sclerotherapy can be treated successfully. Moreover, sclerotherapy of larger veins can be performed in conjunction with treatment with the IPL device (Fig. 21–11).

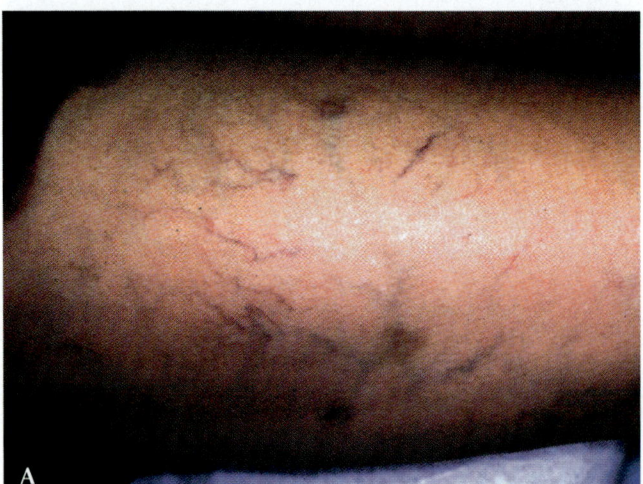
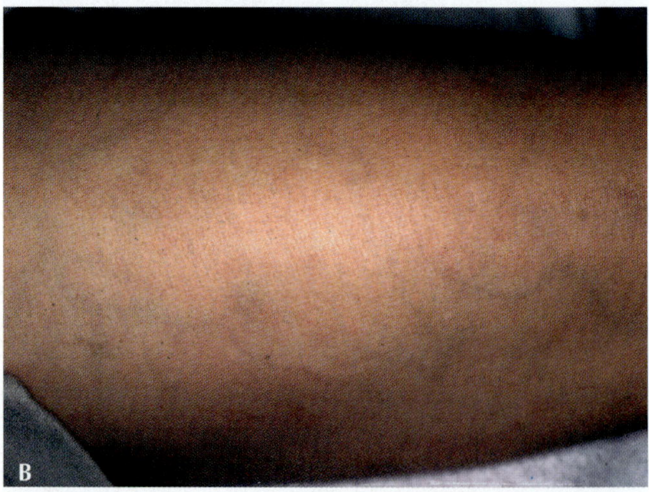

Figure 21–11. Combined treatment with the IPL device and sclerotherapy. (A) The smaller telangiectasias are treated with the IPL device initially. This is rapidly followed by a small injection of sclerosing solution into the associated reticular vein. (B) Occasionally, the solution may be seen going into the telangiectasias. We prefer to perform the IPL treatment first to minimize the possibility of blood contaminating the device crystal.

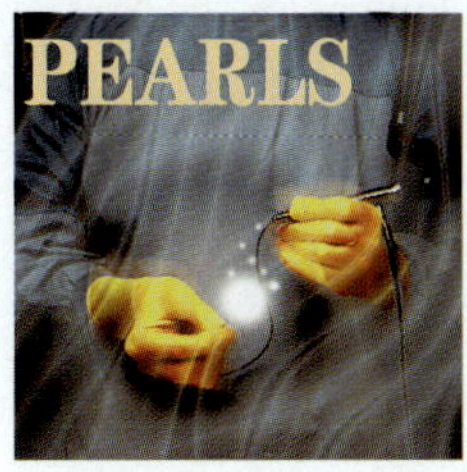

- Because leg telangiectasias vary in size and depth, are under hydrostatic pressure, and differ widely in the degree of oxygenation, treatment of leg veins using laser light is much more difficult than treatment of facial veins.

- In addition to protecting the skin from heat, the water-based gel that directs the laser light enhances optical coupling, minimizes reflections, and maintains continuity of the index of refraction of the skin–air interface. It also may filter some of the higher near-infrared wavelengths.

- Bright red lesions (containing oxyhemoglobin) are better treated with 515- or 550-nm filters, whereas violaceous lesions (containing deoxyhemoglobin) should be treated with 570- or 590-nm filters. The amount of oxygen in the blood vessel helps determine the correct wavelength to use.

- Elongating pulse duration for larger vessels and combining short and long pulse widths may provide better clinical results. More time is required for the heat to pass all the way to the core of a large blood vessel, and additional cooling time is required for the heat conduction from the core to the vessel surface. Small port-wine stains have absorbed higher fluences after double pulses spaced 3 to 10 milliseconds apart before producing purpura.

- Patients undergoing IPL should be screened for the absence of major reverse flow or reflux. If major reflux from the saphenous or lateral venous system is present, ligation with or without stripping, ambulatory phlebectomy, or sclerotherapy is the first treatment.

REFERENCES

1. Braverman IM. Ultrastructure and organization of the cutaneous microvasculature in normal and pathologic states. *J Invest Dermatol.* 1989;93:28.

2. Braverman IM, Keh-Yen A. Ultrastructure of the human dermal microcirculation: IV. Valve-containing collecting veins at the dermal-subcutaneous junction. *J Invest Dermatol.* 1983;81:438–442.

3. Sommer A, Van MP, Neumann HA, Kessels AG. Red and blue telangiectasias: differences in oxygenation? *Dermatol Surg.* 1997;23:55–59.

4. Keijzer M, Jacques SL, Prahl SA, Welch AJ. Light distributions in artery tissue: Monte Carlo simulations for finite-diameter laser beams. *Lasers Surg Med.* 1989;9:148–154.

5. Adrian RM. Treatment of leg telangiectasias using a long-pulse frequency-doubled neodymium:YAG laser at 532 nm. *Dermatol Surg.* 1998;24:19–23.

6. Dierickx CC, Casparian JM, Venugopalan V, Farinelli WA, Anderson RR. Thermal relaxation of port-wine stain vessels probed in vivo: the need for 1–10 millisecond laser pulse treatment. *J Invest Dermatol.* 1995;105:709–714.

7. Kimel S, Svaasand LO, Hammer-Wilson M, et al. Differential vascular response to laser photothermolysis. *J Invest Dermatol.* 1994;103:693–700.

8. Weiss RA, Weiss MA, Marwaha S, Harrington AC. Noncoherent filtered flashlamp intense pulsed light source for leg telangiectasias: long pulse durations for improved results. *Lasers Surg Med.* 1998;10:40.

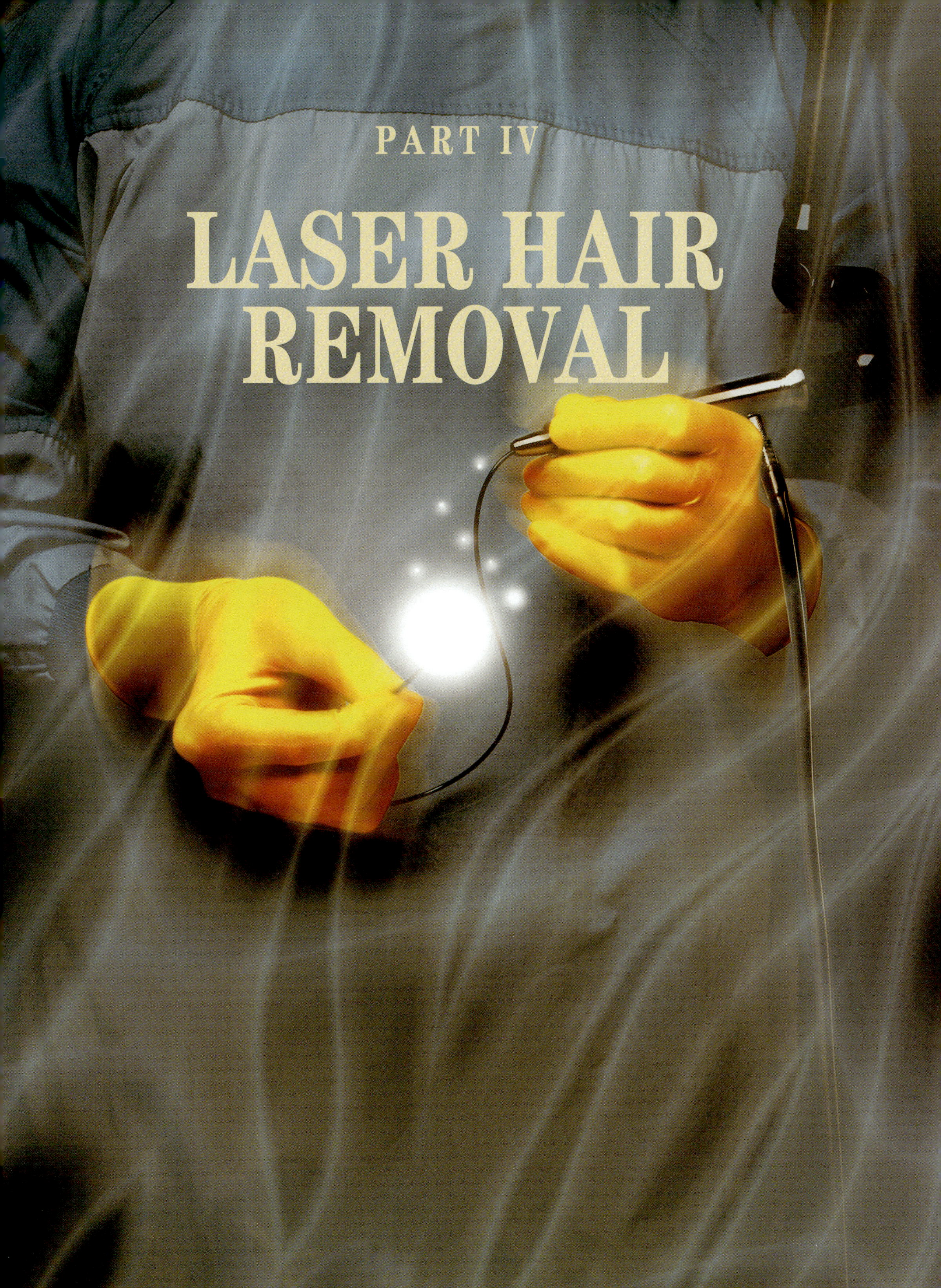
PART IV
LASER HAIR
REMOVAL

A Comparative Study of Intense Light and Laser Sources in Photoepilation

GARY LASK, SHIMON ECKHOUSE, MICHAEL SLATKINE, MICHAEL KREINDEL, AND AMIR WALDMAN

Laser-assisted hair removal has received considerable attention recently because of its noninvasive nature and rapid operating pace. This method is based on selective absorption of light by hair chromophores that damages hair follicles while leaving the skin undamaged. The advantage of this method is its ability to treat instantly large areas of dense hair virtually painlessly.

Pulsed ruby laser systems were used originally to perform melanin-based selective photothermolysis of hair.[1–3] These systems were followed by more advanced systems, such as broad-spectrum intense pulsed-light sources[4] and alexandrite lasers.[5] In addition, a novel approach to laser-assisted hair removal in which an artificial stain serves as the chromophore has also been introduced into the market.[6] At present, however, only short-term results have been achieved with this technique.

This chapter presents a comparative analysis of the three major melanin-based photoepilation technologies: ruby laser, broad-band intense pulsed-light, and alexandrite laser. Furthermore, the rationale for the best use of each system, based on patient population diversity and treatment speed (hair types and skin types), is discussed. As an introduction, the principles of selective photothermolysis in hair removal are discussed. Then, a summary of the results of clinical studies with each technology and an analysis of the practical advantages and limitations of the different systems follow.

SELECTIVE PHOTOTHERMOLYSIS

Photoepilation, which uses intense light energy to selectively damage hair shafts and follicles, is a method of hair removal that is based on the principle of selective photothermolysis. The theory of selective photothermolysis was originally developed for the treatment of vascular lesions,[7] but also applies to hair removal. Selective photothermolysis occurs because the target tissue contains a chromophore that absorbs a specific wavelength of light. During the process of hair removal, light is absorbed by melanin in the hair shaft and hair follicle and converted into heat energy, thereby raising the hair temperature. When the temperature is high enough, irreversible damage occurs to the hair structures, which prevents growth of the hair. To prevent heat flow from the hair to surrounding tissue, pulsed laser or intense-light systems are used.

The light-source parameters used to remove hair by photoepilation have to be selected in such a way that the epidermis, which also contains melanin, is not damaged. This is achieved by proper selection of operating wavelength, temporal profile (or pulse width), fluence level, and, when necessary, the use of epidermal-cooling accessories. The operating principles of hair removal by selective photothermolysis are depicted schematically in Figure 22–1.

Pulsed Beam

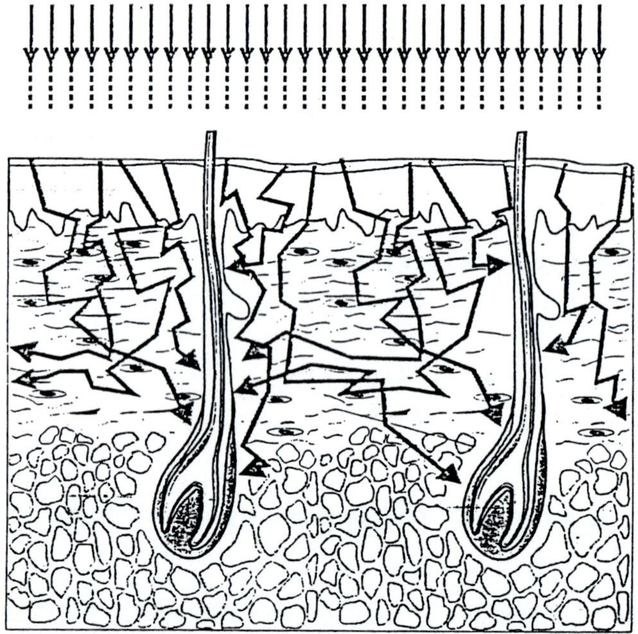

Figure 22–1. Schematic representation of photothermal hair removal. The light on the top that penetrates the epidermis, dermis, and subcutaneous fat is scattered and reaches the hair.

SPECTRAL RANGE

The choice of the optimal wavelengths to ensure the highest degree of hair removal selectivity with minimal epidermal damage requires an understanding of the process of absorption and scattering of light in different tissues. The primary requirement of the wavelength range is that the light must penetrate deeply enough into tissue

to reach the hair bulge and bulb. Depth of light penetration can be estimated with the following equation:[8]

$$ d = \frac{1}{\sqrt{\mu_a[\mu_a + \mu_s(1 - g)]}} \qquad (22–1) $$

where μ_a, is the absorption coefficient of tissue, μ_s is the scattering coefficient, and g is an isotropic factor that is equal to the average cosine of the angle photon scatters.

Absorption and scattering coefficients for dermis with 1% blood content in the wavelength range of 400 to 1000 nm, based on the data of Jacques,[8] Svaasand et al,[9] and Anderson and Parrish,[10] are presented in Figure 22–2A. This figure shows that skin is mostly a scattering medium. In the wavelength range of 400 to 630 nm, the blood content determines dermis absorption. In the range of 630 to 925 nm, dermis absorption is low, but it increases at longer wavelengths due to water absorption. For short wavelengths, the isotropic factor equals 0.8. With longer wavelengths, the isotropic factor increases slightly. Depth of light penetration as a function of wavelength, calculated from Equation 22–1, is presented in Figure 22–2B. Strong light absorption by microvessels prevents light penetration in the spectral range of 400 to 590 nm. At longer wavelengths, light penetration increases mostly due to decreased scattering. The depth of light penetration decreases at 980 nm because of peak water absorption at this wavelength. As is evident in Figure 22–2B, the optimal wavelength range for achieving the deep light penetration necessary to destroy the hair bulb at a typical depth of 2 to 4 mm is 600 to 1000 nm.

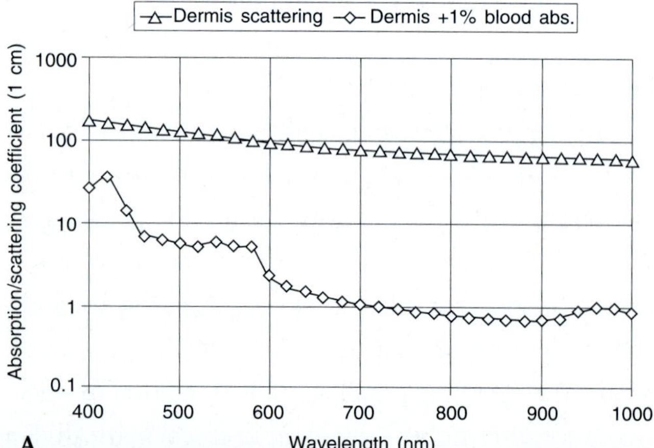

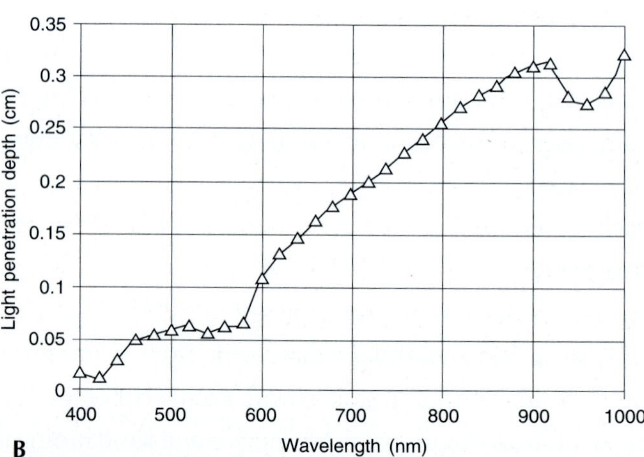

Figure 22–2. (A) Absorption and scattering coefficient of dermis with 1% of blood content in the wavelength range of 400 to 1000 nm. (B) Light penetration depth into the skin as a function of wavelength.

The high concentration of melanin in the epidermis makes the epidermis very sensitive to light irradiation. Consequently, the selectivity level of photothermolysis can be characterized by the ratio between elevation of the hair bulb temperature and that of the epidermis. The characteristic feature of photoepilation is that the absorbing chromophore, melanin, is present in different concentrations in the epidermis and hair. The qualitative differences in hair color between individuals also may be related to the relative concentrations of two types of melanin: eumelanin and phaeomelanin. Cesarini[11] described their relationship for different-colored hair; red and red-blond hairs contain a larger proportion of phaeomelanin, whereas dark hair (e.g., dark brown) contains a larger proportion of eumelanin.

Light absorption coefficients for these two hair types as a function of wavelength are presented in Figure 22–3.[11] These coefficients decrease monotonically with wavelength for all hair colors. The absorption coefficient is related to the darkness of hair, so absorption is much higher for black hair than for blond hair. The ratio of the absorption coefficient at wavelengths of 440 and 650 nm was used by Nicholls[12] as an objective characterization of hair pigmentation. This ratio was found to be approximately 2 for black hair and approximately 4 for blonde hair.

For a short pulse with negligible heat transfer, the temperature of the irradiated tissue is proportional to the light energy fluence. In this case, the temperature of the hair shaft and the epidermis can be calculated by the following equation:

$$T = \frac{N\mu_{am}F_0}{C\rho} e^{-z/d} \qquad (22\text{–}2)$$

where N is melanin concentration, μ_{am} is the absorption coefficient of melanin, c is specific heat, ρ is mass density, F_0 is light energy fluence on the skin surface, and z is the depth of the target in the skin. Taking into account that the depth of epidermis is considerably less than the depth of the hair bulb, the ratio between hair and epidermis temperature elevation is given by

$$\frac{T_H}{T_E} = \frac{N_H c_E \rho_E}{N_E c_H \rho_H} e^{-z/d} \qquad (22\text{–}3)$$

where z is the depth of hair bulb. The ratio of hair bulb temperature (T_H) to epidermal temperature (T_E) has been calculated, based on Equation 22–3, for hair colors that are 10 times darker than the skin (Fig. 22–4). The conditions for effective and safe hair removal are attained when $T_H \gg T_E$.

The spectral range of 690 to 1000 nm can be used to remove hair safely and effectively with a depth up to 4 mm. A similar calculation for darker skin and lighter hair (twice-lower color contrast) is presented in Figure 22–5. The spectral range of 700 to 1000 nm can be used for selective photothermolysis of hair with a depth of less than 3 mm. Wavelengths longer than 800 nm should be used to remove deeper hair with a lower melanin contrast.

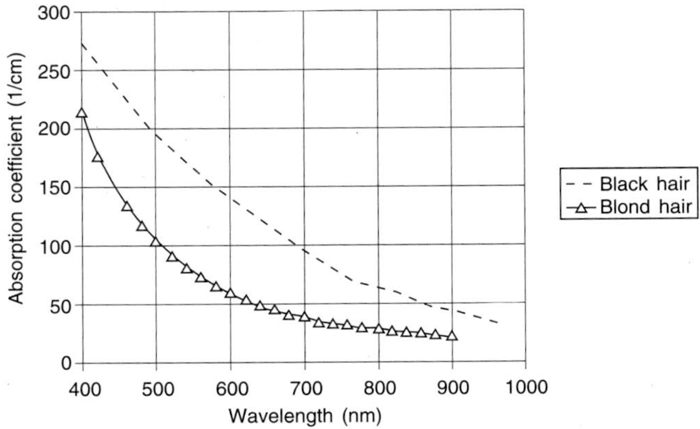

Figure 22–3. Light absorption by black and blond hair as a function of wavelength.

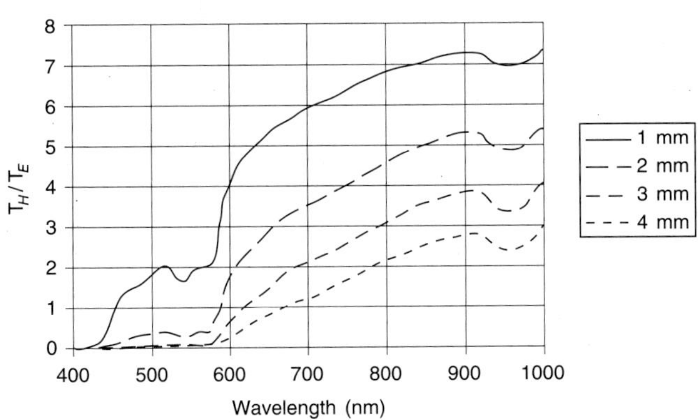

Figure 22–4. Ratio between hair bulb and epidermis temperature as a function of wavelength for different hair depths. Hair-skin contrast is equal to 10 (hair 10 times darker than skin).

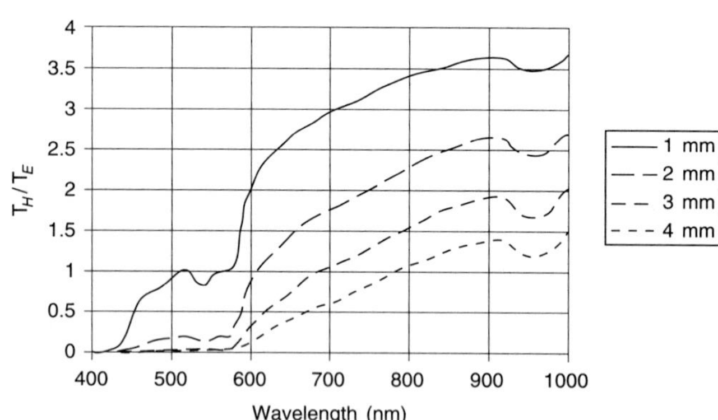

Figure 22–5. Ratio between hair bulb and epidermis temperature as a function of wavelength for different hair depths. Hair-skin contrast is equal to 5 (hair only slightly darker than skin).

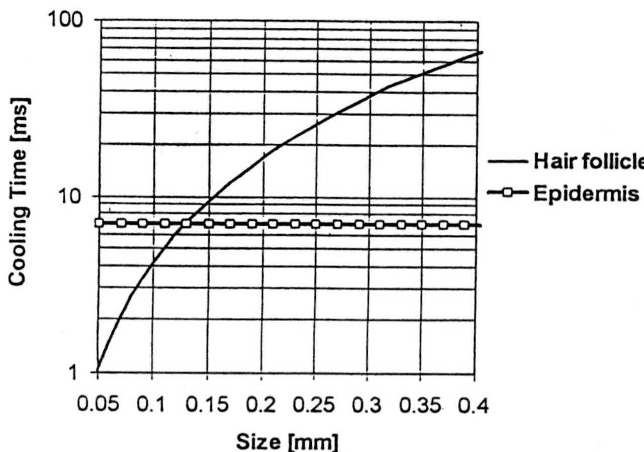

Figure 22–6. Cooling time of hair and epidermis as a function of hair follicle diameter.

In conclusion, it is evident that the contrast between melanin content in the hair and the skin plays a significant role in choosing optimal spectral parameters for the various hair-removal systems. The wavelength range of 690 to 1000 nm is excellent for removing hair that is much darker than the patient's skin, whereas longer wavelengths should be used for the treatment of deep hairs that are not much darker than the patient's skin (as in the case of dark skinned/dark haired or light skinned/light haired patients).

PULSE TIMING

The cooling time (thermal relaxation time) of hair and hair follicles, at temperatures higher than the surrounding tissue, is a function of their size. According to Grossman et al,[2] the thermal relaxation time of a heated object, such as a hair follicle, scales as

$$ t = \frac{d^2}{k\alpha} \qquad (22\text{–}4) $$

where d is the size of the heated object, α is the thermal diffusivity ($\alpha \approx 2 \times 10^{-3}$ cm^2/s for dermis and $\sim 1.5 \times 10^{-3}$ cm^2/s for fat),[13] and k is a geometric factor that is equal to 16 for a cylindrical object.[14] In this study, d is hair follicle diameter, which varies from 150 to 250 μm.

In principle, a pulse duration shorter than the cooling time of the hair but longer than the cooling time of the epidermis should be selected whenever possible. This enables the epidermis and microvessels to cool down during the pulse. Concurrently, the hair bulb and follicle do not cool significantly because of their longer thermal relaxation time. Variations in hair cooling time can be used to fine tune selective photothermolysis conditions by adjusting the pulse duration and delay between pulses when using multiple pulses (Fig. 22–6). For hair follicles that are larger than 130 μm wide, the thermal relaxation time is longer than epidermal thermal relaxation time (approximately 7 milliseconds), so selectivity can be enhanced by selecting longer pulses.

Increased selectivity can be achieved by using a pulse sequence with a total duration longer than the thermal relaxion time of the epidermis but shorter than the thermal relaxion time of the hair follicle. The temperature behavior of the epidermis and hair bulb during a triple pulse is presented in Figure 22–7. One can see that even though the hair bulb and epidermis are heated to the same extent during a single short pulse, selectivity of treatment can still be achieved by using multiple pulses. At the end of the first pulse, the temperature of the epidermis and the temperature of the hair bulb are approx-

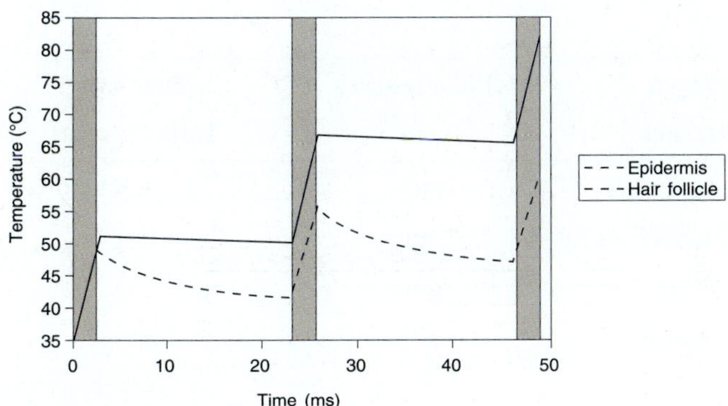

Figure 22–7. Temperature behavior in the epidermis and in the hair bulb during a triple pulse.

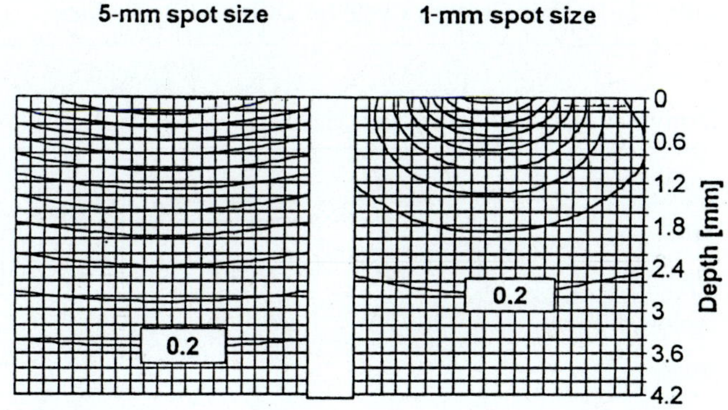

Figure 22–8. 694-nm light fluence distribution at two different spot sizes.

imately the same. In contrast, at the end of a triple pulse, the temperature of the hair bulb has risen three times, whereas photothermolysis of the epidermis is partially compensated by the cooling process.

Spot Size

The geometry of illumination also plays an important role in achieving sufficient light penetration into tissue. When light is applied to the skin using a small spot size, the scatter of photons diffuses the beam rapidly. The fluence decays very quickly as a function of depth, so most of the energy is dissipated radially in the upper layer of the skin and cannot reach hair bulbs. With a large spot size, light penetration is more efficient because the "source" of photons has an almost planar geometry. Keijzer et al[15] used a Monte-Carlo simulation of light behavior in the tissue to demonstrate that a smaller spot size causes stronger light attenuation in the skin. Fluence distribution calculations for 1- and 5-mm spot sizes are presented in Figure 22–8. When a 1-mm spot size is used, the fluence decreases to 20% of its incident value at a depth of 2.6 mm, whereas, on the contrary, the same fluence value is obtained at a depth of 3.5 mm with a spot size of 5 mm.

Consequently, depth of light penetration can be limited by irradiating areas of the skin that are too small. To avoid the effect of radial dissipation of fluence, the spot size should be larger than the light penetration depth into the tissue, namely, 5 to 10 mm.

Physiologic Aspects of Hair Growth

Long-term epilation can occur only with destruction of the hair follicle (the follicle itself or the blood vessels that feed the hair bulb). Destruction of the hair shaft does not lead to long-term epilation because as soon as the new anagen cycle becomes active, a new hair appears. This distinction differentiates photoepilation from traditional methods, such as tweezing and waxing.

For successful noninvasive hair removal, it is necessary to affect hair in the active cycle of growth, particularly during the anagen cycle, because hair can serve as a light-absorbing target only during this phase of the growth cycle. Thus the time between treatments should coincide with the length of the telogen phase.

Table 22–1 presents the percentage of hair in anagen and telogen phases of various body areas.[16] While over 60% of facial hair is in the anagen phase, only 20% of the hair on the legs is in this phase. Therefore, an effective treatment on the legs eliminates fewer follicles compared with a similarly effective treatment on the face. Furthermore, it is unreasonable to expect long-term epilation after one or even two treatments. Table 22–1 also shows that the duration of the resting period for hair follicles depends on the body area. This should be taken into account when treating various body areas so that the time between consecutive treatments is chosen accordingly. Note that the values in the table are statistics and in reality may vary among

Table 22–1. Hair Growth Cycle on Different Body Sites

Body Area	% Telogen Hair	% Anagen Hair	Telogen Duration	Follicle Density $(1/cm^2)$	Depth of Follicle (mm)
Scalp	15	85	3–4 months	350	3–5
Beard	30	70	10 weeks	500	2–4
Upper lip	35	65	6 weeks	500	1–2.5
Axillae	70	30	3 months	65	3.5–4.5
Trunk	—	—	—	70	2–4.5
Pubic area	70	30	12 weeks	70	3.5–4.5
Arms	80	20	18 weeks	80	—
Legs and thighs	80	20	24 weeks	60	2.5–4
Breasts	70	30	—	65	3–4.5

individuals due to differences in age, ethnic origin, and hormonal status.[17]

In recent years, research has been conducted to determine the specific site within a hair follicle that must be destroyed to prevent hair regrowth. The fundamental issue is whether the hair follicle is able to regenerate from the upper portions of the follicle (i.e., the bulge) if the hair papilla is destroyed. Some researchers[18,19] claim that hair follicles can regenerate in the absence of the hair bulb, whereas others[20] maintain that destruction of the hair papilla is essential for permanent epilation.

TREATMENT TECHNIQUES AND EFFECTS

Prior to treatment, the hair is shaved or trimmed very short, and a transparent, water-based gel is applied to the skin to cool the epidermis. When an intense, pulsed-light source is used, the gel also serves as an optimal couplet between the light guide and the skin. The gel should be refrigerated (at 4°C) before treatment with an intense pulsed-light source and kept at room temperature for treatment with a laser source. The skin and hair parameters should serve as a guideline when selecting treatment parameters. With an intense pulsed-light source, the computer software automatically selects the optimal wavelength range and pulse duration after the patient data have been entered. Fluence levels are typically 30 to 40 J/cm^2. When an alexandrite or ruby laser system is used, a fluence level of 20 to 25 J/cm^2 is most common. A 6- to 10-mm-diameter handpiece is used for laser treatment, and a 10 × 45-mm handpiece is used for intense pulsed-light treatment. When a laser is used, a transparent grid with tiny alignment dots is placed on the gel to identify treated and untreated areas (because the laser beam does not leave a visible mark on the skin). The collimated laser is fired at the skin on consecutive dots. Intense pulsed-light systems do not require the use of alignment sheets because the handpiece is held so close to the skin. Immediately after treatment, cold gauze should be applied to the skin to reduce the possibility of short-term erythema.

RUBY LASER

Ruby lasers generate light at a wavelength of 694 nm. Minimal light absorption by microvessels and higher absorption by melanin characterize this wavelength. The ratio of light absorption by the melanin in the epidermis to light absorption by the melanin in the hair is relatively low at this wavelength, which makes this laser useful only for the removal of dark hair on light skin (Fitzpatrick skin types I to III). Moreover, the depth of penetration of the ruby laser is limited to areas with relatively shallow hair follicles (e.g., upper lip and chin). Ruby lasers generate energy pulses with a duration of 3 milliseconds[15] and less, which is more than adequate with the use of room-temperature gel for epidermal heat sinking. The repetition rate of ruby lasers is about 1 pulse per second, and the spot size is 6 to 10 nm. A repetition rate of 1 pulse per second enables fast treatment of small areas (upper lip, 1 minute; chin, 1 to 3 minutes; bikini line, 10 minutes). However, ruby lasers may be considered too slow for larger areas, such as the back.

ALEXANDRITE LASER

The alexandrite laser operates at a wavelength of 755 nm. Light at 755 nm penetrates deeper into tissue than light generated by a ruby laser (see Fig. 22–3), because of lower scattering. Lower absorption by the epidermis enables higher energy fluences to be applied to the skin surface, thus allowing treatment of deeper hair follicles. Alexandrite lasers effectively generate pulses with a duration of approximately 2 to 20 milliseconds, which necessitates the use of room-temperature gel only. The alexandrite laser is operable at a repetition rate of 5 Hz, which, when used with a scanner achieves very fast coverage of large areas. The alexandrite laser is ideal for very fast treatment of the back and legs as long as the skin-type range is Fitzpatrick type I to III and the hairs are fair to dark. Darker skin may be treated with longer pulse durations and lower fluence.

BROAD-BAND INTENSE PULSED-LIGHT SOURCE

A broad-band light source produces radiation in the wavelength range of 590 to 1200 nm, which can be optimized by adjusting the filters according to the skin and hair color of the patient. This potentially allows the device to be used for the removal of hair that has minimal color contrast with the skin. The duration of pulses produced by the system can be varied and the system can generate bursts of two to five pulses enabling full control of the thermal relaxation of the epidermis and follicles. The optimization of wavelength and thermal profile potentially allows the operator to use the system for the treatment of dark-skinned patients (skin types IV and V) at lower fluences. High fluence allows coverage of a 4.5-cm^2 area in one burst. This results in a high treatment speed that is more than adequate for the back and legs.

ADVERSE EFFECTS

Adverse effects with all three systems are minimal and transient if patients are properly screened according to skin type. Patients should be forewarned that the following adverse effects can occur: (1) Light redness may appear after treatment and last a few days; (2) Very superficial burns with occasional blistering are seen. These appear mainly on the bikini line and may last up to 10 days; and (3) Slight transient hypopigmentation may be seen (rarely on the face) that can last 2 to 3 months on average. Usually, facial skin is highly forgiving, whereas arm skin is the least forgiving.

CLINICAL RESULTS

The following criteria were used to compare the clinical results obtained with different light sources for photoepilation:

1. the percentage of clearance observed a few months after a single treatment, and
2. long-term follow-up results after multiple treatments. This comparison is summarized in Table 22–2.

The clinical results obtained with the ruby laser are based on studies published by Grossman et al,[2] Lask et

Table 22–2. Hair-Removal Photoepilation Results: a Comparative Table

	Average Hair Reduction before 2d Treatment	Number of Treatments and Touch-Ups	Hair Reduction 3–6 Months after Last Treatment	Fitzpatrick Skin Type	Hair Color
Intense pulsed light	20–67%	3–6	75–90%	I–V	White, blond, red, brown, black
Alexandrite	20–50%	3–6	75–90%	I–III	Black, dark, brown
Ruby	20–50%	3–6	75–90%	I–III	Black, dark, brown

al,[3] Elman and Noren[21] and Nestor.[22] A summary of hair removal results with the alexandrite laser is based on data presented by Finkel et al.[5] The results obtained with the broad-band intense pulsed-light source are based on clinical studies conducted by Gold (personal communication), Goldman (personal communication), and Schroeter.[23]

EPILATION WITH A RUBY LASER

The Ruby laser studies[21,22] were conducted with a 1-millisecond EpiTouch (Sharplan 5000) system. As many as 400 patients with fair skin (Fitzpatrick skin Types I, II, and III) and brown or black hair were treated for 18 months. Hair growth was measured as a function of fluence and time after treatment. Follow-up sessions after 1 month show approximately 90% clearance for all energy fluences in the range of 20 to 40 J/cm^2 with a 6-mm-diameter spot, while observations after 3 months reveal about 40% hair reduction. When patients underwent three to six treatments, the clearance after 3 months was judged to be 75 to 90%.

EPILATION WITH AN ALEXANDRITE LASER

A 15-month clinical study of hair removal using a 2-millisecond-pulse-duration alexandrite laser was conducted on 126 patients with Fitzpatrick skin type III. The light fluence varied from 20 to 40 J/cm^2, although 25 J/cm^2 was the primary setting. Follow-up sessions 1.5 to 2.5 months after a single treatment showed clearance in the range of 20% to 50% depending on the treatment site. Maximal clearance was obtained for the bikini line, underarms, and sideburns, whereas only minimal clearance was reported for the upper lip and chin. Three-month follow-up sessions after three to six treatments showed 75 to 95% hair reduction.

EPILATION WITH A BROAD-BAND INTENSE PULSED-LIGHT SOURCE

A multicenter U.S. study (five different clinics) evaluated the effectiveness of an intense pulsed-light hair-removal system (EpiLight). A total of 154 patients with all skin types and various hair colors participated in the study, comprising 230 different anatomic sites. The protocol involved a single treatment with follow-up for a period of 12 weeks. During this time, no additional treatments with pulsed light or other epilation techniques were performed on the treatment site. Patients were observed at weeks 2, 4, 8, and 12 to determine hair count and to ascertain any adverse effects.

The results show that an average clearance of 57% was achieved. The amount of clearance was highly dependent on hair color, with black hair showing the best clearance and blond and white hair showing substantially lower clearance (~14%).

Studies of photoepilation in which multiple treatments were conducted showed a much higher degree of clearance, even with long-term follow-up periods. A long-term follow-up of 10 patients treated on the chin for hirsutism[23] showed 95 percent clearance after a period of 7 to 18 months. Another study of 110 patients treated on various body areas showed an average clearance of 30 to 85% after 5 months. Patients underwent four treatments conducted at 2-week intervals (Gold, personal communication).

CONCLUSION

The primary conclusion from the above 3 studies is that the range of hair reduction after multiple treatments is between 75 and 90% with the three different hair removal systems. The key difference between the various systems is the patient population (skin color, hair color) that can be treated and the rate of re-treatment.

CONCLUSIONS

Two years' experience with the ruby laser, high-repetition alexandrite laser, and broad-band intense pulsed-light technologies for noninvasive hair removal reveal that the systems are efficient and safe with proper patient selection. However, given the nature of the hair-growth cycle and the influence of hormonal activity, the success of photoepilation depends greatly on the individual. Patients report that the treatments are virtually painless, and adverse effects are minimal and transient. However, patients should be made aware of these possible adverse effects. Multiple treatments are generally necessary for long-term hair removal, and the clinician must avoid creating expectations of permanent results.

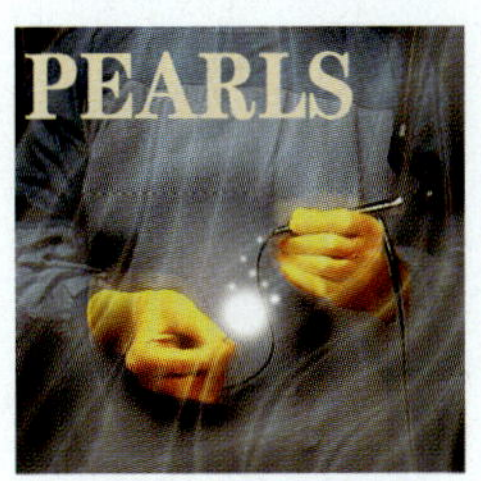

- The relative concentrations of two types of melanin, eumelanin and phaeomelanin, may account for the differences in hair color between individuals (redheads have more phaeomelanin and brunettes have more eumelanin).

- For successful noninvasive hair removal, hair must be affected in the active cycle of growth, the anagen phase, which varies among body areas. Treatments must be "timed" to coincide with the appropriate part of the hair growth phase for hair removal to be effective.

REFERENCES

1. Zaias N, Method of hair depilation. U.S. Patent 5 059 192. October, 1991.
2. Grossman MC, Dierickx C, Farinelli W, Flotte T, Andersson R. Damage to hair follicles by normal mode ruby laser pulses. *J Am Acad Dermatol.* 1996;35:889–894.
3. Lask G, Elman M, Slatkine M, Waldman A, Rozenberg Z. Laser-assisted hair removal by selective photothermolysis. *Dermatol Surg.* 1997;23:737–739.
4. Gold MH, Bell MW, Foster TD, Street S. Long-term epilation using the EpiLight broad-band, intense pulsed light hair removal system. *Dermatol Surg.* 1997;23:909–913.
5. Finkel B, Eliezri YD, Waldman A, Slatkine M. Pulse alexandrite laser technology for noninvasive hair removal. *J Clin Laser Med Surg.* 1997;15:225–229.
6. Goldberg DJ. Topical suspension assisted laser hair removal treatment of axillary and inguinal regions. *Lasers Surg Med Suppl.* 1995;8:34.
7. Laser-tissue interactions. In: Andersan RR, Goldman MP, Fitzpatrick RE, eds. *Cutaneous Laser Surgery.* Mosby; 1994:9.
8. Jacques. The role of skin optics in diagnostics and therapeutic uses of laser. In: Steiner R, Kaufmann R, Landthaler M, Braun-Falco O, eds. *Lasers in Dermatology.* Springer-Verlag: Berlin; 1991.
9. Svaasand LT. Norvang EJ, Fiskerstrand EKS, Stopps MW, Bearns JS, Nelson. Tissue parameters determining the visual appearance of normal skin and port-wine stains. *Lasers Med Sc.* 1995;10:55–65.
10. Anderson RR, Parrish JA. The optics of human skin. *J Invest Dermatol.* 1981;77:13–19.
11. Cesarini JP. Hair melanin and hair color. In: Orfanos CE, Happle R. eds. *Hair and Hair Diseases.* Springer-Verlag, 1990; 165–197.

12. Nicholls EM. The genetics of red hair. *Hum Hered.* 1969; 19:36–42.
13. Svaasand LO, Gomer CJ, Morinalli E. On the physical rationale of laser induced hyperthermia. In: Trelles MA, ed. *Laser Tumor Therapy.* European Community Medical Laser Concerted Action Programme, Second plenary workshop, 1990; 1-65–1-81.
14. Van Gemert MGC, Welch AJ. Time constant in thermal laser medicine. *Lasers Surg Med.* 1989;940:5–21.
15. Keijzer M, Jacques SL, Prahl SA, Welch AJ. Light distribution in artery tissue: Monte Carlo simulations for finite-diameter laser beams. *Lasers Surg Med.* 1989;9:148–154.
16. Richards RN, Meharg GE. *Cosmetic and Medical Electrolysis and Temporary Hair Removal.* Canada: Medrig Ltd.; 1997.
17. Wheeland RG. Laser-assisted hair removal. *Laser Dermatol.* 1997;15:469–477.
18. Oliver RF. The experimental induction of whisker growth in the hooded rat by implantation of dermal papillae. *J Embryol Exp Morphol.* 1967;18:46–51.
19. Costsarelis G, Sun TT, Lavker RM. Label retaining cells reside in the bulge area of pilosebaceous unit: implications for follicular stem cells, hair cycle, and skin carcinogenesis. *Cell.* 1990;61:1321–1327.
20. Holecek BU, Ackerman AB. Bulge-activation hypothesis: is it valid? *Am J Dermatol.* 1993;15:235–257.
21. Elman M, Noren P. Paper presented at: 7th World Congress of Dermatology; June 1997, Sydney, Australia.
22. Nestor MS. Laser hair removal: clinical results and practical applications of selective photothermolysis. *Skin Aging.* 1998; 10:34–39.
23. Schroeter C. Hair removal with the PhotoDerm VL as an intense light source: a histological study. Paper presented at: 18th Annual Meeting of the ASLMS; April 1998, San Diego, CA.

CHAPTER 23

ESC/Sharplan Laser Hair Removal System

VICTOR G. LACOMBE, ISABEL M. THOMPSON, AND GREGORY S. KELLER

When lasers are used for epilation, several practical factors have to be taken into account. Treatment of a variety of body locations, hair colors, and patient skin types requires a device that can lase rapidly, penetrate to the necessary depth, and prevent epidermal damage even in heavily pigmented skin. The physics of laser-pigment interactions was discussed in Chapter 4.

ESC/Sharplan (Allendale, NJ) offers two laser systems designed for removing unwanted hair: the EpiTouch ruby and EpiTouch alexandrite lasers. The ESC/Sharplan philosophy is to apply the energy over the length of time necessary for clinical effectiveness while keeping this time to a minimum to prevent increased collateral damage to the surface epithelium.

EPITOUCH RUBY LASER

The long-pulsed ruby laser was approved by the U.S. Food and Drug Administration (FDA) in 1997 for the treatment of unwanted hair. Its 694-nm wavelength is highly absorbed by melanin and has proven effective for long-term hair removal. The EpiTouch ruby laser is uniquely versatile compared with other ruby lasers in that it can be used in both a Q-switched mode for tattoo and pigmented lesion removal (see Chapter 26) and a long-pulsed mode for epilation. In the long-pulse mode the spot size is 5 to 8 mm, and the system can generate 1 pulse per second. The pulse width is on the order of nanoseconds in the Q-switched mode and 1.2 milliseconds in the long-pulsed mode used for epilation, according to manufacturer specifications. When used for epilation, energies from the ruby laser must be delivered over longer periods of time to allow for heating of hair shaft pigment and thermal conduction to the follicle at the base of the shaft. It is this heating that causes a permanent, or at least long-lasting, change in hair growth.[1]

TREATMENT PROTOCOL
Patient Selection and Preparation

Because of the high melanin absorption, the ruby laser has its greatest efficacy in the treatment of light-skinned individuals, specifically patients with Fitzpatrick skin types I, II, or III. When this system is used on darker-skinned individuals, the energy is more readily absorbed by epidermal melanin, and hyper- or hypopigmentation can occur. Most authors recommend ruby laser treatment for patients with no higher than Fitzpatrick skin type III.[2]

Patients prepare for the procedure by shaving the hair 2 to 3 days prior to laser treatment (Fig. 23–1A). Waxing or plucking should not be done before the treatment because the presence of the hair shaft is necessary for treatment to be effective. A cooling gel at room temperature is spread generously on the treatment site prior to treatment (Fig. 23–1B).

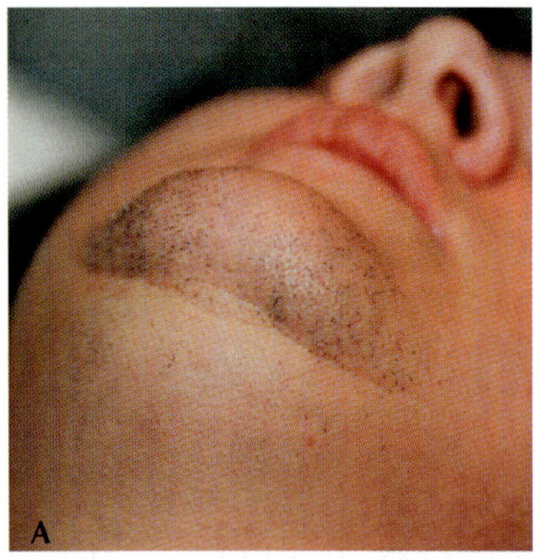 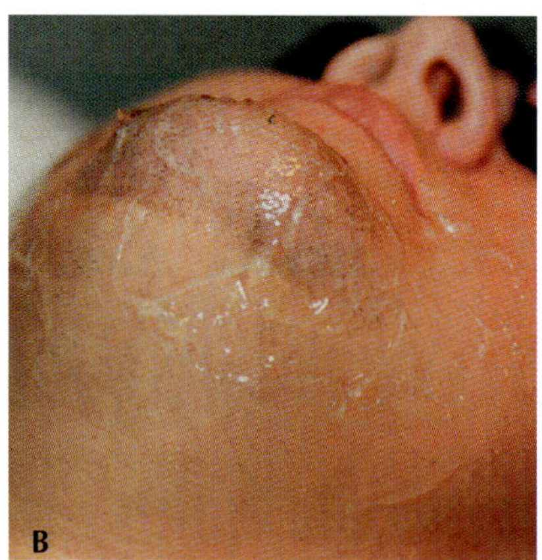 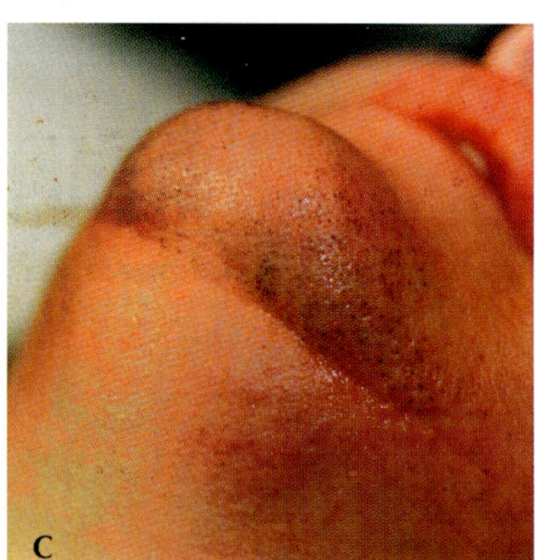

Figure 23–1. (A) Preoperative appearance. The patient has shaved a day or two prior to laser epilation. (B) Application of gel is generous, and the patient is given appropriate eye protection. (C) Follicular edema and mild erythema are seen a few minutes after laser treatment of the chin.

Procedure

The laser is set to the largest beam size available, and energy densities begin at 15 J/cm^2 but can go as high as 40 J/cm^2. The EpiTouch system uses a targeting grid that allows for efficient coverage without overlap. The grid imparts a color change to treated areas, and this is important because the skin itself shows little to no immediate evidence of laser exposure. The endpoint used to determine energy levels for a specific patient is the appearance of mild edema and erythema surrounding a treated follicle (Fig. 23–1C). Some patients with light skin can tolerate higher levels of energy without discomfort or side effects, but patient discomfort also necessitates a decrease in energy density.

Clinical Results and Efficacy

Patients generally need three to six treatments to effect a high percentage of hair reduction over a long period of time. These treatments should be spaced at 3- to 4-week intervals for facial hair and 6- to 8-week intervals for body hair to capture the most number of follicles in the anagen stage.

Clinically, the EpiTouch ruby laser has demonstrated effectiveness in providing long-lasting hair removal in selected patients.[2] Our clinical experience has shown an 85% hair reduction observed 6 months after treatments of the legs, bikini area, and back and a 50 to 75% reduction with five to six treatments of facial hair (Fig. 23–2). The hair that does return is finer, thinner, and lighter. Frequently, this light regrowth is cosmetically acceptable to patients. It should be noted that in general pigmented hairs respond better; blonde, white, and light gray hairs do not respond well.

Complications

For laser-assisted epilation to be considered effective when compared with shaving, waxing, and even elec-

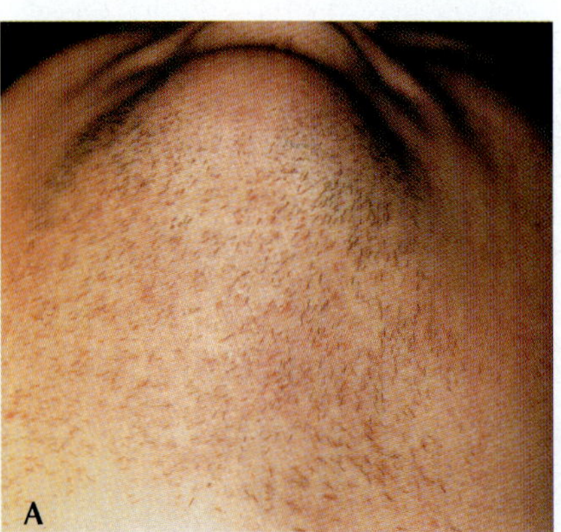 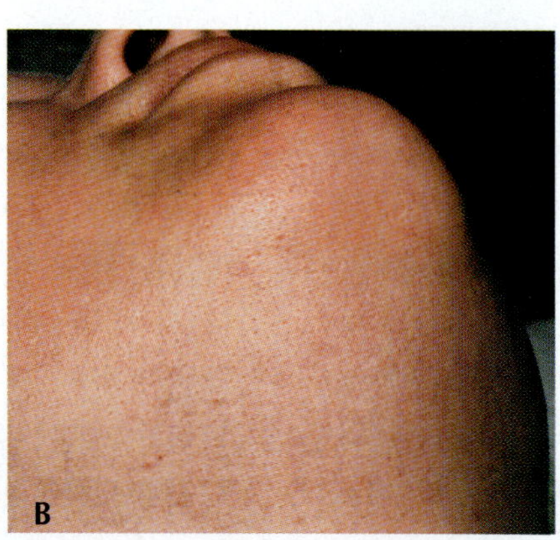

Figure 23–2. (A) Preoperative hirsutism. (B) Postoperative result following six treatments with the long-pulse EpiTouch ruby laser.

trolysis, it must have almost no complications. Overly aggressive treatment with high energy levels in patients with dark skin can result in blistering, peeling, pain, transient hyperpigmentation, and occasionally hypopigmentation. These complications are rare if caution is used. The typical reaction consists of erythema and mild follicular edema that can last from 2 to 24 hours. The application of ice and/or a mild topical anti-inflammatory agent is the recommended posttreatment regimen.

EPITOUCH ALEXANDRITE LASER

The EpiTouch alexandrite laser emits light in the near-infrared spectrum at a wavelength of 755 nm. This wavelength has slightly less absorption by melanin than that produced by the ruby laser but allows deeper penetration to treat a wider variety of hair types. The alexandrite laser also provides more protection for pigment in the epidermal layer. The long pulse of the EpiTouch alexandrite laser has a narrower pulse width compared with the ruby laser (2 millisecond versus 5, 10, and up to 20 millisecond) and a rapid 5-pulse-per-second repetition rate (5 Hz compared with 1 or 0.5 Hz). These qualities allow for rapid and effective treatment of large areas of hair-bearing skin with minimal collateral thermal damage to the epidermis. The EpiTouch alexandrite

laser has a large spot size (10 mm) that also increases energy delivery to deeper structures.

ESC/Sharplan recently made available a scanning device that allows rapid treatment of an area up to 50 × 50 mm (Fig. 23–3). The scanner covers the entire treatment area by firing a random pattern arranged such that no two contiguous spots are treated consecutively. This allows additional cooling time for the epidermis from one spot to the next. Typically, this scanner enables treatment of both legs from ankle to thigh within 25 to 35 minutes. Treatment of an entire back is easily accomplished in a single sitting. The versatility and speed of treatment of this laser-scanner combination are particularly valuable in an office-based practice.

TREATMENT PROTOCOL

The hair is shaved several days prior to treatment so that a fine stubble is present. Waxing or plucking should be avoided because it removes the target hair shaft.

PROCEDURE

As with other lasers, a cooling gel is used as a heat sink; however, this gel need only be at room temperature (Fig. 23–4). Laser treatment begins at an energy density setting of 10 J/cm^2 and is increased when the patient

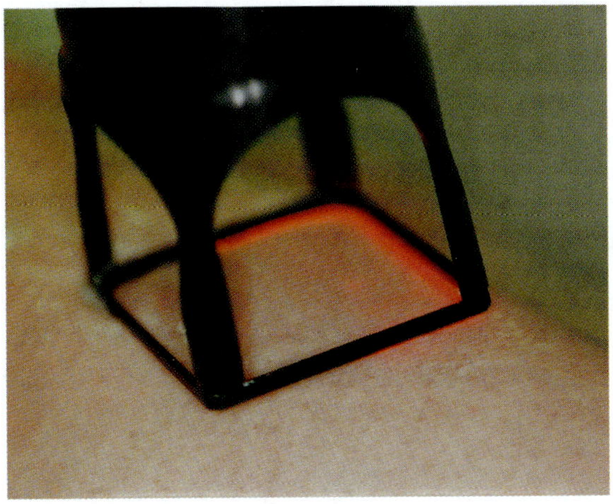

Figure 23–3. Scanner frame that permits rapid treatment of a 50 × 50 mm area.

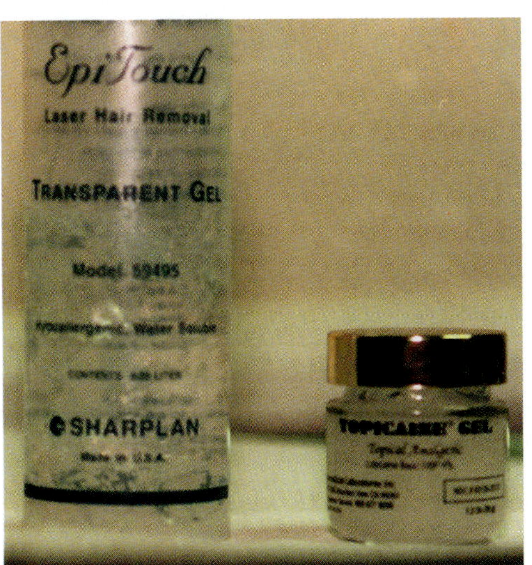

Figure 23–4. Examples of room-temperature cooling gels used as a heat sink.

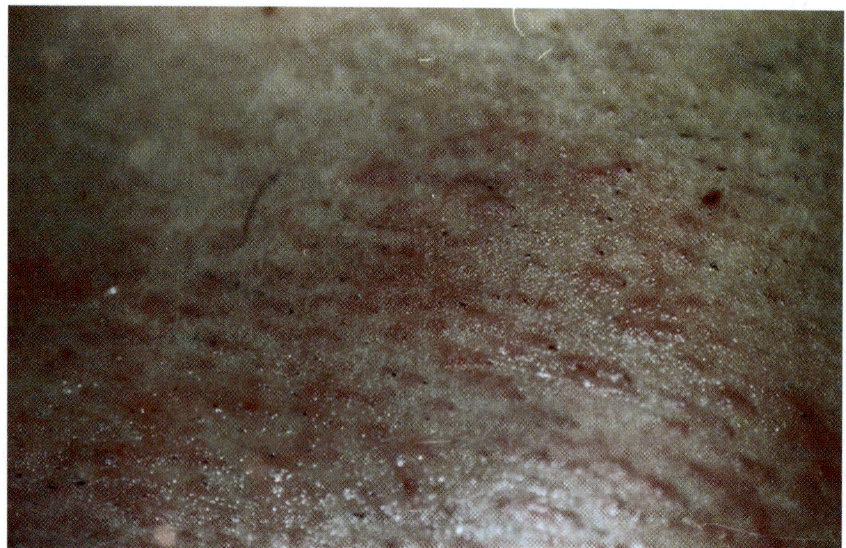

Figure 23–5. Follicular edema following EpiTouch alexandrite laser treatment.

experiences discomfort and/or mild follicular edema and erythema is seen in the treated area (Fig. 23–5). The usual setting for light-skinned patients with dark hair is 15 J/cm^2. Patients with darker skin require fluences in the range of 10 to 13 J/cm^2. As mentioned earlier, the scanning attachment greatly decreases time of treatment for large areas. Overlap and skipped areas of the laser treatment are also minimized with a large scanner because the scanning frame makes a visible print in the cooling gel.

Clinical Results and Efficacy

Patients generally require a minimum of three treatments spaced at 6- to 8-week intervals for body hair. The face, particularly the chin and upper lip, usually requires five to six treatments for satisfactory long-term hair reduction.

Most studies with various alexandrite laser models reveal anywhere from 60 to 95% hair removal at 6 months. Finkel et al[3] reported less than 12% average regrowth 3 months after the last treatment in their series of 126 patients. Some additional regrowth is noted at longer-term follow up, but the hairs are finer and lighter than the original hairs[3] (Figs. 23–6 and 23–7).

Complications

Most patients experience mild erythema for a few hours and a mild folliculitis around the hair shaft. Patients with darker skin are at a greater risk for skin blistering if excessive energy densities are used. There are reports of hypopigmentation occurring as well, but this is uncommon except in very dark-skinned individuals. Mild discomfort or pain is encountered infrequently but can be treated readily with a topical anesthetic or mild pain reliever. Patients should be made aware that the existing hair shaft will be extruded over the next 7 to 10 days and does not represent hair regrowth.

CONCLUSIONS

In summary, it appears that the success of long-term hair removal is similar regardless of whether a ruby or an alexandrite laser system is used. However, the speed of treatment with the EpiTouch alexandrite laser scanner has made this the laser of choice for our practice.

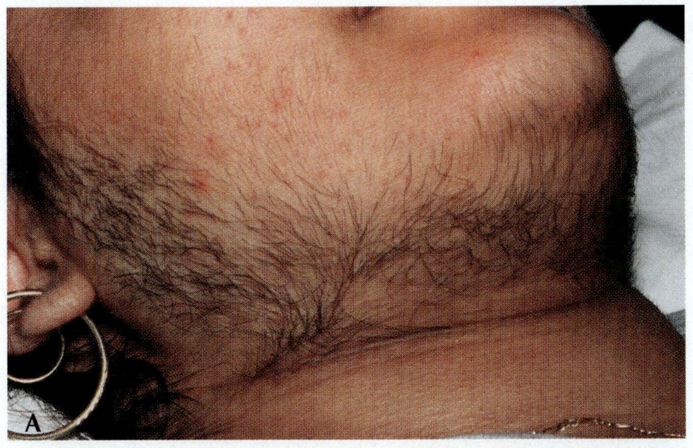
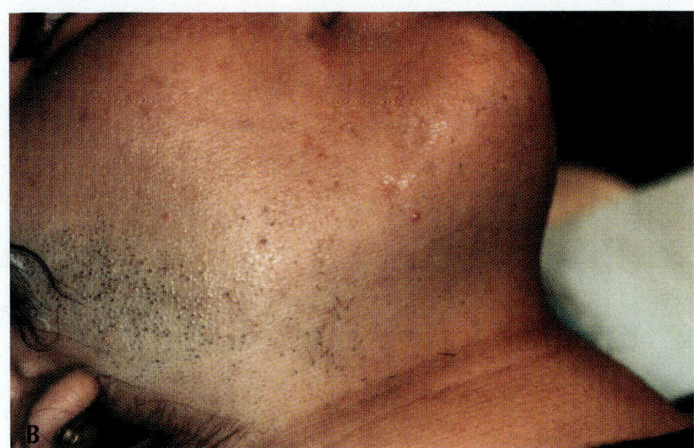
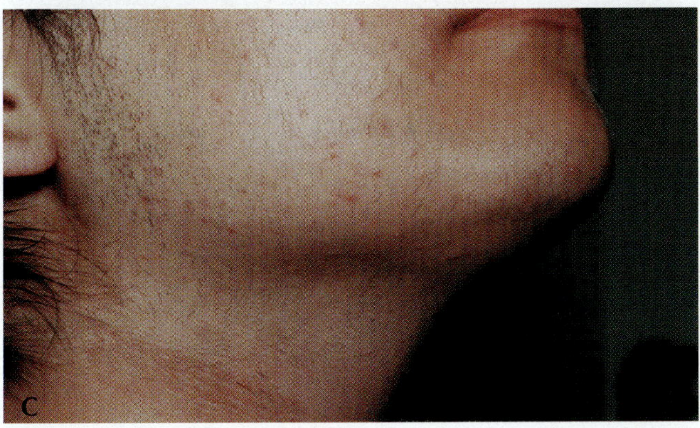

Figure 23–6. (A) Preoperative hirsutism associated with polycystic ovary disease in a 15-year-old Hispanic girl who must shave on a daily basis. (B) Appearance 4 weeks after her third treatment with the EpiTouch alexandrite laser using a 7-mm handpiece at 15 J/cm². (C) Appearance 4 weeks after her fifth treatment. The patient now shaves only once a week.

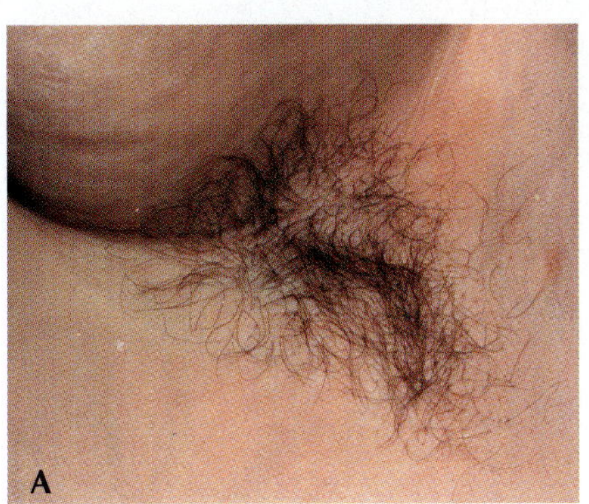
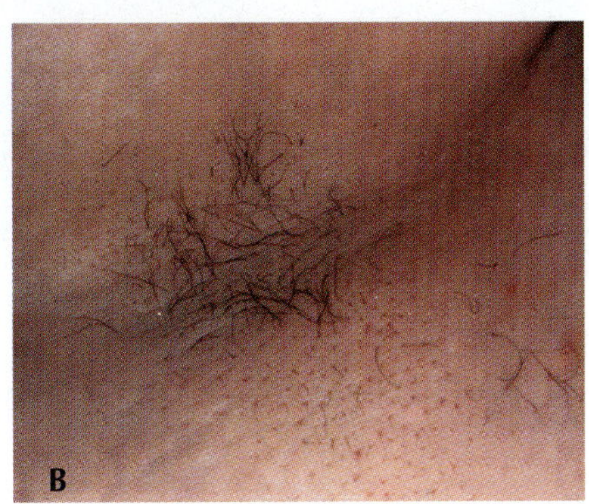

Figure 23–7. (A) Preoperative view of axilla in a patient with Fitzpatrick skin type I. (B) Postoperative view following a single treatment with the EpiTouch alexandrite laser.

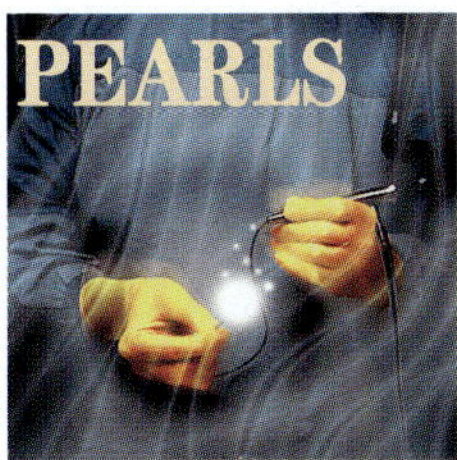

- The EpiTouch ruby laser is more versatile than other ruby lasers because it can be used in both a Q-switched mode for tattoo and pigmented lesion removal and a long-pulse mode for epilation.

- Hair is shaved several days prior to treatment with either EpiTouch laser. Waxing or plucking should not be done because the presence of the hair shaft is necessary for treatment to be effective.

- The EpiTouch system's targeting grid imparts a color change to treated areas, which is important because the skin itself shows little to no immediate evidence of laser exposure.

- The EpiTouch alexandrite laser's wavelength and large spot size allow deeper penetration to treat a wider variety of hair types. The alexandrite laser provides more protection for pigment in the epidermal layer. The EpiTouch's scanner enables treatment of both legs from ankle to thigh within 25 to 35 minutes. Treatment of an entire back is easily accomplished in a single sitting.

- Although most areas of body hair usually require a minimum of three EpiTouch alexandrite laser treatments spaced at 6- to 8-week intervals, the face, particularly the chin and upper lip, may require five to six treatments for satisfactory results.

- It is important for patients to know that after treatments with the EpiTouch alexandrite laser the existing hair shaft will be extruded over the next 7 to 10 days and this does not represent hair regrowth.

REFERENCES

1. Lask GS, Elman M, Slatkine M, Waldman A, Rosenberg Z. Laser-assisted hair removal by selective photothermolysis. Preliminary results. *Dermatol Surg.* 1997;23:737–739.
2. Bjerring P, Zachariae H, Lybecker H, Clement M. Evaluation of the free-running laser for hair removal. A retrospective study. *Acta Derm Venereol.* 1998;78:48–51.
3. Finkel B, Eliezri YD, Waldman A, Slatkine M. Pulsed alexandrite laser technology for noninvasive hair removal. *J Clin Laser Med Surg.* 1997;15:225–229.

CHAPTER 24

Hair Removal with the Long-Pulsed Ruby and Alexandrite Lasers

TINA S. ALSTER AND CHRISTOPHER A. NANNI

The technology of laser hair removal is advancing rapidly. However, the number of lasers currently available for hair removal and their various treatment protocols have created confusion and hype within the field of cutaneous surgery. By exaggerating and distorting the capabilities of these laser systems, the media have helped to create unrealistic public expectations for laser hair removal.

Laser-assisted hair removal is best understood in the context of the theory of *selective photothermolysis*. This theory, proposed by Anderson and Parrish[1] in 1983, states that a particular wavelength of light corresponding to that which is preferentially absorbed by a specified target should remain in contact with the target no longer than its *thermal relaxation time* (the time it takes a target to cool to 50% of its maximum absorbed thermal energy after laser irradiation). For hair removal, the target may be either an endogenous pigment (such as melanin within the hair shaft and follicular epithelium) or an exogenous substance (such as a carbon-based solution placed within the hair follicle).[2-12] The wavelengths of laser light best used to target dermal pigment are in the red and infrared range of the electromagnetic spectrum. The target chromophore within the follicle of unwanted hair absorbs the laser wavelengths, thereby generating heat and/or acoustic waves that disrupt the integrity of the hair follicle and prevent hair regrowth.

Although this is a logical theoretical explanation of laser hair removal, it is far from complete. Many controversies and knowledge gaps in hair biology cloud the field of laser-assisted hair removal. For example, it is unclear which portion of the hair follicle should be injured to prevent hair growth. Both the papilla, deep at the base of the follicle, and the hair bulge, an area closer to the epidermis that is assumed to contain follicular stem cells, are possible targets for laser energy.[13,14] It is also unclear whether gray, blonde, and white hair can be targeted adequately with laser irradiation because of the presence of only minimal amounts of pigment.[14] Lastly, the ideal method to enhance laser damage to the hair follicle by using exogenous pigment or dye has yet to be determined. Indeed, whether the use of exogenous pigment improves the hair-removal process is unproven. (Box 24–1 lists the basic items needed for laser hair removal.)

Box 24–1. Basic Supplies for Laser Hair Removal

Disposable razor

Red marking pen

Cooling gel (EpiTouch), handpiece (EpiLaser, E2000), or cryogen spray (Apogee, Gentle Lase)

4 × 4 gauze pads

Alcohol wipes

Mild topical steroid cream

Safety goggles

RUBY LASER

The EpiLaser (Palomar Medical Technologies, Beverly, MA) was the first long-pulsed ruby laser system approved for hair removal by the U.S. Food and Drug Administration (FDA). Its (694-nm wavelength like its successor, E2000 model) is selectively absorbed by endogenous melanin contained in the hair follicle and shaft. A 7- or 10-mm spot size and a pulse duration of 3 milliseconds generate fluences of 10 to 50 J/cm^2 with a repetition rate of 0.5 Hz (Table 24–1). The 694-nm ruby laser light is avidly absorbed by melanin in the hair follicle and is converted to heat, resulting in thermal damage to the hair follicle.

To protect melanin-containing structures in the epidermis, a cooling sapphire-tipped handpiece is applied to the skin during laser irradiation, thereby decreasing skin surface temperature and preventing unwanted thermal injury to the epidermis.

The sapphire handpiece also serves other functions. During administration of laser pulses, moderate pressure is applied to the skin surface. This external pressure decreases the distance from the epidermal surface to the subcutaneous fat and increases penetration of the 694-nm ruby laser light to deeper follicular structures. As pressure is applied with the handpiece, blood is forced out of the underlying blood vessels, effectively minimizing absorption of laser energy by the nontarget chromophore oxyhemoglobin. The cooling tip also has a mild anesthetic property that allows sensitive areas, such as the

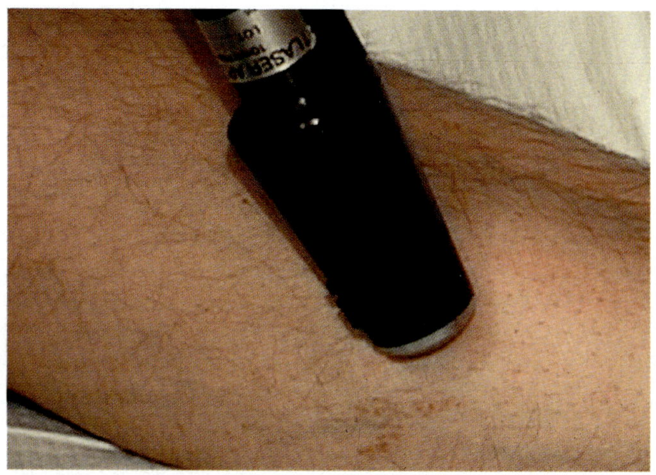

Figure 24–1. Long-pulsed ruby laser (EpiLaser) with sapphire cooling tip applied firmly to a treatment site.

inguinal and upper lip regions, to be treated relatively painlessly. It is important to remember that the cooling tip must be wiped clean after every few laser pulses to avoid accumulation of debris on the lens (Fig. 24–1).

The procedure for hair removal using the EpiLaser long-pulsed ruby system is summarized in Box 24–2. Test sites for individuals with darker or tanned skin tones may be helpful, but guarantees that subsequent treatment sessions will be complication-free should be avoided. Cold compresses or a mild topical corticosteroid may alleviate posttreatment erythema, swelling, and burning.

Table 24–1. Long-Pulsed Ruby Laser Energy Settings (10-mm spot)

Skin type	Low	Average	High
I	15	25–30	40–50
II	12	25	35–40
>II	8–10	12–16	25–30

I: Always burns, never tans (very pale).
II: Sometimes burns, fair tanning (pale)
III: No burning, good tanning (olive tone)

Box 24–2. Epilaser Hair Removal Procedure

1. Shave hair-bearing areas.
2. Draw a treatment grid in red ink to guide the placement of laser spots.
3. Firmly apply the sapphire lens cooling tip to the treatment site.
4. Discharge laser energy to the area with nonoverlapping pulses of a predetermined spot size.
5. Wipe clean the sapphire cooling with alcohol every 5 to 10 pulses to prevent debris from accumulating on the lens.

ADVANTAGES

The 694-nm laser light is ideally suited for the treatment of pigmented birthmarks and acquired pigmented lesions that are also hypertrichotic (e.g., Becker's nevus).[9] Because of its cooling handpiece, the EpiLaser system does not require the use of a cooling gel on the skin's surface, which can be messy and time-consuming. The cooling tip also acts as an anesthetic and can significantly reduce patient discomfort, thereby increasing patient satisfaction. Higher fluences may be tolerated and treatment time reduced because there is no need for frequent intermissions to relieve or prevent pain.

The control panel is operator-friendly and has easy-to-follow instructions displayed on a computer screen. The surgeon has the option of recording patient identification numbers on the laser screen and can obtain a printout of treatment time, number of pulses delivered, and treatment fluences used for each patient.

DISADVANTAGES

Because the laser unit is large and generates a moderate amount of heat, it should be kept in a large room with adequate ventilation. Although the articulated arm is well engineered, it sometimes gets entangled with the peripheral tubing. The sapphire cooling tip may collect hair debris and burn the epidermis if not wiped clean at regular intervals. When a treatment area has not been closely shaved, singed hair shafts adhere to the lens.

It is often difficult to recognize which areas have been lased, even when a treatment grid is used, because of minimal postoperative tissue reaction. The red-ink treatment grid can be difficult to remove, requiring rubbing with alcohol.

Treatment may be uncomfortable and even painful when high fluences are used or when sensitive body areas, such as the bikini line or upper lip, are treated. Blistering, crusting, and hyperpigmentation may occur in patients with dark or tanned skin despite the use of a cooling handpiece. Damaged hair shafts may extrude from the treated hair follicles 5 to 7 days after laser treatment, but do not indicate hair regrowth and may be easily plucked, shaved, or waxed.

ALEXANDRITE LASER

Long-pulsed alexandrite lasers (LPIR; Cynosure, Chelmsford, MA and EpiTouch; ESC/Sharplan) have also been approved by the FDA for laser hair removal. These systems generate light with a wavelength of 755 nm, a 7- or 10-mm spot size (Fig. 24–2), and fluences up to J/cm^2 to target unwanted body and facial hair (Table 24–2). A 5-, 10-, or 20-millisecond pulse duration and repetition rate of 0.5–1 Hz may be used. The relatively long pulse durations allow for the selective thermal destruction of large cutaneous targets, such as hair follicles. Endogenous melanin within the follicle and hair shaft absorbs the 755-nm-wavelength light, resulting in thermal damage

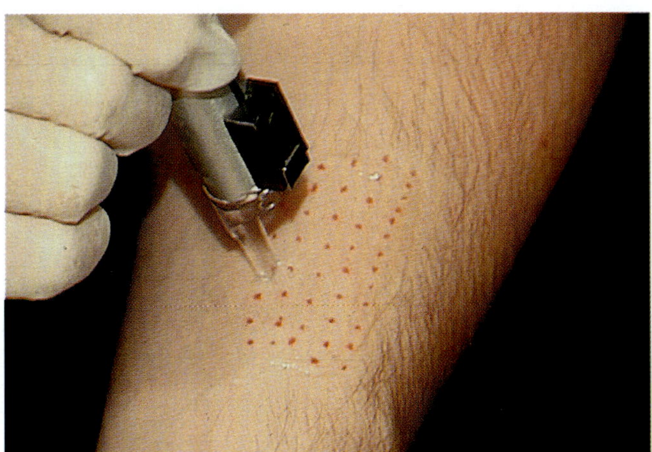

Figure 24–2. Long-pulsed alexandrite (LPIR) laser handpiece adjacent to a treatment site that has been shaved, outlined with red ink, and covered with a cooling water-based gel.

Table 24–2. Long-Pulsed Alexandrite Laser Energy Settings (10-mm spot)

Skin type	Low	Average	High
I	15	20–25	40
II	15	20–25	35–40
III or >	10	15–20	25–30

and delayed hair regrowth. Although the pigment within the follicle is targeted, unwanted epidermal injury also may occur as the alexandrite laser light passes through superficial melanin-containing skin layers. A patient with very fair skin (Fitzpatrick type I) and darkly pigmented hair shafts is the ideal candidate for hair removal with an alexandrite laser. This differential pigmentation is ideal because the dark hair pigment preferentially absorbs laser energy, thus sparing the melanin-poor epidermis.

However, because there are rarely ideal candidates, a cooling gel is typically applied to the skin surface in order to provide a heat sink, thereby decreasing the risk of epidermal injury. Cooling tip handpieces and cryogen spray devices are also available to prevent epidermal injury. Shaving prevents burning of the underlying epidermis, ensuring that most of the laser energy is directed deeper into the hair shaft to effectively remove hair.

The procedure for hair removal using the alexandrite system is summarized in Box 24–3. As with the ruby laser, test sites for patients with darker or tanned skin may be helpful but do not guarantee subsequent treatment sessions will be complication-free. Posttreatment erythema and burning can be alleviated with application of cold compresses or a mild topical corticosteroid.

Box 24–3. Alexandrite Laser Hair Removal Procedure

1. Shave hair-bearing areas.
2. Draw a treatment grid in red ink to guide the laser operator (unless a scanner is used).
3. Apply a cooling water-based gel (e.g., KY Jelly or ultrasound gel), cooling tip handpiece, or cryogen spray to the treatment site.
4. Deliver laser energy to the area with nonoverlapping pulses of a predetermined spot size.

ADVANTAGES

This compact laser may be operated in a small but well-ventilated room; the flexible fiberoptic arm is easy to manipulate and aids access to hard-to-reach body areas. The small laser handpiece is simple to use and allows the operator a clear view of the treatment site. The laser is equipped with a red helium-neon aiming beam that also helps direct handpiece position.

The 10-mm spot size and 0.5–1-Hz repetition rate (and/or use of a scanner device) make the treatment of large areas such as the back or legs more manageable. Theoretically, the 755-nm wavelength is less likely to be absorbed by epidermal melanin than other pigment-specific lasers (e.g., the 694-nm ruby laser) and so may be less damaging to patients with darker skin tones.

DISADVANTAGES

The use of a cooling gel is messy and time-consuming to apply and remove. In larger anatomic locations, it is often difficult to determine which areas have been treated, even when using an inked grid. Treatment may be uncomfortable and even painful when high fluences are used or when sensitive body areas, such as the bikini line or upper lip, are treated. Blistering, crusting, and hyperpigmentation may occur in patients with dark skin types or tanned skin, even when a cooling gel or device is used. Hair shafts that are damaged during laser treatment may be eliminated through the hair follicle 5 to 7 days postoperatively, leading the patient to believe that hair has regrown. This extrusion phenomenon is particularly common in areas where the hair is coarse, such as the bikini line or axilla. These nonviable hairs are easily plucked, shaved, or waxed.

COMPLICATIONS

Perifollicular edema and posttreatment erythema are seen in all patients but resolve rapidly, usually within 1 to 4 hours. Mild transient (burning) pain occurs in 5 to 10% of patients, but there are rare occurrences of moderate pain that require topical or local anesthesia.

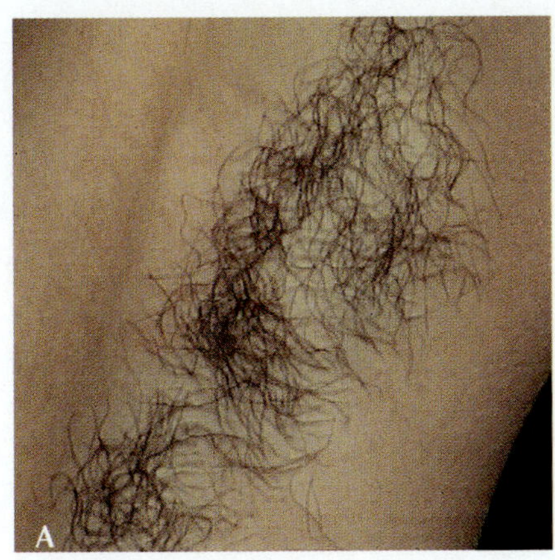
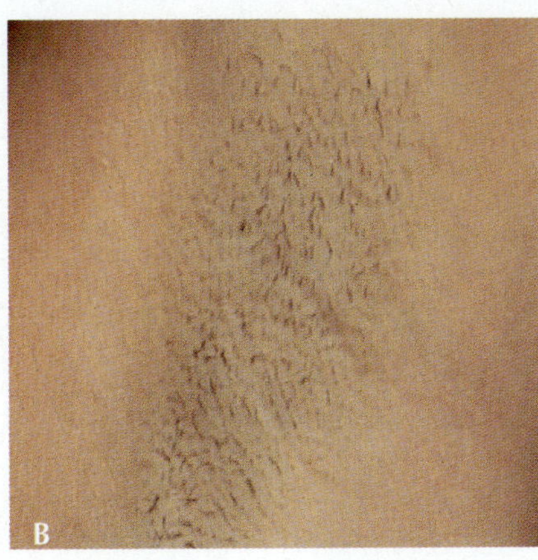

Figure 24–3. Pigmented terminal axillary hair in a woman with type-I skin before laser treatment (A) and 2 months after (B) a second ruby laser treatment.

From 10 to 15% of patients experience blistering and/or fine epidermal crusting, and these effects are significantly more common in patients with Fitzpatrick skin type III and darker or in those with tanned skin.[15] Purpura also may occur in darker-skinned patients or in treatment areas of excessive overlap of laser pulses. Hypopigmentation is seen most commonly in tanned patients. Long-term complications and scarring are rare and avoidable if patients are properly selected and laser protocols are followed.

CLINICAL EFFICACY

Laser hair removal is best viewed as an effective method to delay hair regrowth. Permanent hair removal, loosely defined as an absence of hair growth over the lifetime of the patient, is theoretically possible but not universal. We have personally observed a 50% decrease in hair density that persists for more than 12 months after a single laser session. However, this is an exceptional response, and most patients require multiple monthly or bi-monthly laser sessions (average = 3) with maintenance treatments every 4 to 6 months thereafter to achieve significant and continued hair density reduction.

After a single treatment session with a long-pulsed ruby or alexandrite laser, hair typically regrows in 3 to 6 months. Hair re-growth is often finer and lighter than the original hairs. We tend to use the ruby laser on patients with Fitzpatrick skin types I and II, but use the alexandrite laser without regard to skin type. We find that both laser systems are clinically equivalent in terms of hair removal efficacy and duration (Figs. 24–3, 24–4, and 24–5).

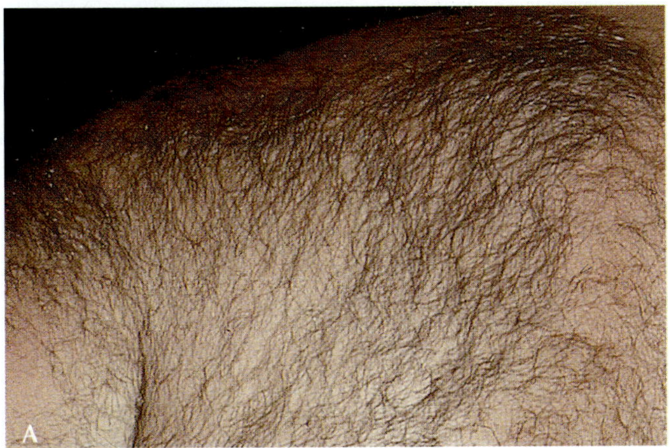
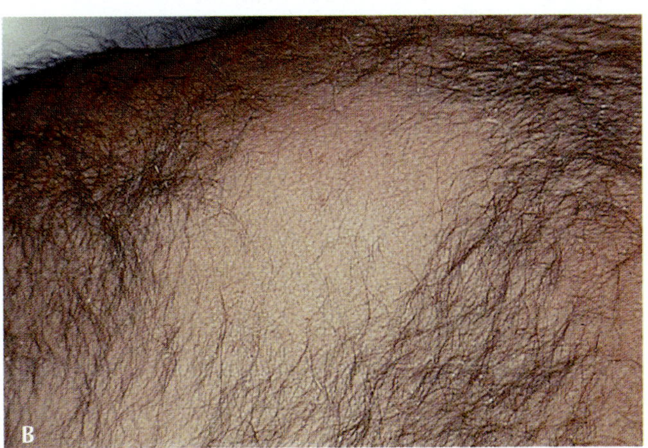

Figure 24–4. Pigmented terminal hairs on the shoulder of a man with type-III skin before (A) and 6 months after (B) a single treatment with a long-pulsed alexandrite laser.

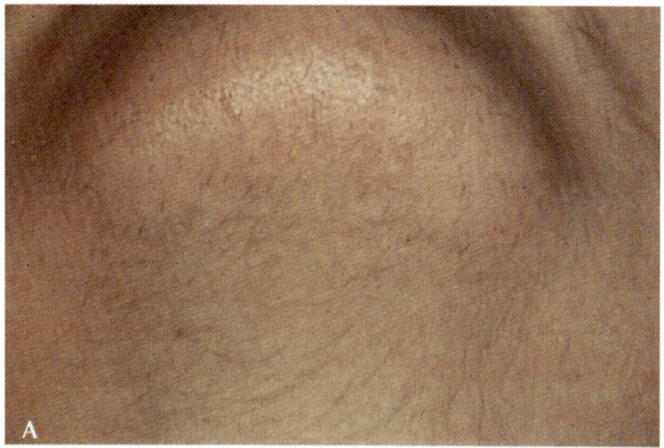

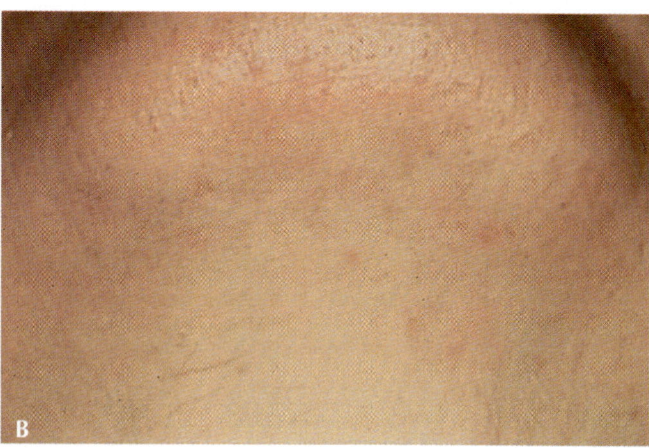

Figure 24–5. Coarse terminal chin hairs in a young woman before laser treatment (A) and 6 months after (B) a third long-pulsed alexandrite laser treatment.

After three laser treatments at 4- to 6-week intervals, most patients experience a prolonged delay in hair regrowth (6–9 months). Following a series of three or more treatment sessions, several patients exhibit a significant and "permanent" decrease in hair density.

CONCLUSIONS

Laser hair removal using the long-pulsed ruby and alexandrite laser systems is a relatively new process. It is too early to predict which treatment protocols, patients, and energy settings are ideal to achieve long-lasting or even permanent hair removal. For now, physicians and patients must be content with a significant delay in hair re-growth. Regardless, laser technology can profoundly affect the quality of patients' lives by providing a safe, rapid, and relatively painless method for long-lasting hair removal.

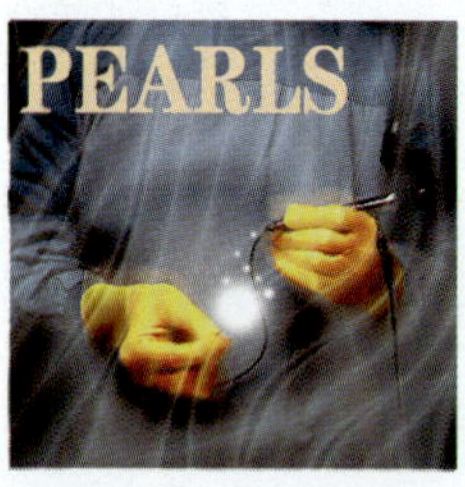

- Do not treat a patient with tanned skin or prior to important social or professional events.
- Increase energy fluences as tolerated, but do not overlap laser pulses.

- Shave or trim hair prior to lasing (do not wax or pluck).
- Draw a treatment grid (in red ink) to guide placement of laser spots.
- Test sites are helpful but not infallible.
- A cooling gel, spray, or handpiece is essential. Keep the lens free of debris (e. g., singed hair) during treatment.
- Topical corticosteroids decrease posttreatment erythema.
- With a cool tip handpiece, application of moderate pressure to the skin surface increases laser penetration and improves the anesthetic effect.

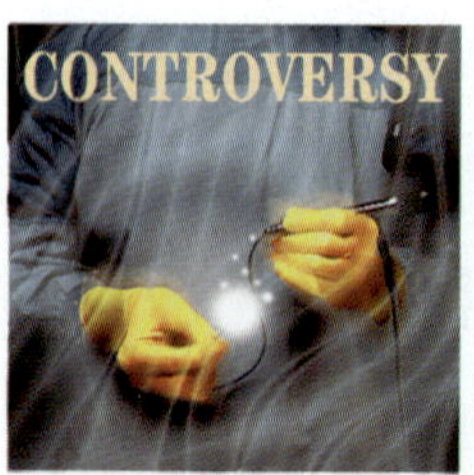

- It is unclear which portion of the hair follicle should be injured to prevent hair growth. Both the papilla and the hair bulge are possible targets for laser energy.
- Gray, blonde, and white hair may not be targeted adequately with laser irradiation because they contain minimal amounts of pigment.
- Optimal use of exogenous pigment or dye to enhance specific laser damage to the hair follicle has yet to be determined, and its efficacy is unproven.

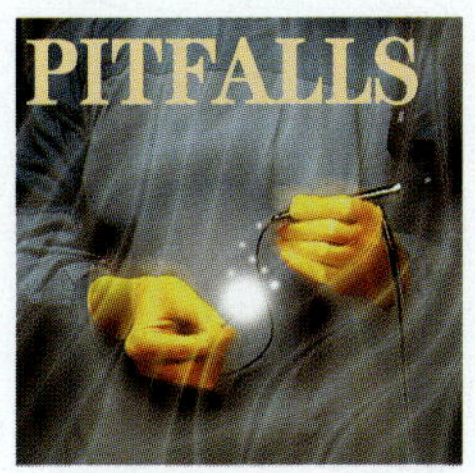

- The ruby laser unit is large, generates a moderate amount of heat, and the articulated arm sometimes gets entangled with the peripheral tubing.
- It is often difficult to recognize intraoperatively which hair-bearing areas have been treated with the ruby or the alexandrite laser, even when an inked treatment grid is used.
- In reality, laser treatment delays hair regrowth but may not completely eliminate it. Patients and physicians must understand that permanent removal of all unwanted hair may not be possible.

REFERENCES

1. Anderson RR, Parrish JA. Selective photothermolysis: precise microsurgery by selective absorption of pulsed radiation. *Science.* 1983;220:524–527.
2. Alster TS. *Manual of Cutaneous Laser Techniques. 2nd Edition.* Philadelphia: Lippincott, Williams & Wilkins; 2000:109–118.
3. Goldberg, DJ, Littler CM, Wheeland RG. Topical suspension-assisted Q-switched Nd:YAG laser hair removal. *Dermatol Surg.* 1997;23:741–745.
4. Grossman MC, Dierickx C, Farinelli W, et al. Damage to hair follicles by normal-mode ruby pulses. *J Am Acad Dermatol.* 1996;35:889–894.
5. Grossman MC, Wimberly J, Dwyer P, et al. PDT for hirsutism. *Lasers Surg Med.* 1995; suppl 7:47.
6. Lask G, Elman M, Slatkine M, et al. Laser-assisted hair removal by selective photothermolysis: preliminary results. *Dermatol Surg.* 1997;23:737–739.
7. Nanni CA, Alster TS. Optimizing treatment parameters for hair removal using a topical carbon-based solution and 1064-nm Q-switched neodymium:YAG laser energy. *Arch Dermatol.* 1997;133:1546–1549.
8. Nanni CA, Alster TS. A pratical review of laser-assisted hair removal using the Q-switched Nd:YAG, long-pulsed ruby, and long-pulsed alexandrite laser systems. *Dermatol Surg.* 1998;1399–1405.
9. Nanni CA, Alster TS. Successful treatment of Becker's nevus using 694 nm long-pulsed ruby laser energy. *Dermatol Surg.* 1998;24:1032–1034.
10. Nanni CA, Alster TS. Long-pulsed alexandrite laser-assisted hair removal: comparisons at 5, 10, 20 millisecond pulse durations. *Laser Surg Med.* 1999;24:332–337.
11. Alster TS. An update on laser options for hair removal. *Skin & Aging.* 1999;15–18.
12. Alster TS. The evolution of laser-assisted hair removal. *Cosmetic Dermatol.* 1999;(Aug)15–18.
13. McKee PH. *Pathology of the Skin.* London: Mosby-Wolfe; 1996:1.20–1.21.
14. Olsen EA. *Disorders of Hair Growth.* New York: McGraw Hill, Inc.; 1994:52–55.
15. Nanni CA, Alster TS. Complications of laser-assisted hair removal using the Q-switched Nd:YAG, long-pulsed ruby, and long-pulsed alexandrite lasers. *J Am Acad Dermatol.* 1999;41:165–171.

CHAPTER 25

Hair Removal with the EpiLight System

ROBERT A. WEISS AND MARGARET A. WEISS

The removal of body hair, whether normally distributed or excessive as a result of medical disease or genetics, has become a popular request by patients over the last few years. This change in attitude probably can be explained by the fact that the modern, streamlined, aerodynamic approach to design in general has translated to human appearance. Public demand therefore has fueled the development of easier and more effective hair-removal methods. Until recently, electrolysis and thermolysis have been the mainstays of treatment. These methods of hair removal typically require about 10 sessions for acceptable results,[1] and regular repeat treatments are commonly required. Electroepilation with metal tweezers reportedly requires significantly more than 10 sessions to obtain even minimal results.[2]

The desired endpoint for truly permanent hair removal is the destruction and fibrosis of peribulbar tissue at the base of the hair follicle. Minimizing accompanying necrosis of the perifollicular dermis above the peribulbar tissue enhances the likelihood of permanent epilation and reduces the probability of scarring.[3] A histologic study of electrothermolysis concluded that surface scarring was minimized by causing a fibrotic scar at the lower follicle but allowing the infundibulum and associated sebaceous glands to regenerate.[3] It is critical to recognize the difference between the desired result of fibrosis at the lower follicle and the undesired result of scarring at the level of the reticular dermis. The use of laser light to remove hair represents a major leap forward in effective hair growth reduction without scarring in fewer sessions than other methods.

LIGHT-BASED HAIR REMOVAL

The light-based removal of hair is based on the principle of selective photothermolysis (see Chapter 4). This principle states that it is possible to selectively target a chromophore without destroying surrounding tissue; it has been successfully applied to treatment of cutaneous vascular lesions. The target chromophore for hair is melanin (rather than hemoglobin, the chromophore for vascular lesions). It is difficult to target melanin because it resides both in the epidermis and in hair follicles, yet melanin absorbs best at lower wavelengths, making deeper penetration to the base of the hair follicle more difficult. However, selectivity may be achieved by targeting the heavy concentrations of melanin in the hair follicles while leaving the low concentrations of melanin in the epidermis unaffected.[4]

Use of light energy rather than electrical energy for epilation was first reported in 1990 when the argon laser was used to treat trichiasis by "thermoablation" with a very small spot size (0.1 mm).[5] In 1996, a study on small superficial eyelid follicles showed a 50% reduction in hair growth with minimal scarring.[6] The concept of using a longer wavelength to reach deep follicles was reported for epilation of hair from grafts employed during urethroplasty for hypospadias repair.[7] Use of the neodymium:yttrium-aluminum-garnet (Nd:YAG) surgical laser (1064 nm) was based on the concept that one could photocoagulate tissue to a depth of up to 5 mm, thus destroying deeper hair follicles. Most recently, the refined 1064-nm laser has been used successfully at extremely short pulse durations for hair removal.[8,9]

The first modern application of selective photothermolysis was the use of a normal-mode ruby laser (694 nm, 270 microseconds, 6-mm beam diameter, at fluences of 30–60 J/cm^2) for selective hair follicle destruction. Grossman et al[10] reported histological evidence of the fluence-dependent selective thermal injury to follicles, which meant that selective destruction of hair follicles by photothermolysis was possible using a normal-mode ruby laser.

Hair removal by selective photothermolysis has also been accomplished by the filtered flashlamp intense pulsed light (IPL) source (EpiLight, ESC Medical, Yokneam, Israel), which produces filtered noncoherent light in the 590- to 1200-nm range divided in millisecond pulses separated by the thermal relaxation time of epidermal melanin. A small spot size leads to rapid scatter and a rapid decay of fluence by depth.[11] Penetration is therefore more efficient with a large spot size. The noncoherent IPL's huge spot size (10 × 45 mm) and emission at wavelengths up to 1200 nm are advantageous because wavelengths above 600 nm are absorbed by hair follicles and penetrate deeply enough to produce selective thermolysis of the follicle bulb.

The first published report of successful long-term hair removal with the IPL device involved terminal beard hair removal in two transsexual (male-to-female) patients.[12] Histologic examination demonstrated atrophy of entire follicles with no scarring at the skin surface. This injury was thought to be a direct thermal effect and/or an indirect photothermolytic effect. Six months after a series of treatments, no pigmentary or skin texture changes and, most important, no recurrence of hair growth was observed. Another recent publication documents approximately 60% hair removal at 12 weeks following IPL device treatment.[13]

CLINICAL EXPERIENCE

Our experience in clinical trials using the EpiLight system have yielded very encouraging results.[14] Our experience indicates a 63% reduction in hair count at 12 weeks, but this falls to 25% at 6 months, which emphasizes the need for caution in interpreting hair removal data over a limited follow-up interval.

PATIENT SELECTION AND PREPARATION

Although patients with Fitzpatrick skin types III to V may be successfully treated with the EpiLight system, the importance of multiple pulsing to allow epidermal cooling becomes paramount in these patients. Patients with Fitzpatrick skin types IV and V may be treated using the 645-nm filter (Fig. 25–1).

For the IPL device to heat the hair follicle sufficiently, a large-diameter dark anagen terminal hair should be selected as the target. Targeting hair follicle stem cells that reside in the bulge in the upper follicle may not produce a response with either a laser or the IPL device because stem cells lack the target chromophore.[15] Therefore, treatment in the telogen phase is unlikely to arrest hair follicle growth. Hair diameter also helps to determine the most effective pulse width; smaller-diameter hair shafts heat up and cool faster, so shorter-duration pulse widths are used for finer hair.

Site preparation such as waxing is unnecessary and actually counterproductive because the target chromophore is eliminated when the hair is removed. Hairs should extend 1 to 3 mm above the skin surface because the protruding hair shaft may act as a "wick" to conduct photons down to the follicle. Moreover, when hair is

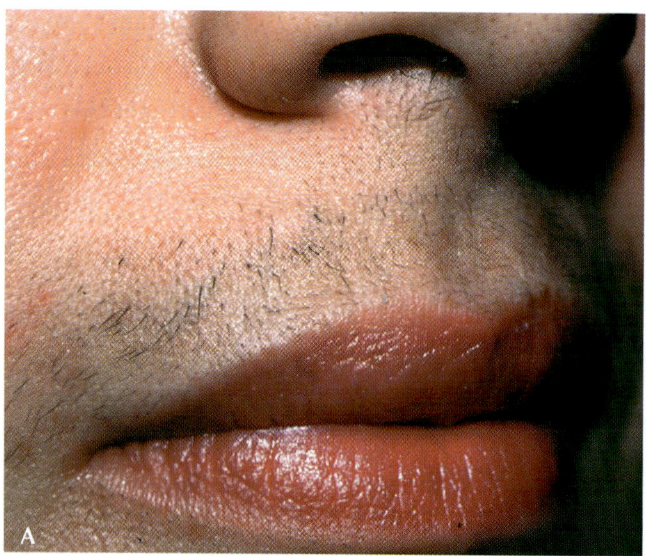

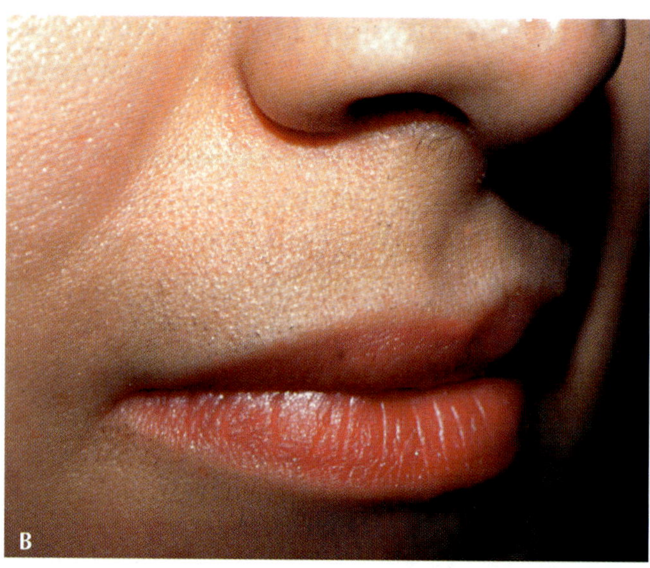

Figure 25–1. (A) Upper lip of woman of Mediterranean background and skin type IV before treatment. (B) Patient at 6 months after two treatments. No discoloration or epidermal injury is evident. The 645-nm filter was used for these treatments.

shaved to the skin surface, it is not possible to immediately see the result, or endpoint, of lasing.

Applying water-based gel (stored in an ice bucket) immediately before pulsing minimizes epidermal injury and enhances patient comfort. During the procedure, the crystal makes contact with the skin through a 2-mm layer of gel, which enhances epidermal cooling while ensuring transmission of large volumes of light from the crystal into the skin (Fig. 25–2).

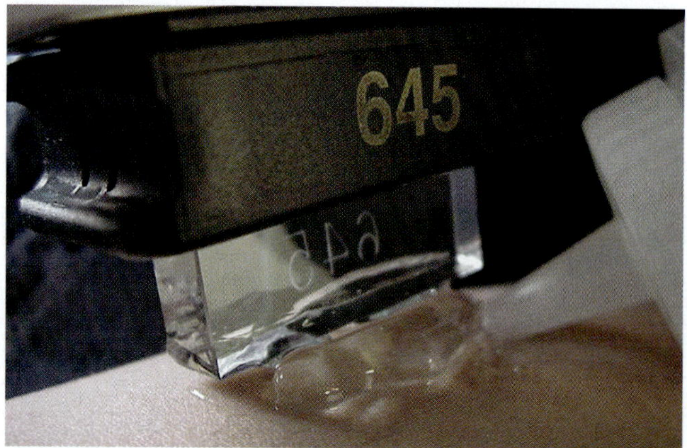

Figure 25–2. Proper application of the gel separating crystal from skin. A 2-mm layer of gel connects the crystal with the skin surface.

PROTOCOL AND PROCEDURES

Parameters include a 645-nm flashlamp cutoff filter that permits noncoherent wavelengths of 645 to 1200 nm to penetrate 4 to 5 mm into the hair follicles. Pulse durations of 3 to 5 milliseconds are separated by 10- to 30-millisecond delay times. Total energy delivered is typically 40 to 50 J/cm^2. The rationale is that a typical hair follicle is a 0.5- to 1.5-mm-diameter cord of pigmented dry protein that absorbs more laser energy that the surrounding tissue and "pulls" it down into the follicle. The initial pulse begins to heat the hair shaft but also heats the epidermis slightly. Because the amount of pigmentation within the hair shaft is several times greater than that in the epidermis, most of the initial photons are absorbed by the hair shaft. Although epidermal melanin absorbs some energy, the relatively short pulse followed by thermal relaxation allows the epidermis to cool sufficiently to avoid thermal damage.

Following the initial light pulse, the hair shaft remains hot because the thermal relaxation time of a 1- to 2-mm-diameter dark cylinder is much longer than that of the epidermis. When the next pulse arrives, the hair follicle is heated further, but the epidermis is only slightly

Ruby laser treatment, 40 J/cm², 3.0 ms

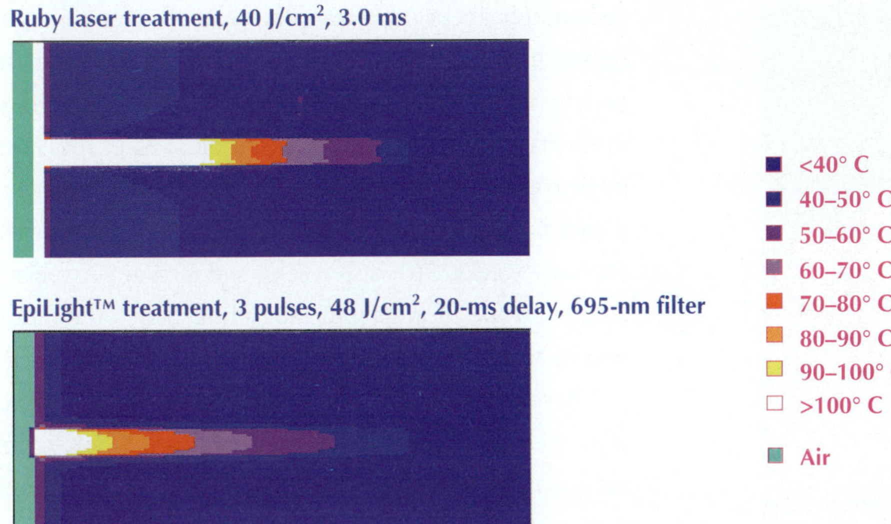

EpiLight™ treatment, 3 pulses, 48 J/cm², 20-ms delay, 695-nm filter

Figure 25–3. Diagram of calculated comparative temperatures in the hair follicle.

reheated after its thermal relaxation cooling period of 10 to 40 milliseconds. Skin temperature remains under 70°C, a temperature at which protein coagulation is unlikely. Typical temperatures reached in a 4-mm-deep hair follicle with the IPL device as compared with ruby and alexandrite lasers are shown in Figure 25–3. This process can be repeated for up to five sequential pulses with the EpiLight system.

ENDPOINTS AND EFFECTS

Our visual endpoint is depigmentation of the treated hairs, as well as shortening, curling, or vaporization to the skin surface of the 1- to 3-mm stubble (Fig. 25–4). The smell of denatured hair protein is another indication of effective treatment. In addition to these signs, there should be very little erythema at the skin surface,

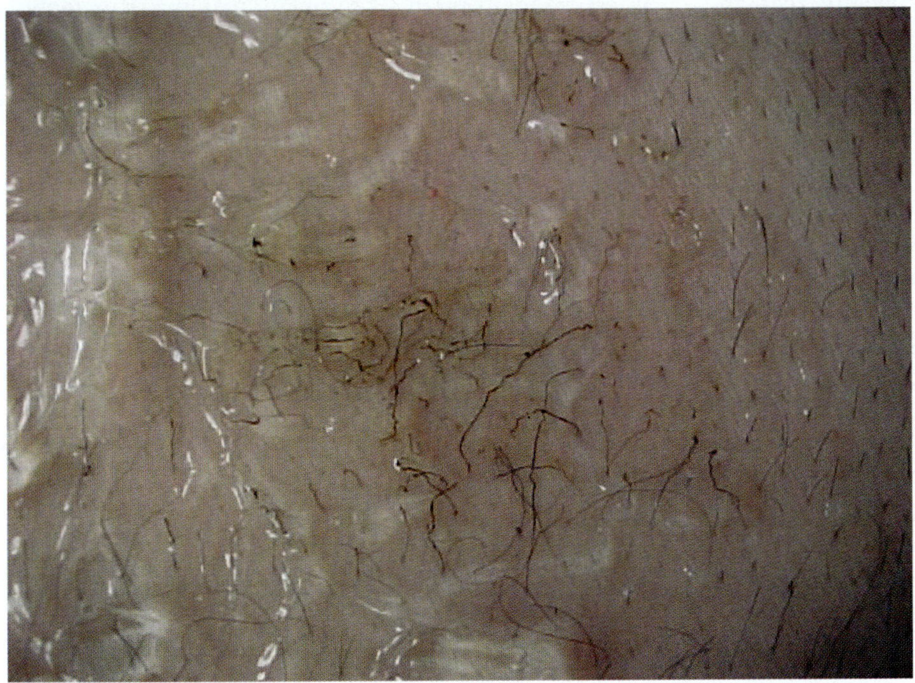

Figure 25–4. Vaporization of hairs to the skin surface following 3 sequential pulses from IPL (3 pulses of 3.2 milliseconds, separated by 20-millisecond delay, 645-nm filter, fluence 42 J/cm²). Some hairs are burned to the surface, others have a frizzled and curly appearance. Some hair stubs have become lighter. Water-based gel is required for treatment and is seen on the skin.

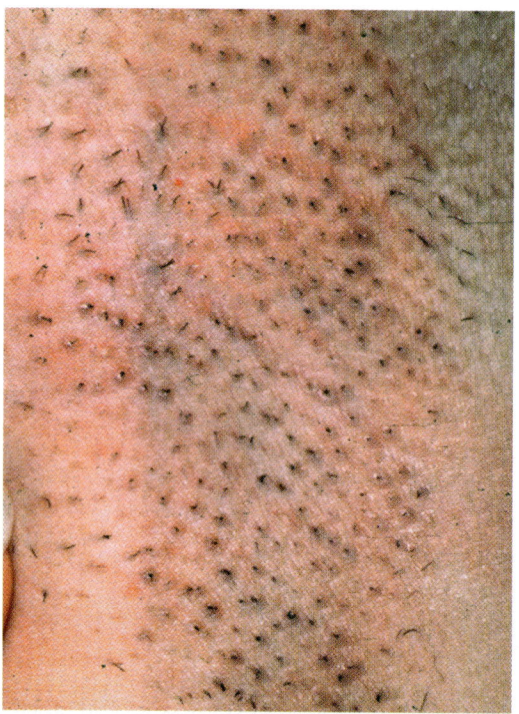

Figure 25–5. Urticarial edema 15 minutes following IPL. Erythema usually accompanies this palpable edema around each follicle.

indicating no damage to the epidermis or dermis immediately below. Within minutes one usually sees an urticarial response surrounding the treated follicles (Fig. 25–5). Our experience has shown us that when we observe these features, long-term (>6 months) reduction in hair count is very likely.

Results

We have treated more than 100 patients with Fitzpatrick skin types I to V and all colors of hair. Initial results from 100 patients enrolled in various protocols consisted of evaluation at 3 months of 28 sites on 23 patients after a single treatment with the IPL device. Parameters included a 2.8- to 5-millisecond pulse, 615- to 695-nm cutoff filters, and thermal relaxation times of 20 to 30 milliseconds between triple-pulse delivery at 40 to 48 J/cm^2. Hair counts were obtained by averaging three square-

centimeter areas on a template placed over the skin. Repeat hair counts and photographs were performed on patients at 2, 4, 8, and 12 weeks. Results included an immediate reduction in hair count of 31%, as measured by disappearance of hairs at the skin surface. This was followed by reductions in hair counts of 54% at 2 weeks, 56% at 4 weeks, 56% at 8 weeks, and 63% at 12 weeks.[14] Follow up at 6 months indicated a final hair count reduction of approximately 25%.

Recent data from four treatments at higher fluence separated by 2-month intervals indicate a hair count reduction of 65% at 1 year. Adverse effects were minimal, with a 92% rate of mild erythema and an 18% incidence of urticarial edema lasting for several hours. Only one site developed a vesicle, which healed uneventfully. Temporary pigmentation changes occurred in approximately 9% of patients. All patients reported far less pain than with electrolysis.

Axilla and Inguinal Regions

The axilla and inguinal regions, which have telogen phases lasting up to 3 months, may require treatment at less frequent intervals to obtain maximal hair reduction (Fig. 25–6). These regions also require the longest wavelengths of light available to penetrate follicles that extend 3 to 4 mm into the skin. For this purpose, the 645- and 695-nm filters are most useful because they remove the shorter, less penetrating wavelengths. Slight erythema is seen, and an urticarial, almost edematous response around individual hair follicles is observed. Within several days, after the follicles are shocked into the resting phase, no further growth is seen, and these hairs may be epilated easily with forceps or are shed spontaneously.

Facial and Bikini Areas

Among cases of excessive hair on the face, our longest follow up is 1.5 years following four treatments (Fig. 25–7).

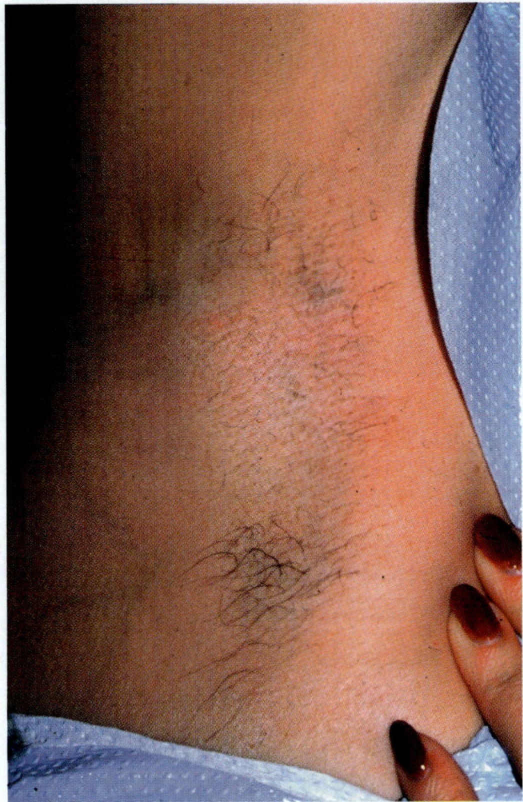

Figure 25–6. Treatment of axilla hairs by IPL. Two months after one treatment most follicles have not yet returned to the active growth phase, giving the impression of total hair removal. The untreated control area shows long hairs. Regrowth of 50% of the hairs occurred within 2 additional months.

This woman had Fitzpatrick type IV skin and hundreds of terminal hairs along her chin despite a dozen electrolysis treatments. Slight erythema was seen following treatment with a 615-nm cutoff filter and a total energy of 40 J

divided into three pulses. We believe that optimal pulse duration for hair removal with the IPL device is between 2.8 and 5 milliseconds. Unlike nanosecond pulses, which cause a photoacoustic effect, the millisecond pulse range results in a thermal effect. Our preliminary histologic data at 6 months to 1 year indicate destruction of peribulbar tissue at the base of the hair follicle without scarring of the more superficial perifollicular dermis. This is seen typically in the bikini area (Fig. 25–8).

Large Body Surfaces

In addition to the increased light penetration of the IPL device, the large spot size allows coverage of large body surfaces relatively rapidly. A grid permits a rapid distribution of pulses in an even fashion (Fig. 25–9). The grid can be used to facilitate treatment of the back as well (Fig. 25–10).

SUMMARY

The advantages of the IPL device include the delivery of many wavelengths simultaneously, the relatively large spot size for larger treatment areas, the ability to adjust pulse duration or width for maximum heating of variable diameter hair shafts, fluences that are easily adjustable, and multiple pulsing of each selected fluence. The exact mechanisms are unknown, but the IPL

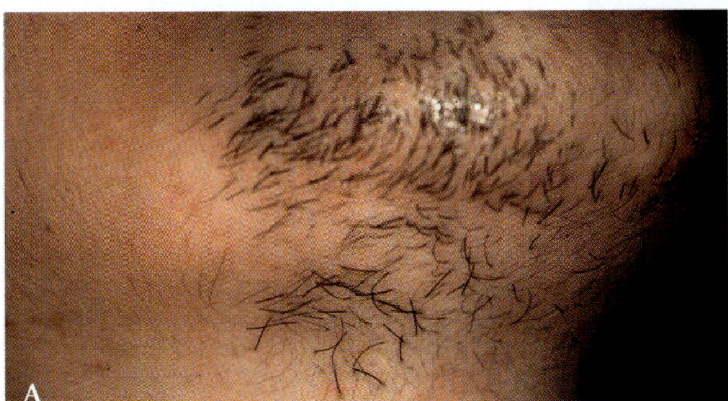

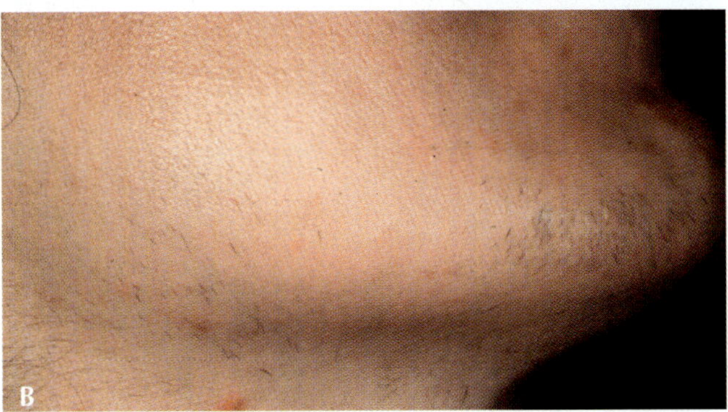

Figure 25–7. Hirsutism of the face of female patient with type-IV skin whose hormonal evaluation reveals no abnormality. A dozen attempts at electrolysis were unsuccessful. (A) Before treatment. (B) Six months after two treatments. Hair reduction of 50% is observed.

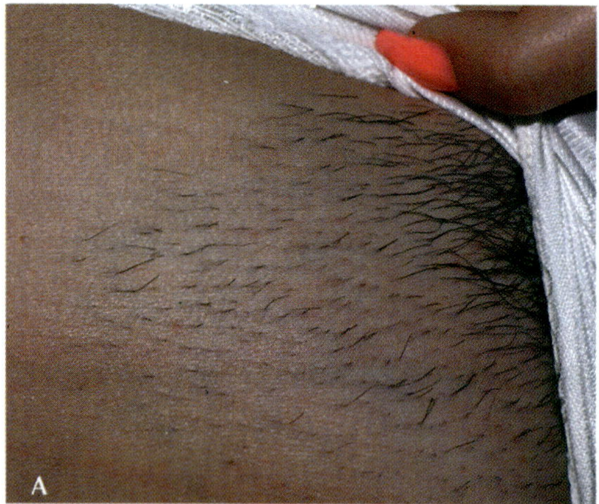

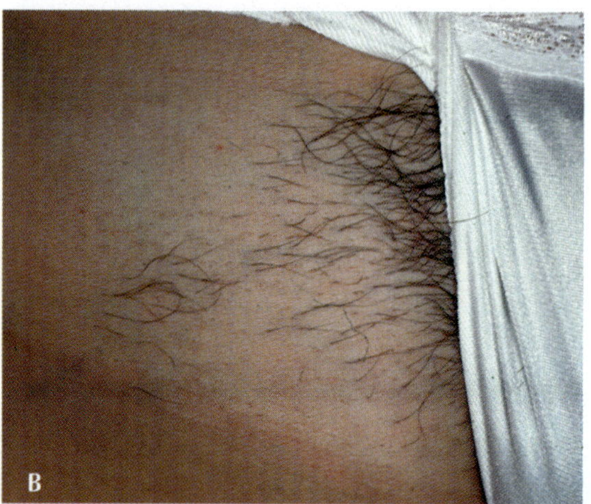

Figure 25–8. (A) Bikini area before treatment. (B) Three months after one treatment, some patchy hair reduction can be seen. These hairs extend deeply and may be resistant to light-based treatment.

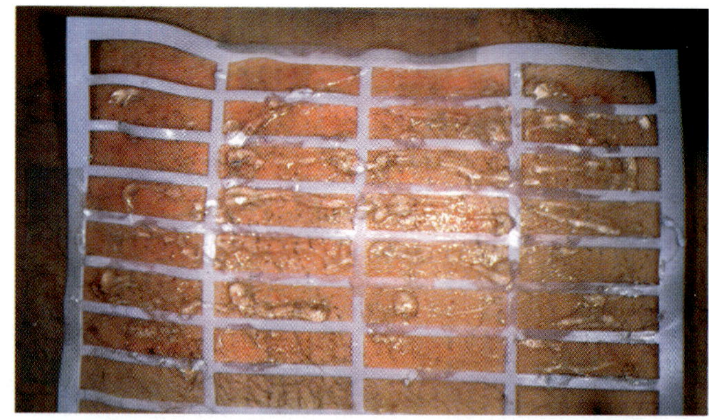

Figure 25–9. Grid used to guide treatment on larger body surfaces, such as the back.

device effectively treats hair-bearing skin with minimal discomfort and low risk of scarring or other complications. Even patients with darker skin types may be treated. Our clinical data on more than 100 patients indicate that it is possible to remove terminal hair for long intervals (>1 year), with a prolonged delay in regrowth of new hairs in many different body regions. Clinical trials using active epidermal cooling to improve efficacy and reduce patient discomfort are in progress. With additional experience and a better understanding of how the IPL device affects the rate and quality of hair growth, IPL-based long-term hair removal will continue to improve.

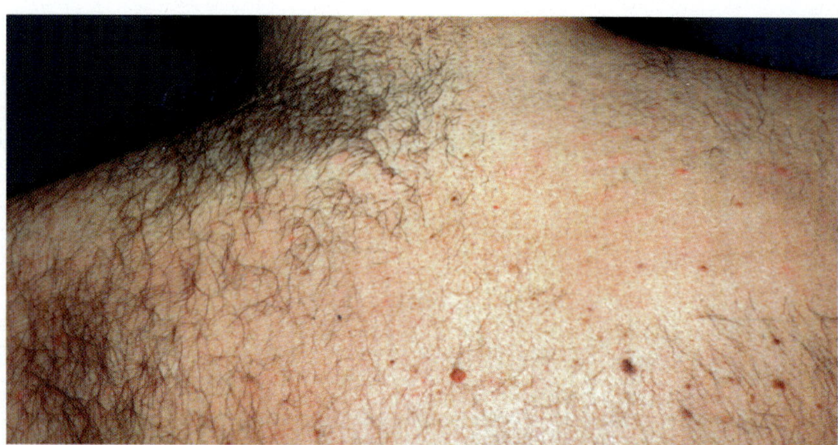

Figure 25–10. Results on the back 6 months after three treatments with IPL of a tanned patient with Fitzpatrick type-III skin. The left side of the back has received no treatment and demonstrates significantly more hair growth. At 1 year follow up, this patient had 50% reduction of hair count with many hairs thinner in diameter than prior to treatment.

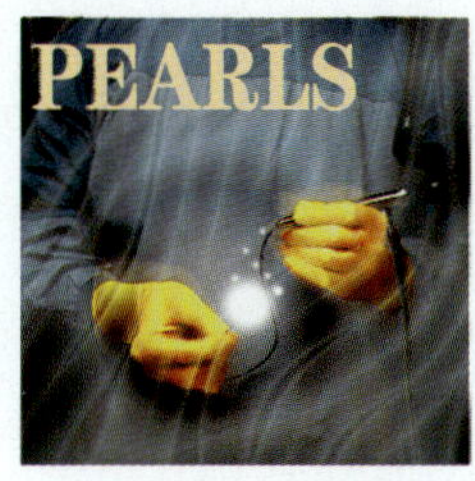

- It is difficult to target melanin because it resides both in the epidermis and in hair follicles, yet melanin absorbs best at lower wavelengths, making deeper penetration to the base of the hair follicle more difficult. However, the noncoherent IPL's huge spot size and emission wavelengths (600–1200 nm) are absorbed by hair follicles and penetrate deeply enough to produce selective thermolysis of the follicle bulb.

- Targeting hair follicle stem cells that reside in the bulge in the upper follicle may not produce a response with the IPL device because stem cells lack the target chromophore (melanin). Therefore, treatment in the telogen phase is unlikely to stop hair follicle growth.

- Hairs should extend 1 to 3 mm above the skin surface before treatment with the IPL device because the protruding hair shaft may act as a "wick" to conduct photons down to the follicle.

- The IPL device's large spot size allows treatment of large areas of the body, including the back. A grid facilitates treatment of the back and other large areas and permits rapid even distribution of light by the IPL.

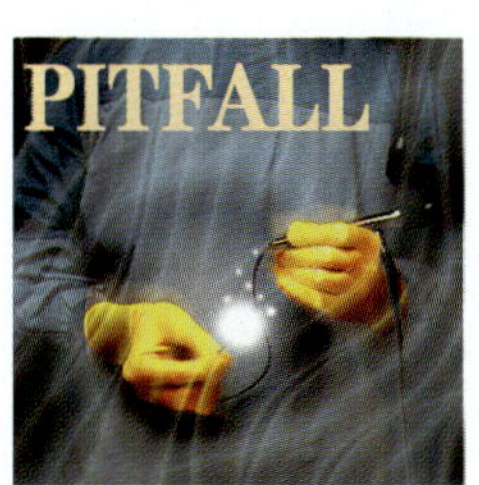

- Although there may be a significant reduction in hair count a few weeks after treatment with EpiLight, some hair regrowth is to be expected as time passes. Therefore, it is important to exercise caution in interpreting hair removal data from a limited follow-up interval.

REFERENCES

1. Urushibata O, Kase K. A comparative study of axillary hair removal in women: plucking versus the blend method. *J Dermatol.* 1995;22:738–742.

2. Verdich J. A critical evaluation of a method for treatment of facial hypertrichosis in women. *Dermatologica.* 1984;168:87–89.

3. Kligman AM, Peters L. Histologic changes of human hair follicles after electrolysis: a comparison of two methods. *Cutis.* 1984;34:169–176.

4. Wheeland RG. Laser-assisted hair removal. *Dermatol Clin.* 1997;15:469–477.

5. Campbell DC. Thermoablation treatment for trichiasis using the argon laser. *Aust N Z J Ophthalmol.* 1990;18:427–430.

6. Elder MJ. The true rate of success in argon laser eyelash thermoablation. *Ophthalmic Surg Lasers.* 1996;27:888–890.

7. Finkelstein LH, Blatstein LM. Epilation of hair-bearing urethral grafts using the neodymium:YAG surgical laser. *J Urol.* 1991;146:840–842.

8. Goldberg DJ, Littler CM, Wheeland RG. Topical suspension-assisted Q-switched Nd:YAG laser hair removal. *Dermatol Surg.* 1997;23:741–745.

9. Nanni CA, Alster TS. Optimizing treatment parameters for hair removal using a topical carbon-based solution and 1064-nm Q-switched neodymium:YAG laser energy. *Arch Dermatol.* 1997;133:1546–1549.

10. Grossman MC, Dierickx C, Farinelli W, Flotte T, Anderson RR. Damage to hair follicles by normal-mode ruby laser pulses. *J Am Acad Dermatol.* 1996;35:889–894.

11. Keijzer M, Jacques SL, Prahl SA, Welch AJ. Light distributions in artery tissue: Monte Carlo simulations for finite-diameter laser beams. *Lasers Surg Med.* 1989;9:148–154.

12. Raulin C, Werner S, Hartschuh W, Schonermark MP. Effective treatment of hypertrichosis with pulsed light: a report of two cases. *Ann Plast Surg.* 1997;39:169–173.

13. Gold MH, Bell MW, Foster TD, Street S. Long-term epilation using the EpiLight broad band, intense pulsed light hair removal system. *Dermatol Surg.* 1997;23:909–913.

14. Weiss RA, Weiss MA, Marwaha S, Harrington AC. Hair removal with a non-coherent filtered flashlamp pulsed light source. *Lasers Surg Med.* 1998;10:190.

15. Wilson C, Cotsarelis G, Wei ZG, et al. Cells within the bulge region of mouse hair follicle transiently proliferate during early anagen: heterogeneity and functional differences of various hair cycles. *Differentiation.* 1994;55:127–136.

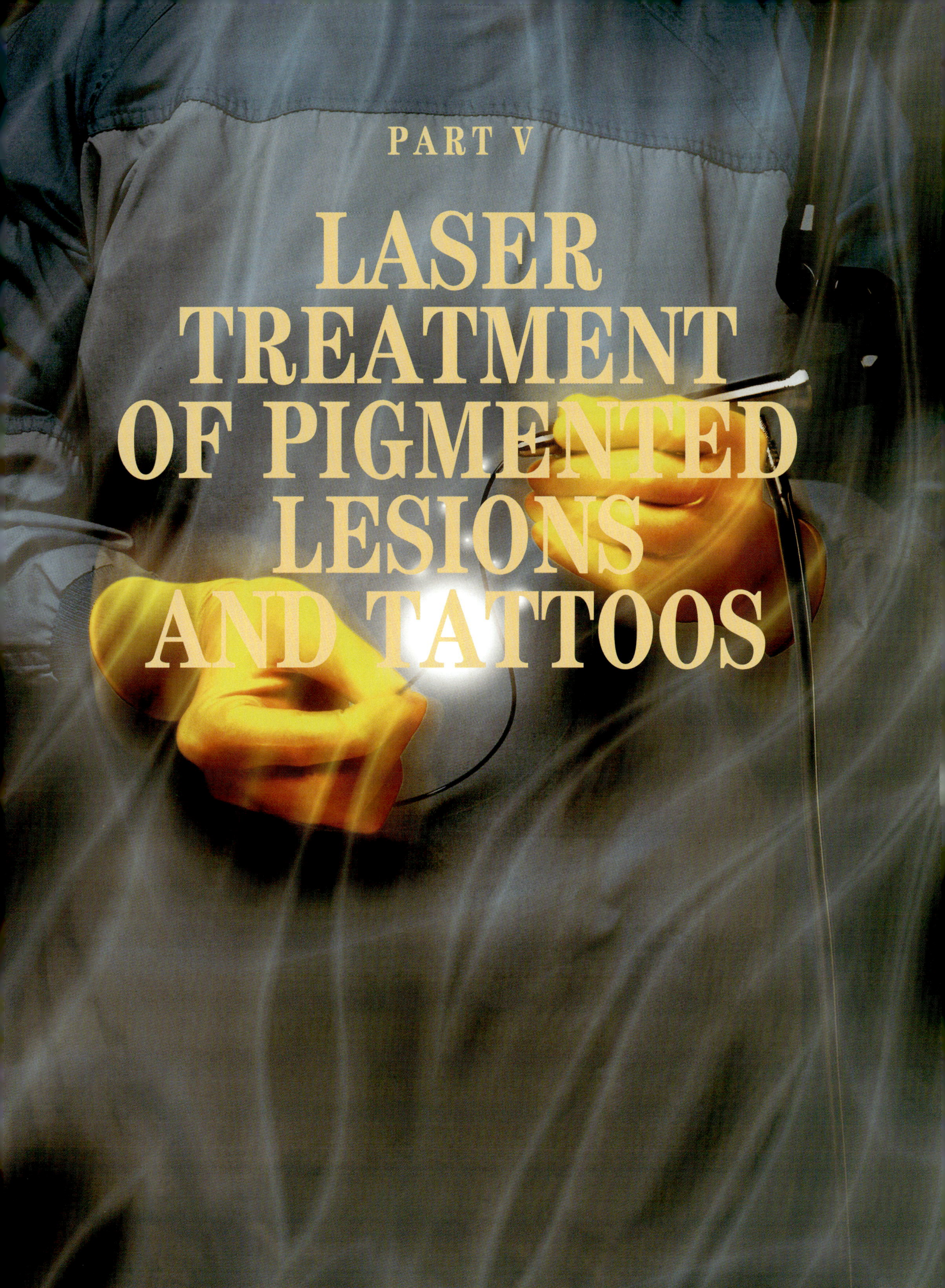
PART V

LASER
TREATMENT
OF PIGMENTED
LESIONS
AND TATTOOS

Laser Treatment of Pigmented Lesions and Tattoos: Use of Q-Switched Ruby Lasers

DAVID SAWYER AND NICHOLAS J. LOWE

PIGMENTED LESIONS

The clinical objectives in the laser treatment of benign pigmented lesions are selective destruction of the offending pigment and preservation of the normal overlying skin without cosmetically unacceptable adverse effects. In 1983, Anderson and Parrish[1] presented their theory of *selective photothermolysis*, which, in principle, involves inducing specific thermal injury in a subcellular chromophore that causes its ultimate removal or destruction without damaging surrounding structures.

For many pigmented lesions, melanin is the ideal chromophore, and it can be targeted uniquely with an understanding of its absorption spectrum and those of other common cutaneous chromophores, such as oxyhemoglobin.[2] Melanin is packed within melanosomes, which are found within melanocytes and pigmented basal keratinocytes.[3,4] Selective injury to these subcellular organelles has been observed with pulsed laser irradiation at many wavelengths, from 351 nm (Excimer laser) to 1064 nm (neodymium:yttrium-aluminum-garnet [Nd:YAG] laser).[5–9]

At wavelengths up to approximately 600 nm, radiation is absorbed significantly in hemoglobin as well as in melanin, the clinical result being an increased incidence of purpura. In addition, such wavelengths penetrate only a short distance into the skin, reaching only the superficial dermis at commonly used fluences.[5,10–12] At longer wavelengths (600 to 1200 nm), there is significant melanin absorption, whereas absorption of hemoglobin is much reduced. At even longer wavelengths (>1200 nm), absorption by both chromophores is reduced, and injury becomes increasingly nonspecific.[2,5,8] Therefore, lasers operating at 600 to 1200 nm can specifically target melanosomes and allow deeper penetration into the dermis at appropriate fluences.[5,8,9]

Neighboring tissue is not damaged at these wavelengths if the pulse width is less than or equal to the target tissue's *thermal relaxation time*, which is the time it takes for induced heat to be dissipated by 50% of its initial value.[1,8,13] The target tissue for pigmented lesions (i.e., melanosomes) has a short thermal relaxation time (hundred[s] of nanoseconds), although the exact value is not known.[12–14]

REMOVAL OF PIGMENTED LESIONS WITH THE Q-SWITCHED RUBY LASER

The Q-switched ruby laser produces very narrow pulse widths (20 to 50 nanoseconds) and operates at a wavelength of 694.3 nm. Therefore, this laser is an obvious choice for selective destruction of epidermal or dermal pigment. In practice, the laser has been shown to be melanin-specific and melanin-dependent. In guinea pig skin, it causes specific melanosome damage at fluences as low as 0.3 J/cm^2 with minimal absorption by oxyhemoglobin.[15]

We use the Spectrum Medical RD-1200 Q-switched ruby laser to treat patients with pigmented lesions. The single synthetic ruby crystal (aluminum trioxide doped with chromium), is optically "pumped" with high-intensity flashlamps. The resulting laser beam is red light with a 694.3-nm wavelength that may be Q-switched with an electrooptical switch (called a *Pockles cell*) to create a pulsed emission of light. The pulse widths achievable with this arrangement are 20 to 50 nanoseconds. Our laser produces an output with 28-nanosecond pulses and high energy fluences from 3 to 10 J/cm^2. The user-controlled pulse repetition rate is 0.5 to 1 Hz. The light energy is transmitted through an articulated-arm delivery system to an optical lens capable of focusing the beam to a spot size of 5 to 6.5 mm at the surface of the skin.

Patient Evaluation and Preparation

Over a 36-month period, 140 patients were selected for treatment. These patients had 307 lesions of four common types: (1) purely epidermal lesions, such as lentigo solaris (Table 26–1; 51 patients, 216 lesions) and café-au-lait macules without neurofibromatosus or Albright's syndrome (Table 26–2; 20 patients, 21 lesions); (2) melasma or epidermal-dermal pigment (Table 26–3; 16 female patients, 16 lesions: 11 centrofacial, four malar, and one mandibular); (3) nevi of Ota (Table 26–4; 18 patients, 19 nevi. One patient had bilateral involvement.); and (4) postinflammatory hypopigmented (PIHP) lesions (35 patients).

In a separate 8-month study,[16] pigmented infraorbital dark circles were treated (15 female and 2 male patients). The average age was 44.4 years (range, 32 to 75 years). Three women were taking oral contraceptives, and four were taking progesterone and estrogen as hormone replacement therapy. Skin types were Fitzpatrick type II (8 patients), III (6 patients), IV (1 patient), and V (2 patients) (mean, 2.5 patients).

All patients were treated on an outpatient basis, and none had had any previous treatments of their respective conditions. Patients were photographed before the initial treatment and at each subsequent visit. At re-treatment sessions, outcome was assessed, and patients were examined and questioned about adverse sequelae by an independent observer not involved in treatment and unaware of the stage of treatment or fluences used.

Table 26–1. Treatment of Lentigo Solaris

Location	Response Grade*	Average No. of Treatments (range)	Mean Fluence (J/cm²; range, 5–7.5)	Mean Treatment Interval (range, 6–26 W)
Head and neck	4	1.5 (1–3)	6.8	8
	3	1.8 (1–3)	6.7	7
Trunk	4	1.3 (1–2)	6.9	9
	3	2.0 (2)	6.5	10
Upper limb	4	1.2 (1–2)	6.5	18
	3	2.0 (1–3)	6.3	16
Lower limb	4	1.6 (1–2)	6.9	15
	3	2.0 (2)	6.6	18
All sites	4	1.44 (1–3)	6.8	11
	3	1.88 (1–3)	6.7	12
	1, 2	—	—	—
Overall	—	1.5 (1–3)	6.8	11.5

*Response scores: 1, 0–25% improvement; 2, 26–50% improvement; 3, 51–75% improvement; 4, 76–100% improvement.

Table 26–2. Treatment of Café-au-Lait Patches

Response Grade*	Average No. of Treatments (range)	Mean Fluence (J/cm^2; range, 6–10)	Mean Treatment Interval (range, 6–26 w)
4	2.2 (1–4)	7.0	12
3	2.3 (1–4)	7.3	10
2	2.0 (1–3)	7.1	11
1	2.3 (1–3)	7.2	13
Overall	2.2 (1–4)	7.1	11

*Response scores: 1, 0–25% improvement; 2, 26–50% improvement; 3, 51–75% improvement; 4, 76–100% improvement.

Table 26–3. Treatment of Melasma

Response Grade*	Average No. of Treatments (range)	Mean Fluence (J/cm^2; range, 6–10)	Mean Treatment Interval (range, 6–26 w)
4	—	—	—
3	2.5 (1–6)	6.9	13
2	1.5 (1–2)	6.3	20
1	2.3 (1–5)	6.6	9
Overall	2.3 (1–6)	6.7	12

*Response scores: 1, 0–25% improvement; 2, 26–50% improvement; 3, 51–75% improvement; 4, 76–100% improvement.

Table 26–4. Treatment of Nevus of Ota

Response Grade*	Average No. of Treatments (range)	Mean Fluence (J/cm^2; range, 6–10)	Mean Treatment Interval (range, 6–24 w)
4	5.3 (3–9)	9.3	10
3	2.9 (1–5)	9.0	12
2	2.5 (2–3)	10.0	8
1	1.0 (1)	10.0	—
Overall	3.9 (1–9)	9.3	10

* Response scores: 1, 0–25% improvement; 2, 26–50% improvement; 3, 51–75% improvement; 4, 76–100% improvement.

Results

The immediate response to treatment was an ash-white discoloration of the irradiated area. This occurred at fluences above the "threshold response;" below this threshold, no such reaction was seen. This discoloration resolved within 30 minutes to 2 hours, occasionally leaving some erythema and edema that subsided gradually over 24 hours. Postoperative pain was limited to a transient burning sensation that lasted 60 to 80 minutes. At higher fluences, scaling and some minor bleeding occurred, often followed by crusting that resolved in 3 to 6 days.

The maximum improvement in most patients with infraorbital pigmented lesions occurred 3 to 4 months following laser treatment; in some patients, maximum improvement was noted 6 months after the treatment. Six of 17 patients (35%) had a grade-1 response after one treatment, 7 (41%) had a grade-2 response after one treatment, and 4 (24%) had a grade-3 response after one treatment. Nine patients had at least two treatment sessions. Responses, irrespective of lesion, were graded on a scale of 1 to 4: grade 4, greater than 75% improvement; grade 3, 50 to 75% improvement; grade 2, 25 to 49% improvement; grade 1, less than 25% improvement. One of 9 patients (11%) achieved a grade-2 response, 6 (67%) achieved a grade-3 response, and 2 (22%) achieved a grade-4 response. Of those patients treated once, 23.5% achieved a grade-3 or -4 response. Of those treated twice, 88% achieved a grade-3 or -4 response (Table 26–5). We have since treated a total of 25 additional patients with this problem. The results seem long-lasting.

Adverse effects included transient hyperpigmentation in 29.4% of patients, which resolved in 4 to 8 weeks with application of 4% hydroquinone solution. Transient hypopigmentation was seen in 5.9% of patients. No permanent textural changes or scarring was noted.

Postoperative Treatments and Re-Treatments

Routine postoperative treatments included topical polymyxin-bacitracin ointment and a broad-spectrum sunscreen. All patients were advised to continue antibiotic treatment as long as any scaling or crusting remained (at least 5 days) and to use the sunscreen for at least 1 month. After application of the ointment, treated areas were covered with a nonadherent dressing. Re-treatments were performed at a minimum of 6 weeks (range, 6 to 26 weeks), except for infraorbital pigmented lesions, which were treated at 4-week intervals.[16]

Table 26–5. Melanocytic-Type Infraorbital Pigmentation

Patient No.	Age (y)	Fitzpatrick Skin Type	No. of Treatments	Response Score after Last Treatment*
1	49	V	1	3
2	75	II	1	1
3	32	II	3	4
4	48	II	2	2
5	55	II	2	3
6	66	II	2	4
7	36	III	1	1
8	39	III	2	3
9	39	IV	2	3
10	37	V	2	4
11	36	II	1	2
12	42	III	1	1
13	37	III	2	3
14	34	III	2	3
15	48	II	1	2
16	41	II	1	3
17	41	III	1	1

*Response scores: 1, 0–25% improvement; 2, 26–50% improvement; 3, 51–75% improvement; 4, 76–100% improvement.
Reproduced from Lowe NJ, Wieder JM, et al. Infraorbital pigmented skin. Dermatol Surg. 1995;21:767–770.

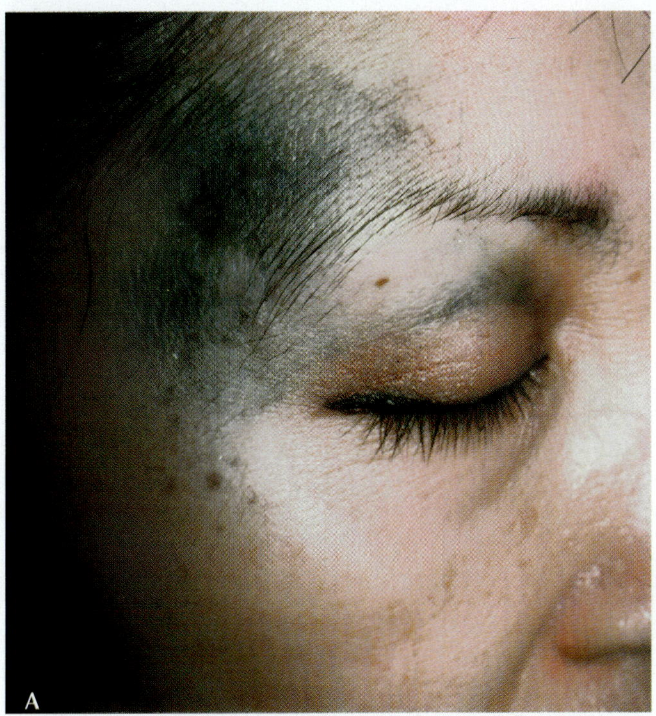

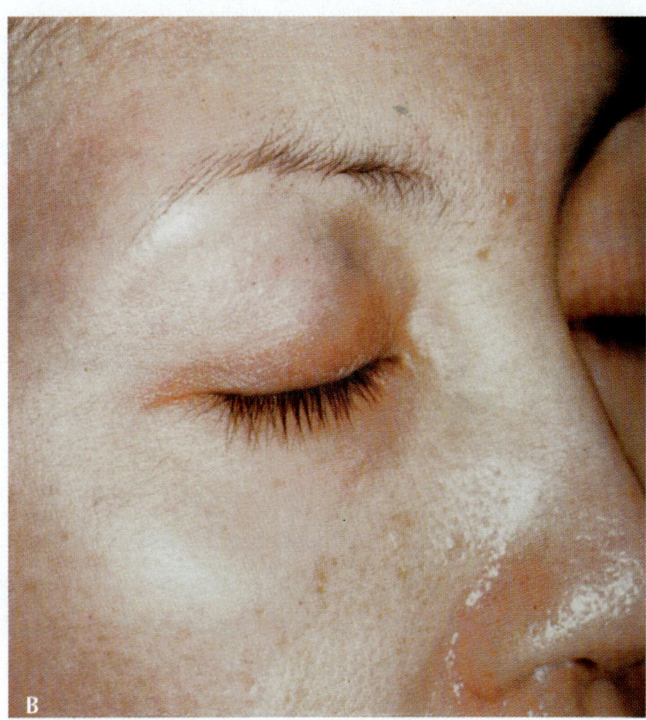

Figure 26–1. (A) Nevus of Ota before treatment. (B) After five treatment sessions with the Q-switched ruby laser.

Conclusions

The Q-switched ruby laser has been shown to be effective in the treatment of nevus of Ota (Fig. 26–1),[17,18] a benign dermal melanocytosis. It appears that patients having this type of melanin-containing infraorbital skin darkening may be suitable candidates for treatment with this laser. Other lasers that may be potentially effective for this category of patients include the Q-switched, frequency-doubled Nd:YAG laser and the Q-switched alexandrite laser. However, one advantage of the Q-switched ruby laser is the lack of permanent textural changes or scarring.

The Q-switched ruby laser is a highly effective tool for the treatment of a whole gamut of other benign pigmented lesions. Although other pulsed lasers may produce comparable or slightly better results for some epidermal lesions, the flexibility of this laser, which can be used to treat epidermal-dermal and purely dermal lesions, is noteworthy.

TATTOOS

The application of decorative or ceremonial tattoos dates back thousands of years; there is evidence of tattooing as early as the Bronze Age and observation of tattoos on Egyptian mummies.[19–21] The practice has become quite sophisticated and continues to be widespread, with particular emphasis on new tattoos among teenagers and young adults. Some tattoos are primarily for cultural identity, whereas others may be considered purely decorative. Tattoos may be of a strictly amateur design and application or a more elaborate, usually more colorful, professional design and application. Other tattoos have medical purposes (e.g., delineation of radiation fields), whereas others may result from trauma (e.g., material embedded under the skin as a result of an accident) or exposure to various metals used in dentistry (e.g., an amalgam tattoo). This section focuses primarily on professional and amateur skin tattoos.

TATTOO COMPOSITION AND TISSUE INTERACTIONS

Both amateur and professional tattoos that are primarily black generally involve carbon-based pigments, although iron-oxide pigments can also create a black tattoo. Professional tattooists, with their ever-increasing array of colors, generally use different metal ions to create various colors. Red ink may contain mercury, cadmium, or iron; yellow ink generally contains cadmium or ochre; black ink, as mentioned, contains carbon or iron oxide; blue ink contains cobalt; green ink contains chromium; and white ink usually contains titanium.[22,23] These pigments, because of their granule size, composition, and absorption and reflection properties, are amenable to fairly specific destruction using several laser modalities.

Tattoo ink particles generally reside in dermal fibroblasts and often are in a perivascular location. Approximately 2 months after application, there is some degree of fibrosis in the area, and the particles remain fairly stable for an indefinite period.[24] Professional tattoo ink tends to localize predominantly in the upper or papillary dermis, whereas amateur tattoos are highly variable, and the tattoo ink may reside in the papillary or reticular dermis and occasionally as deep as the subcutaneous tissue.[25,26] Tattoo ink particle size has been studied and has been measured at an average 4.42 $\pm$ 0.72 μm.[27] Particle size is important in the laser treatment of tattoos because it determines the thermal relaxation time of the particles, which ranges from approximately 30 nanoseconds to 1 millisecond.[28] Ink particle size, shape, and location vary more in amateur tattoos than in professional tattoos, and the depth and density of tattoo ink varies greatly in both amateur and professional tattoos.[29]

History of Tattoo Removal

Many people, often years after acquiring a tattoo, seek removal of the tattoo by various methods. It has been estimated that 50% or more of people in Western culture who acquire tattoos eventually wish to have them removed.[30,31]

Numerous methods have been developed over the years for tattoo removal. These have met with varying degrees of success, and most have carried a risk of scarring or permanent pigment change. Attempts at tattoo removal date from ancient Greece ($\sim$1400 years ago).[32] There are four categories of tattoo removal: (1) mechanical methods, such as dermabrasion or salabrasion; (2) excisional methods, using full-thickness or tangential excisions; (3) chemical methods, using acids, such as trichloroacetic acid (TCA), or caustic chemicals, such as phenol or cryotherapy; and (4) thermal methods, which include electrodesiccation or

cautery, the infrared coagulator, and continuous-wave (CW) lasers such as the ruby, carbon dioxide (CO_2), or argon laser. The most recent method, which overlaps partly with thermal treatments, involves a more specific destruction of pigmentation using laser systems that exploit the principle of selective photothermolysis.

Mechanical Methods

The oldest method, salabrasion, or the use of abrasive salt preparations, has been used for tattoo removal for at least 1400 years.[32] A modern variation on this type of mechanical destruction involves the use of dermabrasion with either a diamond fraise or a wire brush. More recently, a series of shallow dermabrasions has been recommended to minimize scarring and pigment changes.[33]

Excisional Methods

Small, very limited tattoos can be excised successfully with a resulting scar that may be very subtle or barely noticeable depending on the tattoo's location and size. Staged excisions may be necessary for larger tattoos, and tissue expansion can be used as well to minimize stretchback. With this method, some scarring is inevitable, but it may be cosmetically acceptable and preferable to the original tattoo.[34,35]

Chemical Methods

Chemical methods, in one form or another, have been around for more than 100 years[36] and have involved the use of tannic acid or silver nitrate and, more recently, phenol or TCA.[37,38] Both approaches have been associated with significant scarring and pigmentary changes, although they can be relatively successful. Cryotherapy, another chemical method, has been reported to be successful but is not currently recommended because results are highly unpredictable, and significant scarring is a risk.[39]

Thermal Methods

Thermal destruction of tattoos can be accomplished with electrodesiccation or electrocautery under local anesthesia; however, scarring is a common occurrence. For very small tattoos, this may be an acceptable approach, but scarring or pigmentary changes generally result. The infrared coagulator is a noncoherent light source[40] that emits wavelengths in the infrared range (approximately 900 to 960 nm) and has been used fairly extensively for tattoo removal. This method can be effective, but it frequently results in nonspecific tissue destruction and scarring.

Another method of thermal destruction of tattoos involves one of the earliest applications of lasers in medical therapy. In particular, the CW ruby laser, emitting a wavelength of 694 nm, was first used to remove tattoos in the mid-1960s.[41] In addition, an early version of the Q-switched ruby laser was also used for tattoo removal, as described in 1967 and 1968.[26,42] These early laser methods were largely dismissed or ignored until the advent of the modern Q-switched ruby laser in the last decade. The CW Nd:YAG laser has also been used in the thermal destruction of tattoos[43] with moderate success but frequent scarring.

Much more widely employed in thermal destruction of tattoos were the CW argon and CO_2 lasers. Use of the argon laser for tattoo removal was reported in 1979 with relatively complete tattoo removal and "acceptable" cosmetic results in 29 to 33% of patients.[44,45] However, the tissue destruction of the argon laser is relatively nonspecific, and hypertrophic scars resulted, as well as incomplete removal.[29] The CW CO_2 laser was also used for tattoo removal beginning in 1978.[46,47] This laser vaporizes the tissue overlying and involving the tattoo, resulting in fairly extensive dermal damage and tissue necrosis of a nonspecific nature. Atrophic and hypertrophic scarring have been relatively common with this laser, as have permanent pigmentary changes.[29]

Tattoo Removal with the Q-Switched Ruby Laser

Use of high-energy, rapidly pulsed or Q-switched lasers to specifically destroy or fragment tattoo ink particles has revolutionized the treatment of tattoos and allowed complete or partial removal with minimal risk of scarring. Typical spot sizes employed with the Q-switched ruby laser range from 3 to 8 mm with fluences ranging from 4 to 10 J/cm^2.

Goldman et al first reported the technique of Q-switching in 1965,[48] and as early as 1967 and 1968, use of the Q-switched ruby laser for removal of dermal pigmentation was reported.[26,42] In 1983, Reid et al[49] reported excellent results using the Q-switched ruby laser on tattoos, and recently they have reported an extensive 9-year experience.[50] Since these early reports, many authors have documented the efficacy of the Q-switched ruby laser in tattoo removal.

The parameters and wavelengths of the lasers discussed here are selected on the basis of the theory of selective photothermolysis.[1,51] Q-switching is accomplished with an electrooptical switch that changes the quality of resonance of the laser light so that it is emitted in very brief high-energy pulses, usually in the range of nanoseconds.[52] Generally speaking, each pulse is shorter than the thermal relaxation time of the target tissue. This allows virtually all the energy of the laser pulse to be absorbed by the chromophore with minimal opportunity for thermal conduction and nonspecific peripheral damage. The mechanism of tattoo pigment destruction involves rapid absorption of the laser energy by the pigment with vaporization and/or rapid thermal expansion of the pigment particles with a concomitant shockwave effect and fragmentation of the pigment particles. The residual pigment then can be absorbed by phagocytic cells, eliminated by exudation through breaks in the epidermis, or possibly chemically changed so that its optical properties are altered, resulting in clinical lightening.[29,53]

Patient Selection and Preparation

The Q-switched ruby laser, with a wavelength of 694 nm and a pulse width of 20 to 40 nanoseconds, has been shown to be effective in eradicating professional, amateur, traumatic, medical, and chemical tattoos of the skin and mucosa. Blue and black pigments appear to respond best to the Q-switched ruby wavelength, and many types of green tattoo pigments also respond well.[54] Other colors, particularly red, are fairly resistant to Q-switched ruby laser treatments.

Micropigmented (cosmetic) tattoos include blue-black tattoos for eyeliners or eyebrows and red-brown tattoos for lip lines. Laser removal of these pigments is unpredictable. The pigment particles may be oxidized by the laser, resulting in a darker tattoo. However, some blue-black tattoos can be removed successfully.

It should be noted that the energy of the Q-switched ruby laser is also strongly absorbed by melanin. Thus, the overlying skin pigmentation of the patient may play a role in laser efficacy. Posttreatment hypopigmentation is fairly common, although usually transient.[55,56]

Treatment of tattoos can be performed with or without anesthesia. Patient pain levels vary with the energy levels delivered and subjective patient tolerance. Some patients require or request either topical anesthesia such as EMLA cream (eutectic mixture of local anesthetics) or infiltration with lidocaine or other local anesthetic. Particular care must be taken with disinfecting agents, particularly alcohol, to avoid potential ignition.

Safety

As with all medical lasers, laser safety is paramount, and proper precautions must be taken before and during laser treatment. Appropriate goggles or eye protection for the operator, all personnel in the room, and the patient is critical to avoid retinal damage. Combustible materials, such as gauze in the field, the patient's hair or skin, and other equipment, including anesthesia tubing and oxygen delivery systems, must be appropriately guarded from the laser beam and any potential sparks. In addition, the Q-switched ruby laser is a high-voltage machine, and care must be taken to avoid electric shock and contact with water and the machine at the same time. Virtually all Q-switched lasers have a potential to aerosolize tissue and splatter viable debris; therefore, masks, eye shields, and splatter shields or clear biologic dressings should be employed to avoid or contain tissue splatter. Although the latter technique of biologic dressing may result in a 10% drop in energy, it is an effective method of containing potentially infectious material.[57]

Endpoint and Postoperative Care

Clinically, a uniform whitening of the area, which appears almost immediately, is the usual endpoint. This tissue whitening is usually transient and may resolve after 10 to 20 minutes. In addition, there may be some moderate purpura or pinpoint bleeding at higher energy levels. Some erythema and edema will also be seen. A scale or crust often forms in the 2 weeks following laser treatment, and it may exude pigment particles. The patient may also experience vesiculation at the treatment site. Postoperative wound care consists of cleansing the wound and applying topical antibiotic or bland ointments. Sun protection is also necessary once the epidermis is intact. In general, multiple treatment sessions are required, ranging from approximately 2 to 10 sessions at 4- to 8-week intervals.

Results

In 1990, Taylor et al[25] reported treatment of 35 amateur and 22 professional tattoos with the Q-switched ruby laser. After three or four treatments, 74% of the amateur tattoos and 22% of the professional tattoos showed 75 to 100% clearance. The incidence of scarring was minimal. Another 1990 report[58] of 101 amateur and 62 professional tattoos documented very similar results and superior response with amateur tattoos. Reid et al,[50] in Scotland, reported a cumulative 9-year experience in 418 patients with comparable results. Ashinoff and Geronemus[59] reported a series of traumatic and medical tattoos that were also treated successfully without scarring or permanent pigmentary changes. In a case report involving an amalgam tattoo of the gingiva,[60] the Q-switched ruby laser achieved successful lightening of the lesion. Another very large series reported by Levins et al[57] in 1991 on 200 tattoos treated with the Q-switched ruby laser showed superior responses in black, blue, green, and brown pigments.

In general, amateur tattoos respond somewhat more quickly than professional tattoos. Kilmer et al[56] reported good clearing with the Q-switched ruby laser at 6 to 8 J/cm^2 after an average of 4 to 6 treatments for amateur tattoos and 6 to 10 treatments for professional tattoos. Other reports have documented good to excellent clearing of amateur tattoos in 4 to 6 sessions at fluences of 4 to 20 J/cm^2 and professional tattoos in 6 to 12 sessions at 8 to 10 J/cm^2. The treatment frequency was every 3 to 4 weeks.[57] The most responsive colors were blue-black, black, green, and brown. Lowe et al[61] reported average fluences of 10 J/cm^2 and an average of 5 treatments at 6- to 8-week intervals. With this regimen, 22 of 28 patients experienced greater than 75% clearing.[61] Similar responses have been reported by numerous authors.[29,59,62]

Complications

The incidence of complications with Q-switched ruby laser tattoo removal appears to be quite low overall and is related to energy level, the patient's skin color, and overall number of treatments. Early reports showed scarring to be quite rare with fluences of 4 J/cm^2 or less. Of 57 patients, one had localized scarring of approximately 2 cm^2 in a professional tattoo treated at 7 J/cm^2.[48,53,58] A more recent large study reported transient textural changes early on that resolved within a couple of months, with less than 5% of patients showing permanent textural changes. This same study showed true hypertrophic scarring in approximately 0.5% of patients.[57]

The most common reported complication or adverse effect is a transient, possibly prolonged, or possibly permanent confetti-like hypopigmentation at the treatment site. In an early study, 39% of patients treated at or below 4 J/cm^2 and 46% treated above 5 J/cm^2 demonstrated this adverse effect 1 month postoperatively.[25] Often the hypopigmentation resolves in 4 to 12 months, although one report showed up to 40% of patients with some degree of hypopigmentation after 1 year. Another study reported a high incidence of transient hypopigmentation lasting 4–6 months in more than 50% of patients undergoing an average of five treatments; in some patients, the hypopigmentation was permanent.[56,57] One very limited study of five dark-skinned patients (Fitzpatrick skin types V and VI) reported complete depigmentation with the Q-switched ruby laser at one test site in one patient.[63] Hyperpigmentation appears to be very uncommon and usually transient in nature in perhaps 2 to 3% of patients, with a somewhat increased frequency in darkly pigmented patients.[25,53]

Of particular note is the phenomenon sometimes observed in cosmetic tattoos of darkening of the pigment on laser treatment. The Q-switched ruby laser, the Q-switched Nd:YAG laser, the alexandrite laser, and in particular the 510-nm PDPL all can cause red rouge or lip tattooing to turn black. In addition, some white or flesh-colored pigments may turn dark after treatment. It is prudent to spot test small areas of any cosmetic tattoos, particularly lip liner or rouge, flesh-, or white-colored tattoos, before treating larger areas. The darkening is quite immediately observed. The resulting dark pigment may or may not be amenable to further laser treatment,[29] which has been successful in some patients.

Darker-skinned patients, such as those with Fitzpatrick skin types V and VI, may be more prone to hypertrophic scarring, keloids, or pigmentary changes. One very limited initial study has shown that tattoos can be treated successfully in these patients with minimal adverse effects. Grevelink et al[63] in 1996 reported treating five dark-skinned patients on the face, neck, and chest with no significant scarring using the Q-switched Nd:YAG laser. Use of the Q-switched ruby laser in this study was abandoned early on because of some depigmentation seen at test sites. Thus, treating very dark-skinned patients with the Q-switched ruby laser appears to be relatively contraindicated. Grevelink et al recommend using the Q-switched Nd:YAG laser for tattoo removal in darker-skinned patients, which showed fewer adverse effects.[63]

CONCLUSIONS

Clearly, the advent of Q-switched and flash-lamp pumped lasers has revolutionized the treatment of tattoos while minimizing risks and long-term complications. The systems clear tattoos with minimal risk of complications when used prudently. No single laser system can treat all tattoo pigments and colors; however, all the Q-switched systems are excellent at clearing blue and black tattoos. The ideal laser system may combine the properties of the alexandrite or ruby laser with those of the Nd:YAG laser and its frequency-doubling capacity or with those of the 510-nm PDPL. Such a system could treat the most common tattoo pigments (i.e., blue, black, red, and green) along with other, less common colors. Although the Q-switched ruby laser may clear some tattoos more rapidly than other systems, there is a higher risk of hypopigmentation, particularly in darker-skinned patients. The Nd:YAG and alexandrite lasers appear to cause less long-lasting hypopigmentation. The alexandrite laser, perhaps because of its longer pulse width, may result in less tissue splatter and potential for spread of viable tissue. Each laser carries its advantages and liabilities.

SUMMARY

Ideally, a practitioner has access to a number of lasers and treats various tattoos and pigments by considering the wavelength, the pulse width, and the patient's overlying pigmentation. The proliferation of laser centers at private and university facilities should make possible access to all the appropriate laser systems. It is important to remember—and to make patients aware—that not all lesions can be cleared completely, even with multiple treatments; however, most lesions are amenable to significant, if not complete, clearing with the various laser systems now available.

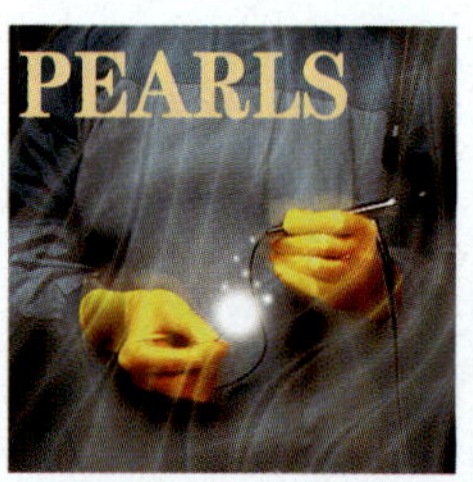

- The Q-switched ruby laser's very narrow pulse width (20 to 25 nanoseconds) and 694.3-nm wavelength make it ideal for selective destruction of epidermal or dermal pigment because it is melanin-specific and melanin-dependent.

- The frequency-doubled ND:YAG laser and the Q-switched alexandrite laser are also effective in treating nevus of Ota; the Q-switched ruby laser has a long track record of treatment.

- Despite continued popularity of tattoos, it is estimated that more than 50% of people who get tattoos eventually want them removed.

- Salabrasion, the use of an abrasive salt preparation, is the oldest method of tattoo removal. Although results are variable, the method's modern incarnation involves dermabrasion with a diamond fraise or wire brush.

- The CW ruby laser was first used for tattoo removal in the mid-1960s, but it was the advent of the modern Q-switched ruby laser that dispelled doubts about using the ruby laser for tattoo removal.

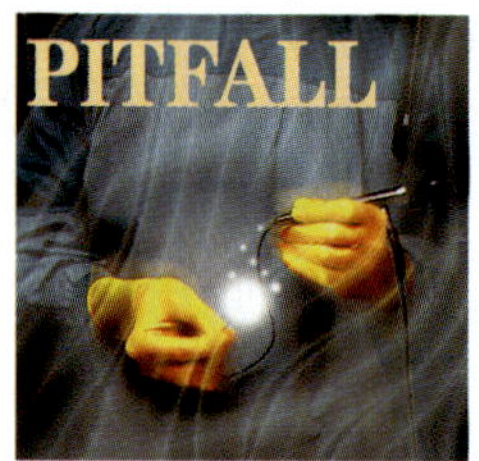

- Laser removal of micropigmented tattoos is unpredictable; sometimes the pigment particles are oxidized by the laser and actually become a darker tattoo.

REFERENCES

1. Anderson RR, Parrish JA. Selective photothermolysis: precise microsurgery by selective absorption of pulsed radiation. *Science.* 1983;220:524–527.
2. Anderson RR, Parrish JA. The optics of human skin. *J Invest Dermatol.* 1981;77:13–19.
3. Habif T. *Clinical Dermatology: A Colour Guide to Diagnosis and Therapy.* St. Louis: Mosby; 1990.
4. Lever WF, Schaumburg-Lever G. *Histopathology of the Skin.* 7th ed. Philadelphia: Lippincott; 1990.
5. Sherwood K, Murray S, Kurban K, et al. Effects of wavelength on cutaneous pigment using pulsed irradiation. *J Invest Dermatol.* 1989;92:717–720.
6. Anderson RR, Margolis RJ, Watanabe S, et al. Selective photothermolysis of cutaneous pigment by Q-switched Nd:YAG laser pulsed at 1064, 532, and 355 nm. *J Invest Dermatol.* 1989;93:22–28.
7. Ara G, Anderson RR, Mandel KG, et al. Irradiation of pigmented melanoma cells with high intensity pulsed irradiation generates acoustic waves and kills cells. *Lasers Surg Med.* 1990;10:52–59.
8. Murphy GF, Shepard RS, Paul BS, et al. Organelle specific injury to melanin containing cell in human skin by pulsed irradiation. *Lab Invest.* 1983;49:680–685.
9. Margolis RJ, Dover JS, Polla LL, et al. Visible action spectrum for melanin specific selective photothermolysis. *Lasers Surg Med.* 1989;9:389–397.
10. Nelson JS, Applebaum J. Treatment of superficial cutaneous pigmented lesions by melanin specific selective photothermolysis using the Q-switched ruby laser. *Ann Plast Surg.* 1992;29:231–237.
11. Fitzpatrick RE, Goldman MP, Ruiz-Esparza J. Laser treatment of benign pigmented epidermal lesions using a 300-ns pulse and 510-nm wavelength. *J Dermatol Surg Oncol.* 1993;18:341–347.
12. Grekin RC, Shelton RM, Geisse JK, et al. 510-nm pigmented lesion dye laser. *J Dermatol Surg Oncol.* 1993;19:380–387.
13. Kurban AK, Morrison P, Trainor S, et al. Pulse duration effects on cutaneous pigment. *Lasers Surg Med.* 1992;12:282–287.
14. Watanabe S, Anderson RR, Bruson S, et al. Comparative studies of femtosecond to microsecond laser pulses on selective pigmented cell injury in skin. *J Photochem Photobiol.* 1991;9:389–397.
15. Polla LL, Margolis RJ, Dover JS. Melanosomes are a primary target of Q-switched ruby laser irradiation in guinea pig skin. *J Invest Dermatol.* 1987;89:281–286.

16. Lowe NJ, Wieder JM, et al. Infraorbital Pigmented Skin. *Dermatol Surg.* 1995;21:767–770.

17. Lowe NJ, Wieder JM, Sawcer DE, et al. Nevus of Ota: treatment with high energy fluences of the Q-switched ruby laser. *J Am Acad Dermatol.* 1993;29:997–1001.

18. Goldberg DJ, Nychay SG. Q-switched ruby laser treatment of nevus of Ota. *J Dermatol Surg Oncol.* 1992;18:817–821.

19. Scutt R, Gotch C. *Tattooing.* Cranbury, NJ: AS Barnes; 1974.

20. Grumet GW. Psychodynamic implications of tattoos. *Am J Orthopsychiatr.* 1983;53:482.

21. Ebensten H. *Pierced Hearts and True Love.* London: Derek Verschoyle; 1953.

22. Rostenberg A, Brown RA, Caro MR. Discussion of tattoo reactions with report of a case showing a reaction to a green color. *Arch Dermatol Svoh.* 1950;62:540.

23. Everett MA. Tattoos: abnormalities of pigmentation. In: *Clinical Dermatology.* Vol 2, units 11–21. Hagerstown, Md: Harper & Row; 1980.

24. Mann R. Klingmuller G. Electron-microscope investigation of tattoos in rabbit skin. *Arch Dermatol Res.* 1981;271:367.

25. Taylor CR, et al. Treatment of tattoos by Q-switched ruby laser. *Arch Dermatol.* 1990;126:383–389.

26. Laub DR, et al. Preliminary histopathological observation of Q-switched ruby laser radiation on dermal tattoo pigment in man. *J Surg Res.* 1968;8:220–224.

27. Lea PJ, Pawlowski A. Human tattoo: electron microscopic assessment of epidermis, epidermal-dermal junction and dermis. *Int J Dermatol.* 1987;26:453–458.

28. Anderson RR, Parrish JA. The optics of human skin. *J Invest Dermatol.* 1981;77:13–19.

29. Goldman MP, Fitzpatrick RE. *Cutaneous Laser Surgery.* St. Louis: CV Mosby; 1994.

30. Pers M, von Herbst T. The demand for removal of tattoos: a plea for regulations against tattooing of minors. *Acta Chir Scand.* 1996;131:201.

31. Goldstein N. Psychological implications of tattoos. *J Dermatol Surg Oncol.* 1979;5:883.

32. Scutt RWB. The chemical removal of tattoos. *Br J Plast Surg.* 1972;25:189.

33. Clabaugh W. Removal of tattoos by superficial dermabrasion. *Arch Dermatol.* 1968;98:515.

34. Bunke HJ, Conway H. Surgery of decorative and traumatic tattoos. *Plast Reconstr Surg.* 1957;20:67.

35. Goldstein N. Tattoo removal. *Dermatol Clin.* 1987;5:349.

36. Variot G. Nouveau procede de destruction des tatouages. *Compte Rendu de la Societe de Biologie (Paris).* 1888;8:836.

37. Piggot TA, Norris RW. The treatment of tattoos with trichloroacetic acid: experience with 670 patients. *Br J Plast Surg.* 1988;41:112.

38. Lindsay DG. Tattoos. *Dermatol Clin.* 1989;7:147.

39. Colver GB, Dawber RPR. The removal of digital tattoos. *Int J Dermatol.* 1985;24:567.

40. Colver GB, Jones RL, Cherry GW, et al. Precise dermal damages with an infrared coagulator. *Br J Dermatol.* 1986;114:603.

41. Bailey BN. Treatment of tattoos. *Plast Reconstr Surg.* 1976;40:3Gl.

42. Yules RB, Laub DR, Honey R, et al. The effect of Q-switched ruby laser radiation on dermal tattoo pigment in man. *Arch Surg.* 1967;95:179.

43. Goldman L, et al. Laser treatment of tattoos: a preliminary survey of three years' clinical experience. *JAMA.* 1967;201:841.

44. Apfelberg DB, Maser MR, Lash H. Argon laser treatment of decorative tattoos. *Br J Plast Surg.* 1979;32:141.

45. Apfelberg DB, Rivers J, Maser MR, et al. Update on laser usage in treatment of decorative tattoos. *Lasers Surg Med.* 1982;2:169.

46. Brady SC, Blokmanis A, Jewett L. Tattoo removal with the carbon dioxide laser. *Ann Plast Surg.* 1978;2:482.

47. McBurney EI. Carbon dioxide laser treatment of dermatologic lesions. *South Med J.* 1978;71:795.

48. Goldman L, et al. Radiation from a Q-switched ruby laser. *J Invest Dermatol.* 1965;44:69.

49. Reid WH, et al. Q-switched ruby laser treatment of black tattoos. *Br J Plast Surg.* 1983;36:455.

50. Reid WHI, et al. Q-switched ruby laser treatment of tattoos: a nine-year experience. *Br J Plast Surg.* 1990;43:663.

51. Anderson RR, Parrish JA. Microvasculature can be selectively damaged using dye lasers: a basic theory and experimental evidence in human skin. *Lasers Surg Med.* 1981;1:263.

52. Lipow M. *Laser Physics Made Simple.* Chicago: Year Book; 1986.

53. Glassberg E, et al. Lasers in dermatology. In: Lask GP, Moy RL, eds. *Principles and Techniques of Cutaneous Surgery.* New York: McGraw-Hill; 1996.

54. Lowe NJ, et al. Q-switched ruby laser: further observations on treatment of professional tattoos. *J Dermatol Surg.* 1994;20:307.

55. Levins PC, Anderson RR. Q-switched ruby laser for the treatment of pigmented lesions and tattoos. *Clin Dermatol.* 1995;13:75.

56. Kilmer SL, Anderson RR. Clinical use of the Q-switched ruby and the Q-switched Nd:YAG (1064-nm and 532-nm) lasers for treatment of tattoos. *J Dermatol Surg Oncol.* 1993;19:330.

57. Levins PC, et al. Q-switched ruby laser treatment of tattoos. *Lasers Surg Med.* 1991;(suppl 3):255.

58. Scheibner A, et al. A superior method of tattoo removal using the Q-switched ruby laser. *J Dermatol Surg Oncol.* 1990;16:1091.

59. Ashinoff R, Geronemus RG. Rapid response of traumatic tattoos to treatment with the Q-switched ruby laser. *Lasers Surg Med.* 1992;(suppl 4):71.

60. Ashinoff R, Tanenbaum D. Treatment of amalgam tattoo with the Q-switched ruby laser. *Cutis.* 1994;54:269.

61. Lowe NJ, et al. Q-switched ruby treatment of professional tattoos. *Lasers Surg Med.* 1993;(suppl 5):54.

62. Geronemus RG, Ashinoff R. Use of the Q-switched ruby laser to treat tattoos and benign pigmented lesions of the skin. *Lasers Surg Med Suppl.* 1991;3:64.

63. Grevelink JM, et al. Laser treatment of tattoos in darkly pigmented patients: efficacy and side effects. *J Am Acad Dermatol.* 1996;34:653.

CHAPTER 27

Q-Switched Neodymium:YAG Laser Treatment of Tattoos

JAMES P. WATSON

Tattooing of the skin for decorative purposes is an old custom that is increasing in popularity. Estimates indicate that more than 10 million people in the United States have tattoos. Most professional tattoo pigments are a heterogeneous mixture of heavy metal dyes, including mercury, cadmium, cobalt, and chromium. Organic pigments more recently have been used by artists to produce bright, multicolored tattoos. Amateur tattoos are more likely to be made with India ink, which is a simple carbon-based pigment. These tattoo particles vary in size from 2 to 400 μm and are introduced into the dermis by multiple needle punctures. There is a great deal of variation in the depth of dye penetration and the tattoo particle size in both amateur and professional tattoos, making it difficult to clearly distinguish differences between them. During the healing process, part of the dye leaches out of the skin until the basement membrane seals off the external loss of dye. The remaining pigment is gradually phagocytosed by tissue macrophages and can be seen as intracellular particles on histologic examination.

Although there is a high level of enthusiasm and acceptance for tattoos by people who get them, many choose to have them removed later, most commonly for social reasons. Tattoo removal has been performed for nearly as long as tattoo placement has been practiced. Older methods of tattoo removal include surgical excision and grafting, chemical destruction with tannic acid or urea, thermal destruction with coagulators or cigarette butts, cryotherapy with liquid nitrogen, salabrasion with salt, and dermabrasion. All these techniques, unfortunately, violate the dermis, almost always resulting in a scar and often hypopigmentation or hypertrophic changes more noticeable than the original tattoo. Although primary excision of small tattoos is still a useful alternative, modern lasers designed for tattoo removal have largely supplanted these techniques because of the lower risk of scarring.

LASER TATTOO REMOVAL

Although the work of Goldman in the early 1960s included use of a Q-switched ruby laser, technical difficulties at that time prevented this concept from further development. Instead, the early lasers used clinically were mostly continuous-wave (CW) argon, carbon dioxide (CO_2), and ruby lasers. These lasers effectively removed dermal pigment through thermal necrosis but almost always resulted in a scar. Consequently, laser tattoo removal was not widely accepted until many years later when pulsed lasers were developed.

With time, it became clear that by shortening the pulse duration, higher fluences could be used to more effectively clear tattoo pigment. By limiting time of exposure to the laser light to less than the thermal relaxation time of the skin, the thermal effects of the laser are confined only to the targeted tissue without heat being conducted to surrounding tissue. With the advent of the *Q-switch*, an electronic switch that is much faster than electromechanical switches, lasers were developed that delivered pulse durations in the nanosecond range. This technological breakthrough dramatically reduced the incidence of scarring and paved the way for development of the lasers used for tattoo removal today.

In 1983, Anderson and Parrish described the concept of selective photothermolysis (see Chapter 4), which paved the way for development of lasers that targeted specific substances or tissues. For tattoos, the desired target was tattoo ink, and the undesired targets were melanin, hemoglobin, and other biological skin chromophores. Because these undesired targets had higher absorption coefficients in the ultraviolet and visible light spectrum, red and infrared lasers were developed to target tattoo pigment, thereby minimizing damage to melanin, hemoglobin, etc. Although most laser experts still believe that laser light destroys pigment primarily by thermolysis, photoacoustic and possibly photobiochemical effects probably also account for the effectiveness of these ultrashort-wavelength lasers.

Although the exact mechanism of laser tattoo removal is not fully understood, histologic evidence suggests that the extremely short, high-energy pulses of light from Q-switched lasers fragment the tattoo particles that reside within macrophages into smaller pieces of pigment. Some of these tattoo particles can leach out of the skin, but most are either carried away by the reticuloendothelial system or phagocytosed again by tissue macrophages. This partly accounts for why multiple treatment sessions are required to remove most tattoos.[1]

TREATMENT EFFICACY

To date, no laser system has been designed that will remove most tattoos in one session. It is also difficult to predict if a particular tattoo can be eliminated completely and, if so, how many treatment sessions will be required to clear all pigment from the skin. Nevertheless, there are a few generalizations that can help clinicians counsel patients.

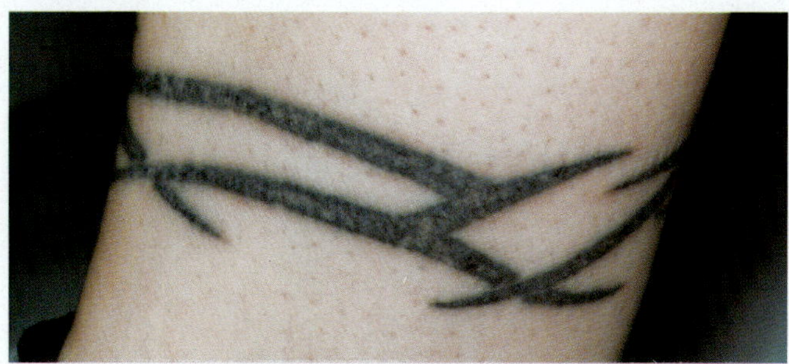

Figure 27–1. A 2-year-old professional tattoo. Note the very dense, thick pigmentation.

In general, tattoos that are made with a motorized gun require more treatment sessions than those made by hand-held needles. Professional tattoos are often more densely pigmented (Fig. 27–1) and may require 6 to 10 treatment sessions. Multicolored tattoos are particularly hard to remove and may require more than 10 treatment sessions. Amateur tattoos are usually less dense and often contain only India ink pigment (Fig. 27–2). These tattoos respond readily to laser treatments and can often be cleared in four to six treatments. Traumatic tattoos occur from abrasions that epithelialize over debris caught in the dermis (Fig. 27–3). These "accidental tattoos" usually have a minimal amount of pigment and can be cleared with one or two treatments. Amalgam tattoos are similar in that they have very little pigment. The efficacy of laser tattoo removal also varies with the age of a tattoo. In general, older tattoos are easier to clear than fresh, new tattoos (Fig. 27–4).

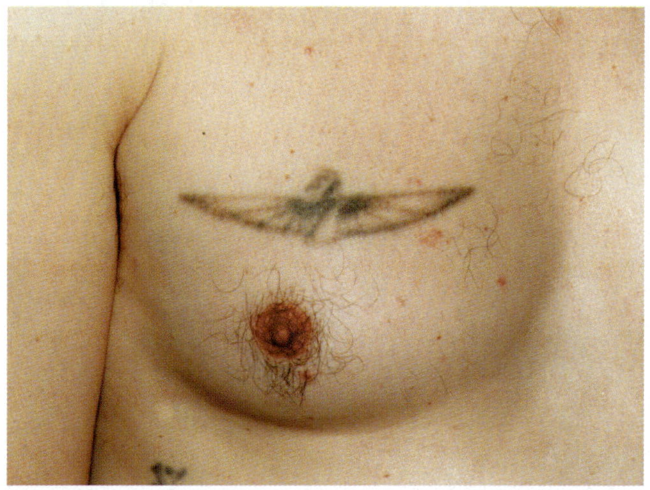

Figure 27–2. An amateur tattoo made with black India ink, 5 years old.

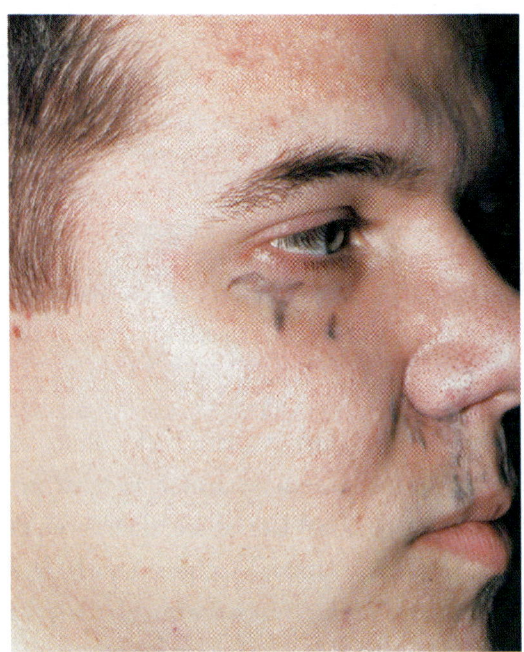

Figure 27–3. Example of a traumatic tattoo caused by incomplete debridement of an asphalt burn.

The laser wavelength and absorption spectrum of the tattoo pigment also determine treatment prognosis. Red tattoos are red because they absorb the opposite color, green, and vice versa. For this reason, red ink tattoos are removed most effectively with green-light lasers such as the 510- or 532-nm Q-switched lasers (e.g., argon laser). Green tattoos, on the other hand, are removed most

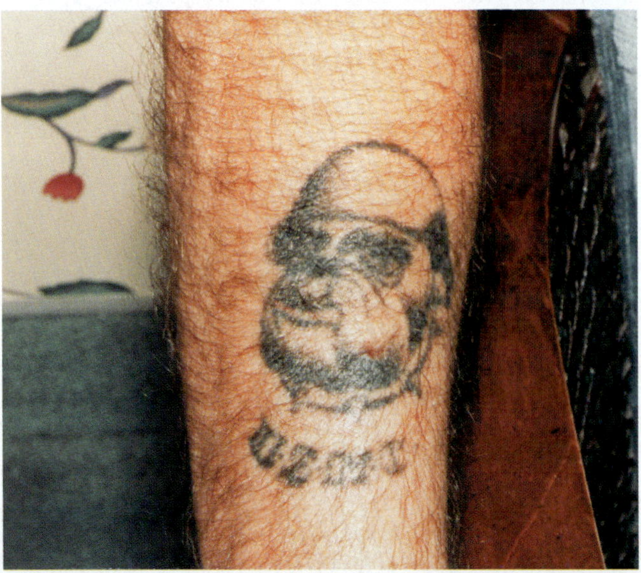

Figure 27–4. A 20–year-old professional tattoo.

effectively with red-light lasers, such as the 694-nm ruby laser or the 755-nm alexandrite laser. Black ink can be removed by lasers of most visible and infrared wavelengths because black ink absorbs all colors of the visible and invisible spectrum.[2] For this reason, black ink tattoos respond well to almost all Q-switched lasers. As the wavelength of the laser increases, so does the depth of penetration. The depth of penetration is often reduced by other competing chromophores with absorption spectra that overlap that of the target chromophore. For example, melanin can reduce the effectiveness of green-light lasers to treat tattoos because both tattoos and melanin have overlapping absorption spectra. As a consequence, although green-light lasers can be used for removing black tattoos, lasers with red or infrared wavelengths can treat the same tattoos and will not be absorbed by melanin, because melanin does not absorb much red or infrared light.

Depth of penetration is also due in part to the spot size of the laser beam. Larger spot sizes usually result in deeper penetration, which can be important in tattoo removal.

CONTINUOUS-WAVE RUBY LASERS

The CW ruby laser was the first laser used for medical applications by Goldman et al[3] in the early 1960s. This solid-state laser source emitted a wavelength of 694 nm, which was absorbed by both melanin and tattoo pigment. This early work suggested that the ruby laser could remove dermal pigment from nevi, melanomas, and tattoos.[4] Because of technical problems, however, the ruby laser did not develop into a clinically useful tool. In subsequent years, CW argon and CO_2 lasers were advocated as effective ways of removing tattoos but were still associated with high rates of scarring.[5,6] Today, the CW ruby laser has largely been abandoned for treating tattoos for the same reason, but it is still used by some to treat congenital nevi as a non Q-switched pulsed laser.[7]

Although development of the Q-switched ruby laser was a major breakthrough in treating tattoos with minimal risk of scarring, there were still problems with this tool. Because of the strong absorption by melanin of the 694-nm wavelength of light, the ruby laser had a high incidence of transient hypopigmentation that could take months to resolve. More important, cases of permanent depigmentation were also reported. These risks reduced the utility of the ruby laser in darker-skinned patients. Most physicians also noted that there was a small percentage of Q-switched ruby laser–resistant tattoos that would not resolve with 10 or more laser treatments. Some of these were tattoos with deeper pigment that could not be eradicated because of the shallow penetration of the 694-nm ruby laser wavelength. Others were tattoos with red pigment that could not be eradicated with red light. For these reasons, efforts were made to develop lasers with wavelengths outside the absorption spectrum of melanin, to find lasers that would treat deeper tattoos, and to find lasers that would treat tattoos with red pigment effectively.

FREQUENCY-DOUBLED Q-SWITCHED NEODYMIUM:YAG LASER

The solid-state neodymium:yttrium-aluminum-garnet (Nd:YAG) crystal emits light at two wavelengths, 1064 and 532 nm. With the Q-switch, the pulse durations can be shortened to 5 to 10 nanoseconds, which is even shorter than the pulse widths of the Q-switched ruby and alexandrite lasers. Current models come with spot sizes in the range of 1.5 to 4 mm, which is comparable with the spot size of the alexandrite laser. With the 1064-nm wavelength, fluences in the range of 6 to 18 J/cm^2 are produced, depending on the spot size. With the 532-nm wavelength, fluences of 2 to 4 J/cm^2 are effective in treating pigmented lesions and red and orange tattoo pigments. Because of the properties of the Nd:YAG crystal, these lasers can have repetition rates of up to 10 Hz. For this reason, the Q-switched Nd:YAG laser can treat large tattoos much faster than the Q-switched ruby laser (1-Hz repetition rate), despite having a smaller spot size.

Although the 1064-nm wavelength Nd:YAG laser had already been used extensively for years in ophthalmology, the Q-switched Nd:YAG laser was not developed for tattoo removal until the late 1980s. Early reports showed it to be effective in the treatment of amateur and professional tattoos.[8] Not only did the Q-switched Nd:YAG laser reduce the risk of hypopigmentation and depigmentation, it was also more effective for tattoos with deeper pigment due to the deeper penetration of the infrared Nd:YAG laser wavelength. Using a system of filters, the Q-switched Nd:YAG laser could also be "frequency doubled," thereby emitting a green-light wavelength of 532 nm. This second wavelength was very useful in treating epidermal pigmented lesions, which increased its versatility. The 532-nm wavelength was also noted to be effective in treating tattoos with red ink, because green is the complement of red.

Laser-Tissue Interactions

Target chromophores for the 1064-nm wavelength of the Q-switched Nd:YAG laser include decorative and traumatic tattoo pigments. With the 1064-nm wavelength, the Q-switched Nd:YAG laser light penetrates deeper into the skin than the ruby or alexandrite lasers and is most effective for treating black tattoos in patients with dark skin.

Target chromophores for the 532-nm wavelength, using the frequency-doubled mode, include melanin, oxyhemoglobin, and red and orange tattoo pigments. With the 532-nm wavelength, the skin penetrance is the least of the three Q-switched lasers. Nevertheless, because red tattoo pigment selectively absorbs the complement color (green) the most, this frequency is well suited to treating red and orange tattoos. Likewise, the 1064-wavelength has the least absorption by melanin and the 532-nm wavelength has the highest melanin absorption, which parallels their risk for producing hypopigmentation (Fig. 27–5).

Because the Q-switched Nd:YAG laser has the shortest pulse duration of the three Q-switched lasers, it has the most tissue splatter. This can be controlled with protective eyewear (Fig. 27–6), plastic shields on the handpiece, or light transparent dressings on the skin during

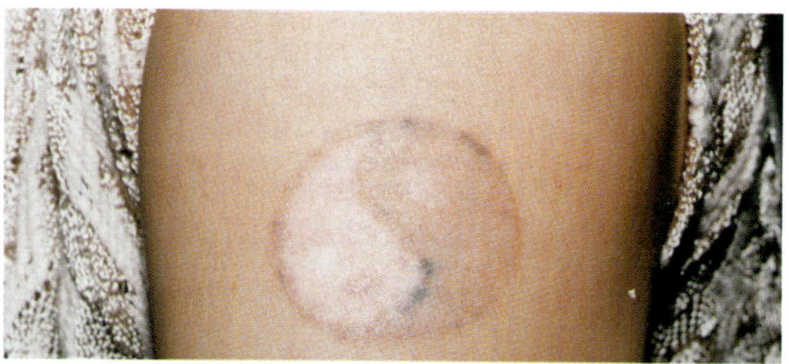

Figure 27–5. An amateur tattoo originally of red and black ink treated with both 532- and 1064-nm Nd:YAG laser light. Note the hypopigmentation where the red ink was removed.

treatment sessions. Use of larger spot sizes (3–4 mm) also reduces tissue splatter.

Clinical Use

The ideal situation in which to use a Q-switched Nd:YAG laser is in treating dark amateur or professional tattoos (Figs. 27–7 through 27–9). Because of the low melanin absorption, even dark-skinned patients can be treated effectively with a low risk of permanent hypopigmentation or depigmentation.[9–11] All dark-skinned patients are still at risk for postinflammatory hyperpigmentation, however. Therefore, patients with Fitzpatrick skin types III, IV, and V should be pretreated with topical hydroquinone and resume hydroquinone use 1 to 2 weeks after

the treatment to reduce this adverse effect. Patients with a history of herpes simplex eruptions in the skin area to be treated should be prescribed acyclovir for 1 to 2 days before treatment, as well.

With the Q-switched Nd:YAG laser, most amateur tattoos can be cleared in four to six treatments, and most professional tattoos can be cleared in 8 to 12 treatment sessions. Certain tattoos cannot be cleared completely, however, especially brightly colored tattoos or flesh-colored tattoos. Although red tattoo pigment absorbs the frequency-doubled (532-nm) wavelength the most, even these tattoos are difficult to clear.

The expected tissue response to the Q-switched Nd:YAG laser is immediate whitening of the skin. With the 1064-nm wavelength, this is followed by pinpoint bleeding, which increases with fluency. With the 532-nm wavelength, pinpoint bleeding does not occur; the treated area develops a purpura that lasts for 7 to 10 days.

Universal precautions should be taken by the physician and staff during both the treatment and postoperative wound care because of probable transient bleeding. Topical antibiotics with nonadherent dressings are the most commonly used form of wound care, but hydrophylic clear dressings such as Vigilon (C. R. Bard, Inc., Covington, GA) have also been used during treatment to reduce splatter and left in place as a postoperative dressing. Dressings

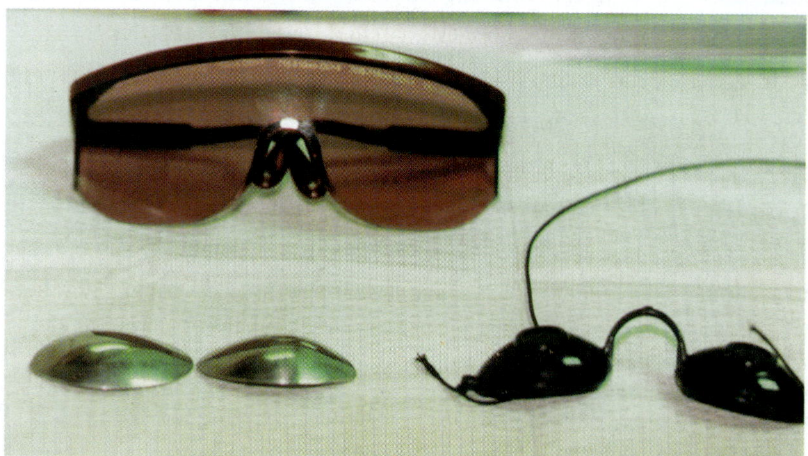

Figure 27–6. Protective eyewear for patients and clinicians.

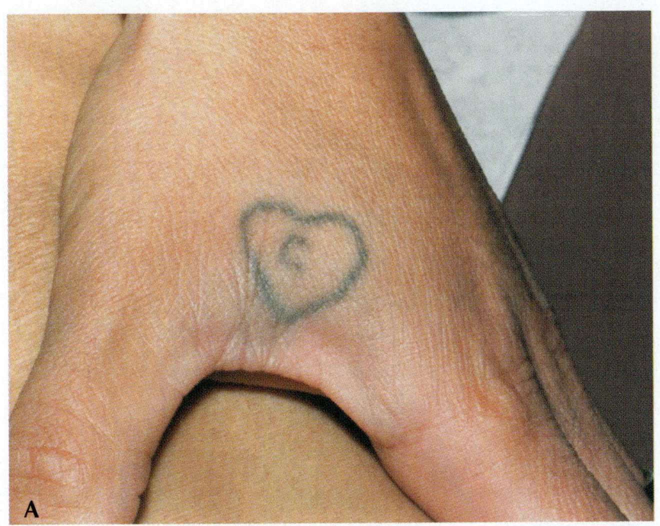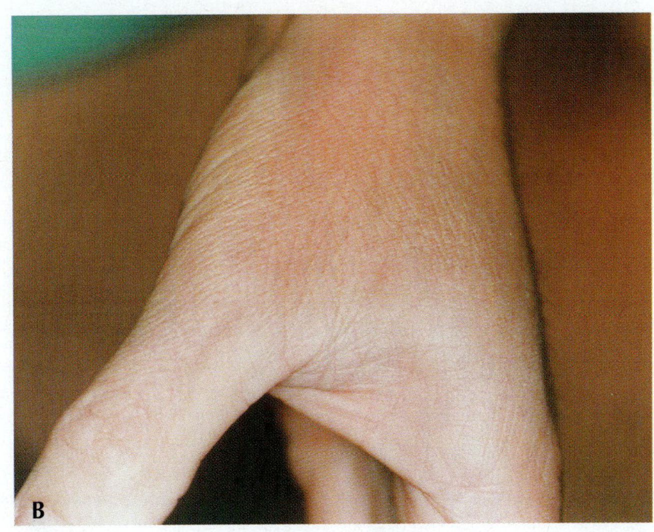

Figure 27–7. Amateur tattoo before (A) and after (B) two treatments with the 1064-nm Nd:YAG laser.

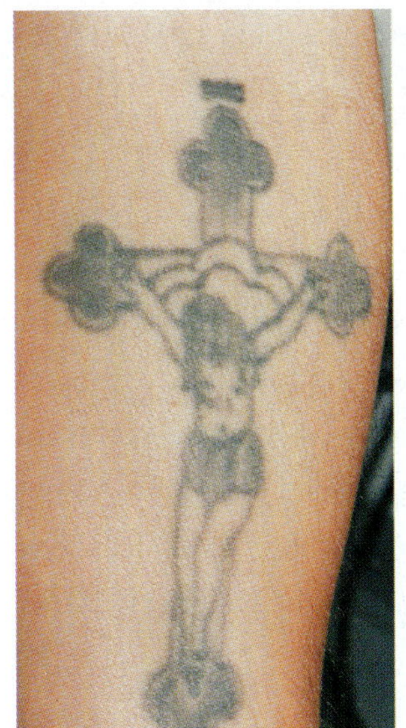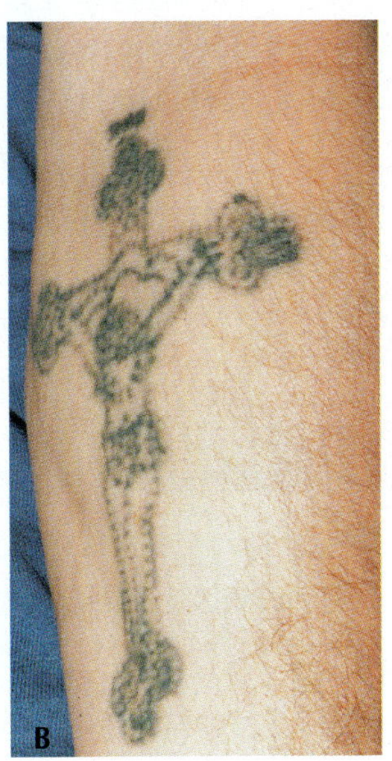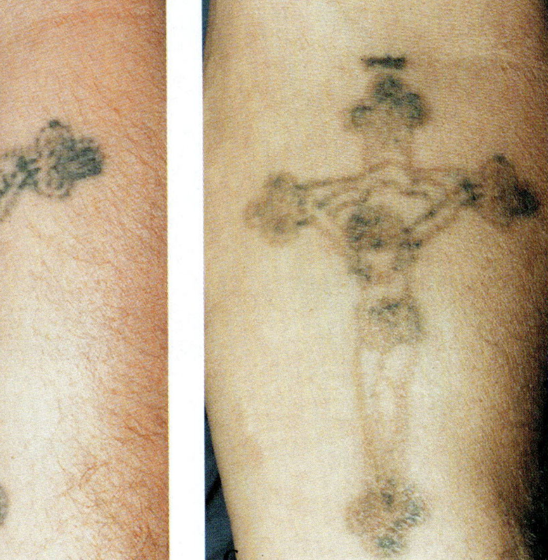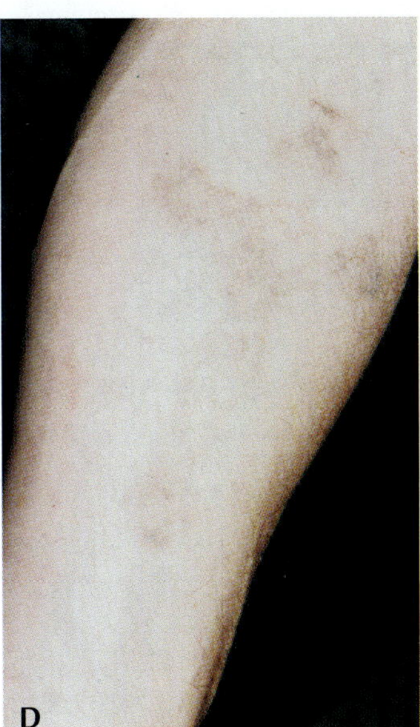

Figure 27–8. (A) Amateur tattoo of black India ink that is 20 years old. (B) Appearance after one treatment with the Nd:YAG laser. (C) Appearance after four treatments with the Q-switched Nd:YAG laser. (D) Appearance after five treatments with the Nd:YAG laser. This tattoo probably requires one additional treatment.

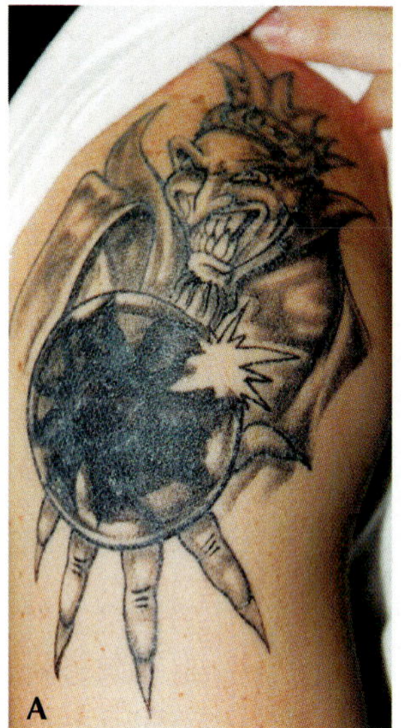
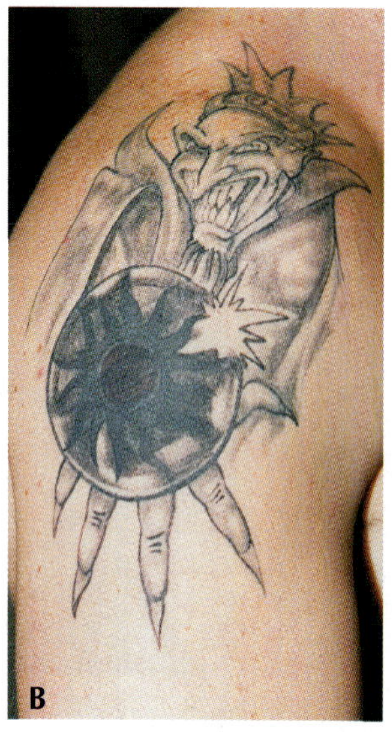
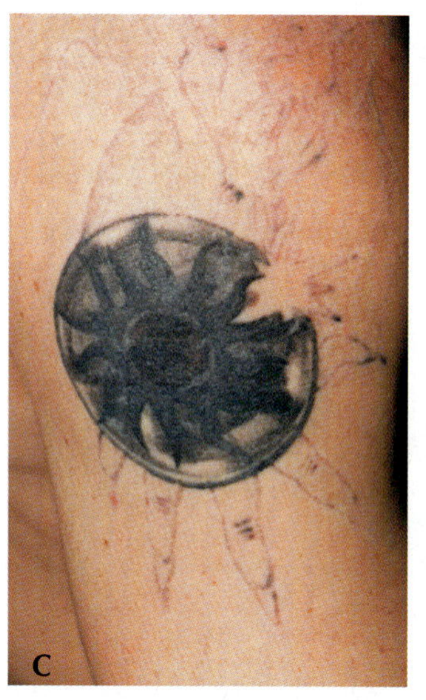
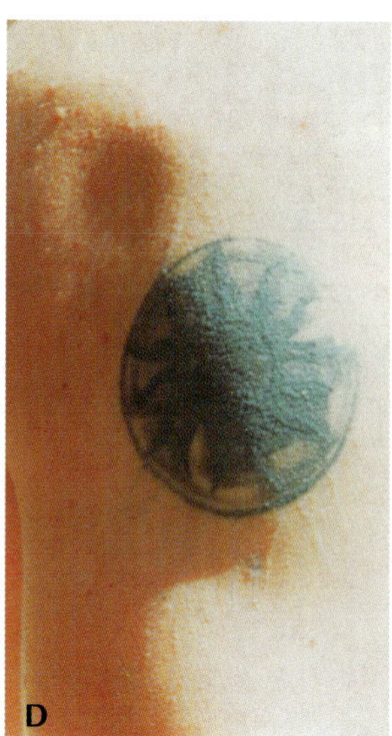
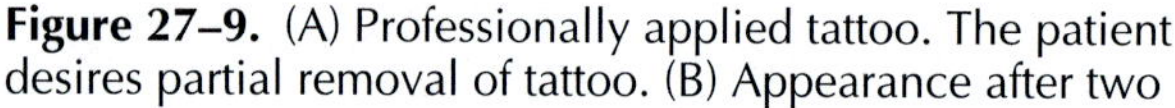

Figure 27–9. (A) Professionally applied tattoo. The patient desires partial removal of tattoo. (B) Appearance after two treatments. (C) Appearance after six treatments. (D) Appearance after 10 treatments, final result.

can be changed after 24 hours and the wound cleansed with soap and water. Avoidance of sun exposure is imperative in all tattoo-treated patients for up to 6 months to reduce the risk of postinflammatory hyperpigmentation.

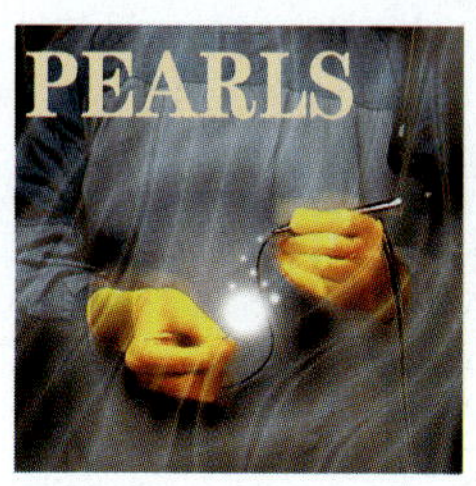

- For tattoos, the desired target is tattoo ink, and the undesired targets are biological skin chromophores. Because these undesired targets have higher absorption coefficients in the ultraviolet and visible light spectrum, red and infrared lasers were developed to target tattoo pigment.
- The exact mechanisms of laser tattoo removal are not fully understood. Histologic evidence suggests that Q-switched lasers fragment tattoo particles in macrophages. Some of these smaller tattoo particles can leach out of the skin, but most are taken care of by the body. This is why multiple treatment sessions are required to remove most tattoos.
- Depending on the method of tattoo application and the type and quantity of ink used, patients may require just a couple laser treatments (accidental tattoos with debris or amateur tattoos of India ink) or more than 10 sessions (multicolored professional tattoos) to achieve acceptable results.
- Because of the properties of the Nd:YAG crystal, Nd:YAG lasers can have repetition rates of up to 10 Hz and can treat large tattoos much faster than the Q-switched ruby laser (1-Hz repetition rate), despite having a smaller spot size.

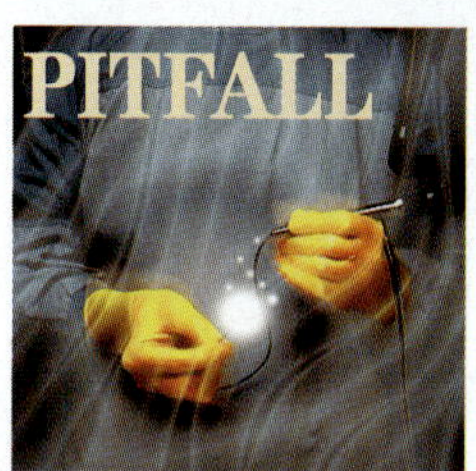

- Because the Q-switched Nd:YAG laser has a shorter pulse duration than other Q-switched lasers, it splatters more tissue. Protective eyewear, plastic shields on the handpiece, light transparent dressings on the skin, and even larger spot sizes may help control splatter during a treatment session.

REFERENCES

1. Ferguson JE, Andrew SM, Jones CJ, August PJ. The Q-switched neodymium:YAG laser and tattoos: a microscopic analysis of laser-tattoo interactions. *Br J Dermatol.* 1997;137:405–410.

2. Zelickson BD, Mehregan DA, Zarrin AA, et al. Clinical, histologic, and ultrastructural evaluation of tattoos treated with three laser systems. *Lasers Surg Med.* 1994;15:364–372.

3. Goldman L, Ingelman JM, Richfield DF. Impact of the laser in nevi and melanomas. *Arch Dermatol.* 1964;90:71–74.

4. Goldman L, Rockwell RJ, Meyer R, et al. Laser treatment of tattoos: a preliminary survey of three years of clinical experience. *JAMA.* 1967;201:841–846.

5. Bailin PL, Ratz JR, Levine HL. Removal of tattoos by CO_2 laser. *J Dermatol Surg Oncol.* 1980;6:997–1002.

6. Apfelberg DB, Maser MR, Lash H, et al. Comparison of the argon and carbon dioxide laser treatment of decorative tattoos: a preliminary report. *Ann Plast Surg.* 1985;14:6–10.

7. Ueda S, Imayam S. Normal-mode ruby laser for treating congenital nevi. *Arch Dermatol.* 1997;133:355–359.

8. Ferguson JE, August PJ. Evaluation of the Nd/YAG laser for treatment of amateur and professional tattoos. Br J Dermatol. 1996;135:586–591.

9. Jones A, Roddey P, Orengo I, Rosen T. The Q-switched ND:YAG laser effectively treats tattoos in darkly pigmented skin. *Dermatol Surg.* 1996;22:999–1001.

10. Leuenberger ML, Mulas MW, Hata TR, Goldman MP, Fitzpatrick RE, Grevelink JM. Comparison of the Q-switched alexandrite, Nd:YAG, and ruby lasers in treating blue-black tattoos. *Dermatol Surg.* 1999;25:10–14.

11. Grevelink JM, Duke D, van Leeuwen RL, Gonzalez E, DeCoste SD, Anderson RR. Laser treatment of tattoos in darkly pigmented patients: efficacy and side effects. *J Am Acad Dermatol.* 1996;34:653–656.

CHAPTER 28

Alexandrite Laser Treatment of Pigmented Lesions and Tattoos

TINA S. ALSTER

Several types of lasers are currently available that specifically target pigmented lesions and tattoos, including red- and green-light lasers (e.g., the 755-nm alexandrite, 694-nm ruby, 1064-nm neodymium:yttrium-aluminum-garnet [Nd:YAG] 532-nm frequency-doubled Nd:YAG, and 510-nm pulsed dye lasers). The availability of such a wide range of applicable lasers is a function of the broad absorption spectrum of melanin. Similarly, tattoo inks absorb light at a number of wavelenghs because of their different and varied absorption spectra.

Lasers that produce pulses of light that are shorter than the thermal relaxation time of melanosomes and tattoo ink particles are used to selectively destroy targeted melanin and tattoos in a process called *selective photothermolysis*.[1] The targeted melanosome or tattoo ink selectively absorbs the laser light, and the resulting increase in temperature induces thermal ablation of the melanosome or ink granule. This selective destruction produces little collateral damage to surrounding tissue structures because the damage occurs over a shorter period than the time it takes for the absorbed heat to be conducted to the adjacent normal skin.

The Q-switched (QS) alexandrite laser emits a 755-nm wavelength with a pulse duration of 50 to 100 nanoseconds. Its mechanism of action on melanosomes and melanocytes as well as on tattoo ink involves selective photothermolysis, photoacoustic mechanical disruption, and chemical alteration.[2,3] Photoacoustic mechanical disruption results from rapid thermal tissue expansion, creating pressure waves that fragment pigment particles in the dermis. Absorption of the laser energy by melanin-rich stage-III and -IV melanosomes or by blue, black, or green tattoo inks causes selective tissue or ink granule destruction.

PIGMENTED LESIONS

The QS alexandrite laser can be used to treat epidermal and dermal pigmented lesions without purpura formation because of the relative lack of hemoglobin absorption at 755 nm. Thus, solar lentigines, café-au-lait spots, nevi of Ota, and benign melanocytic nevi can be treated successfully (Figs. 28–1 and 28–2).[4–8] The clinical response of melasma to laser treatment is highly variable, with repigmentation or pigmentary worsening occurring commonly.[4,8]

Fluences of 6 to 7 J/cm^2 with a 3-mm spot size are used to treat nevi of Ota, melanocytic nevi, and infraorbital hyperpigmentation. Treatment sessions are scheduled at 6- to 8-week intervals, and an average of five treatments are required to clear a nevus of Ota.[5] Three treatments produce significant clearing of melanocytic nevi,[6,7] whereas two sessions can significantly lighten infraorbital hyperpigmentation.[9] Café-au-lait macules and melasma respond variably to alexandrite laser irradiation at fluences ranging 6 to 7 J/cm^2, with recurrence rates as high as 100%.[4,8]

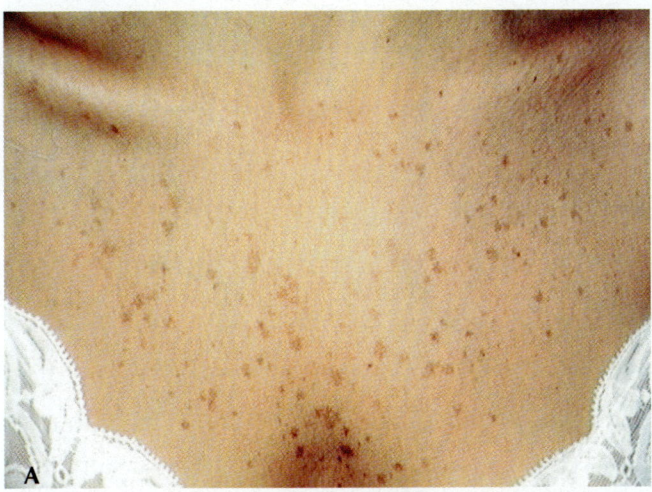

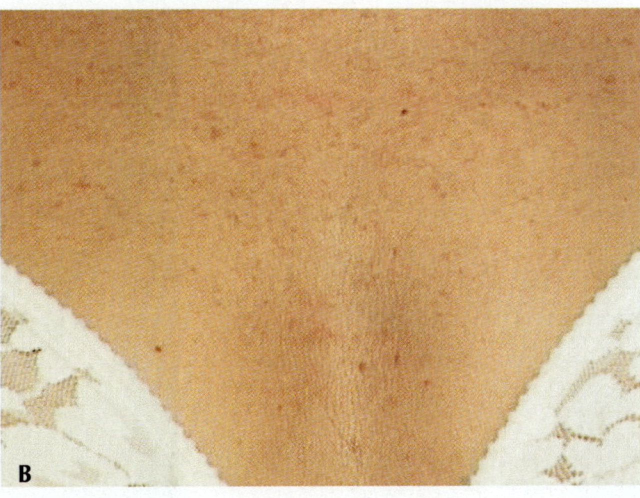

Figure 28–1. Solar lentigines on the anterior chest before (A) and 2 months after (B) a second QS alexandrite laser treatment (average fluence, 6 J/cm^2).

Long-pulsed alexandrite laser systems with pulse durations of 10 to 20 milliseconds that are now available for long-term or even permanent hair removal are being investigated for the eradication of pigmented lesions, particularly those not amenable to previously available treatments (e.g., café-au-lait spots, Becker's nevi).

TATTOOS

The QS alexandrite laser can also be used to treat tattoos.[10–15] Professional tattoos are composed of multicolored organometallic dyes, whereas amateur tattoos contain carbon-based ink or graphite. Compared with amateur tattoos, professional tattoos are more difficult to remove, requiring additional laser treatments because of increased tattoo ink burden and deeper dermal deposition of the ink. The alexandrite laser is used to selectively treat blue, black, and green tattoo inks. It is less useful in eliminating yellow and red tattoo inks.[4,8] Even traumatic tattoos that occur after mechanical penetration of the skin by such foreign body particles as asphalt or other carbon-containing materials can be treated effectively with QS alexandrite irradiation.[15] Cosmetic tattoos, however, may be difficult to remove because they often contain iron or titanium-oxide ink particles. These ink types may form an insoluble pigment with resulting tattoo darkening immediately after QS alexandrite laser irradiation.[16]

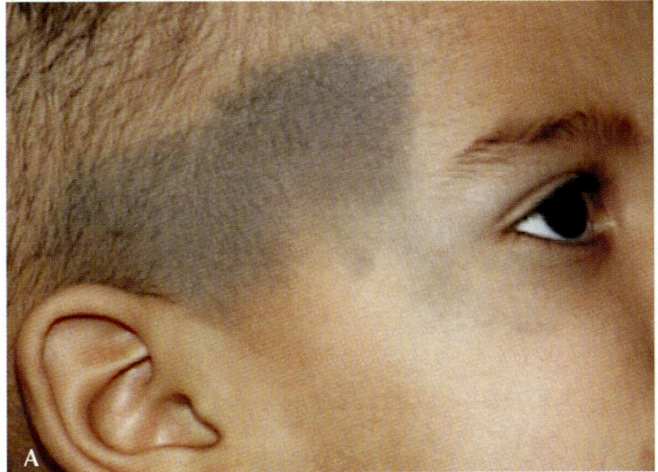

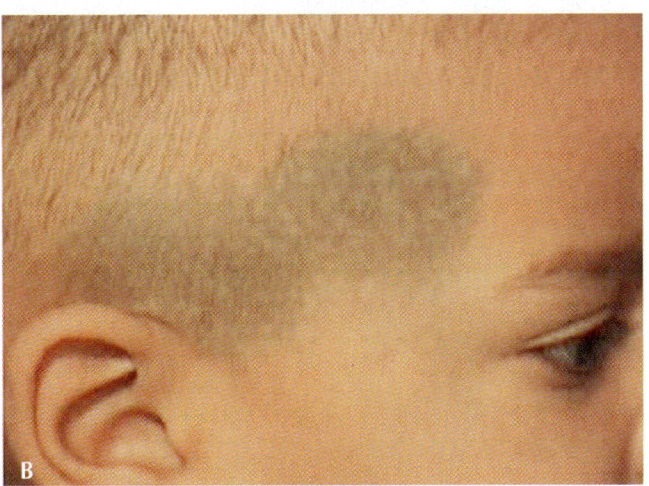

Figure 28–2. Nevus of Ota before (A) and 3 months after (B) four QS alexandrite laser treatments (average fluence, 6.75 J/cm^2).

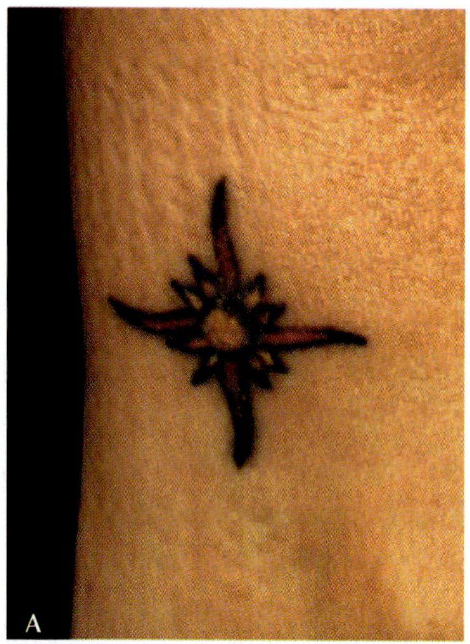
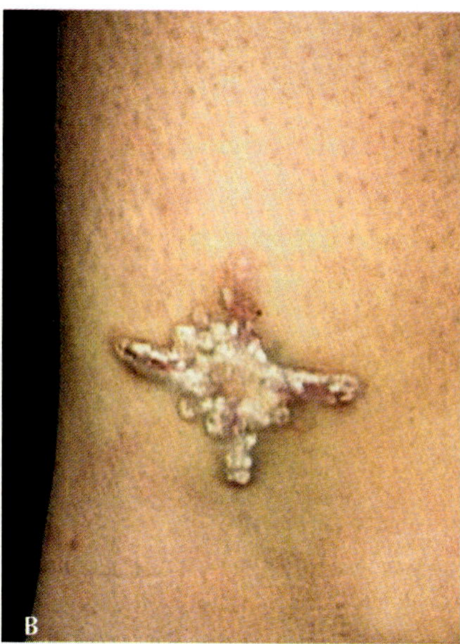
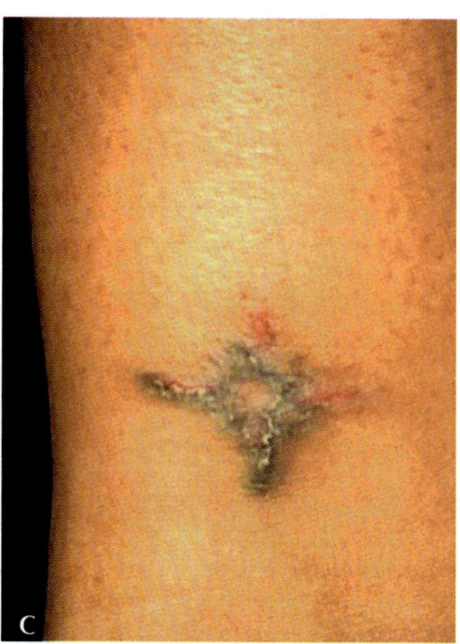

Figure 28–3. Professional tattoo before (A) and immediately after (B) QS alexandrite laser irradiation showing ash-white tissue response without bleeding. (C) Marked tattoo fading was achieved after six laser sessions.

Fluences of 6 to 8 J/cm^2 with a 3-mm spot size are used to treat decorative and traumatic tattoos at bimonthly intervals. Professional tattoos require an average of eight to ten laser treatments, whereas amateur tattoos require four to six treatments (Figs. 28–3 through 28–5).[10,12,14] Traumatic tattoos are treated with slightly higher fluences (ranging from 7 to 8 J/cm^2) and demand a variable number of sessions (range, one to four) depending on the amount of pigment granules imbedded in the skin.[15]

CONCLUSIONS

The QS alexandrite laser can effectively treat epidermal and dermal pigmented lesions and various tattoos without complications using the basic principles of selective photothermolysis. Although pigmented lesions such as solar lentigines and nevi of Ota are relatively easy to treat using this pigment-specific laser technology, café-au-lait macules and melasma show variable responses to treatment. Laser treatment of tattoos can be difficult when

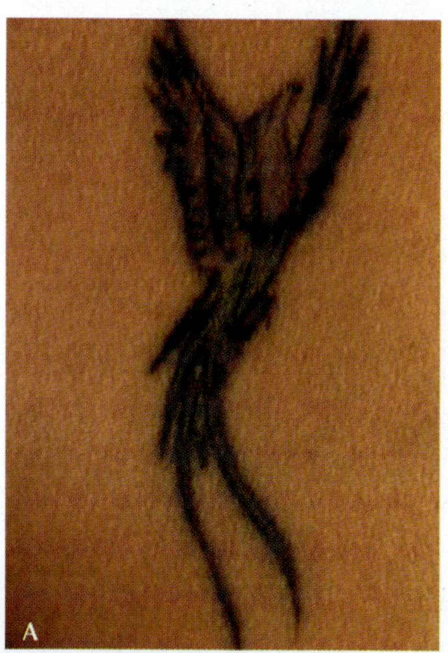
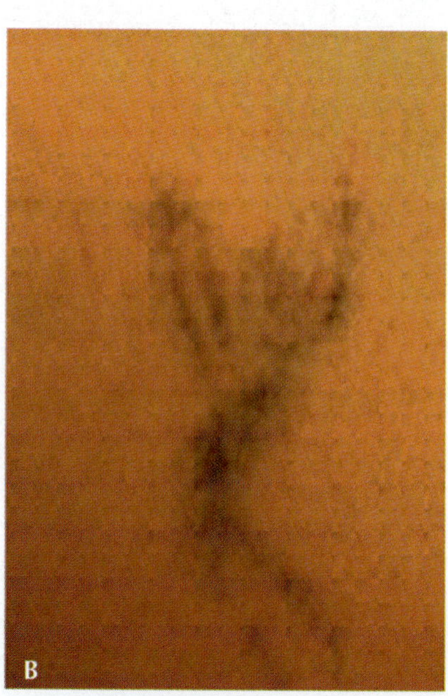

Figure 28–4. Multicolored professional tattoo before (A) and 8 weeks after (B) 10 QS alexandrite laser treatments (average fluence, 7 J/cm^2). A green-light laser (510-nm pulsed dye laser) was used to eliminate the red and yellow tattoo inks.

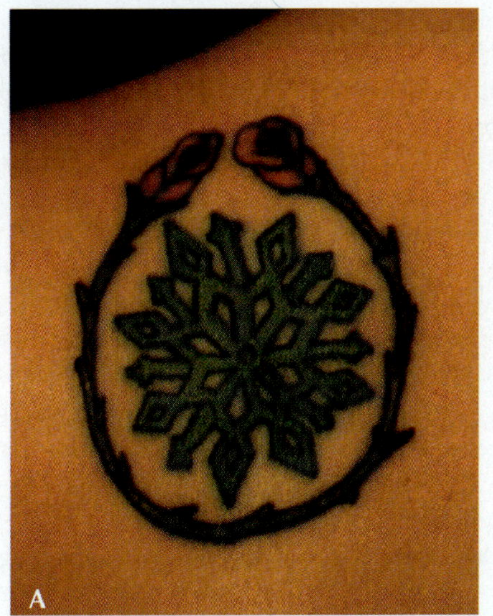
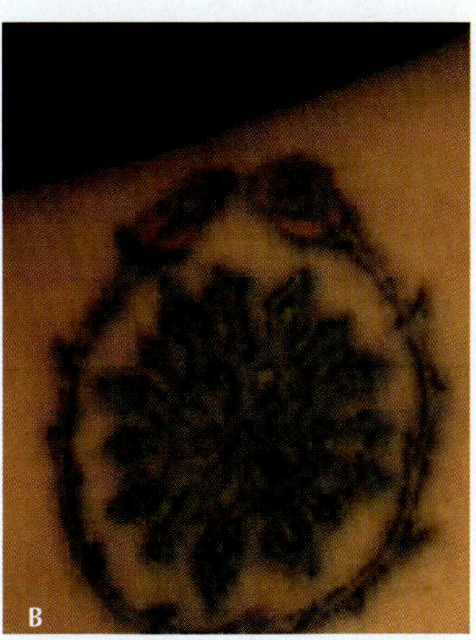

Figure 28–5. Multicolored professional tattoo before (A) and after (B) three sessions with a QS alexandrite laser to treat the green and blue-black pigment and a 510-nm pulsed dye laser to treat the red ink portion.

iron or titanium-oxide inks have been used in the tattooing process. Newer long-pulsed, pigment-specific lasers may prove to further enhance the clinical results obtained in resistant pigmented lesions and other conditions.

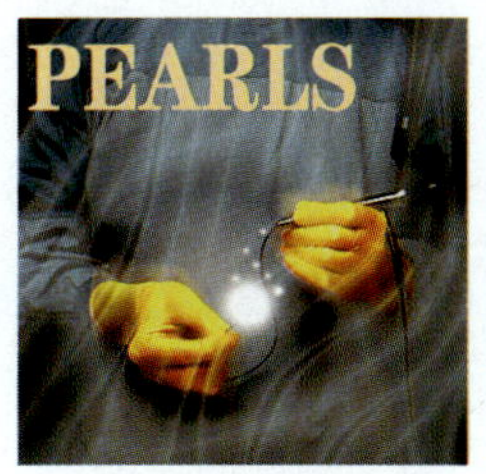

- The QS alexandrite laser can be used to treat epidermal and dermal pigmented lesions without purpura formation because of the relative lack of hemoglobin absorption. Appropriate fluences should produce tissue whitening without bleeding or tissue splatter.
- Use the largest spot size and shortest pulse duration available to optimize results.
- Compared with amateur tattoos, professional tattoos are more difficult to remove because of increased tattoo ink burden and deeper dermal deposition of the ink. The alexandrite laser is less useful in eliminating yellow and red tattoo inks, but works well on black, blue, and green inks.
- Cosmetic tattoos may be difficult to remove because they often contain iron or titanium-oxide ink particles. These ink types may form an insoluble pigment with resulting tattoo darkening immediately after QS alexandrite laser irradiation.

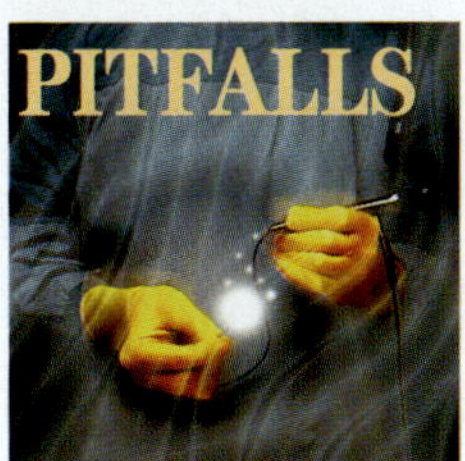

- Possible adverse effects of QS alexandrite laser treatment include hypopigmentation, hyperpigmentation, vesiculation, textural changes, and tattoo ink darkening.
- The clinical response of melasma to QS alexandrite laser treatment is highly variable, with repigmentation or pigmentary worsening occurring commonly.
- Café-au-lait macules respond variably to alexandrite laser irradiation, with recurrence rates as high as 50 to 100%.

REFERENCES

1. Anderson RR, Parrish JA. Selective photothermolysis: precise microsurgery by selective absorption of pulsed irradiation. *Science.* 1983;22:524–527.
2. Ara G, Anderson RR, Mandel KG, et al. Irradiation of pigmented melanoma cells with high intensity pulsed radiation generates acoustic waves and kills cells. *Lasers Surg Med.* 1990;10:52.
3. Margolis R, Dover J, Polla L, et al. Visible action spectrum for melanin-containing cells in human skin by pulsed laser irradiation. *Lab Invest.* 1983;49:680–685.
4. Alster TS. *Manual of Cutaneous Laser Techniques.* Philadelphia: Lippincott, Williams & Wilkins; 2000:53–87.
5. Alster TS, Williams CM. Treatment of nevus of Ota by the Q-switched alexandrite laser. *Dermatol Surg.* 1995;21:592–596.

6. Rosenbach A, Alster TS. Laser treatment of pigmented lesions. *J Geriatr Dermatol*. 1996;4:195–196.

7. Rosenbach A, Alster TS. Comparison of the Q-switched alexandrite (755 nm) and Q-switched Nd:YAG (1064 rim) lasers in the treatment of benign melanocytic nevi. *Dermatol Surg*. 1997;23:239–245.

8. Kilmer SL, Alster TS. Laser treatment of tattoos and pigmented lesions. In: Alster TS, Apfelberg DB, eds. *Cosmetic Laser Surgery*. New York: John Wiley & Sons, Inc.; 1996:111–128.

9. Kovak S, Alster TS. Comparison of the Q-switched alexandrite (755 nm) and Q-switched Nd:YAG (1064 nm) lasers in the treatment of infraorbital dark circles. *Dermatol Surg*. 2000 (In press).

10. Alster TS. Q-switched alexandrite (755 nm) laser treatment of professional and amateur tattoos. *J Am Acad Dermatol*. 1995;33:69–73.

11. Dozier SE, Diven DG, Jones D, et al. The Q-switched alexandrite laser's effects on tattoos in guinea pigs and harvested human skin. *Dermatol Surg*. 1995;21:237–240.

12. Fitzpatrick RE, Goldman MP. Tattoo removal using the alexandrite laser. *Arch Dermatol*. 1994;130:1508–1514.

13. Fitzpatrick RE, Goldman MP, Ruiz-Esparza J. Use of the alexandrite laser (755 nm, 100 nsec) for tattoo pigment removal in an animal model. *J Am Acad Dermatol*. 1993; 28:745–750.

14. Stafford TJ, Lizek P, Boll J, Tan OT. Removal of colored tattoos with the Q-switched alexandrite laser. *Plast Reconstr Surg*. 1995;95:313–320.

15. Alster TS. Successful elimination of traumatic tattoos by the Q-switched alexandrite (755 nm) laser. *Ann Plast Surg*. 1995;34:542–545.

16. Anderson RR, Geronemus R, Kilmer SL, et al. Cosmetic tattoo ink darkening: a complication of Q-switched and pulsed laser treatment. *Arch Dermatol*. 1993;129:1010–1014.

CHAPTER 29

Treatment of Pigmented Lesions with Copper Bromide and Copper Vapor Lasers

SUE E. McCOY

The ablative process of copper lasers is selective only inasmuch as these wavelengths are more strongly absorbed by pigmented tissue than normal (nonpigmented or lightly pigmented) skin. The mechanism of destruction is thermal necrosis, the degree and depth of which are controlled by the pulse duration, the pulse repetition, and the total number of exposures (i.e., the total energy absorbed by the lesion). (See Chapter 18 for detailed information about specifications and parameters of these lasers.)

Histologically, lesions irradiated with the copper bromide laser (CBL) appear somewhat similar to those treated with the carbon dioxide (CO_2) laser, with ablation of the epidermal component of the lesion and thermal necrosis of the lesion in the upper dermis. A cuff of perilesional damage is usual, and it varies with the pathology of the treated lesion. In general, the thicker and/or deeper the lesion into the dermis, the higher the total energy that must be used and the greater the margin of tissue destruction. However, unpublished histologic data gathered by me confirms that CBL thermolysis of most cellular pigmented lesions results in substantially less injury to nonlesional surrounding skin than either cryosurgery or electrocautery.

Because copper lasers have a minimum pulse duration of 7 milliseconds, selective photothermolysis of structures the size of melanocytes, not to mention melanosomes, is not possible. Nonetheless, benign pigmented lesions composed of a mass of nevus cells or melanocytes can be ablated effectively using the green or combined dual-color wavelengths. Neither the CBL nor the copper vapor laser (CVL) is suited to treating problems of hyperpigmentation (e.g., ephelides, melasma, postinflammatory hyperpigmentation). However, in lesions composed of basal or benign melanocyte proliferation such as solar lentigines, in which there is elongation of the rete ridges and increased pigmentation in both basal cells and melanocytes, the pigmentation is an appropriate chromophore for green light. Treatment is less selective than with Q-switched green-light lasers, but it can give very satisfactory long-term results.

TREATABLE LESIONS
ACQUIRED BENIGN PIGMENTED NEVI

Junctional, compound, and intradermal nevi are so morphologically and histologically diverse that it is impossible to generalize about treatment of them with a laser. In principle, copper lasers can only ablate a nevus by first destroying the epidermis, which means that a healing phase must follow. If the depth of tissue necrosis is superficial to the skin appendages, then reepithelialization follows. If the nevus extends deep into the dermis, then healing by secondary intention necessarily follows ablation, unless the lesion has been incompletely necrosed (Fig. 29–1). In such cases, recurrence of the lesion is common.

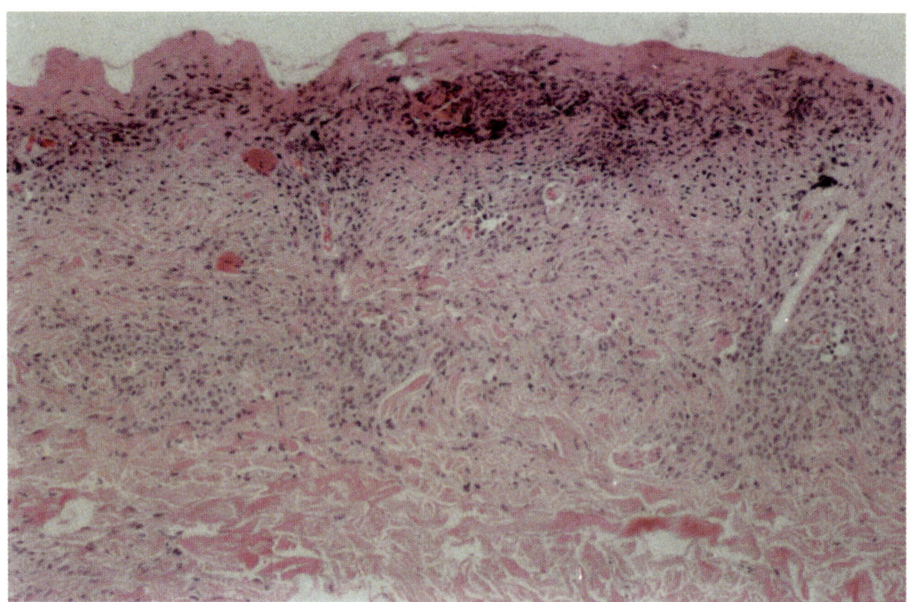

Figure 29–1. Histology of a compound nevus treated with the combined green-yellow light of a CBL using 8.1 W and 50-millisecond exposures. The epidermis has been completely ablated, and the papillary dermis shows marked coagulative necrosis; however, the deeper nevus cells extending into the reticular dermis are preserved.

For reasons that can only be theorized, the final cosmetic result of treatment of most nevi is better if they are laser irradiated on several occasions about 8 weeks apart until no further nevus is visible macroscopically. Clinically evident recurrence is uncommon after such treatment, although it is likely that a degree of mild dermal fibrosis overlying the remaining deep dermal nevus cells masks the residual lesion macroscopically. However, it should be noted that if a laser-treated nevus does reappear and is subsequently excised or biopsied, the histopathologic features may resemble dysplasia or even melanoma (termed *pseudomelanoma*), although the behavior of such lesions remains benign.

The method of treatment uses both wavelengths of the laser combined to maximize the total power available. Exposures sufficient to cause immediate graying and visible shrinkage of the nevus are used. After the entire nevus has been irradiated, the surface can be wiped away easily with saline-soaked gauze, and the procedure is repeated until the lesion base is flush or just below the level of the surrounding skin. This process is the most painful of all treatments using copper lasers. Unless the lesion is very small and treatment can be completed in a few seconds, local anesthetic infiltration is usually necessary.

A scab necessarily forms in the days following treatment, and healing time varies depending on the region of the body treated. A small hypopigmented scar is common, although the cosmetic result is usually considerably better than that resulting from excision and suture or other tissue-destructive methods.

SKIN TAGS (ACROCHORDONS), SEBORRHEIC KERATOSES, AND PAPULOSA NIGRA

These extremely common, predominantly epidermal exophytic or pedunculated lesions are easily removed using the method described for nevi. The full thickness of the epidermis must be ablated to effect permanent cure, but the skin appendages remain intact for rapid reepithelialization (Fig. 29–2). Skin tags need not be wiped but simply treated to the point of gray-white discoloration. This reduces pain and permits treatment without anesthesia (Fig. 29–3).

SOLAR LENTIGINES

The combination of fair skin, sun exposure, and age almost invariably results in the appearance of these epidermal blemishes, which are only cosmetically significant once differentiated from lentigo maligna (melanoma

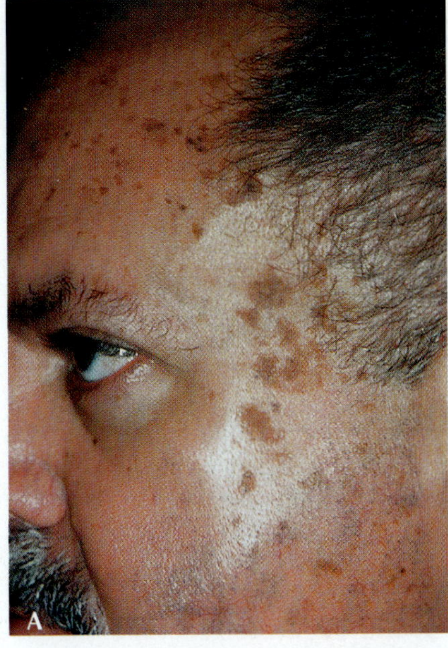
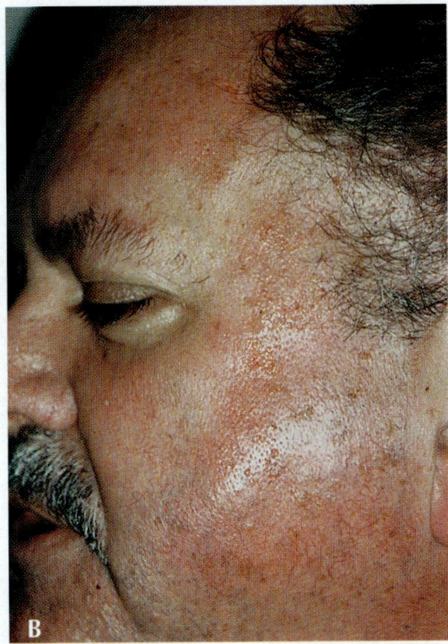
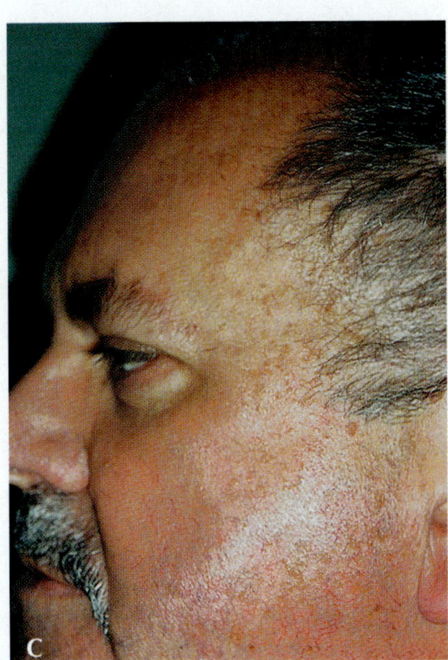

Figure 29–2. (A) A 57-year-old man with multiple seborrheic keratoses. (B) Appearance immediately after treatment with a CBL using combined green-yellow light at 7.8 W with 50-millisecond exposures. A local anesthetic block of the temporal branch of the mandibular nerve was used. Scab formation for 7 to 10 days ensued following treatment. (C) Appearance 18 months after a single treatment.

in situ). Because they are thin lesions involving only the epidermis, precise laser thermolysis of the affected epidermis usually gives permanent and satisfactory results.

Green light only is recommended for these pigmented lesions in an attempt to limit energy absorption to the targeted tissue in the epidermis rather than the dermis. Because the green wavelength of copper lasers provides higher power than yellow light, shorter exposures than those used for vascular lesions are effective. The shortest exposure that will give immediate slight gray discoloration

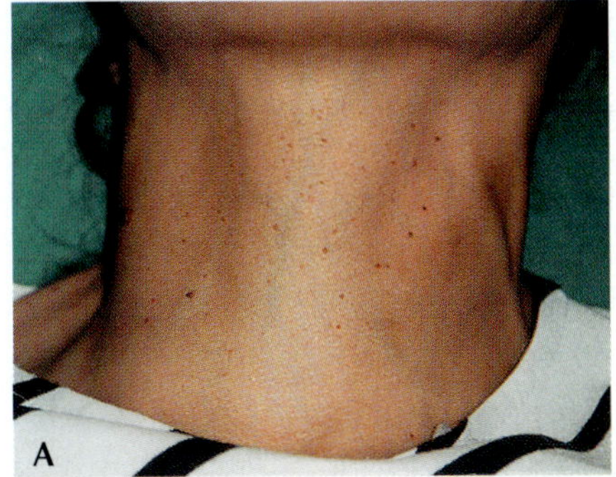
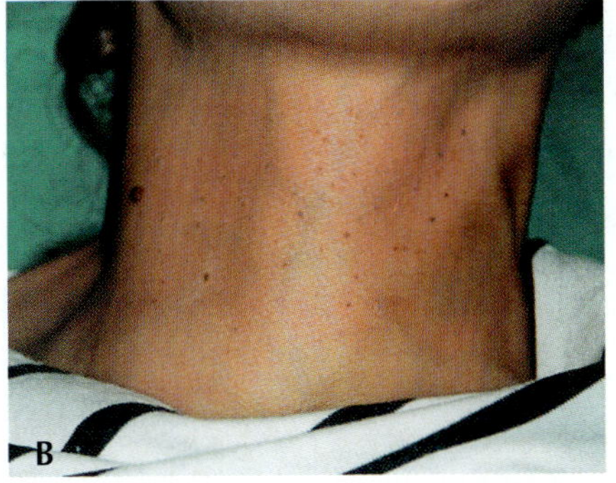
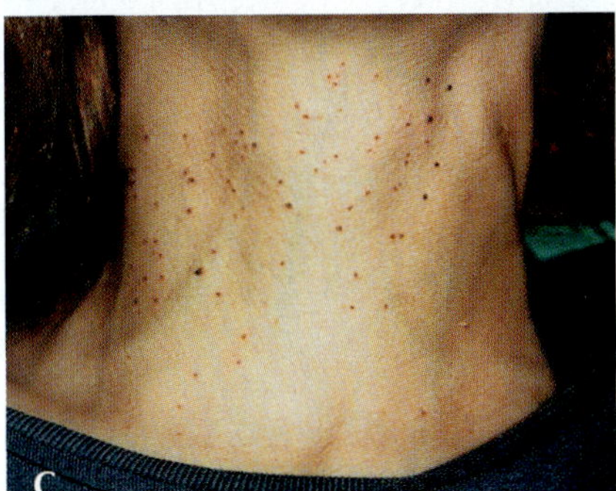
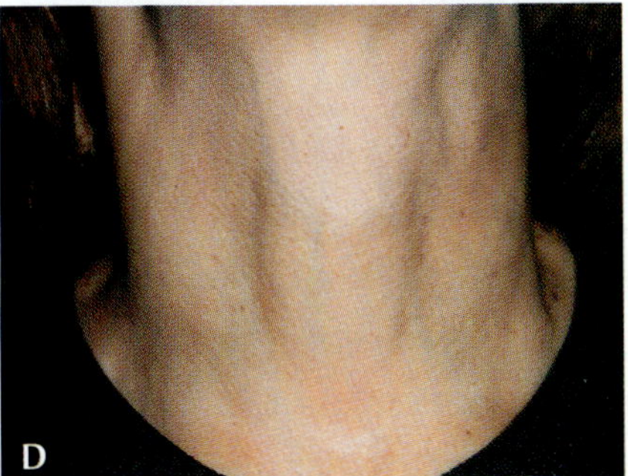

Figure 29–3. (A) A 49-year-old woman with skin tags (acrochordons) and small seborrheic keratoses of the neck. (B) Appearance immediately after CBL treatment using combined green-yellow light at 8.2 W with 30-millisecond exposures. The erythema typically lasts 2 to 3 hours. (C) One day later the lesions show darkening and shrinkage. The area is completely painless. (D) Two months later, 90% of the lesions have cleared without scarring or hypopigmentation.

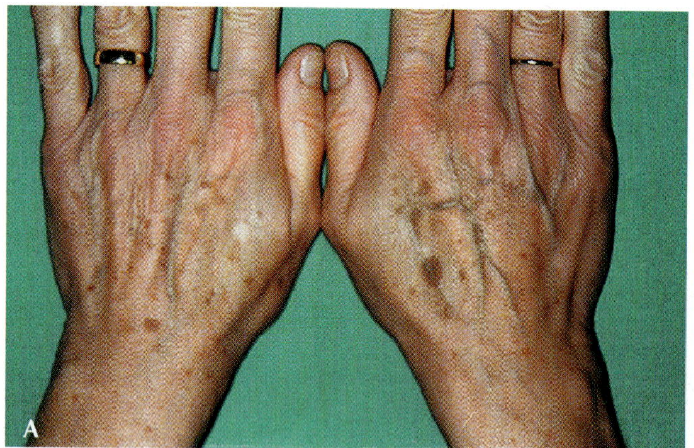

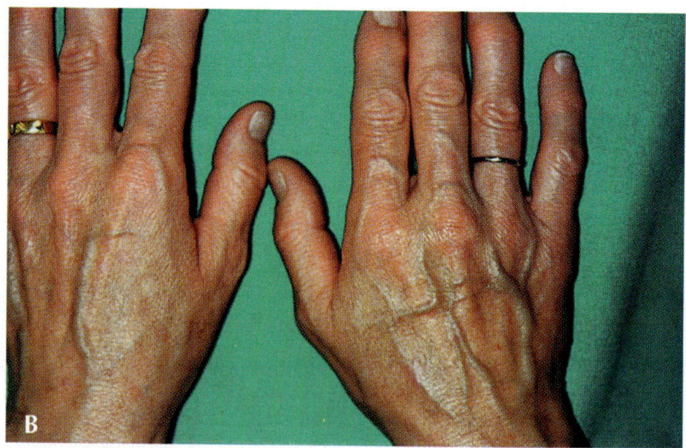

Figure 29–4. (A) Solar lentigines on the hands of a 52-year-old woman. (B) Appearance 4 months after CBL treatment using green light at 3.8 W with 20-millisecond exposures. Note that the right hand shows one lesion with residual erythema. This will show mild hypopigmentation with time.

of the skin should be used, increasing the energy only if the epidermis cannot be easily wiped away with saline-soaked gauze. There should then be no further laser irradiation of the exposed papillary dermis unless areas of pigmented lesion remain. Treatment of most lentigines can be effected without anesthesia, although where large numbers of lesions are concentrated (e.g., the backs of the hands) topical anesthetic creams are useful.

Light scab formation more akin to dry skin than a thick crust follows. Facial lesions heal in 5 to 7 days; hands and forearms heal in 10 to 14 days. Longer healing phases suggest that too-high energies have been used. Patients should expect slight erythema of the treated skin for several weeks (Fig. 29–4). Hypopigmentation may be a late event but, again, it usually reflects overzealous treatment.

SEBACEOUS HYPERPLASIA

Confluent hyperplasia such as rhinophyma should not be treated with copper lasers because the minimum exposure times are many times greater than the thermal relaxation time of skin. However, the more discrete papules that typify the common presentation of this benign skin condition can be treated successfully with copper lasers using a method similar to that described for nevi. The small spot size of copper lasers allows precise thermal necrosis of the hypertrophic

sebaceous glands, and although the process is nonselective and therefore must first ablate the overlying thinned epidermis, careful use of a copper laser can give results comparable with those of a microsecond-pulsed CO_2 laser.

CONTRAINDICATED LESIONS
DERMAL LESIONS

Lesions located in the dermis (e.g., syringoma, xanthelasma, dermatofibroma, neurofibroma, lipoma, epidermoid cysts, and blue nevus) with a normal overlying epidermis, cannot be treated selectively with a copper laser—or any other laser. Exposures that could necrose a composite structure the size of a small pea inevitably cause significant and unacceptable thermal damage to the perilesional dermis as well as the overlying and neighboring epidermis. Surgery remains the treatment of choice for such lesions.

NEVUS OF OTA, CAFÉ-AU-LAIT MACULES, AND MELASMA

Although the higher power of the CBL permits minimum effective exposures in tens of milliseconds, selective destruction of structures the size of organelles or single cells (melanosomes, melanocytes) requires pulses in the tens of nanoseconds. Because other lasers fulfilling these criteria are in common clinical use, copper lasers have no place in the management of these blemishes.

MALIGNANT LESIONS

I believe that copper lasers should not be used in the management of skin malignancies. Exceptions to this generalization may arise in the palliative treatment of symptomatic cancers in the very elderly or the terminally ill or in the field of photodynamic therapy.

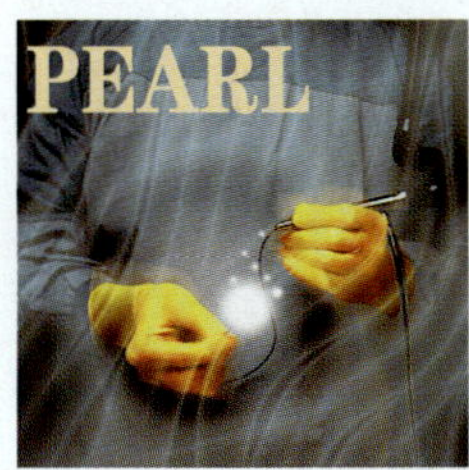

- Although a small hypopigmented scar is common after treatment for a pigmented nevus, the cosmetic result is usually considerably better than that resulting from excision and suture or other tissue-destructive methods.

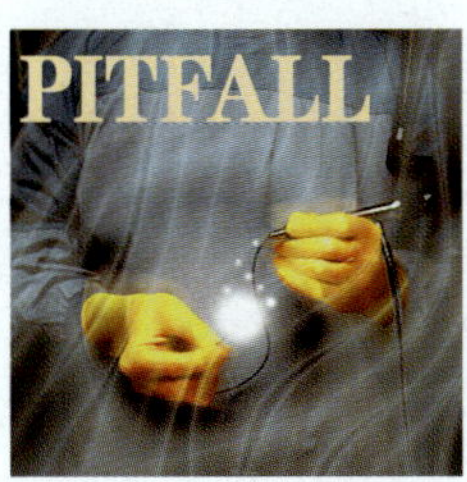

- Selective photothermolysis of structures the size of melanocytes, not to mention melanosomes, is not possible using a copper laser. However, benign pigmented lesions composed of a mass of nevus cells or melanocytes can be ablated.

- Neither the CBL nor the CVL is suited to treating problems of hyperpigmentation. However, in lesions composed of basal cell or benign melanocyte proliferation (e.g., solar lentigines) in which there is elongation of the rete ridges and increased epidermal melanin, the pigmentation is an appropriate chromophore for the green light of the copper laser.

- Copper lasers can only ablate a nevus by first destroying the epidermis, which means that a healing phase must follow. Unless the lesion has been completely necrosed, recurrence of the lesion is common.

- The process of removing a benign pigmented nevus is the most painful of all treatments using copper lasers. Unless the lesion is very small and treatment can be completed in a few seconds, local anesthetic should be used. However, treatment of most lentigines can be effected without anesthesia, unless there are large numbers of concentrated lesions.

- Syringoma, xanthelasma, dermatofibroma, neurofibroma, lipoma, epidermoid cysts, and blue nevus cannot be treated selectively with a copper laser—or any other laser. Likewise, copper lasers have no place in the management of nevus of Ota, café-au-lait macules, or melasma. Copper laser treatment of malignant lesions should be limited to palliative measures in the very elderly or terminally ill.

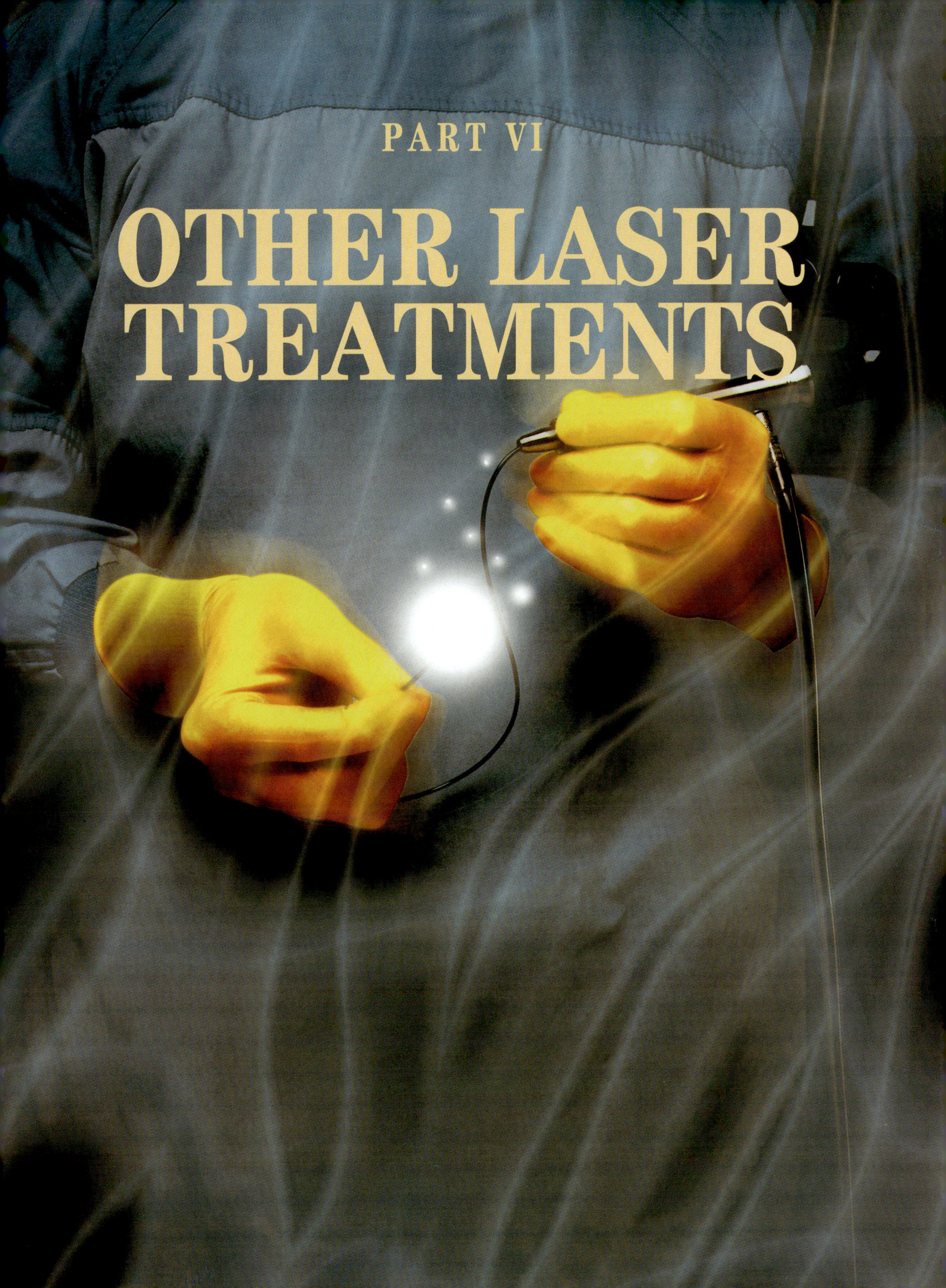

PART VI
OTHER LASER TREATMENTS

CHAPTER 30

Cutaneous Surgery with the Carbon Dioxide Laser*

FRED J. STUCKER AND TIMOTHY LIAN

The carbon dioxide (CO_2) laser can be used effectively in cutaneous surgery to cut or incise the skin, plane the skin's surface, and vaporize tissue masses. The same biological effects seen with laser skin resurfacing and laser treatment of various lesions (the instantaneous boiling of intracellular water and immediate vaporization of tissue) enable the CO_2 laser to be used successfully in cutaneous laser surgery. Clinical applications involve varying the spot size, power, and duration of action of the laser while minimizing thermal damage to surrounding cells. Because of its potential for multimodal use, the CO_2 laser possesses great potential for elegant, precise surgery, but because it instantaneously vaporizes tissue, it has equally significant potential for tissue damage or complications.

Obviously, surgical challenges should not wait for technological advances to address a clinical problem or dilemma. It would seem that those who engage in the injudicious hype of laser technology and the early proponents who often acted without critical animal research or clinical evaluation question this approach. Existing instrumentation is capable of satisfactorily incising, dermabrading, and debulking, so the CO_2 laser appears to offer no unique benefits in this respect. However, in certain circumstances the CO_2 laser has clear advantages over existing methods, and those circumstances are outlined in this chapter and accompanied by comments about the CO_2 laser's legitimate place in a surgeon's armamentarium. The CO_2 laser is used successfully in many clinical areas for cutting, planing, and debulking, but the cost of this technology needs to be placed in perspective when considering the replacement of much less expensive instrumentation.

New technology must simplify surgery; decrease costs, operating time, and morbidity; or provide a more functional or superior cosmetic result to justify replacing current techniques. Because the CO_2 laser is capable of dangerous consequences as well as desired surgical goals, the surgeon must constantly arbitrate the value of this instrumentation. Avoidance of surgical disadvantages from lack of proper consideration in any or all of the major areas of surgery—patient selection, preoperative evaluation, and preparation; surgical technique; and postoperative care—is imperative. No technology, however elegant, can ensure success without proper attention to each of these areas. Proper patient selection is the hallmark of successful surgery, because selection of an inappropriate patient frequently precludes any chance for desirable surgical outcome. The CO_2 laser's indications for use ultimately determine if this technology should replace conventional methods; perhaps my experiences with CO_2 laser surgery will allow more informed decisions.

---

*Editor's note: This is a chapter that was first published in 1989. While most authors would not treat all but the most hypertrophic port-wine stains with the carbon dioxide laser, the chapter presents unique and valuable solutions for the unusual situation.

CUTTING THE SKIN

The CO_2 laser set at a high power density and moved across the skin in continuous mode can function as a very precise cutting instrument. I routinely use a 0.2-mm spot size and power setting of 10 W, and over the past several years, I have never varied the power setting from 10 W. Moving the handpiece to achieve the appropriate depth of the incision involves the same surgical skill one employs with a scalpel.

The "no touch" technique feels somewhat unnatural and requires experience before one can precisely and consistently cut through only the full thickness of skin. Constantly varying the power only prolongs the learning curve by introducing yet another variable while the operator acquires this experience. For this reason, I do not advocate deviation from the 10-W power setting when using the CO_2 laser for cutaneous surgery. When using a hand-held scalpel, one learns very quickly the natural skill of applying enough force to incise exactly through the dermis without plunging deeper and severing critical structures. Acquiring surgical facility with the CO_2 laser is comparable to learning scalpel technique if extraneous variables, such as power variance, are eliminated. In fact, it may be prudent to lower the wattage, say, to 5 or 7 W, while learning proper laser technique.

The CO_2 laser is commonly used for resection of skin malignancies and benign tumors (including keloids) and for bloodless skin incisions. There may be an advantage to resecting cancers with a laser because it seals small lymphatic and vascular channels and eliminates the potential for surgery-related tumor spread, but I do not routinely resect skin malignancies with the CO_2 laser. Cure rates of skin cancers are excellent with conventional modalities, so any improvement in results with the CO_2 laser is difficult to verify. I do use the laser for skin cancer patients if epinephrine is contraindicated as an addition to local anesthesia. In such instances, hemostasis is clearly better than that achieved with scalpel incision that follows infiltration of local anesthesia without epinephrine. However, resection of benign or malignant tumors can usually be done more expeditiously with the CO_2 laser than with conventional surgery. Surgical preparation is essentially unnecessary, and skin-only resections are remarkably bloodless. Uncomplicated resection of benign or malignant lesions requiring no reconstruction other than direct closure of the wound edges can be finished before epinephrine begins to have an effect on hemostasis (Fig. 30–1).

I routinely use the CO_2 laser to resect keloids because it is my experience that the CO_2 laser yields superior results compared with conventional techniques. The keloid scar is laser resected in a plane just beneath the dense collagen collections in the dermis, and the resultant open wound is managed as if it were a full-thickness burn. Sulfamethazine is used until the wound has reepithelialized, but the speed of reepithelialization varies greatly, depending on the size and location of the resected keloid. The immediate effect of laser treatment is that the open wound is approximately 50% larger than the base of the resected keloid. Over 7 to 10 days, the wound contracts to the original size of the resected lesion. From this point on, the wound narrows and orients itself in the direction of the relaxed skin tension lines and ultimately reepithelializes to just 10 to 30% of the size of the original lesion. Intralesional steroid injections control recurrence, which in my experience has never been seen prior to complete reepithelialization.

Occasionally, I use the CO_2 laser to incise skin if there is the potential for excessive bleeding. Blood dyscrasias, hemophilia, bleeding disorders, severe anemia, and a total auriculectomy are all relative indications.

PLANING THE SKIN

The CO_2 laser may also be used to plane the epidermis and dermis and is done most frequently for reconstructive

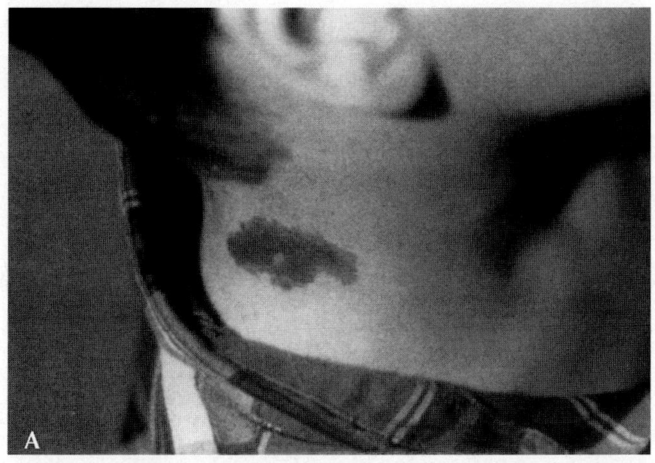

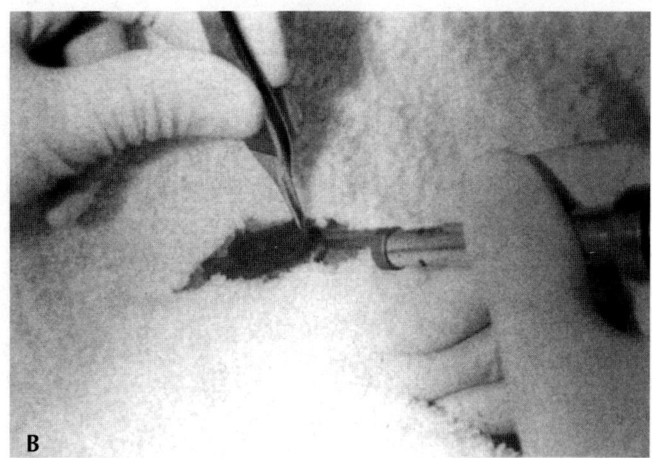

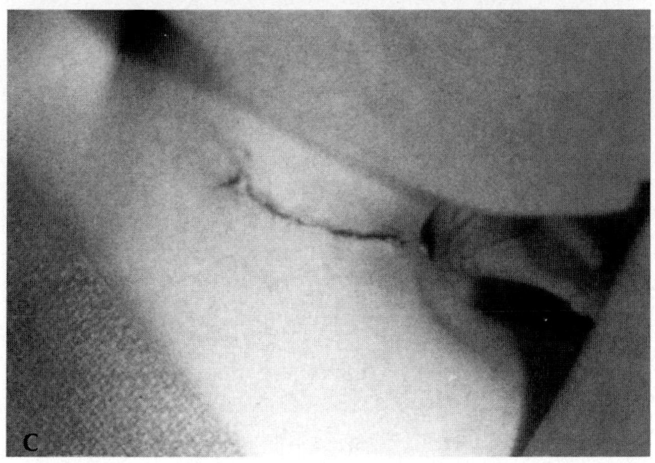

Figure 30–1. (A) Nevus on the neck of a 6-year-old child. (B) CO_2 laser resection. (C) Postresection and running 4.0 nylon subcuticular closure. The entire procedure was completed in 12 minutes with no blood loss. (Reproduced by permission from Stucker FJ. Cutaneous laser surgery. *Facial Plast Surg.* 1989;6:144–150.)

purposes (Fig. 30–2). Flaps and grafts of skin are de-epithelialized so they can be buried and used later for reconstruction. The facility with which the CO_2 laser can shave superficial cells, thus enabling the remaining dermis to be buried, enhances the reconstructive capabilities of local flaps and free grafts. After planing, the deepithelialized tissue has absolute hemostasis and can be buried immediately and safely. The speed and efficacy of the CO_2 laser for this indication essentially renders all other techniques obsolete.

Other indications that may benefit from use of the CO_2 laser as a planer are port-wine stains and tattoos. In these situations, one scar is "traded" for another, which results from burns caused by laserbrading. The port-wine stain is improved by superficial scar contraction and emp-

tying of deeper dilated, vascular channels. The clinical goal is improvement that allows camouflaging of the residual port-wine stain by makeup.

Professional tattoo artists place different-colored pigments at different preset depths under the skin depending on how deep the pigment needs to be to show optimally through the overlying skin. The outline of the tattoo image is usually drawn first with dark blues and blacks, and these pigments are always placed deepest in the skin. When attempting removal of a tattoo, it is important to avoid traumatizing the entire tissue (skin) affected by the tattoo just to get to the depth of the dark pigment. Lighter colored pigments (blue, white, pink, red, and yellow) need significantly less planing for removal because they are much more

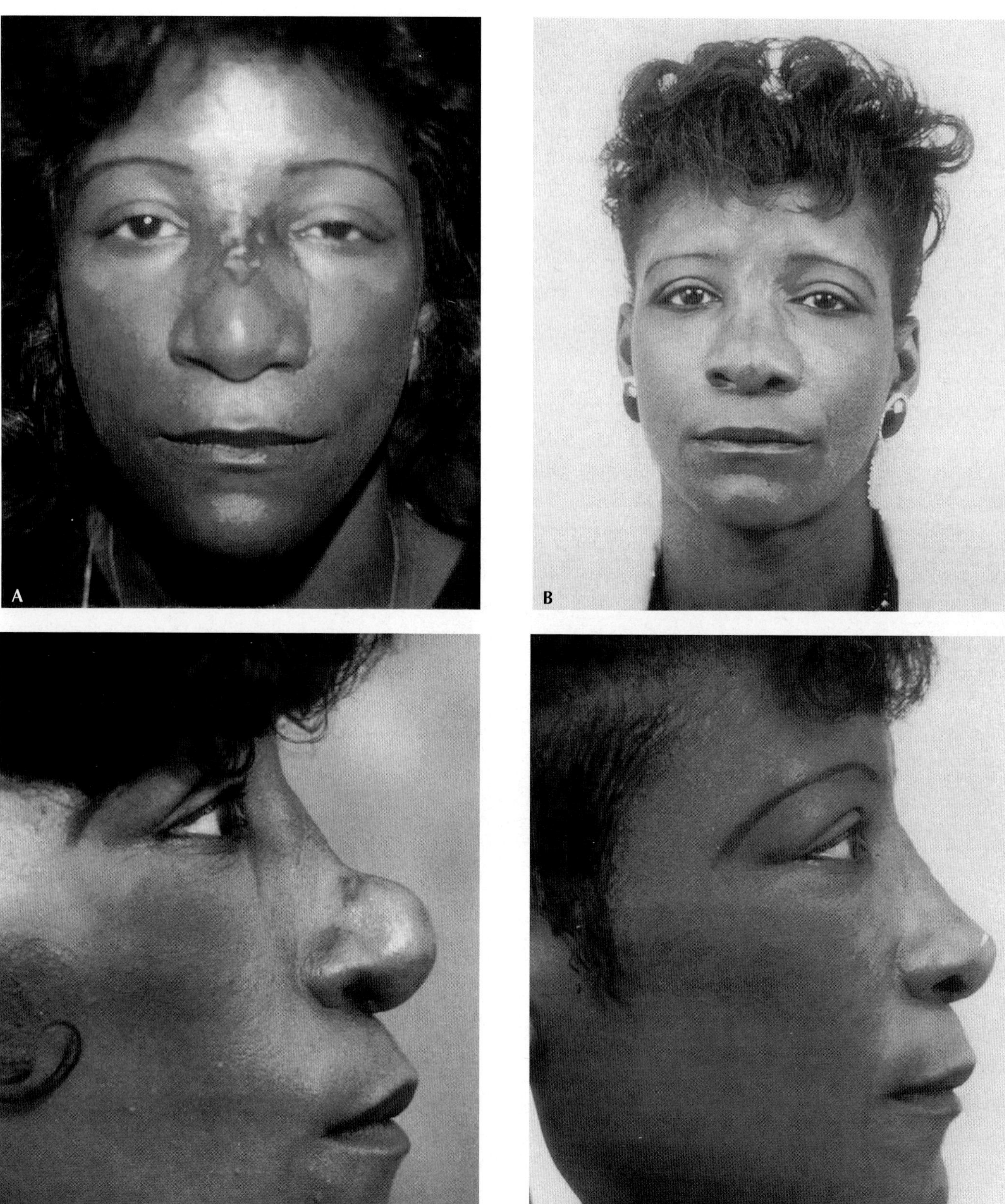

Figure 30–2. (A) Preoperative full-face view. (B) Frontal view 1 year after second procedure. (C) Preoperative lateral view. (D) Lateral view 1 year after second procedure. (Reproduced by permission from Stucker FJ. Cutaneous laser surgery. *Facial Plast Surg.* 1989;6:144–150.)

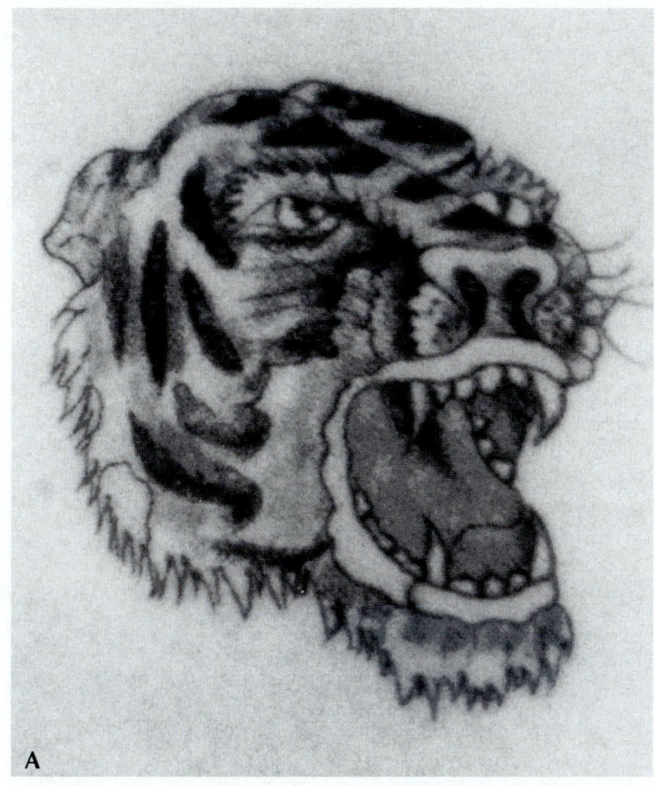

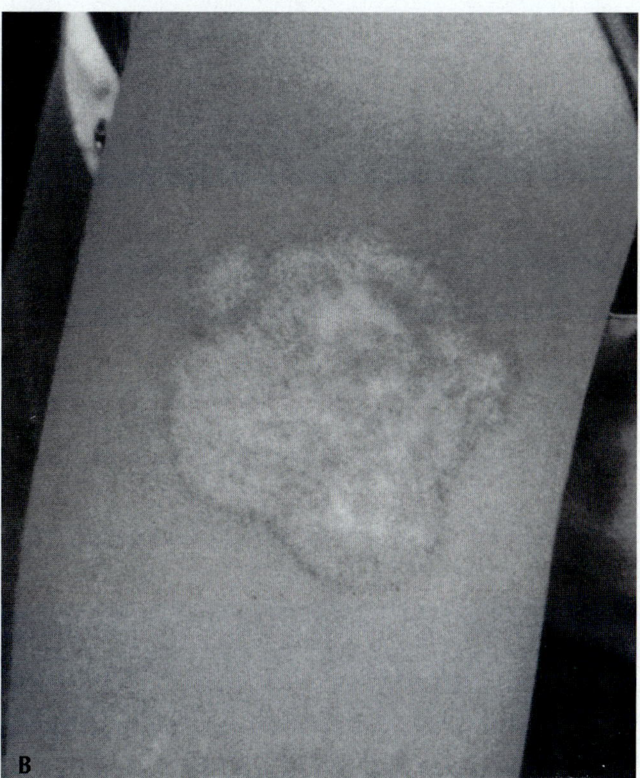

Figure 30–3. Tattoo on upper arm before (A) and 1 year after (B) CO_2 laser treatment. (Reproduced by permission from Stucker FJ. Cutaneous laser surgery. *Facial Plast Surg.* 1989;6:144–150.)

superficially placed. Knowledge of tattoo application procedures and depth of pigment penetration allows significantly less trauma and scarring, thus resulting in a much more acceptable scar than uniformly planing to the deepest level of pigment (Fig. 30–3).

VAPORIZING TISSUE

The CO_2 laser may also be used to vaporize large amounts of tissue that are not amenable to resection. I employ the CO_2 laser in a vaporizing mode for removing pyogenic granulomas or other grossly infected lesions, palliating multiple skin cancers, and managing rhinophyma (Fig. 30–4). The need for hemostasis usually requires a 1-mm spot size. This method of treatment usually results in a dry wound (no weeping) that can accept a physiologic dressing.

CONCLUSIONS

The CO_2 laser has many surgical uses; some add nothing but cost, but some possess clear advantages over other modalities. The CO_2 laser is superior to any other current method for treatment of rhinophyma, removal of multiple shallow, benign lesions (<5 mm thick), and de-epithelialization of flaps and grafts. I employ the CO_2 laser in many other situations, but the indications are more relative. Because my laser is always available for any surgical procedure and my nursing staff is thoroughly familiar with its uses, I may use it more in cutaneous surgery.

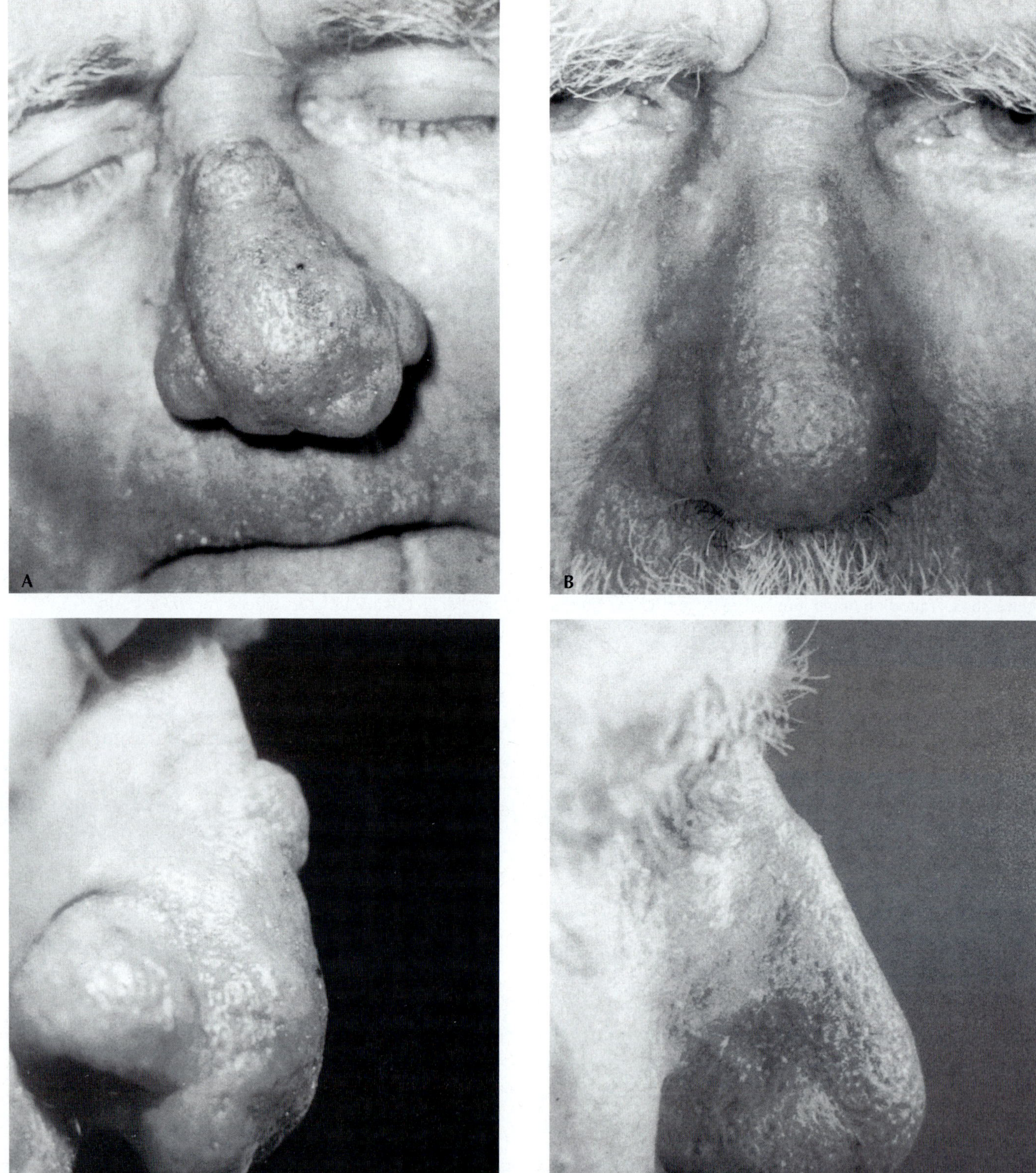

Figure 30–4. Frontal view of rhinophyma before (A) and 2 months after (B) CO_2 resection. Lateral view of same patient before (A) and 2 months after (D) CO_2 resection. (Reproduced by permission from Stucker FJ. Cutaneous laser surgery. *Facial Plast Surg.* 1989;6:144–150.)

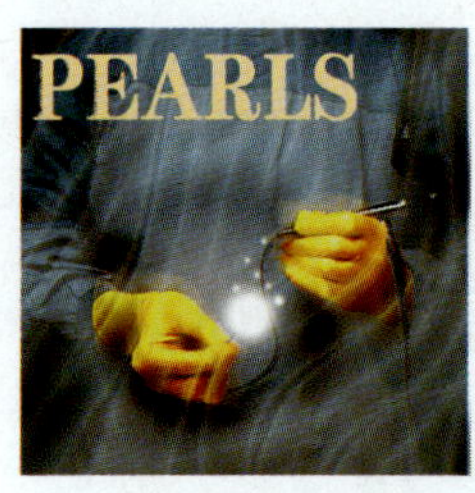

- The author does not vary the power setting of the CO_2 laser from 10 W but recommends actually lowering the wattage to 5 or 7 W while learning proper laser technique. This allows the surgeon to properly focus on learning the basics of the technique without worrying about another variable.
- Resecting cancers with a laser may be beneficial because it seals small lymphatic and vascular channels and eliminates the potential for surgery-related tumor spread. However, any advantage of the CO_2 laser is difficult to verify because of the success rates of other modalities. The CO_2 laser is known to decrease the time spent on resection and is a remarkably bloodless procedure.
- Although the immediate effect of laser treatment of a keloid is an open wound approximately 50% larger than the base of the resected keloid, over 7 to 10 days the wound contracts and ultimately reepithelializes to just 10 to 30% of the size of the original lesion.

- The speed and efficacy of the CO_2 laser for shaving superficial cells enhances the reconstructive capabilities of local flaps and free grafts. After planing, the deepithelialized tissue has absolute hemostasis and can be buried immediately and safely.
- When using the CO_2 laser to remove tattoos, it is important to remember that different tattoo inks are placed at different depths in the skin. Adjust the depth of planing depending on the color of the pigment, which reflects the depth of the pigment under the skin.

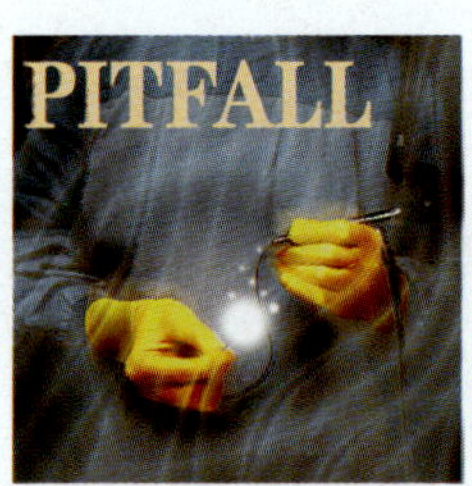

- Existing instrumentation is capable of satisfactorily incising, dermabrading, and debulking, so the CO_2 laser appears to offer no unique benefits in this respect. The cost of CO_2 laser technology needs to be placed in perspective when considering the replacement of much less expensive instrumentation.

CHAPTER 31

Expanded Applications of the Carbon Dioxide Laser: Use of Magnification for the Removal of Facial Lesions*

LOUIE L. PATSEAVOURAS

Lasers are almost universally accepted by most medical and surgical specialties. In facial plastic surgery, the laser can be used to cut or vaporize tissue. When used in conjunction with the operating microscope, lasers can remove cutaneous lesions with unique precision that results in minimal scarring.

Lasers affect tissues largely through the transformation of light energy into thermal energy. The tissue effects of each type of laser are determined by the wavelength of the emitted light and the optical characteristics of the target tissue. In the treatment of cutaneous disorders, argon and carbon dioxide (CO_2) lasers are most commonly used (Table 31–1).

With the CO_2 laser, energy absorption results in the instantaneous conversion of intracellular and extracellular water to steam and smoke with minimal conduction of thermal energy to adjacent tissue. Thus, the energy of the CO_2 laser is absorbed nonselectively by all types and colors of living tissue, because no one chromophore absorbs the laser's wavelength. Therefore, the CO_2 laser is versatile in treating a variety of lesions.

CLINICAL APPLICATION

Clinical applications of the CO_2 laser are based on several variables. First, the laser beam can be focused or defocused (Table 31–2), which controls spot size and power density. Second, the laser beam can be transmitted in a continuous or intermittent fashion. Third, the power setting can be changed depending on the desired effect.

Table 31–1. Lasers for Treatment of Skin

Argon	CO_2
Thermal destruction of chromophores: melanin and hemoglobin	Conversion of intra- and extra cellular water to steam
Specific selective	Nonspecific

Table 31–2. Carbon Dioxide Laser

	Focused	Defocused
Spot size	0.1–0.2 mm	Up to 2 mm
Power	Higher	Lower
Action	Scalpel	Vaporization

Reproduced by permission from Patseavouras LL. Expanded applications of carbon dioxide laser in facial plastic surgery. *Facial Plast Surg.* 1989;6:15–57

*Editor's note: This is an unusual solution to a problem that the author has used for a decade and a half with exceptional results that rival more conventional technologies.

If the laser beam is defocused by moving the handpiece away from the target tissue, the spot size enlarges to an impact diameter of approximately 2 mm, which results in a lower power density that produces rapid vaporization of tissues in an "airbrush" fashion. A low power setting (usually 3 to 6 W) is sufficient for airbrush vaporization. In the focused mode, the spot size on the targeted tissue is 0.1 to 0.2 mm in diameter, which is ideal for cutting. A higher power setting (9 to 12 W) ablates rhinophymas and port-wine stains.

VISUALIZATION

Spot size, power setting, and depth of penetration determine the completeness of lesion removal and the cosmetic result; insufficient penetration may incompletely remove the lesion, whereas too deep penetration could result in scarring. The only way to control these variables is through maximum visualization.

The operating microscope changed the CO_2 laser from a tool reserved for tissue vaporization to a precise surgical instrument by allowing total control over all variables. Maximum visualization of the lesion being treated is accomplished with concomitant use of the operating microscope during the laser removal of all lesions (of the face and neck). When the CO_2 laser is used in the vaporizing mode and the vaporization is visualized under the operating microscope, one can see precisely the difference between vaporization of abnormal and normal tissue. This allows abnormal tissue to be ablated without sacrificing normal tissue, which results in less scarring. The lesions described in this chapter are treated with the CO_2 laser in the defocused mode using the airbrush technique under the operating microscope. The cutting mode is reserved for large basal or squamous cell carcinomas.

Using the free handpiece, the helium-neon guiding beam is visualized under the operating microscope to precisely control delivery of the laser beam, which results in excellent cosmetic results. Other modalities employed without the microscope have yielded less than desirable cosmetic results.

INDICATIONS FOR USE

Through continuous refinement of technique and control of parameters such as power setting and exposure time, the CO_2 laser soon became the method of choice for the removal of most facial lesions. Lesions amenable to CO_2 laser treatment now include proliferative disorders such as warts, actinic chelitis, syringoma, trichoepithelioma, adenoma sebaceum, neurofibroma, epidermal nevi, xanthelasma, eruptive vellus hair cysts, seborrheic keratosis, actinic keratosis, and rhinophyma. Treatable vascular conditions include port-wine stain, senile (cherry) angioma, pyogenic granuloma, lymphangioma, and telangiectasia. In addition, basal cell and squamous cell skin cancers can be treated effectively, and decorative and traumatic tattoos can be removed with minimal scarring.

ADVANTAGES

When justifying the use of a new modality, advantages must be weighed against disadvantages. The prime advantage of the CO_2 laser is its precise delivery of a beam of light to the target tissue or lesion, which minimizes the potential damage inflicted on surrounding tissue. The heat generated by the laser seals small vascular channels (0.5 to 1.5 mm in diameter), lymphatic channels, and sensory nerve endings of skin and mucous membranes. Therefore, the laser produces little or no bleeding, resulting in a better visual field, reduced swelling, and decreased pain. Because of this lack of bleeding, patients taking warfarin can be treated successfully without discontinuing the drug. In the incisional mode, the laser can be used with little difficulty to harvest tissue that can be examined histologically. The rapidity with which lesions can be removed has made it possible to treat even those patients in wheelchairs. Moreover, the precision of microscope-directed laser treatment results in less residual scarring, especially in places where scarring and deformity are

---

Box 31–1. Advantages of the CO_2 Laser

Precise control

No scatter or heat conduction

Energy totally absorbed in 100 μm of water
   in living tissue

Bloodless field offers better visibility

Permits surgery in tight locations

Hemostasis

Seals lymphatics to decrease postoperative swelling

Works in anticoagulated patients

Decreased postoperative pain

No effect on pacemakers

Box 31–2. Disadvantages of the CO_2 Laser

Does not provide tactile sensation of the scalpel

Requires additional manual dexterity due to
   anticipated handpiece

Expensive

Noisy

Requires extra safety precautions

Procedurally slower as an incisional tool

---

likely to occur, such as the tip of the nose and the lips. Finally, the laser has no effect on pacemakers. Box 31–1 summarizes the advantages of the CO_2 laser.

DISADVANTAGES

Disadvantages of the CO_2 laser include the surgeon's loss of tactile sensation because he or she cannot "feel" the laser touching the skin, as is possible with a scalpel. Because of this lack of feedback, some increase in manual dexterity may be required. A period of adjustment may be necessary because of the bulky nature of the laser itself and the limitations of handpiece positioning. Moreover, the laser is slower in the cutting mode than in the vaporizing mode. There is even evidence that CO_2 laser incisions and vaporization wounds heal more slowly than those created with a scalpel, usually requiring 3 weeks to obtain comparable tensile strength and cosmetic appearance. Although unrelated to performance or technique, the CO_2 laser is also expensive and noisy. Box 31–2 summarizes the disadvantages of the CO_2 laser.

Adherence to safety precautions is essential because even while vaporizing small lesions there is the potential for laser accidents (see Chapter 3). Potential hazards include ignition of surgical drapes and other flammable materials, eye injury, contaminants in the laser plume, and equipment failure or accidental discharge of the laser beam.

TECHNIQUE

When a lesion is to be removed, the area is marked with a suitable marking agent (such as gentian violet) and then blocked with a local anesthetic (usually 1% lidocaine with or without epinephrine). Safety precautions are instituted (see Chapter 3). The operating microscope is brought into the field, and the lesion is viewed under $10\times$ or $16\times$ magnification (Fig. 31–1).

For removal of small lesions, the power setting of the CO_2 laser is 3–6 W. In the ocular region, no more than 3 W is needed. For removal of larger lesions, such as port-wine stains or rhinophyma, 8 to 10 W of power is usually sufficient. However, as the base of the lesion is reached after initial passes, the power setting may be decreased. The operator then uses the free CO_2 laser handpiece to airbrush the lesion in a defocused, continu-

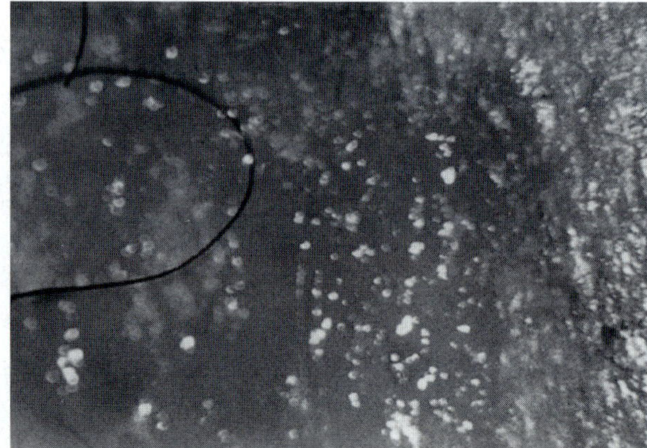

Figure 31–1. Basal cell carcinoma ($\times 10$). (Reproduced by permission from Patseavouras LL. Expanded applications of carbon dioxide laser in facial plastic surgery. *Facial Plast Surg.* 1989;6:151–157.)

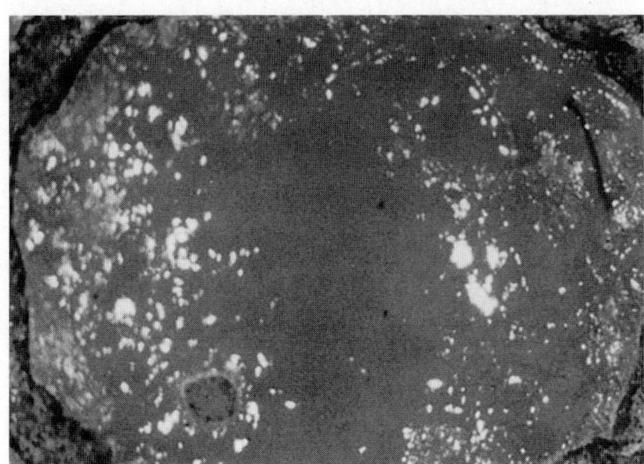

Figure 31–2. Beginning CO$_2$ laser vaporization. Margins are vaporized first. (Reproduced by permission from Patseavouras LL. Expanded applications of carbon dioxide laser in facial plastic surgery. *Facial Plast Surg.* 1989;6:151–157.)

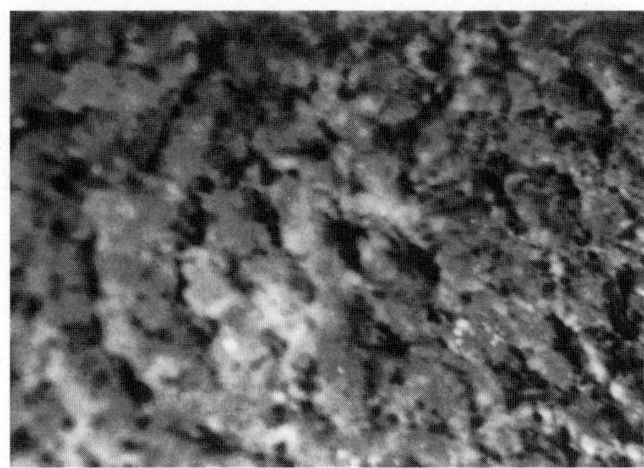

Figure 31–3. Initial airbrushing of lesions. (Reproduced by permission from Patseavouras LL. Expanded applications of carbon dioxide laser in facial plastic surgery. *Facial Plast Surg.* 1989;6:151–157.)

ous mode with a spot size of 1 mm. Single bursts of energy can be created by pulsing the foot switch.

Initially, airbrushing is performed on the lesion or portion of the lesion that lies within the microscopic field (Fig. 31–2), and then an entire layer of the lesion is treated in this manner. With vaporization, a carbon residue forms (Fig. 31–3), which is removed with cotton swabs saturated with 3% hydrogen peroxide and then wiped dry with a sponge (Fig. 31–4). (If not dried, residual moisture on the lesion interferes with vaporization on the next pass.) Under magnification, any remnants of the lesion are easily identified because lesions differ in texture, water content, and color compared with normal

surrounding tissue. Residual tissue of pigmented lesions is identified by the small areas of pigment that remain, although sometimes the char from vaporization resembles residual pigment and vice versa. Repeated airbrushing (Fig. 31–5) with the same or a reduced power setting is performed until all visible evidence of the lesion is eliminated (Fig. 31–6). With pigmented lesions or suspected basal cell carcinoma, a biopsy is performed prior to removal. If verified as carcinoma, the base of the lesion is excised (Fig. 31–7), and the tissue is sent for laboratory analysis to determine if there are any residual basal cells; the test is similar to a Papanicolaou smear. Box 31–3 summarizes the technique.

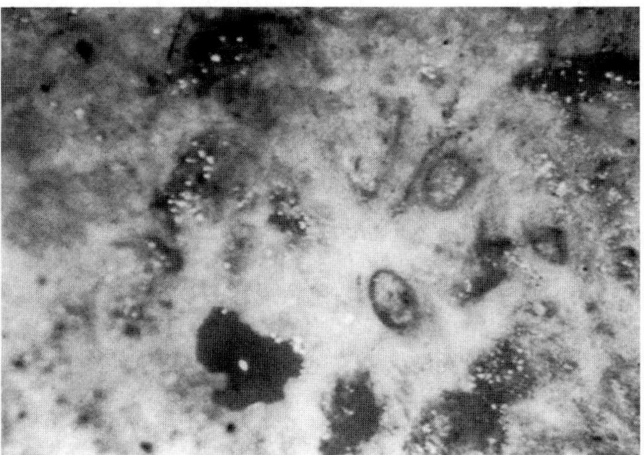

Figure 31–4. Cleansed with hydrogen peroxide. (Reproduced by permission from Patseavouras LL. Expanded applications of carbon dioxide laser in facial plastic surgery. *Facial Plast Surg.* 1989;6:151–157.)

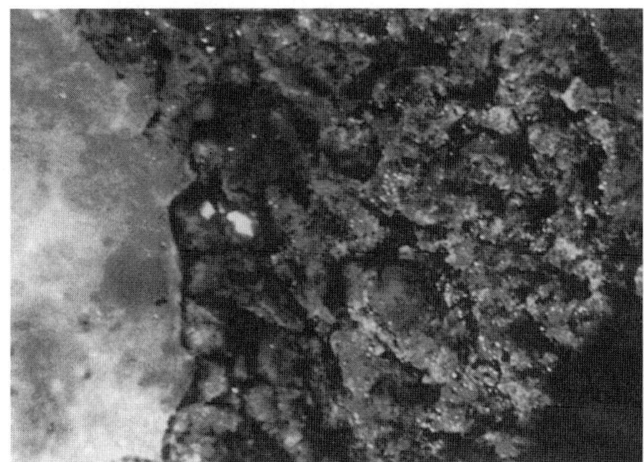

Figure 31–5. Beginning second airbrush vaporization. (Reproduced by permission from Patseavouras LL. Expanded applications of carbon dioxide laser in facial plastic surgery. *Facial Plast Surg.* 1989;6:151–157.)

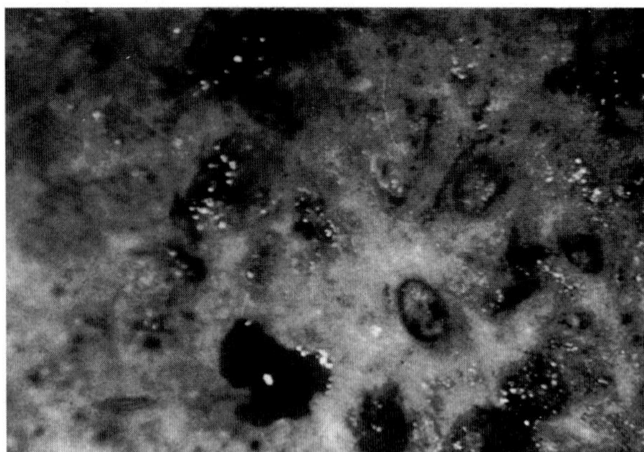

Figure 31–6. Vaporization of lesion completed. (Reproduced by permission from Patseavouras LL. Expanded applications of carbon dioxide laser in facial plastic surgery. *Facial Plast Surg.* 1989;6:151–157.)

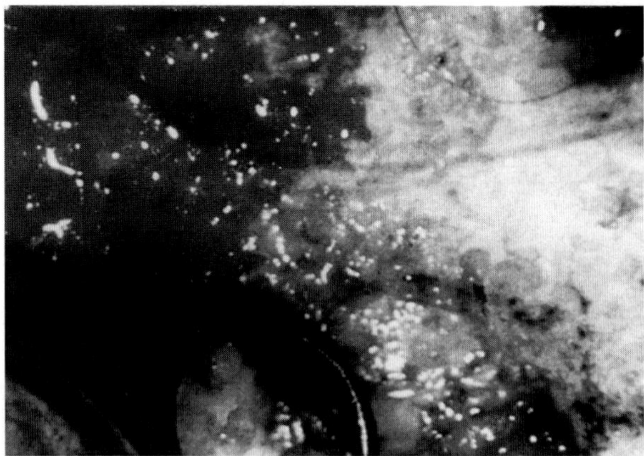

Figure 31–7. Curetting of base of lesion. (Reproduced by permission from Patseavouras LL. Expanded applications of carbon dioxide laser in facial plastic surgery. *Facial Plast Surg.* 1989;6:151–157.)

Box 31–3. Technique

1. Apply local anesthetic
2. Follow safety precautions
3. Bring operating microscope into the field
4. Set up the CO_2 laser in defocused mode with appropriate power setting
5. Airbrush lesion
6. Cleanse wound with hydrogen peroxide
7. Repeat airbrushing

A small amount of polysporin ointment is applied to the wound after the treatment session, and the area is covered with a telfa pad. The patient is instructed to cleanse the area twice a day with hydrogen peroxide and then apply polysporin ointment. Lesions normally reepithelialize after approximately 2 to 3 weeks and remain slightly erythematous for 3 weeks to 3 months. Pain is virtually nonexistent. The incidence of hypertrophic scar formation, hypopigmentation, and, in the case of basal cell carcinoma, recurrence (Fig. 31–8) are negligible with CO_2 laser treatment.

CONCLUSIONS

Clinical application of lasers is now well accepted. Previous methods of removing facial lesions (excision, electrodesiccation and curettage, Mohs' histographic surgery, cryosurgery, radiation, topical 5-fluorouracil application, or any combination of these) often resulted in hypertrophic scars or hypopigmentation. In addition, these modalities often required multiple treatments, produced excessive pain and postoperative bleeding, and resulted in prolonged wound care.

The CO_2 laser, when used in vaporization mode with the lesion visualized under the operating microscope, avoids most of these unsatisfactory results. The microscope-directed CO_2 laser also rapidly and easily removes lesions with the airbrush technique. The operating microscope allows excellent visualization in the bloodless field. Pain is minimal, and there is decreased swelling. Although reepithelialization may occur more slowly, patients undergoing CO_2 laser treatment have not complained and, generally, are extremely pleased with the excellent cosmetic results (Figs. 31–9 through 31–12)—especially patients who have had facial lesions removed by other modalities.

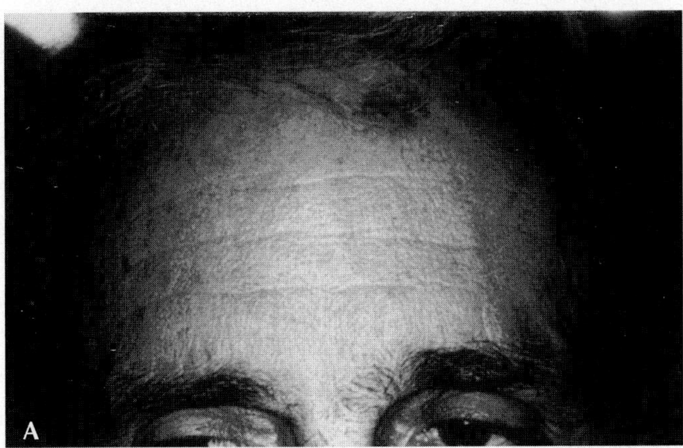

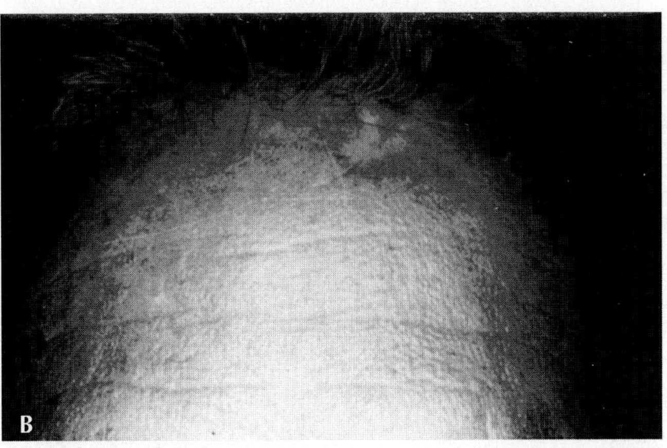

Figure 31–8. (A) Before removal of basal cell carcinoma of forehead. (B) Four months after laser excision. (Reproduced by permission from Patseavouras LL. Expanded applications of carbon dioxide laser in facial plastic surgery. *Facial Plast Surg.* 1989;6:151–157.)

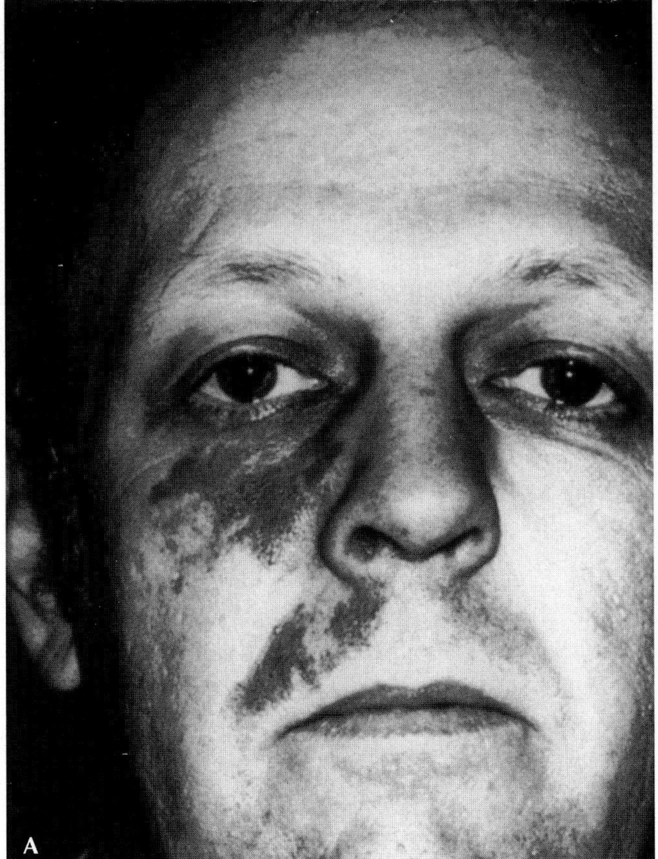

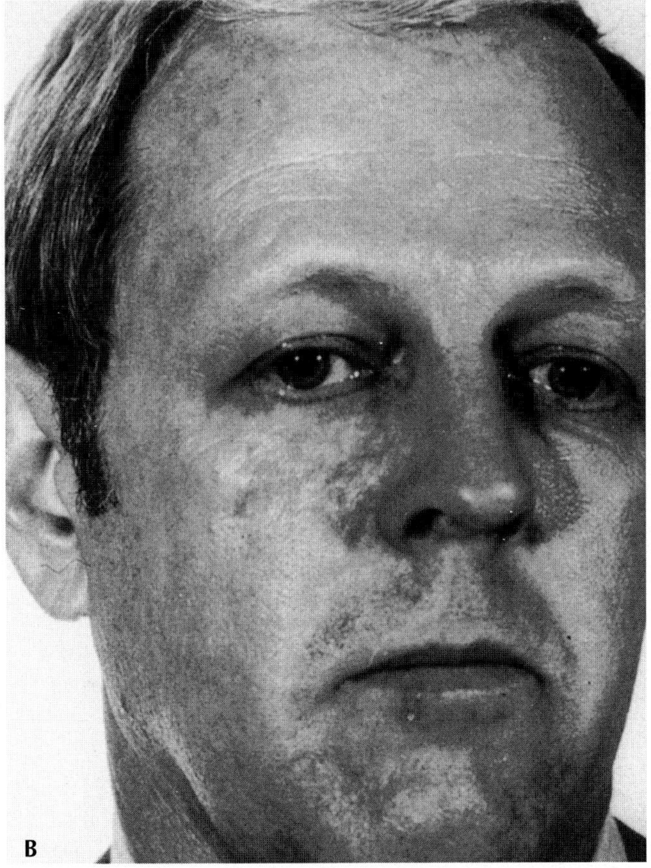

Figure 31–9. (A) Before laser removal of port-wine stain. Also showing test spot. (B) After CO$_2$ laser removal of port-wine stain. (Reproduced by permission from Patseavouras LL. Expanded applications of carbon dioxide laser in facial plastic surgery. *Facial Plast Surg.* 1989;6:151–157.)

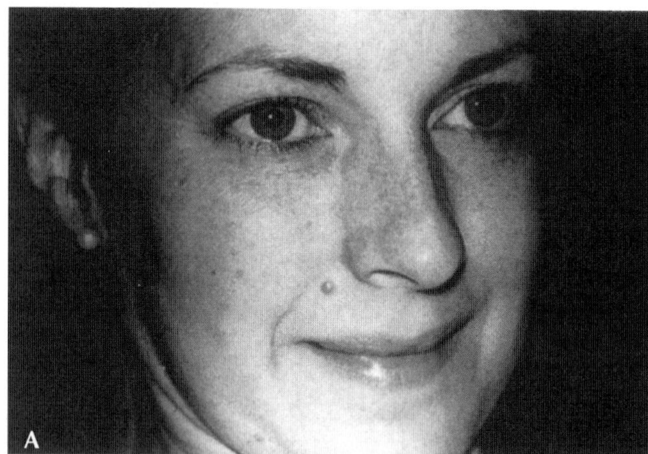
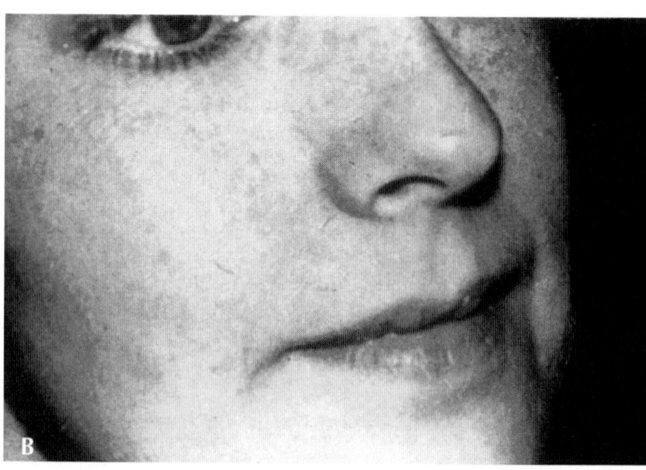

Figure 31–10. (A) Before removal of pigmented nevus of nasolabial fold. (B) After laser removal of pigmented nevus. (Reproduced by permission from Patseavouras LL. Expanded applications of carbon dioxide laser in facial plastic surgery. *Facial Plast Surg.* 1989;6:151–157.)

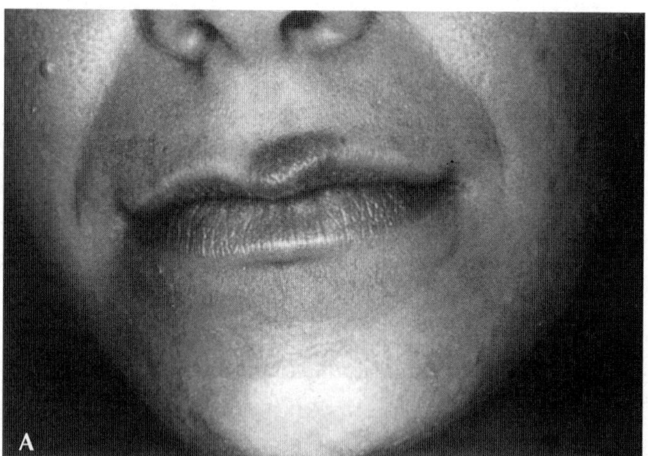
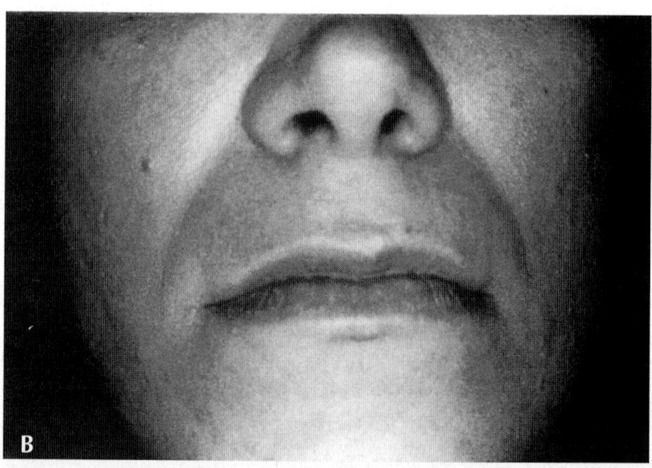

Figure 31–11. (A) Before removal of nevus of the lip. (B) After laser removal of nevus of the lip. (Reproduced by permission from Patseavouras LL. Expanded applications of carbon dioxide laser in facial plastic surgery. *Facial Plast Surg.* 1989;6:151–157.)

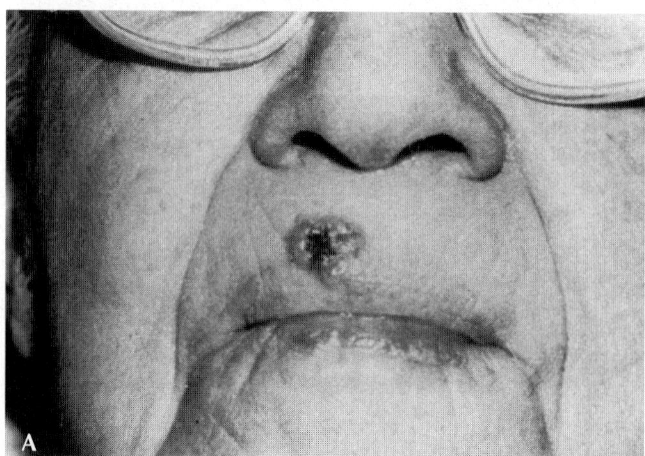
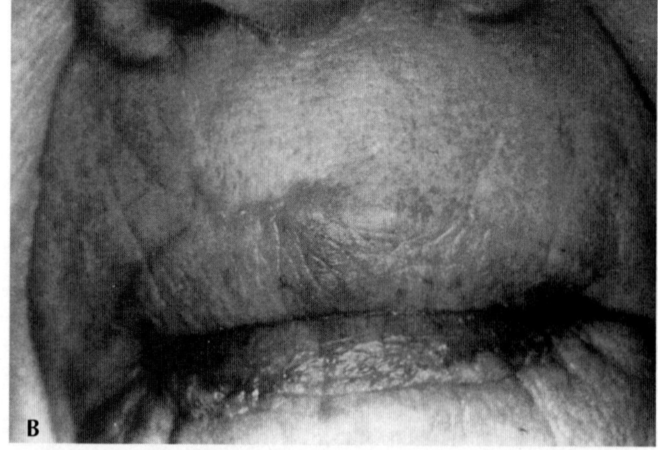

Figure 31–12. (A) Before removal of basal cell carcinoma of the lip in a 93–year-old woman who wanted no surgery. (B) After laser removal of basal cell carcinoma of the lip. (Reproduced by permission from Patseavouras LL. Expanded applications of carbon dioxide laser in facial plastic surgery. *Facial Plast Surg.* 1989;6:151–157.)

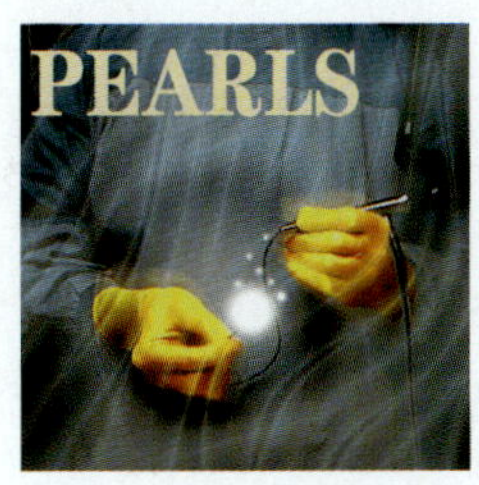

PEARLS

- The operating microscope has changed the CO_2 laser from a tool reserved for tissue vaporization to a precise surgical instrument by allowing maximum visualization of the lesion being treated. Especially during vaporization, one can see precisely the difference between vaporization of abnormal and normal tissue, which results in less thermal damage and scarring.

- The heat generated by the CO_2 laser seals small vascular channels, thereby producing little or no bleeding. Because of this, patients on warfarin can be treated successfully without discontinuing the drug.

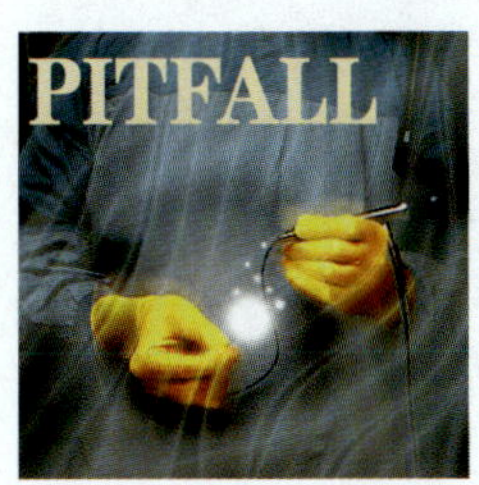

PITFALL

- The surgeon loses tactile sensation because he or she cannot "feel" the laser touching the skin, so increased manual dexterity may be required. In addition, a period of adjustment may be necessary because the laser itself is cumbersome and the handpiece has limited positioning capabilities.

- There is evidence that CO_2 laser incisions and vaporization wounds heal more slowly than those created with a scalpel, usually requiring 3 weeks to obtain comparable tensile strength and cosmetic appearance.

REFERENCES

Apfelberg DB, Maser MR, Lash H. Extended clinical use of the argon laser for cutaneous lesions. *Arch Dermatol.* 1979;115:719–721.

Apfelberg DG, Maser MR, Lash H, White D. Treatment of xanthelasma palpebarum with the carbon dioxide laser. *J Dermatol Surg Oncol.* 1987;13:149–151.

Arndt K. Adenoma sebaceum: successful treatment with argon laser. *Plast Reconstr Surg.* 1982;70:1–93.

Bailin P. The carbon dioxide laser treatment of keloids. Presented at: Fourth International Congress on Dermatologic Surgery; 1983; Granada, Spain.

Buecker JW, Ratz JL, Richfield D. Histology of port-wine stain treated with carbon dioxide laser. *J Am Acad Dermatol.* 1984;10:94–101.

David L, Sanders G. CO_2 laser blepharoplasty: a comparison to cold steel electrocautery. *J Dermatol Surg Oncol.* 1987;13:110–114.

Eisen RH, Katz AE, Bohigian RK, et al. Surgical treatment of rhinophyma with the Shaw scalpel. *Arch Dermatol.* 1986;122:307–309.

Goldman L, Dreffer R, Rockwell RJ, Perry E. Treatment of port-wine marks by an argon laser. *J Dermatol Surg Oncol.* 1976;2:385–388.

Henning JPH, van Gemert MJC. Rhinophyma treated by argon laser. *Lasers Surg Med.* 1983;2:211–215.

Kantor G, Wheeland R, Bailin P, Walker N, Ratz J. Treatment of earlobe keloids with carbon dioxide laser excision: a report of 16 cases. *J Dermatol Surg Oncol.* 1985;11:1063–1067.

McBurney E, Rose D. Carbon dioxide laser treatment of verrucae vulgares. *J Dermatol Surg Oncol.* 1984;10:45–48.

Ratz J, Bailin P, Levine H. CO_2 laser treatment of port-wine stains: a preliminary report. *J Dermatol Surg Oncol.* 1982;8:1039–1044.

Roenigh RK, Ratz JL. CO_2 laser treatment of cutaneous neurofibromas. *J Dermatol Surg Oncol.* 1987;13:187–190.

Wheeland RG, Bailin PL, Ratz JL, Roenigh RK. Carbon dioxide laser vaporization and curettage in the treatment of large or multiple superficial basal cell carcinoma. *J Dermatol Surg Oncol.* 1987;13:119–124.

Wheeland RG, Bailin R, Ratz JL. Combined carbon dioxide laser excision and vaporization in the treatment of rhinophyma. *J Dermatol Surg Oncol.* 1987;13:172–176.

Wheeland RG, Bailin P, Kronberg E. Carbon dioxide laser vaporization for the treatment of multiple trichoepithelioma. *J Dermatol Surg Oncol.* 1984;10:470–475.

Wheeland R, Bailin P. Dermatologic application of the argon and carbon dioxide laser. *Curr Concepts Skin Disord.* 1984;5:5–11.

CHAPTER 32

Laser Revision of Scars

TINA S. ALSTER

Laser treatment of scars was first reported in the 1980s using a variety of available continuous-wave (CW) laser systems, but scar recurrences were similar to those observed after traditional surgical excision. Subsequent advances and refinements in laser technology have led to a better understanding of laser-tissue interaction, allowing identification of the appropriate laser systems for different scar types without the complications and recurrences noted previously.

SCAR CATEGORIZATION

The etiology and pathogenesis of excessive scar formation remain poorly understood despite the fact that the first documentation of an abnormal scar (keloid) occurred more than 1,000 years ago.[1] The term *keloid* was introduced in 1817 by Alibert[2] and is often used synonymously with the term *hypertrophic scar*, even though the two lesions are significantly different. Because scar response depends on the type of laser used, proper categorization of the scar is paramount to achieving optimal treatment results.

Hypertrophic scars usually develop within the first 1 or 2 months after surgery or trauma. They commonly present as erythematous, firm, and raised linear bands over the mediastinum, upper back, and deltoid regions, but they can occur in any area.[3] Hypertrophic scar tissue usually occurs within wound margins[4] and is symptomatic (i.e., pruritic and dysesthetic) in up to one third of patients.[5] Increased collagen synthesis and reduced collagen lysis during the remodeling phase of wound repair are the most plausible explanations for the formation of hypertrophic scars.

Keloids, unlike hypertrophic scars, grow beyond the original wound margins.[3,4,6–8] They are seen most commonly on the earlobes, shoulders, chest, upper back, and nuchal region in patients with darker skin tones. However, any patient can develop keloids. The proliferative phase of wound repair is so prolonged that keloids have been described as being representative of incomplete tumors.[9] Histologically, keloids reveal thick bundles of hyalinized collagen in a nodular arrangement.

Atrophic scars appear as indented or pitted areas that are limited to previous areas of inflammation, trauma, or surgery. They are particularly common on the face, chest, upper back, and shoulders of individuals who have suffered repeated episodes of inflammatory or cystic acne. Early in their course, atrophic scars are typically erythematous, but over time, they become hypopigmented. Variable amounts of fibrosis and inflammation are observed on histologic examination of these scars.

LASER TREATMENT OF SCARS

The first reports on the use of lasers to treat hypertrophic scars and keloids appeared in the medical literature in the mid-1980s. The vaporizing systems used, such as the CW carbon dioxide (CO_2), argon, and neodymium:yttrium-aluminum-garnet (Nd:YAG) lasers, all led to early scar improvement followed by scar recurrence or worsening within 1 year of treatment.[10–19]

In the early 1990s, the first reports on a series of experiments using a vascular-specific pulsed dye laser on hypertrophic scars and keloids were published.[20–26] It was evident early on that the 585-nm pulsed dye laser could affect more than its intended microvascular target. Scars treated with pulsed dye lasers become more pliable with significantly less hypertrophy, erythema, and pruritus. These clinical observations have been substantiated by skin surface textural analyses, erythema reflectance spectrometry readings, scar height measurements, and pliability scores, all showing significant improvement after pulsed dye laser irradiation.[22]

Histopathologic examination of pulsed dye laser-irradiated scars reveals finer and more fibrillar-appearing collagen. In addition, an increase in the number of tissue mast cells has been noted in laser-treated areas, suggesting the possible etiologic mechanism of scar clearance. Since histamine has been shown to alternately influence collagen synthesis in a positive and a negative manner, its role in laser-induced scar improvement is yet to be determined. In addition, the fact that mast cells elaborate a wide variety of cytokines may account in some way for the clinical improvement seen: microvasculature destruction is affected, tissue factors are released, and collagen remodeling occurs. Other etiologic mechanisms include the possibility of collagen stimulation through dermal heat conduction from laser-targeted blood vessels or lack of tissue oxygenation leading to collagen catabolism and release of collagenase.[25]

Atrophic scars were also treated initially with CW and superpulsed CO_2 laser systems, but the clinical results were operator-dependent and generally were unfavorable except in the most experienced operator's hands.[27,28] Now that high-energy pulsed CO_2 laser systems have become available, atrophic scars from acne, chickenpox, surgery, and trauma can be improved in a more controlled manner with fewer significant side effects.[29–33]

The newest resurfacing laser to become available is the 2940-nm erbium:YAG (Er:YAG) laser, and it is exceptionally effective at ablating tissue with minimal collateral thermal damage (thereby limiting side effects such as scarring).[34] The long wavelengths of the Er:YAG and CO_2 lasers (in the infrared range) allow for specific absorption by water-containing tissue such as the epidermis and dermis. The Er:YAG laser is useful for mild atrophic scars,[35,36] whereas deeper scars typically require CO_2 laser treatment to achieve deeper tissue vaporization, collagen shrinkage (from heat conduction), and subsequent collagen remodeling.[37]

PREOPERATIVE PATIENT EVALUATION

Patients should be evaulated by an initial screening to ascertain whether their scars, skin types, and expectations can be accommodated by laser treatment. The appropriate laser system is determined based on the scar type (Table 32–1). Scar categorization also allows the

Table 32–1. Laser Treatment of Scars

Scar Type	Laser	No. of Treatments Required
Hypertrophic	585-nm pulsed dye	2–4
Keloid	585-nm pulsed dye	2–6
Atrophic	High-energy, pulsed CO_2	1
	Er:YAG	1–2

physician to discuss with the patient information relevant to the laser being used, including the anticipated number of treatments to achieve the desired clinical effect.

The age of the scar and its developmental history should also be determined. Younger scars (<1 year old) are typically more erythematous than older scars. While younger scars are amenable to pulsed dye laser irradiation, they may not need laser treatment because they typically continue to improve spontaneously for the first year after injury or surgery. In patients whose scars worsen, however, it is best to advise earlier laser intervention to prevent further abnormal scar proliferation and to effect speedier improvement.[31,38]

Whether the scar has been treated previously is also important because additional fibrosis may be present within a treated scar, making it even more difficult to achieve improvement. Atrophic scars that have been dermabraded, for example, may not be able to be vaporized as readily with the CO_2 or Er:YAG laser, possibly reducing the final clinical result. However, hypertrophic scars and keloids that have received intralesional corticosteroid injections do not show a significant reduction in response to subsequent pulsed dye laser treatment.

Patients with hypertrophic scars and keloids may report symptoms such as pruritus and dysesthesia within their scars, requiring the use of oral antihistamines. Pulsed dye laser irradiation of these scars may produce an improvement in symptoms within one or two treatment sessions.

In patients with darker skin tones (Fitzpatrick skin type IV and higher), and thus more epidermal melanin, less energy may be effectively delivered to the dermal scar tissue because of the selective absorption of 585-nm light by melanin. Lighter-skinned patients, therefore, are expected to respond most favorably to pulsed dye laser irradiation.

A complete skin examination should be performed to assess for keloid tendencies. In patients who are known to be keloid-prone, a laser test site should be considered prior to laser resurfacing of atrophic scars because laser vaporization could lead to a hypertrophic tissue response. There does not appear to be an increased risk of scar worsening or new scar development using the pulsed-dye laser to treat scars in patients who are keloid-prone; however, patients who have taken oral isotretinoin within the preceding 6 months are at increased risk of developing hypertrophic scars. Thus, it is prudent to delay laser treatment for at least 6 months after a course of isotretinoin.

Patients who expect their scars to totally disappear after laser treatment face uniform disappointment with their clinical results, regardless of the amount of improvement actually achieved. If a patient continues to voice unrealistic expectations after an adequate explanation has been given regarding the laser procedure and its anticipated effect, then laser treatment should not be performed.

LASER PROTOCOL

The number of laser treatments necessary to achieve significant scar improvement depends not only on the type of scar present but also on each patient's tissue response and collagen remodeling capability. In general, two or more pulsed dye laser sessions are needed to improve hypertrophic scars and keloids, whereas a single laser resurfacing treatment is typically needed with the CO_2 or Er:YAG laser. Whereas atrophic scars can be vaporized effectively with the CO_2 and Er:YAG lasers without recurrence, hypertrophic scars and keloids will recur universally with these lasers.

Pulsed Dye Laser

A 585-nm flashlamp-pumped pulsed dye laser is best used at average fluences of 6.0 to 7.0 J/cm^2 with a 5- or 7-mm spot size and at 4.5 to 5.0 J/cm^2 with a 10-mm spot size when treating hypertrophic scars and keloids (Table 32–2 and Fig. 32–1). Adjacent, nonoverlapping laser pulses are delivered to the entire scar because when

Table 32–2. Laser Parameters

Laser Type	Wavelength	Pulse Width	Energy or Power	Spot Size (mm)	Scars Treated
Pulsed Dye	585 nm	450–1500 μs	4.5–7.0 J/cm^2	5–10	Hypertrophic Keloid
CO$_2$	10,600 nm	<1 ms	300–500 mJ		
			5–7 W	3	Atrophic
			60 W	3–12 (scan)	
Er:YAG	2940 nm	150–600 μs	1.0–3.0 J	5–7	Atrophic

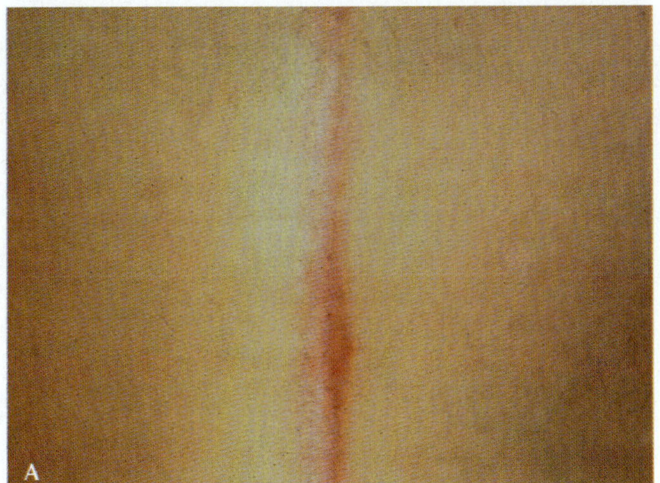

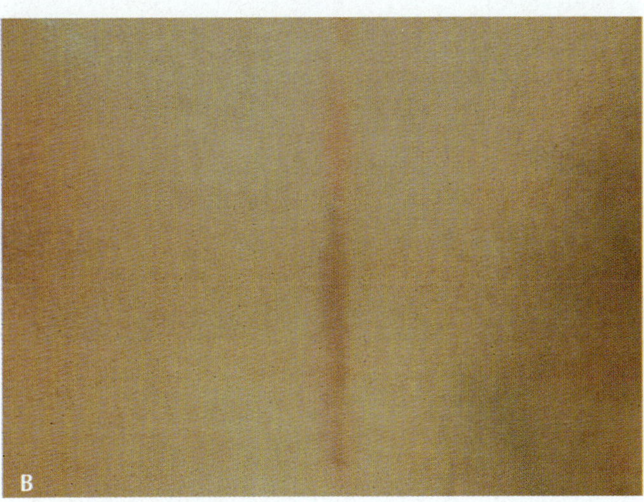

Figure 32–1. Hypertrophic median sternotomy scar of 2 years' duration in a 5-year-old girl before (A) and 1 year after (B) second 585-nm pulsed dye laser treatment (average fluence, 6.5 J/cm^2; pulse duration, 450 microsecond; spot size, 7 mm) showing marked improvement in scar color and height.

laser spots overlap, excessive heat (thermal damage) is produced in the treated skin, causing a significant risk of vesiculation, textural changes, and scarring.

Immediately after pulsed dye laser irradiation, a variable amount of tissue purpura is produced. The purpuric response is most evident (darker) in scars that are more erythematous (Fig. 32–2). A lesser degree of purpura is seen when using the 10-mm spot size at the proper fluences. Purpura typically resolves within 7 to 10 days, during which time the patient applies antibiotic ointment to the irradiated areas and avoids exposure to sunlight.

Patients are evaluated 6 to 8 weeks postoperatively. Depending on the clinical result obtained, another laser treatment at the same or slightly higher fluence can be delivered. If the previously irradiated areas are hyperpigmented (indicating hemosiderin deposition or postinflammatory hyperpigmentation), it is necessary to wait an additional 2 to 4 weeks to allow sufficient time for healing before reassessing the scar for further treatment.

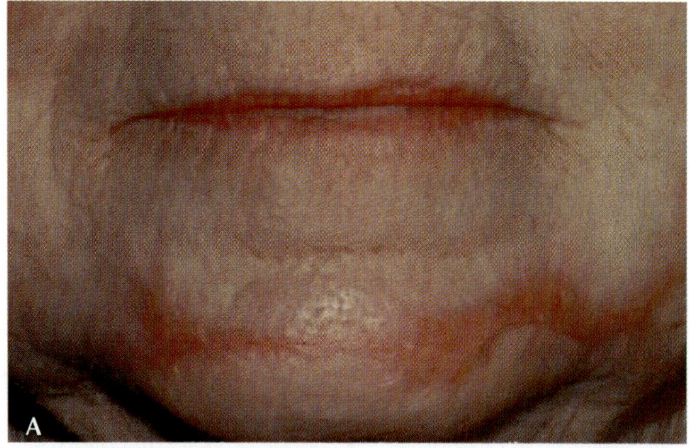

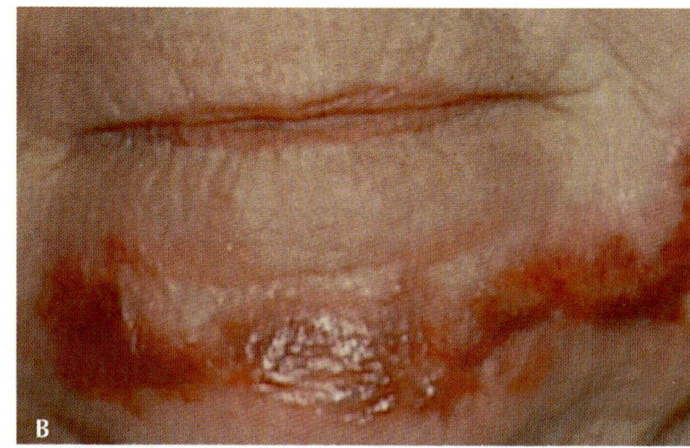

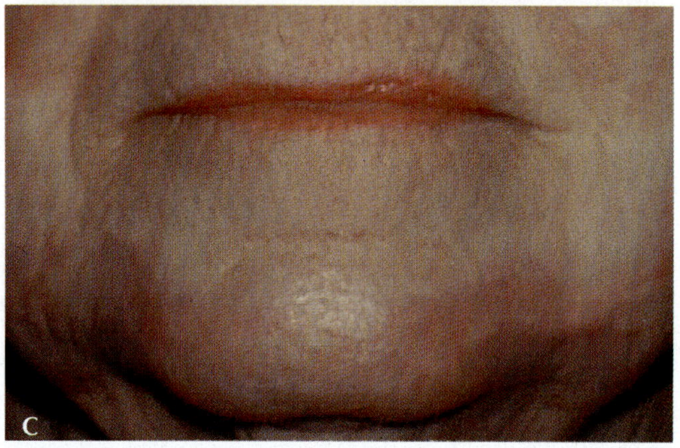

Figure 32–2. Hypertrophic burn scars in a 55-year-old woman before (A) and immediately after (B) 585-nm pulsed dye laser treatment showing expected purpuric tissue response. (C) Improvement of scars noted 8 weeks following second laser treatment (fluence, 4.5 to 5.0 J/cm^2, pulse duration, 1.5 millisecond, spot size 10 mm).

High-Energy, Pulsed, or Scanned CO$_2$ Laser

The new pulsed or scanned CO$_2$ lasers can ablate or vaporize thin layers of skin layer by layer, enabling "sculpting" of atrophic scars (Fig. 32–3). As described earlier, a much narrower zone of cutaneous thermal damage is produced by the new pulsed systems compared with the older CW systems. Several pulsed and scanned CO$_2$ laser systems are currently available for cutaneous resurfacing, and they have separate guidelines for use. When used properly, each of these laser systems has been shown to yield clinically equivalent results despite differences in depth of vaporization and levels of residual thermal damage.[39]

In general, each laser system can be used at maximum energy (up to 500 mJ) with short pulse widths ($<$ 1 millisecond) to achieve tissue vaporization with minimal residual thermal damage to the surrounding skin. After each laser pass, during which the laser light interacts with the skin and produces a puff of steam (vaporized tissue), the partially desiccated, residual tissue is removed with saline-soaked gauze. Additional laser passes are delivered until the desired clinical result is obtained. In addition to bloodless tissue vaporization, CO$_2$ laser resurfacing has been noted to produce immediate skin tightening due to the thermal denaturation of type-I collagen. It is believed that the combination of tissue ablation and collagen shrinkage accounts for the extensive collagen remodeling and improvement in surface irregularities seen after laser resurfacing.[32]

The entire cosmetic unit should be treated to reduce the possibility of skin texture, color, or tonal irregularities. When an isolated atrophic scar is present, spot resurfacing can be performed. First, scars are deepithelialized across their entire breadth (including the atrophic por-

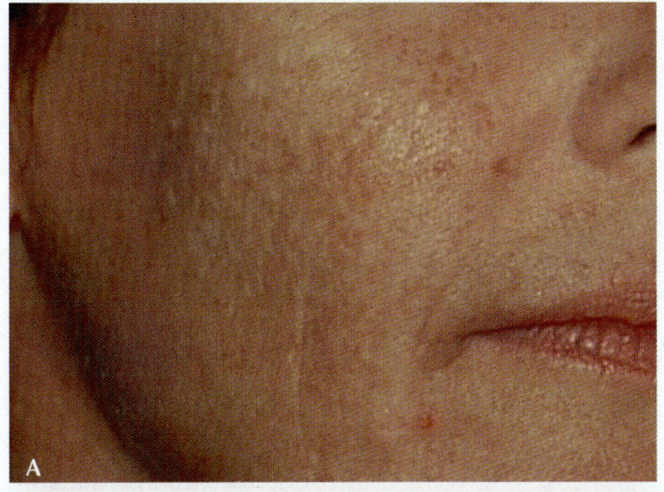
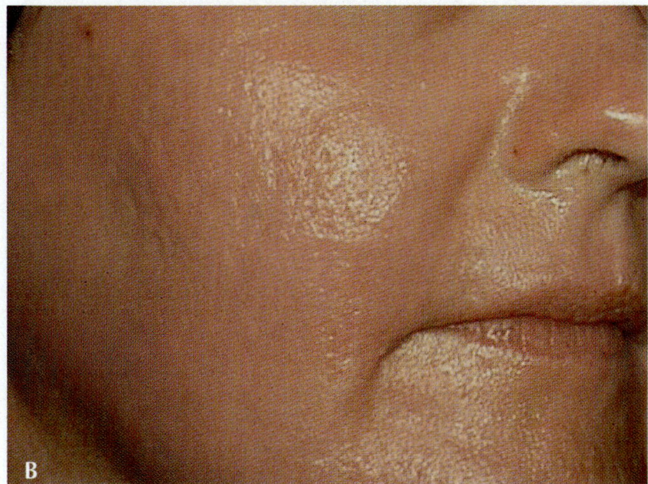
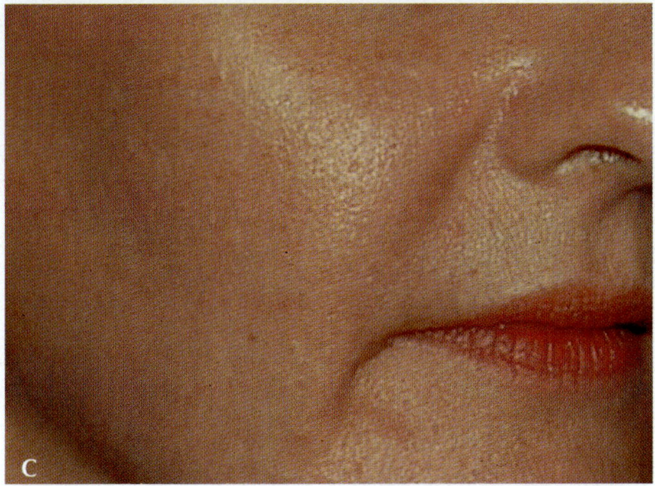

Figure 32–3. Atrophic facial acne scars in a 38-year-old woman before (A) and 1 month after (B) full-face high-energy, pulsed CO_2 laser resurfacing showing typical postoperative erythema. (C) Significant improvement of scars and resolution of erythema 6 months after laser treatment.

tions), followed by "sculpting" of the scar edges with a smaller spot or scan size. When large skin areas require resurfacing, such as atrophic acne scars on the cheeks, it is best to use the largest scanning handpiece available to reduce the time of the procedure.

Immediately after resurfacing, the treated skin appears pale pink and slightly edematous. The erythema and edema intensify over the next 48 to 72 hours. Patients are encouraged to keep the laser-treated areas moist, either with continuous application of healing ointments or with hydrogel wound dressings. Frequent ice pack application and use of antiinflammatories help to minimize swelling. After extensive resurfacing procedures, oral antiherpetics and antibiotics are often prescribed.

Close follow-up of all patients is necessary during the first week after surgery to assess the skin for infection, poor wound healing, or irritation, and treatment should be immediate and aggressive if problems arise. After the first week, patients are instructed in the use of camouflage makeup and maintenance skin care, and subsequent follow-up visits are scheduled on a regular basis (at least monthly) to assess further healing.

Erbium: Yttrium-Aluminum-Garnet Laser

Atrophic scars are resurfaced with the Er:YAG laser in the same manner as with the CO_2 laser. However, wiping the skin between laser passes is not always necessary because of the relative lack of partially desiccated tissue remaining on the skin. The Er:YAG laser is typically used at energies ranging 1 to 35, repetition rates of 7 to 15 Hz, and pulse durations of 200 to 300 milliseconds with a 5- to 7-mm spot size.

Because the Er:YAG laser has a reduced residual thermal effect on the skin and therefore produces less intraoperative pain, intravenous sedation may not be required for superficial procedures. Topical and/or local anesthesia with nerve blocks is usually sufficient. In addition, the postoperative recovery period is shortened, with the time to complete healing reduced from several months to a few weeks. Patients are often able to return to their regular activities within a week of surgery with minimal erythema.

Combination Laser Treatment

A combined approach using a high-energy, pulsed CO_2 laser for scar deepithelialization followed by 585-nm pulsed dye laser irradiation has been shown to improve hypertrophic scars that are not erythematous.[40] One or two CO_2 laser passes are made over the scar using a pulse energy of 500 mJ and 5 W of power with a 3-mm collimated handpiece followed immediately by 585-nm pulsed dye laser irradiation to achieve collagen tightening or tissue shrinkage rather than total scar vaporization, which could lead to scar recurrence.

CONCLUSIONS

Lasers successfully treat a variety of scars. To optimize treatment results, scars need to be identified properly so that the correct laser technology can be employed. Hypertrophic scars and keloids respond best to the 585-nm pulsed dye laser, whereas atrophic scars can be ablated with high-energy, pulsed or scanned CO_2 and Er:YAG laser systems.

When properly used, lasers can achieve significant clinical improvement of such recalcitrant lesions as hypertrophic scars and keloids. Future advances in laser technology as well as the addition of concomitant therapies may further improve clinical results. It appears that by enhancing the remodeling phase of wound healing, scars can be favorably influenced and may even be prevented. Laser surgery may best be able to accomplish this goal using both direct (vaporization, collagen shrinkage) and indirect (microvascular destruction).

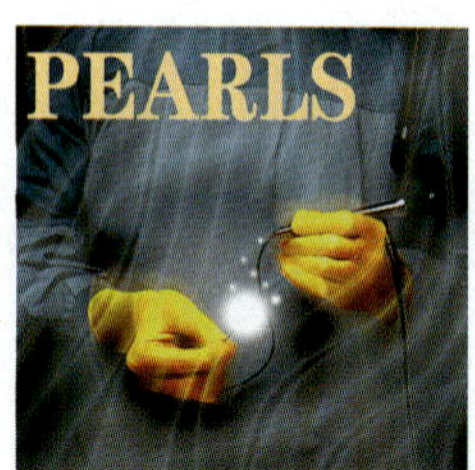

- Although the term *keloid* is often used synonymously with the term *hypertrophic scar*, the two lesions are significantly different. For example, keloids grow beyond the original wound margins, whereas hypertrophic scar tissue usually occurs within wound boundaries.
- Easily controlled, high-energy, pulsed. CO_2 laser systems have improved the treatment of atrophic scars from acne, chickenpox, surgery, and trauma with fewer significant side effects than older CW CO_2 systems. The newer Er:YAG lasers also show promise for the treatment of shallow atrophic scars.
- A patient's keloid tendencies need to be evaluated. If a patient is known to be keloid-prone, a laser test site should be considered prior to laser resurfacing of atrophic scars. Treatment should be delayed at least 6 months after a course of oral isotretinoin to avoid hypertrophic scarring. There is no increased risk of scar worsening or new scar development using the pulsed-dye laser on keloid-prone patients.

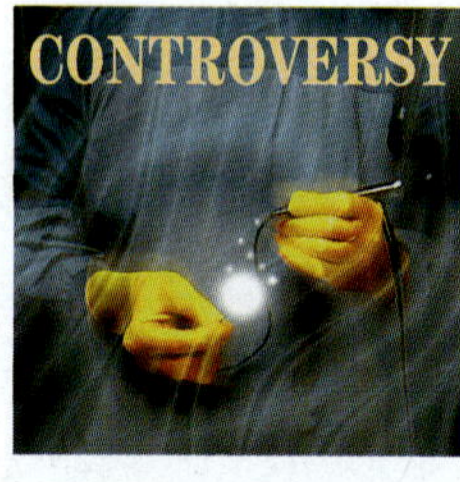

- The etiologic mechanisms of scar clearance after laser treatment are still unknown. However, the increase in the number of tissue mast cells in pulsed dye laser-treated areas suggests one possible explanation for scar clearance. Also, histamine's role in laser-induced scar improvement is yet to be determined but has been shown to alternately influence collagen synthesis in a positive and a negative manner.

REFERENCES

1. Omo-Dare P. Yoruban contributions to the literature on keloids. J Natl Med Assoc. 1973;65:367–372.

2. Alibert JLM. Quelques recherches sur la cheloide. Mem Soc Medicale d'Emulation. 1817:744.

3. Rockwell WB, Cohen IK, Ehrlich HP. Keloids and hypertrophic scars: a comprehensive review. Plast Reconstr Surg. 1989;84:827–837.

4. Rudolph R. Wide spread scars, hypertrophic scars, and keloids. Clin Plast Surg. 1987;14:253–260.

5. Alster TS. Laser treatment of hypertrophic scars. Facial Plast Surg Clin North Am. 1996;4:267–274.

6. Datubo-Brown DD. Keloids: a review of the literature. Br J Plast Surg. 1990;43:70–77.

7. Muir IFK. On the nature of keloids and hypertrophic scars. Br J Plast Surg. 1990;43:61–69.

8. Murray JC, Pollack SV, Pinnell SR. Keloids and hypertrophic scars. Clin Dermatol. 1984;2:121–133.

9. Russell JD, Witt WS. Cell size and growth characteristics of cultured fibroblasts isolated from normal and keloid tissue. Plast Reconstr Surg. 1976;57:207–212.

10. Apfelberg DB, Maser MR, Lash H, et al. Preliminary results of argon and carbon dioxide laser treatment of keloid scars. Lasers Surg Med. 1984;4:283–290.

11. Henderson DL, Cromwell TA, Mes LG. Argon and carbon dioxide laser treatment of hypertrophic and keloid scars. Lasers Surg Med. 1984;3:271–277.

12. Kantor GR, Wheeland RG, Bailin PL, et al. Treatment of earlobe keloids with carbon dioxide laser excision: a report of 16 cases. J Dermatol Surg Oncol. 1985;11:1063–1067.

13. Hulsbergen-Henning JP, Roskam Y, van Gemert[B5]MJ. Treatment of keloids and hypertrophic scars with an argon laser. Lasers Surg Med. 1986;6:72–75.

14. Apfelberg DB, Smith T, Lash H, et al. Preliminary report on use of the neodymium-YAG laser in plastic surgery. Lasers Surg Med. 1987;7:189–198.

15. Sherman R, Rosenfeld H. Experience with the Nd:YAG laser in the treatment of keloid scars. Ann Plast Surg. 1988;21:231–235.

16. Apfelberg DB, Maser MR, White DN, et al. Failure of carbon dioxide laser excision of keloids. Lasers Surg Med. 1989;9:382–388.

17. Stern JC, Lucente FE. Carbon dioxide laser excision of earlobe keloids: a prospective study and critical analysis of existing data. Arch Otolaryngol Head Neck Surg. 1989;115:1107–1111.

18. Lim TC, Tan WT. Carbon dioxide laser for keloids. Plast Reconstr Surg. 1991;88:111.

19. Norris JE. The effect of carbon dioxide laser surgery on the recurrence of keloids. Plast Reconstr Surg. 1991;87:44–49.

20. Alster TS, Kurban AK, Grove GL, et al. Alteration of argon laser-induced scars by the pulsed dye laser. Lasers Surg Med. 1993;13:368–373.

21. Alster TS. Improvement of erythematous and hypertrophic scars by the 585-nm pulsed dye laser. Ann Plast Surg. 1994;32:186–190.

22. Alster TS, Williams CM. Treatment of keloid sternotomy scars with 585-nm flashlamp-pumped pulsed dye laser. Lancet. 1995;345:1198–1200.

23. Alster TS, McMeekin TO. Improvement of facial acne scars by the 585-nm flashlamp-pumped pulsed dye laser. J Am Acad Dermatol. 1996;35:79–81.

24. Alster TS, Nanni CA. Pulsed dye laser treatment of hypertrophic burn scars. Plast Reconstr Surg. 1998;102:2190–2195.

25. Dierickx C, Goldman MP, Fitzpatrick RE. Laser treatment of erythematous/hypertrophic and pigmented scars in 26 patients. Plast Reconstr Surg. 1995;95:84–90.

26. Goldman MP, Fitzpatrick RE. Laser treatment of scars. Dermatol Surg. 1995;21:685.

27. Garrett AB, Dufresne RG, Ratz JL, Berlin AJ. Carbon dioxide laser treatment of pitted acne scarring. J Dermatol Surg Oncol. 1990;16:737–740.

28. Fitzpatrick RE, Goldman MP, Ruiz-Esparza J. Clinical advantages of the CO_2 laser superpulsed mode. J Dermatol Surg Oncol. 1994;20:449–456.

29. Ho CH, Nguyen Q, Lowe NJ, et al. Laser resurfacing in pigmented skin. J Dermatol Surg Oncol. 1995;21:1035–1037.

30. Alster TS, West TB. Resurfacing of atrophic facial scars with a high-energy, pulsed carbon dioxide laser. Dermatol Surg. 1996;22:151–155.

31. Alster TS. Laser scar revision. In: Alster TS, Apfelberg DB, eds. Cosmetic Laser Surgery (2nd Edition). New York: John Wiley & Sons; 1999:227–244.

32. Walia S, Alster TS. Prolonged clinical and histological effects from CO_2 laser resurfacing of atrophic acne scars. Dermatol Surg. 1999;25:926–930.

33. Alster TS. Laser revision of scars. In: Harahap M., ed. Surgical Techniques for Cutaneous Scar Revision. New York: Marcel Dekker, Inc.; 2000:171–184.

34. Alster TS. Clinical and histologic evaluation of six erbium:YAG lasers for cutaneous resurfacing. Laser Surg Med. 1999;24:87–92.

35. Kaufmann R, Hibst R. Pulsed erbium:YAG laser ablation in cutaneous surgery. Lasers Surg Med. 1996;19:324–330.

36. Nemeth AJ, Miller I, Glass LF, et al. Erbium:YAG laser for acne scarring/resurfacing. Lasers Surg Med. 1997; suppl 9:32.

37. Alster TS. Cutaneous resurfacing with CO_2 and erbium:YAG lasers: preoperative, intraoperative, and postoperative considerations. Plast Reconstr Surg. 1999;103:619–632.

38. McCraw JB, McCraw JA, McMellin A, Bentacourt N. Prevention of unfavorable scars using early pulsed dye laser treatments: a preliminary report. Ann Plast Surg. 1999;42:7–14.

39. Alster TS, Nanni CA, William CM. Comparison of four CO_2 resurfacing lasers: a clinical and histopathologic evaluation. Dermatol Surg. 1999;25:153–159.

40. Alster TS, Lewis AB, Rosenbach A. Laser scar revision: comparison of CO_2 laser vaporization with and without simultaneous pulsed dye laser. Dermatol Surg. 1998;24:1299–1302.

CHAPTER 33

Treatment of Stretch Marks

W. GREGORY CHERNOFF

Cutaneous striae, more commonly known as *stretch marks*, are a cosmetically undesirable common skin condition that rarely causes significant medical morbidity but can be a source of distress to patients. The most common areas for which patients seek improvement are the breast, abdomen, hips, and thighs. Although common, striae remain poorly understood clinically.

There is a significant amount of literature on the pathophysiology of stretch marks. Troisier and Menetrier first described the clinical condition in 1889.[1] In the early 1900s, it was observed that striae often were associated with such debilitating conditions as rheumatic fever, typhoid fever, tuberculosis, and other chronic infections.[2] Therefore, the etiology of striae was questioned, and hypotheses associating them with malnutrition, protein loss, toxic states, and general debilitation arose. Striae occurred most commonly during pregnancy and became known generally as *striae gravidarum*.[3] Observations that adolescents of both sexes developed striae not necessarily associated with obesity provoked more questions concerning etiology.[4,5] In 1976, Moretti noted striae in cachectic states such as tuberculosis and typhoid fever, reinforcing what had been noticed in the early 1900s.[6] Striae were also seen with intense slimming diets.

Regardless of the etiology, stretch marks, once initiated, undergo clinically recognizable stages of evolution. Early on, they are pink to violaceous in color without noticeable surface depression. As the color fades, the lesions develop a normal skin color or often appear lighter than normal skin and are accompanied by depression of the surface and the development of linear surface wrinkles. Once striae reach this stage, they are termed *atrophic*.

The clinical evolution of stretch marks can be likened histologically to that of scar formation or of wound healing. Dermal collagen and elastic fibers normally provide strength, resiliency, and elasticity to the skin, and it has been suggested that the extracellular matrix is somehow altered or damaged in stretch marks. However, the cellular and extracellular matrix alterations that mediate the clinical appearance of stretch marks remain poorly understood.

ANATOMY

Stress rupture of the connective tissue framework commonly has been given as an explanation of striae,[7–11] and parallel arrangement of elastic fibers was noted by Ebert in 1933.[12] Modern authorities have published contradictory views on the microscopic anatomy. Chernosky and Knox in 1964 considered that elastic fibers were entirely absent in the centermost point of the stria.[8] They found the elastic fibers to be coiled periph-

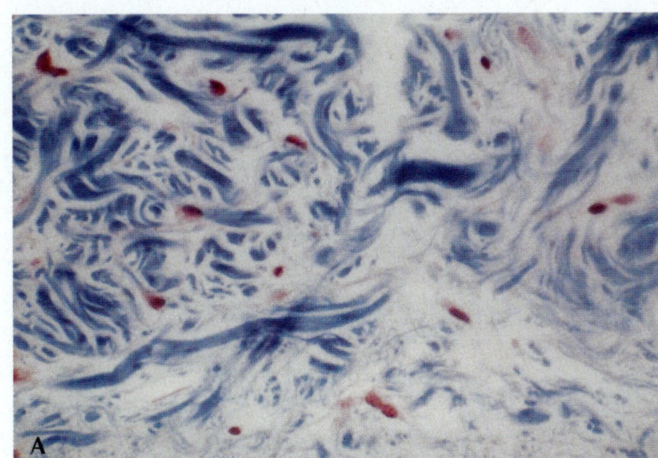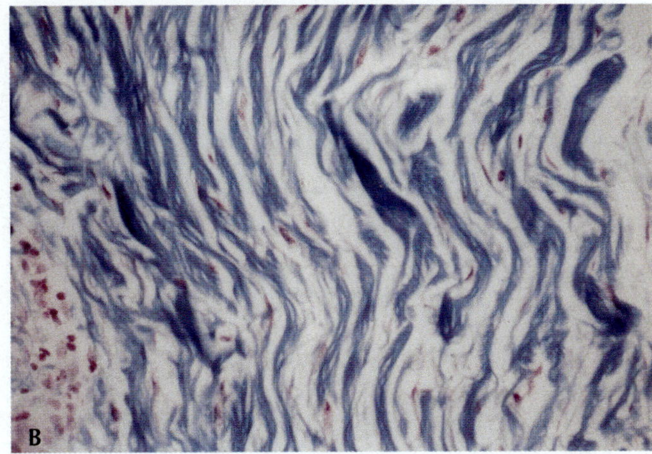

Figure 33–1. (A) Appearance of collagen before CO_2 laser treatment. Note haphazard arrangement. (B) Appearance 1 year after CO_2 laser treatment with a 3-mm spot, 350 mJ, 5 W, and two passes. Note collagen realignment.

erally and clumped in the deeper dermis with gradual transition to normal skin and the elastic fibers becoming more superficial near the margin. Montgomery believed that rupture of the elastic fibers caused the fragmented and curled appearance.[9] Pinkus et al. in 1966 described numerous thin elastic fibers that were qualitatively altered but present.[13]

While many authors were focusing on degradation of the elastic fiber network, others emphasized the changes in collagen.[13] Reports described numerous compact, thin bundles of collagen arranged parallel to the surface. This was a striking deviation from the normal organization of collagen bundles. In 1976, Burg questioned whether striae were a type of scar, representing the healed phase of earlier disintegration of connective tissue.[14]

In 1980, Arem and Kischer performed a scanning electron microscopic study of striae revealing many tight, layered bundles of collagen arranged in variable sheets.[15] No mention was made of the electron microscopic appearance of elastic fibers. By light microscopy, however, the elastic fibers were found to be greatly reduced and fragmented. The authors speculated that striae were a form of scarring that followed the rupture and separation of collagen, with the resulting void being filled by newly synthesized, realigned collagen (Fig. 33–1).

Recent light and electron microscopic studies revealed the following histologic characteristics: The epidermis directly over the stria consistently appears flattened and thinned. There is a generalized loss of rete pegs. The area occupied by the stria shows a loose bundling of thin, isosynophnic collagen in disarray. The collagen bundles appear to replace the papillary dermis beneath the epidermis. Typically, the lower depth of the stria is at the midpapillary dermis. There is rarely a sharp transition zone between the stria and normal tissue. Blood vessels, sweat glands, and hair follicles are not apparent. Elastic fibers, while normally numerous and close together, are usually fine and straight, mimicking the pattern of the collagen bundles. The normal curling appearance seen in non-strial skin is absent.[16]

LASER TREATMENT

Therapy for stretch marks generally has been unsatisfactory. There is no widely accepted surgical procedure for improving the appearance of stretch marks, and studies using topical tretinoin have yielded variable results.[17–19]

Recent advances in multiwavelength laser therapy have renewed interest in the treatment of stretch marks. The most common laser wavelengths used have been those of the exfoliating carbon dioxide (CO_2) and erbium:yttrium-aluminum-garnet (Er:YAG) lasers, vascular lasers, and now the nonablative, nonexfoliating lasers.[20,21] On average, treatments are spaced 6 weeks apart, regardless of location on the body. Box 33–1 lists the most commonly used laser parameters for each wavelength and the appropriate treatment regimens for immature striae.

While the histologic appearance of stretch marks is bewildering, all striae appear to follow a similar clinical pattern. Early on, they are similar in appearance to an early scar with increased vascularity and erythema. If striae are seen at an early stage, it is beneficial to begin therapy with a vascular laser. I have used either a 585- or a 532-nm laser (Fig. 33–2). The stretch marks are treated aggressively in an effort to decrease the vascularity to the region. Repeated treatments have produced some softening of the striae as well as improvement in skin tone and texture. However, hypopigmentation of the involved area has been a problem with vascular laser therapy.

If the striae are mature or in the atrophic state, it is possible to induce a hypervascular state by using an exfo-

liating laser such as the Er:YAG or CO_2 laser. Box 33–2 outlines laser therapy for mature striae. With fluences similar to those used for the treatment of atrophic scars, the epidermis is removed, and usually a second pass is

Box 33–1. Lasers for Immature Striae (Reddened, Rich Vasculature)	
532-nm green	Pulse width: 50 ms
	Fluence: 18–30 J/cm²
	4-mm spot
	Endpoint: erythema, purpura
	or
585-nm yellow	Fluence: 10–12 J/cm²
	5 × 7 mm oval spot
	Endpoint: erythema, purpura
	or
1320-nm Nd:YAG	Dynamic cooling-20-ms duration with 30-ms delay
	Fluence: 32 J/cm²
	Endpoint: surface temp 45°C

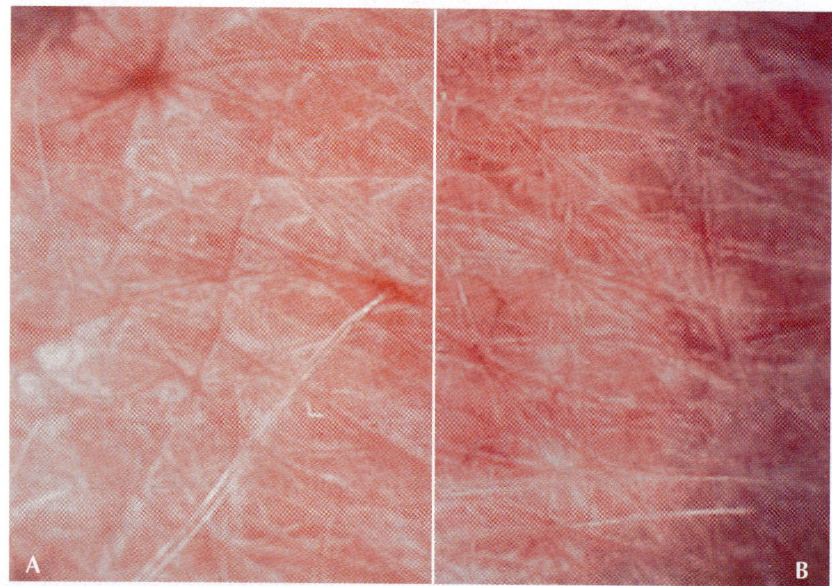

Figure 33–2. (A) Cosmax camera view of preoperative immature striae. Note increased vascularity. (B) Appearance after treatment with a 532-nm laser with a 4-mm spot size, 50-millisecond pulse width, 24 J/cm², and two passes. There were four treatments spaced 6 weeks apart.

<table>
<tr><td colspan="2">Box 33–2. Laser Treatment for Mature Striae
(Stepladder, No Redness)</td></tr>
<tr><td>1. Isolagen</td><td>Three injections; then wait 6 weeks.</td></tr>
<tr><td>2. 1320-nm Nd:YAG</td><td>Dynamic cooling for 20 ms duration then 30 ms delay
Fluence: 32–36 J/cm^2
Endpoint: erythema</td></tr>
<tr><td>3. If no response:
   Erbium YAG

   CO$_2$</td><td>1 J/cm^2
2 passes
Endpoint: removal of epidermis
150 mJ; 100 watts
Square pattern; density 5 (30%)
Endpoint: removal of epidermis; visible shrinkage.</td></tr>
<tr><td>4. When re-epithelialized</td><td>Utilize immature striae protocol (see Box 33–1).</td></tr>
</table>

performed, yielding immediate contracture of the treatment region (Figs. 33–3 and 33–4). Additional treatment with a vascular laser during the prolonged erythematous stage can create further softening of the region (Figs. 33–5 and 33–6). The patient must be advised that the resulting erythema can be prolonged, at times lasting 6 months to 1 year. Once again, however, hypopigmentation has been a problem in this patient population. Patients are also advised that an acceptable endpoint involves softening of the atrophic "stepladder" appearance of the stretch mark and that complete resolution of the area is not a realistic expectation.

The recent advent of the nonexfoliating, nonablative laser, such as the 1320-nm CoolTouch YAG laser (NewStar Lasers, Auburn, CA) and the 980-nm diode laser, has provided an interesting alternative in the ongoing management of striae (Figs. 33–7 and 33–8). The nonablative lasers stimulate fibroblast growth by creating a wound-healing response. This is done by heating dermal collagen to 80°C at a depth of 100 mm while keeping surface temperature between 40 and 45°C. This induces a permanent healing response, and subsequent new collagen formation yields a softening of the stria similar to that produced by the vascular laser or the ablative exfoliating lasers.

Much has been learned over the past 5 years about how to soften striae. Continued research is required on the histopathology of striae, their etiologic basis, and the fine-tuning of therapeutic regimens. Multiwavelength laser therapy has a promising role in the treatment of this common condition.

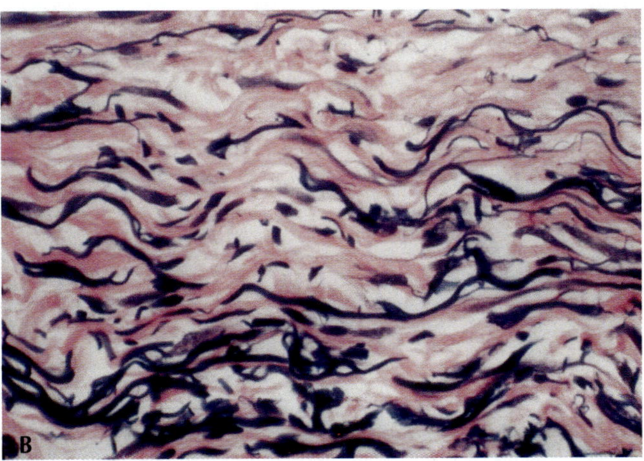

Figure 33–3. (A) Appearance of elastin before CO$_2$ laser treatment. (B) Appearance 1 year after CO$_2$ laser treatment with a 3-mm spot, 350 mJ, 5 W, and two passes. Note elastin realignment.

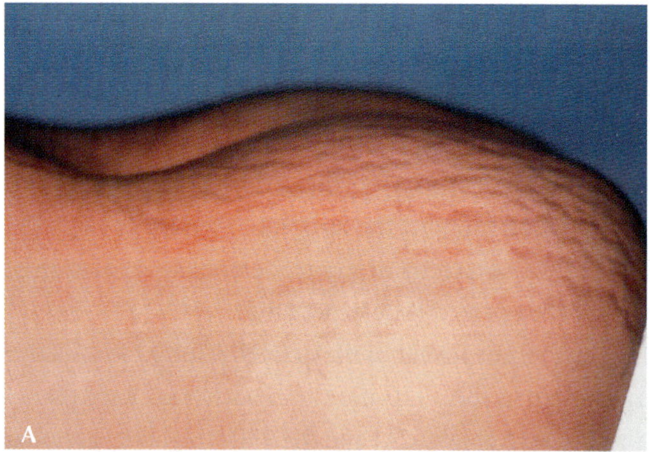

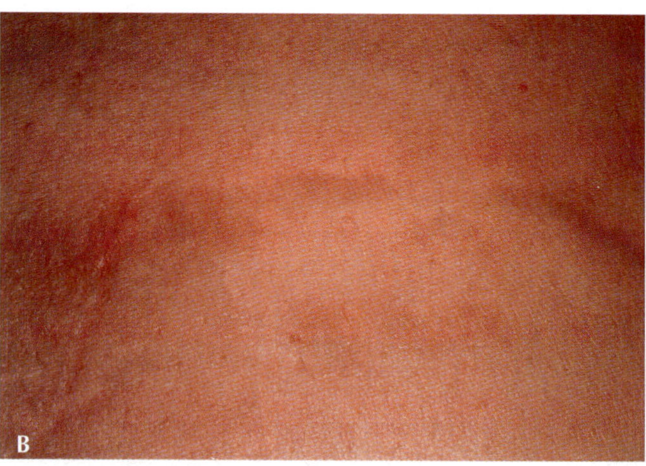

Figure 33–4. (A) Appearance before treatment. (B) Appearance 1 year after CO_2 laser treatment with a 3-mm spot, 350 mJ, 5 W, and two passes.

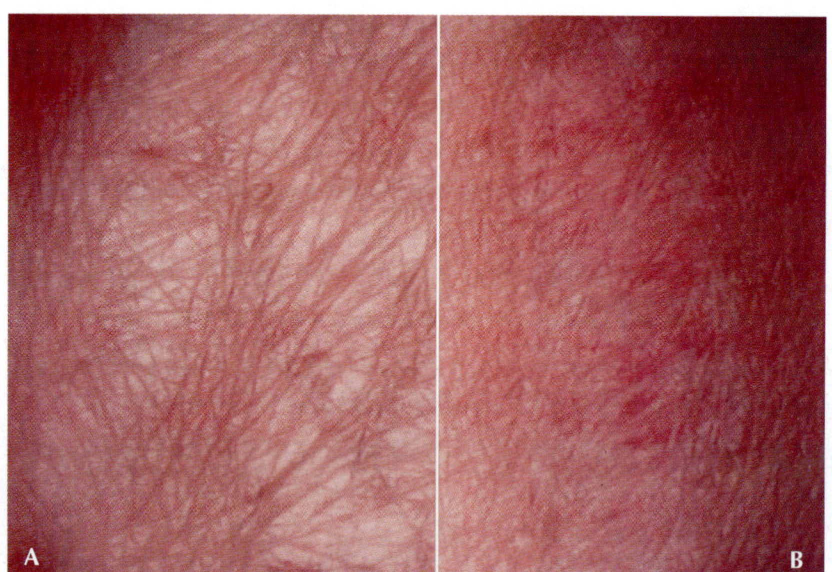

Figure 33–5. (A) Cosmax camera view 3 months after CO_2 laser treatment and before vascular laser treatment. (B) Appearance 3 months after vascular laser treatment.

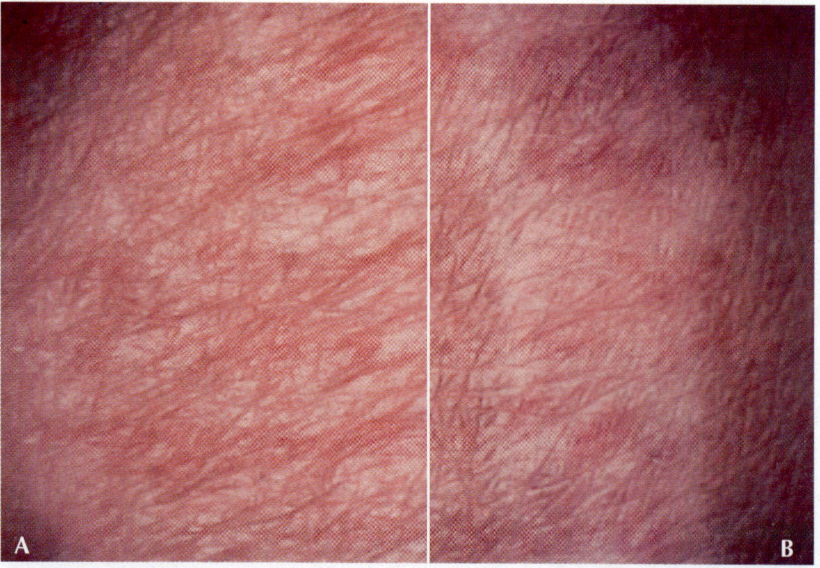

Figure 33–6. (A) Appearance 6 months after vascular laser treatment. (B) Appearance 1 year after vascular laser treatment.

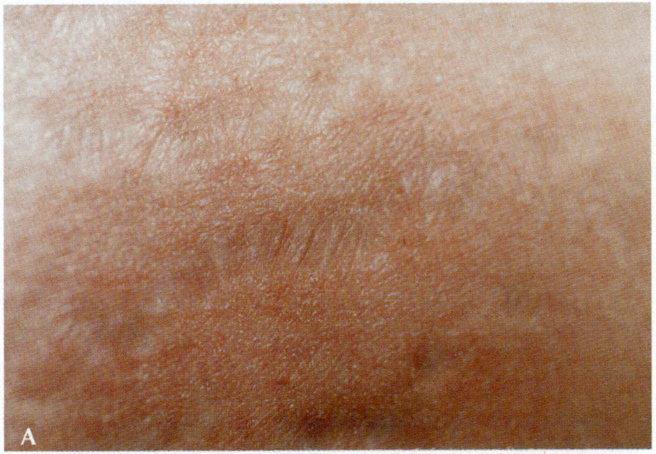

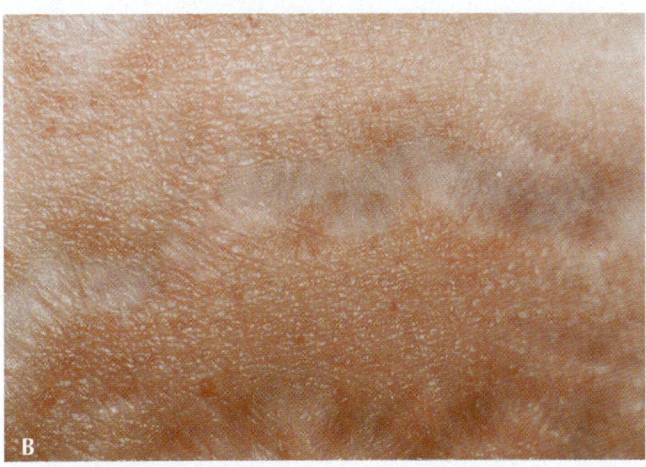

Figure 33–7. (A) Preoperative appearance. (B) Appearance 1 year after CoolTouch laser treatment. The CoolTouch is a

1320-nmYAG laser used with a 5-mm spot size, 32 J/cm^2, and two passes. There were four treatments spaced 6 weeks apart.

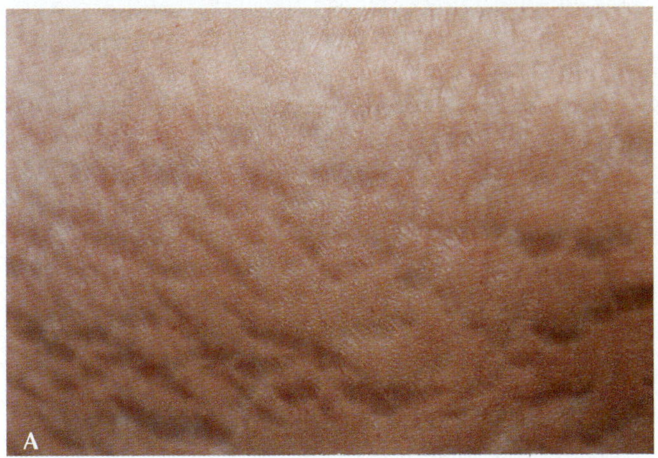

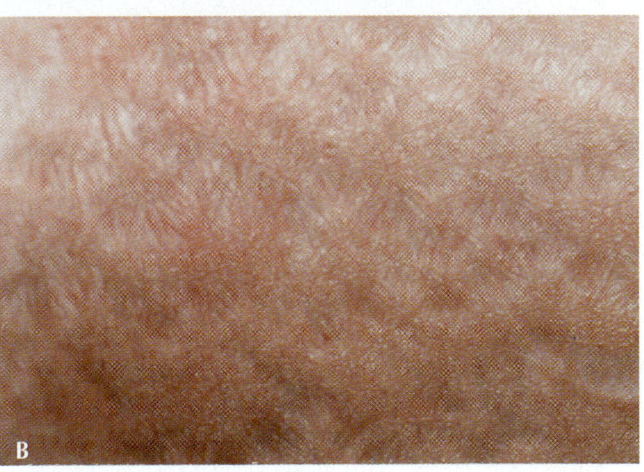

Figure 33–8. (A) Preoperative appearance. (B) Appearance 1 year after Isolagen injections and CoolTouch laser treatment. There were three Isolagen injections spaced 2 weeks apart.

The CoolTouch laser employed a 5-mm spot size at 32 J/cm with two passes. There were four treatments spaced 6 weeks apart.

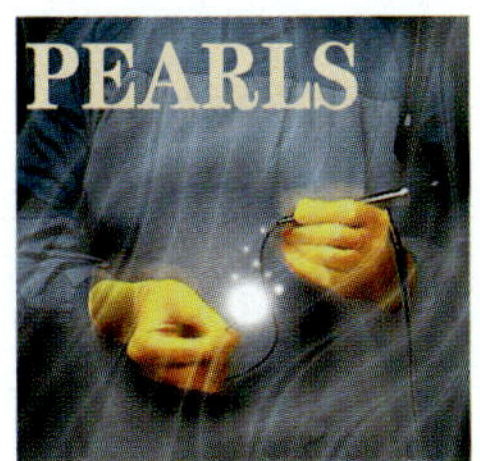

- Dermal collagen and elastic fibers provide strength, resiliency, and elasticity to the skin. Although the alterations of these tissues that mediate the appearance of stretch marks remain poorly understood, the histological nature of striae may be compared with that of scar formation or wound healing.

- There is rarely a sharp transition zone between the stria and normal tissue, but blood vessels, sweat glands, and hair follicles are not apparent in striated tissue.

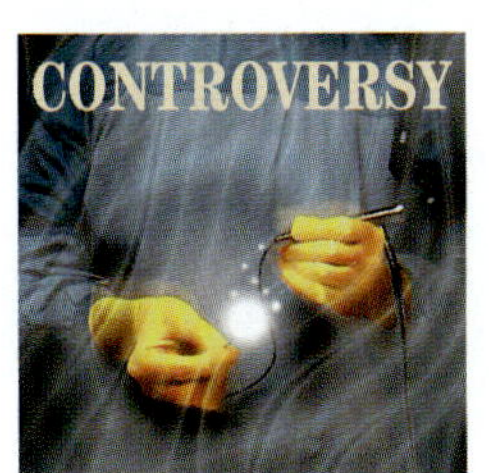

- There are contradictory views on the microscopic anatomy of stretch marks. Some studies have found that elastic fibers were entirely absent in the centermost point of the stria, whereas others have found peripherally coiled and clumped elastic fibers in the deeper dermis with gradual transition to normal skin. Some believe that rupture of the elastic fibers causes the fragmented and curled appearance.

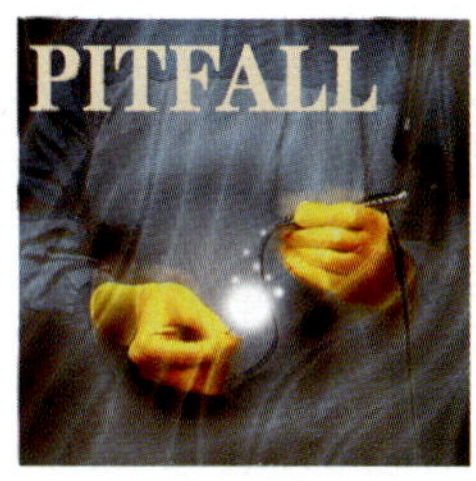

- Erythema can be prolonged, sometimes lasting up to a year, and complete removal of stretch marks is not a realistic expectation. Patients need to realize that the goal is a softening of the atrophic "stepladder" appearance of the stretch mark.

- Hypopigmentation of the striated area has been a problem with vascular laser therapy, as well as with Er:YAG and CO2 laser therapy.

REFERENCES

1. Troisier E, Menetrier P. Histologie des vergetures. *Ann Gynecol.* 1889;31:206.
2. Sibley WK. Striae atrophiae. *Proc R Soc Med.* 1923–1924;17:44.
3. Poidevin LOS, Sydney MB. Striae gravidarum—their relation to adrenal cortical hyperfunction. *Lancet.* 1959;2:436.
4. Sisson WR. Colored striae in adolescent children. *J Pediatr.* 1954;45:520.
5. Simkin B, Arce R. Steroid excretion in obese patients with colored abdominal striae. *N Engl J Med.* 1962;266:1031.
6. Moretti G, Rebora A, Guarrera M. Striae distensae: How and why they are found. In: Moretti G, Rebora A, eds. *Striae Distensae.* Milan: Brocades; 1976:9.
7. Gans O, Steigleder GH. *Histologie der Hautkrankheiten.* 2nd ed. Vol. I. Berlin: Springer; 1925:24.
8. Chernosky ME, Knox JM. Atrophic striae after occlusive corticosteroid therapy. *Arch Dermatol.* 1964;90:15.
9. Montgomery H. *Dermatopathology.* New York: Harper & Row;1967:776.
10. Agache P, Ovide MT, Kienzler JL, Laurent R. Mechanical factors in striae distensae. In: *Striae Distensae.* Moreti G, Rebora A, eds. Milan: Brocades; 1976:87.
11. Shuster S. The cause for striae distensae. In: Moretti G, Rebora A, eds. *Striae Distensae.* Milan: Brocades; 22. 1976:97.
12. Ebert MH. Hypertrophic striae distensae. *Arch Dermatol Physiol.* 1933;28:825.
13. Pinkus H, Krech MK, Megregan AH. Histopathology of striae distensae, with special reference to striae and wound healing in the Marfan syndrome. *J Invest Dermatol.* 1966;46:283.
14. Burg G. Histochemistry and cytochemistry of striae distensae. In: Moretti G, Rebora A, eds. *Striae Distensae.* Milan: Brocades; 1976:23.
15. Arem AJ, Kischer CW. Analysis of striae. *Plast Reconstr Surg.* 1980;65:22.
16. Watson RE, Parry EJ, Humphries JD, et al. Fibrillin microfibrils are reduced in skin exhibiting striae distensae. *Brit J Dermatol.* 1998;138(6):931–937.
17. Ash K, Lord J, Zukowski M, McDaniel DH. Comparison of topical therapy for striae alba (20% glycolic acid/0.05% tretinoin versus 20% glycolic acid/10% L ascorbic acid). *Dermatol Surg.* 1998;24(8):849–856.
18. Kang S, Kim KJ, Griffiths CE, et al. Topical tretinoin (retinoic acid) improves early stretch marks. *Arch Dermatol.* 1996;132(5):519–526.
19. Grossman MC. What is new in cutaneous laser research? *Dermatol Clin.* 1997;15(1):1–8.
20. Dzubow LM. Leg veins and stretch marks: Have they seen the light? *Dermatol Surg.* 1996;22(4):321.
21. McDaniel DH, Ash K, Zukowski M. Treatment of stretch marks with the 585-nm flashlamp-pumped pulsed dye laser. *Dermatol Surg.* 1996;22(4):332–337.

CHAPTER 34

Photodynamic Therapy of Skin Cancer

BRUMMETTE DALE WILSON, THOMAS J. DOUGHERTY, AND ALLEN J. OSEROFF

In *photodynamic therapy* (PDT) a patient is given a photosensitizing drug that is activated by light in the presence of oxygen to destroy malignant tumors or other diseased tissues.[1] A number of light sources have been used to activate photosensitizers for PDT, including lasers, light-emitting diodes, and noncoherent light sources.[2] The photosensitizer absorbs light and is excited initially to a singlet state, which converts to a triplet state that transfers its energy to endogenous oxygen, producing cytotoxic singlet oxygen. Photobleaching inactivates the photosensitizer in normal skin, compared with the target tissue, allowing a higher therapeutic ratio.[3]

Although others had experimented in some of the early aspects of PDT,[4,5] the studies by Dougherty et al[6] of the photochemical response of malignant tumors to hematoporphyrin derivatives (HPDs) provided the sustained impetus for the development of effective therapeutic regimens using PDT.

PORFIMER SODIUM

Purification of HPDs led to isolation of an oligomeric ether, porfimer sodium (Photofrin), that accumulates more selectively in tumor compared with normal skin (e.g., ratios of 10:1 for basal cell carcinomas).[1] Light activation causes tumor destruction with relative sparing of normal tissue. Benzoporphyrin derivative (BPD,

Verteporfin) has demonstrated similar selectivity with a tumor-to-normal-skin ratio of 5:1.[7]

Porfimer sodium is administered intravenously, followed by light exposure in 24 to 72 hours.[1] Its absorption peak of 630 nm allows it to penetrate tissue effectively. The primary target with porfimer sodium is the vascular endothelium, resulting in blood flow stasis and thrombosis.[8,9] Because porfimer sodium is relatively selectively retained by both tumor cells and vasculature, tumor ablation occurs by direct tumor destruction and disruption of its vascular supply.[8–13]

CLINICAL RESULTS

Using a porfimer sodium dose of 1 mg/kg and 630-nm laser irradiation with 215 J/cm^2 at 150 mW/cm^2, we have treated more than 980 superficial and nodular basal cell carcinomas. Because of the length of the healing process and because we found further destruction of residual carcinoma over a 3- to 4-month interval after treatment, the initial responses were determined at least 6 months after PDT (Figs. 34–1 and 34–2). For patients with nevobasal cell carcinoma syndrome (NBCCS), the initial complete response (CR) rate was 95% (Fig. 34–3). For the unselected group of carcinomas as a whole, the CR rate was 92%.

We also examined lower porfimer sodium doses of 0.875 and 0.75 mg/kg because decreasing the dose

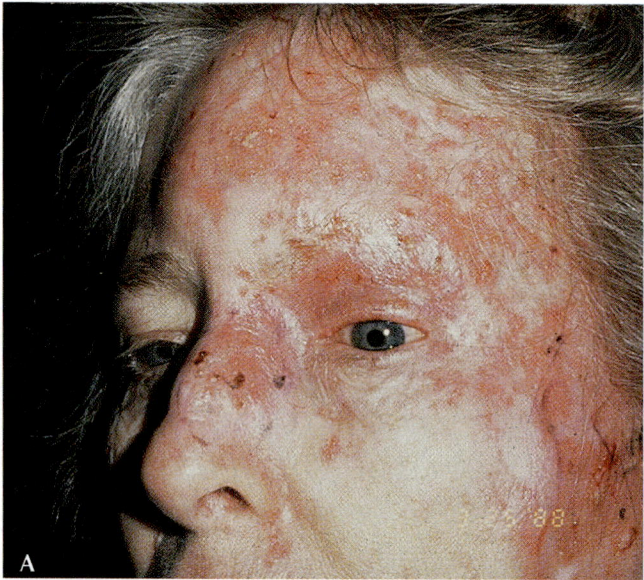

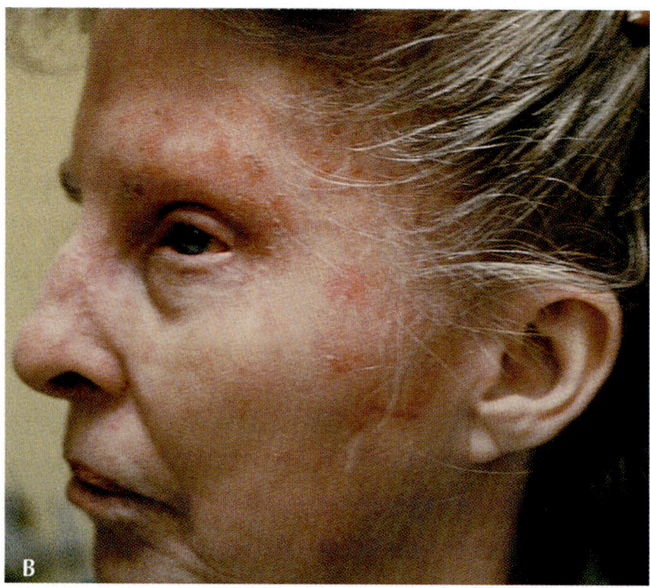

Figure 34–1. (A) Appearance of a 62-year-old patient before PDT with porfimer sodium at the Roswell Cancer Institute Dermatology Clinic. The patient had had a basal cell carcinoma removed from the left forehead 20 years previously. Subsequently, the patient developed extensive areas of superficial basal cell carcinomas on the left forehead, nose, preauricular cheek, and eyebrow. (B) Appearance after multiple treatment sessions. Although small areas of recurrences at the left lateral canthus and left parietal scalp were treated by Mohs' surgery, this patient was tumor free for over 5 years.

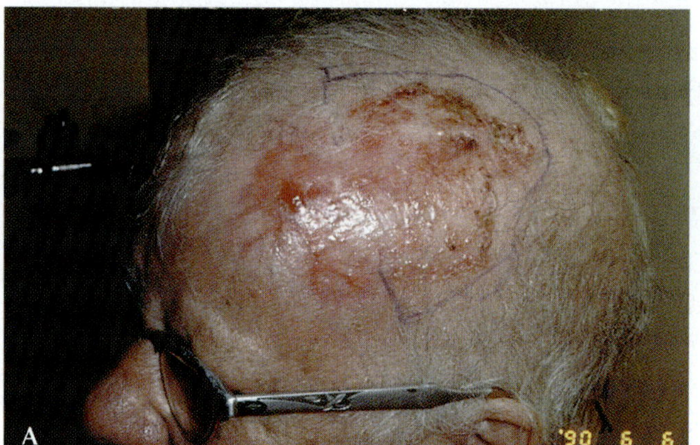

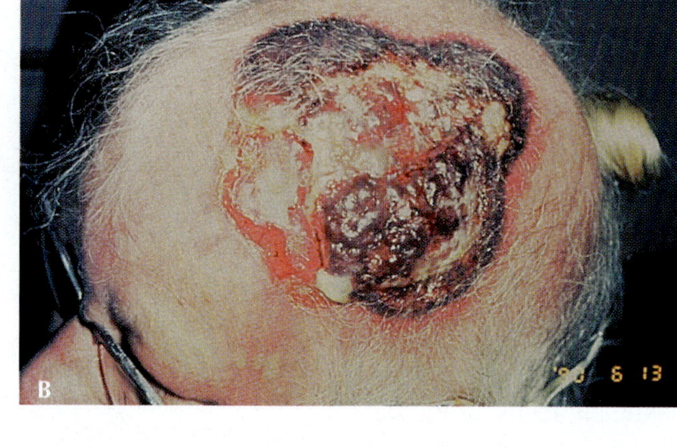

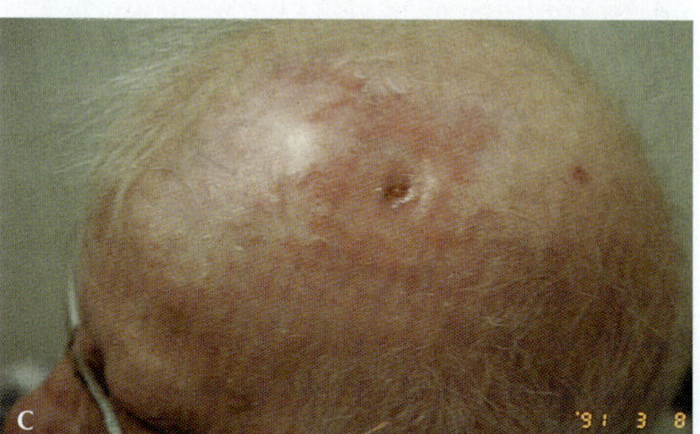

Figure 34–2. (A) Pretreatment appearance of a 72-year-old woman with an extensive morpheaform basal cell carcinoma in the left frontal parietal scalp. Two sessions of PDT with porfimer sodium were performed. (B) There was an extensive phototoxic response with necrosis of the tumor. (C) The patient has been tumor-free for over 5 years.

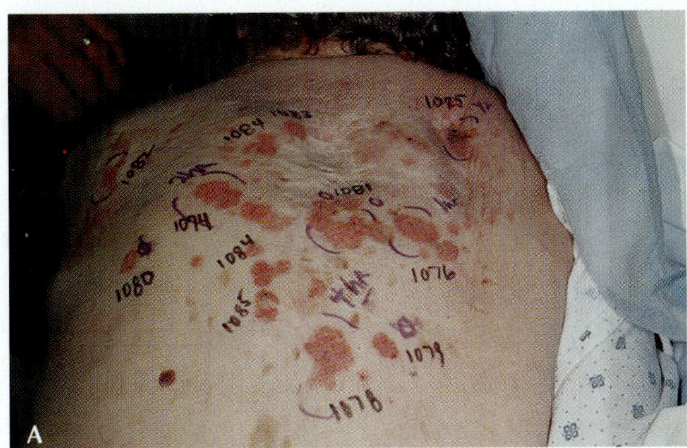

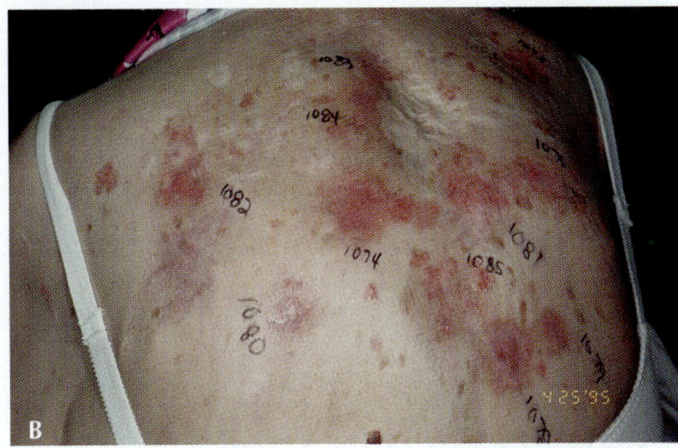

Figure 34–3. (A) Pretreatment appearance of extensive basal cell carcinomas on the back of a patient who presented with nevobasal cell carcinoma syndrome that had been treated over the years by multiple modalities. We treated the numerous basal cell carcinomas on the face, neck, and trunk with PDT with porfimer sodium. (B) Erythematous scars are present 3 months after PDT.

seems to improve selectivity and lower cutaneous phototoxicity. Unfortunately, efficacy also decreased, with initial CR rates of 87% and 72% for doses of 0.875 and 0.75 mg/kg, respectively. Bowen's disease also responds to PDT with porfimer sodium (Fig. 34–4), and the treatment parameters are the same as those for superficial and nodular basal cell carcinomas.[14]

We monitored patients for as long as 5 years after PDT and performed a Kaplan-Meier analysis to establish the recurrence rates. For the entire group of lesions, the

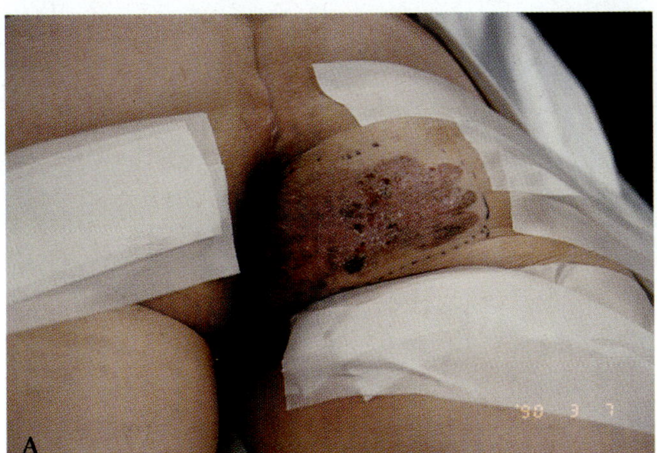

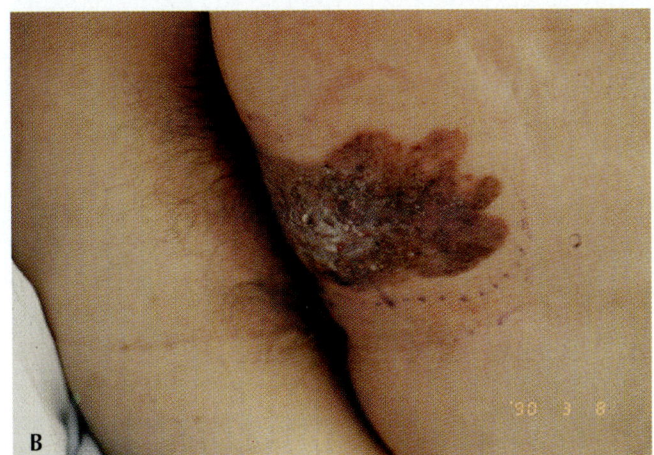

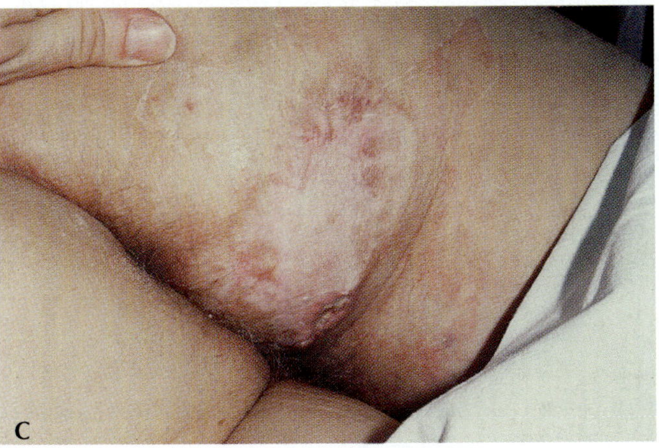

Figure 34–4. (A) Preoperative appearance of extensive Bowen's disease of the buttocks extending to the anus. The perianal region was treated by Mohs' micrographic surgery, and the remaining tumor was treated with PDT using porfimer sodium. (B) Appearance 48 hours after PDT. (C) Appearance 1 year after PDT.

recurrence rate was approximately 5% at 3 years and 10% at 4 years. Again, the NBCCS patients did somewhat better.[14–17]

Thus, the lowest recommended treatment parameters involve 1 mg/kg of porfimer sodium used with fluences of 215 J/cm^2, and this approach gives results that are comparable with those of conventional destructive or excisional modalities but with superior cosmesis and maintenance of function.[15–19]

5-AMINOLEVULINIC ACID

5-Aminolevulinic acid (ALA) is a precursor of the endogenous photosensitizer protoporphyrin IX (PpIX), the penultimate step in the heme synthetic pathway. Because it is bioconverted to heme, the endogenous PpIX produced by exogenous ALA has a short accumulation time in tissue, so there are few problems with cutaneous photosensitization.[20–23] When applied topically, ALA is highly selective for both carcinomas and actinic keratoses because damaged stratum corneum is more permeable to ALA and because dermal connective tissue contains PpIX. The relatively small amount of dermal damage leads to minimal scarring and excellent cosmesis. The drawbacks to PDT with ALA are related to the uncertain and variable depth of penetration in thick lesions and to pain during treatment that generally requires local anesthesia (personal observations).[20–23]

For skin lesions, ALA has been administered topically at various concentrations (10 to 40%), usually with occlusion (3 to 24 hours). Subsequently, the ALA is activated by red light (630 to 635 nm), the peak absorption spectrum of PpIX.[21–26] In addition, irradiated protoporphyrin forms photoproducts that are active in vivo at 670 nm.[27] Published results of ALA use in the treatment of nonmelanoma skin tumors demonstrated recurrence rates ranging from 3 to 41%.[2] The use of different light and drug doses (10 to 40%) as well as different light sources by various investigators contributes to the variation. Oral and gastrointestinal lesions as well as basal cell carcinomas have been treated successfully with systemic ALA.[28–30] Similar to BPD, ALA administration is less dependent on the blood supply than porfimer sodium.[31]

CLINICAL RESULTS

We have examined the use of PDT with topical ALA in patients with basal cell carcinoma, Bowen's disease, and cutaneous lymphoma using 4- to 6-hour and 18- to 24-hour ALA applications under occlusion followed by 635-nm laser irradiation or irradiation with broader-band (590 to 700-nm) light from a filtered halogen lamp.

BASAL CELL CARCINOMA

The largest experience has been with superficial basal cell carcinoma (sBCC), where more than 500 lesions have been treated at the two application times with up to 5 years of follow up (Fig. 34–5). Using 20% ALA, the light doses have ranged from 100 to 300 J/cm^2 at 150

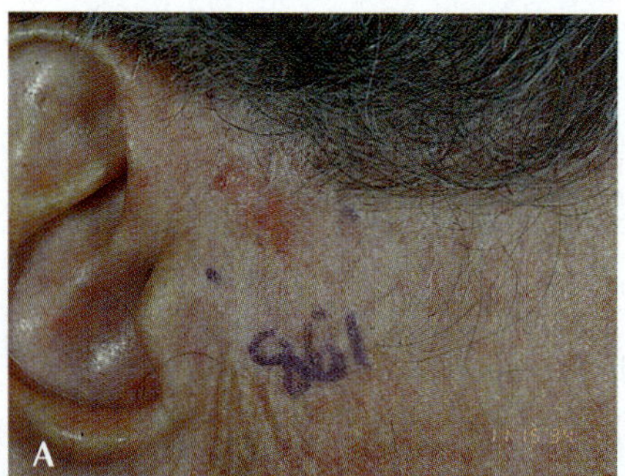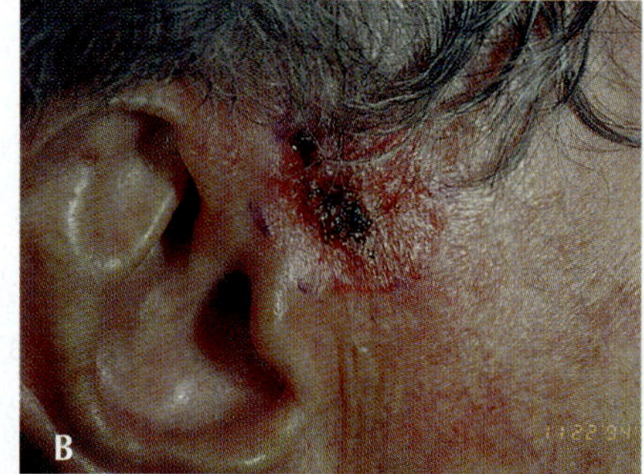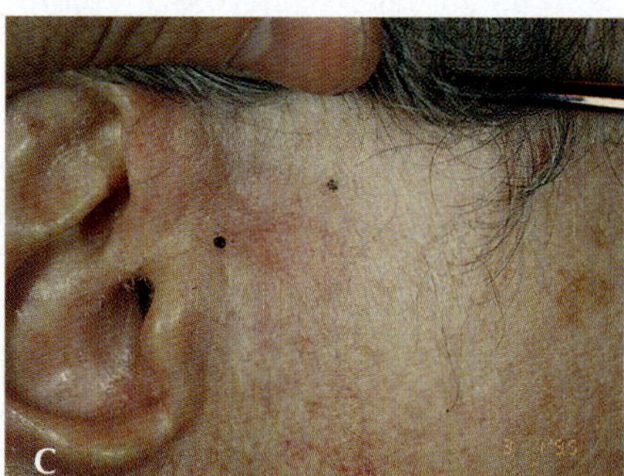

Figure 34–5. (A) Pretreatment appearance of preauricular superficial basal cell carcinoma. (B) Appearance 1 week after PDT with ALA. (C) Appearance 3 months after PDT. The patient has been tumor-free for 3 years.

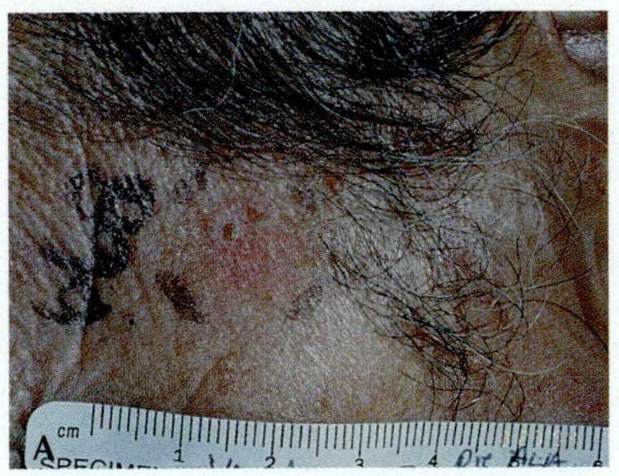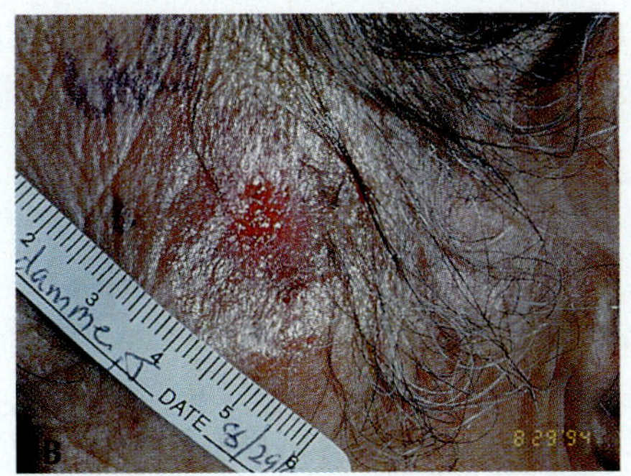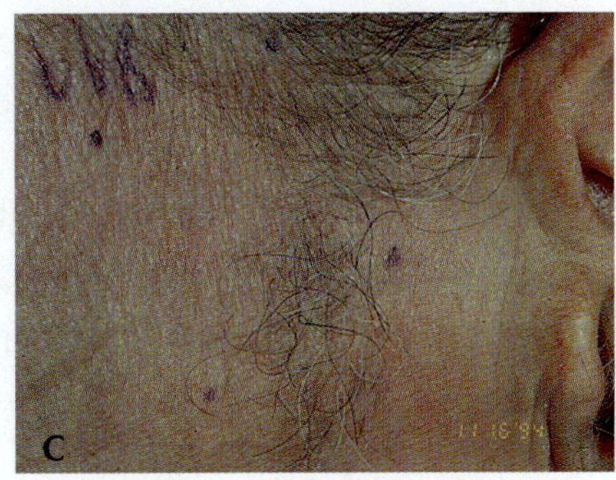

Figure 34–6. (A) Pretreatment appearance of left temporal Bowen's disease. (B) Appearance 1 week after PDT with ALA. (C) Appearance 3 months after PDT. Patient has been tumor-free for 3 years.

mW/cm^2 at 635 nm. Light doses of at least 200 J/cm^2 appear to be necessary for satisfactory responses.

Under these conditions, the median CR rates 6 months after treatment are 100%. The two ALA application times had comparable recurrence rates of less than 5% over the first year, but the 4- to 6-hour application time produces responses that are more durable. Recurrence rates with this application time were about 10 to 15% at 3 years.

Thus, PDT with ALA appears to be not quite as effective as PDT with porfimer sodium or conventional surgery, but it has very high patient acceptance because of the convenience, lack of scarring, and absence of skin photosensitivity. Possibly, more optimized treatment conditions or additional treatments of recurrent disease will produce more durable responses.

Bowen's Disease

Photodynamic therapy with topical ALA for Bowen's disease also appears promising (Fig. 34–6), particularly for large lesions and those in areas such as the shins, where slow healing from surgery or PDT with porfimer sodium may be a concern.

In a series of about 50 lesions, the initial CR rate was about 90%, with all lesions having greater than 90% clearance. The recurrence rate was comparable with that for sBCC. Similar results were reported by Morton et al in a comparison of PDT with cryotherapy in the treatment of Bowen's disease.[14]

Other Cancers

With the current PDT treatment protocol with topical ALA, nodular basal cell carcinomas show typical initial CR rates of less than 90% and comparably high recurrence rates. For thick lesions in particular and those located on the scalp, systemic PDT appears to be a better choice.

Using multiple treatments with PDT doses that spare the epidermis, topical ALA shows promise in the treatment of cutaneous T- and B-cell lymphomas.[32] The results suggest that PDT may have promise as an immunomodulator.

OTHER PHOTOSENSITIZERS

Benzoporphyrin derivative (BPD), which has also been used to treat skin cancers, is injected intravenously and has a rapid uptake in tissue. In fact, treatment can be started on the same day as the injection.[2,33] Benzoporphyrin derivative is activated at an absorption peak of 690 nm, which makes it somewhat more tissue penetrating than porfimer sodium.[2] Administered in liposomes, BPD has been reported to be effective in skin lesions in preliminary studies.[2,33,34] Benzoporphyrin derivative clears the system within a few days, thus minimizing cutaneous phototoxicity. Photosensitization of the skin usually lasts less than a week.

Tin ethiopurpurin ($SnET_2$) is a synthetic chlorophyll analogue that is activated at 660 nm.[2,18,35–37] Photosensitivity is generally short (2 weeks), although some patients have experienced periods of photosensitization lasting much longer (4 to 6 weeks).[10,11]

Other photosensitizers that have been studied include mesotetrahydroxyphenylchlorin (MTHPC), zinc phalocyanine, mono-L-aspartylchlorin-N-Pe6,[38] 2-(1-hexyloxyethyl)-2-devinyl pyropheophorbide-A (HPPH-photochlor),[39] and lutetium texaphyrin PCl 1-0123 (Lu-Tex).[19]

CONCLUSIONS

Photodynamic therapy has proven to be an effective treatment modality. The results obtained when PDT is used appropriately in the treatment of basal cell carcinomas and squamous cell carcinomas in situ[40] appear comparable with those of other standard modalities. In addition, PDT for Kaposi's sarcoma associated with acquired immunodeficiency syndrome has shown limited palliative results. It should be noted, however, that although the U.S. Food and Drug Administration has approved porfimer sodium for use in esophageal cancer and early lung cancer, at present it is still considered an investigational therapy for nonmelanoma skin cancers.

Photodynamic therapy can be used in conjunction with other treatment regimens, including Mohs' surgery, excisional surgery, and radiation therapy, to treat large and multiple tumors, as seen in patients with NBCCS and those with widespread disease. Advances involving the development of new potential sensitizers and light sources will expand the availability and usefulness of PDT as a standard treatment modality.

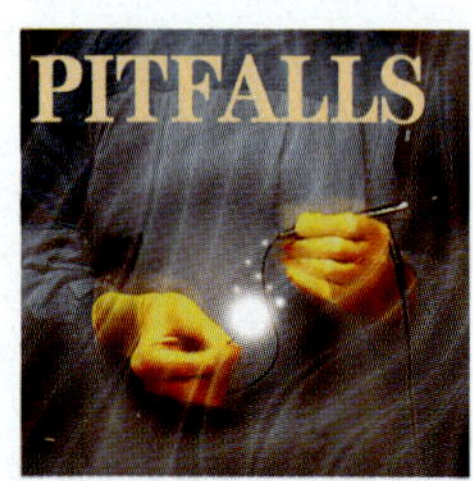

- Lowering the dose of porfimer sodium to 0.875 or 0.75 mg/kg seems to improve selectivity and lower cutaneous phototoxicity but also reduces efficacy. A dose of 1 mg/kg gives results that are comparable with those of conventional destructive or excisional modalities but with superior cosmesis and maintenance of function.

- Drawbacks to PDT with ALA are related to the uncertain and variable depth of penetration in thick lesions and to pain during treatment that generally requires local anesthesia.

- The U.S. Food and Drug Administration has approved porfimer sodium for use in esophageal cancer and early lung cancer, but it is still considered an investigational therapy for nonmelanoma skin cancers.

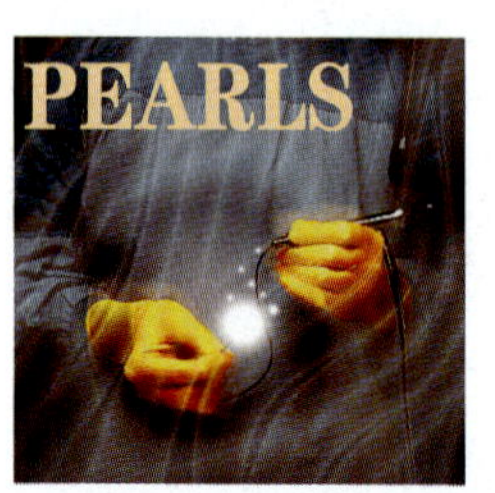

- Because it is bioconverted to heme, ALA has a short accumulation time in tissue, so there are few problems with cutaneous photosensitization. Topical ALA is highly selective for both carcinomas and actinic keratoses because damaged stratum corneum is more permeable to ALA and because dermal connective tissue contains PpIX.

- Although PDT with ALA appears to be not quite as effective as PDT with porfimer sodium or conventional surgery, it has very high patient acceptance because of the convenience, lack of scarring, and absence of skin photosensitivity.

REFERENCES

1. Dougherty TJ, Marcus SL. Photodynamic therapy. *Eur J Cancer.* 1992;28A:1734–1742.
2. Bissonnette R, Lui H. Current status of photodynamic therapy in dermatology. *Dermatol Clin.* 1997;15:507–516.
3. Mang TS, Dougherty TJ, Potter WR, et al. Photobleaching of porphyrins used in photodynamic therapy and implications for therapy. *Photochem Photobiol.* 1987;45:501–506.
4. Daniell MD, Hill JS. A history of photodynamic therapy. *Aust NZ J Surg.* 1991;61:340–348.
5. Lui H, Anderson RR: Photodynamic therapy in dermatology: recent developments. *Dermatol Clin.* 1993;11:1–13.
6. Dougherty TJ, Kaufmann JE, Goldfarb A. Photoradiation therapy for the treatment of malignant tumors. *Cancer Res.* 1978;38:2628–2635.
7. Lui H, Zeng H, McLean DI, et al. In vivo fluorescence spectroscopy monitoring of BPD verteporfin concentration changes in skin tissue during photodynamic therapy of skin cancers. *J Dermatol SC.* 1996;12:87.
8. Henderson BW, Dougherty TJ. How does photodynamic therapy work? *Photochem Photobiol.* 1992;55:145–157.

9. Korbelik M, Krosl P, Olive L, et al. Distribution of Photofrin between tumour cells and tumour associated macrophages. *Br J Cancer*. 1991;64:508–512.

10. Wilson BD. Photodynamic therapy in the treatment of basal cell carcinomas: mechanism of action. Presented at: Photomedicine Society, Annual AAD Meeting; December 1993; Washington DC.

11. Wilson BD, Bernstein Z, Sommer C, et al. Photodynamic therapy for the treatment of Kaposi's sarcoma: a comparison study utilizing Photofrin and tin ethyl-ethiopurpurin. *Lasers Surg Med Suppl*. 1995;7:45.

12. Nelson JS, Liaw LH, Orenstein A, et al. Mechanism of tumor destruction following photodynamic therapy with hematoporphyrin derivative, chlorin phenocyanine. *J Natl Canc Inst*. 1988;80:1599–1605.

13. Luo Y, Chan CK, Kessel D. Rapid initiation of apoptosis by photodynamic therapy. *Photochem Photobiol*. 1996;63:528–534.

14. Morton CA, Whitehurst C, Moseley H, et al. Comparison of photodynamic therapy with cryotherapy in the treatment of Bowen's disease. *Br J Dermatol*. 1996;135:766–771.

15. Wilson BD, Mang TS, Stoll HL, et al. Photodynamic therapy for the treatment of basal cell carcinoma. *Arch Dermatol*. 1992;128:1597–1601.

16. Wilson BD, Mang TS. Photodynamic therapy for cutaneous malignancies. *Clin Dermatol*. 1995;13:91–96.

17. Buscaglia DA, Shanler SD, Mang TS, Wilson BD, et al. Photodynamic therapy with photofrin II successfully treats basal cell carcinomas in patients with basal cell nevus syndrome. Presented at: Society for Investigative Dermatology, annual meeting; September, 1994; Toronto, Canada.

18. Sommer CA, van Leengoed H, Conti CM, et al. Photodynamic therapy (PDT) for cutaneous carcinomas using the second generation photosensitizer tin ethyl etiopurpurin (SnET2). *Lasers Surg Med Suppl*. 1995;7:45.

19. Renschler A, Yuen TS, Panella TJ, et al. Photodynamic therapy trials with lutetium texaphyrin PCI-0123 (LU-TEX). Presented at: 25th Annual ASP Meeting; July 5–10; St. Louis, MO.

20. Loh CS, MacRobert AJ, Bedwell J, et al. Oral versus intravenous administration of ALA for photodynamic therapy. *Br J Cancer*. 1993;68:41–51.

21. Kennedy JC, Pottier RH, Pross DC. Photodynamic therapy with endogenous protoporphyrin IX: basic principles and present clinical experience. *J Photochem Photobiol B*. 1990;6:143–148.

22. Wolf P, Rieger E, Kerl H. Topical photodynamic therapy with endogenous porphyrins after application of 5-aminolevulinic acid. *J Am Acad Dermatol*. 1993;28:17–21.

23. Lui H, Salasche S, Kollias N, et al. Photodynamic therapy of nonmelanoma skin cancer with topical aminolevulinic acid: a clinical and histologic study. *Arch Dermatol*. 1995;131:737–738.

24. Svanberg K, Andersson T, Killander D, et al. Photodynamic therapy of nonmelanoma malignant tumours of the skin using topical delta-amino levulinic acid sensitization and laser irradiation. *Br J Dermatol*. 1994;130:743–751.

25. Cairnduff F, Stringer MR, Hudson EJ, et al. Superficial photodynamic therapy with topical 5-aminolevulinic acid for superficial primary and secondary skin cancer. *Br J Cancer*. 1994;69:605–608.

26. Warloe T, Peng Q, Heyerdahl J, et al. Photodynamic therapy with 5-aminolevulinic acid induced porphyrins and DMSO/EDTA for basal cell carcinoma. *Proc SPIE*. 1995;2371:226–235.

27. Gudgin Dickson EF, Pottier RH. On the role of protoporphyrin IX photoproducts in photodynamic therapy. *J Photochem Photobiol B*. 1995;29:91–93.

28. Gossner L, Stroka R, Hahn EG, et al. Photodynamic therapy: successful destruction of gastrointestinal cancer after oral administration of aminolevulinic acid. *Gastrointest Endosc*. 1995;41:55–58.

29. Grant WE, Hopper C, MacRobert AJ. Photodynamic therapy of oral cancer: photosensitisation with systemic aminolevulinic acid. *Lancet*. 1993;342:147–148.

30. Regula J, MacRobert AJ, Gorchein A, et al. Photosensitisation and photodynamic therapy of oesophageal, duodenal, and colorectal tumors using 5 aminolaevulinic acid induced protoporphyrin IX—a pilot study. *Gut*. 1995;36:67–75.

31. Korbelik M, Krosl G. Cellular levels of photosensitizers in tumors: the role of proximity to the blood supply. *Br J Cancer*. 1994;70:604–610.

32. Babich B, Whitaker J, Conti C, et al. Treatment of all stages of cutaneous T cell lymphoma with fractionated photodynamic therapy using topical β-aminolevulinic acid (ALA-PDT). *J Invest Dermatol*. 1996.

33. Levy JG. Photosensitizers in photodynamic therapy. *Semin Oncol*. 1994;21:4–10.

34. Korbelik M, Krosl G. Accumulation of benzoporphyrin derivative in malignant and host cell populations of the murine RIF tumor. *Cancer Lett*. 1995;97:249–254.

35. Wilson BD. Photodynamic therapy in the treatment of cutaneous malignancies. In: Wheeland RG, ed. *Cutaneous Surgery*. Philadelphia, PA: W.B. Saunders Co; 1994:1104–1111.

36. Razum NJ, Snyder AB, Doiron DR. SnET2: clinical update. *Proc SPIE*. 1996;2675:43–46.

37. Divaris DXG, Kennedy JC, Pottier RH. Phototoxic damage to sebaceous glands and hair follicles of mice after systemic administration of 5-aminolevulinic acid correlates with localized protoporphyrin IX fluorescence. *Am J Pathol*. 1990;136:891–897.

38. Dougherty TJ. Photodynamic therapy. *Photochem Photobiol*. 1993;58:895–900.

39. Dougherty TJ, Oseroff AR, Wilson BD, et al. Phase I and II trials utilizing 2-(1-hexyloxethyl)-2 devinyl pyropheophorbide A (HPPH-photochlor). (In progress)

40. Jones C, Stoll HL, Mang TS, et al. Photodynamic Therapy in the treatment of Bowen's disease. *J Am Acad Dermatol*. 1992;27:979–982.

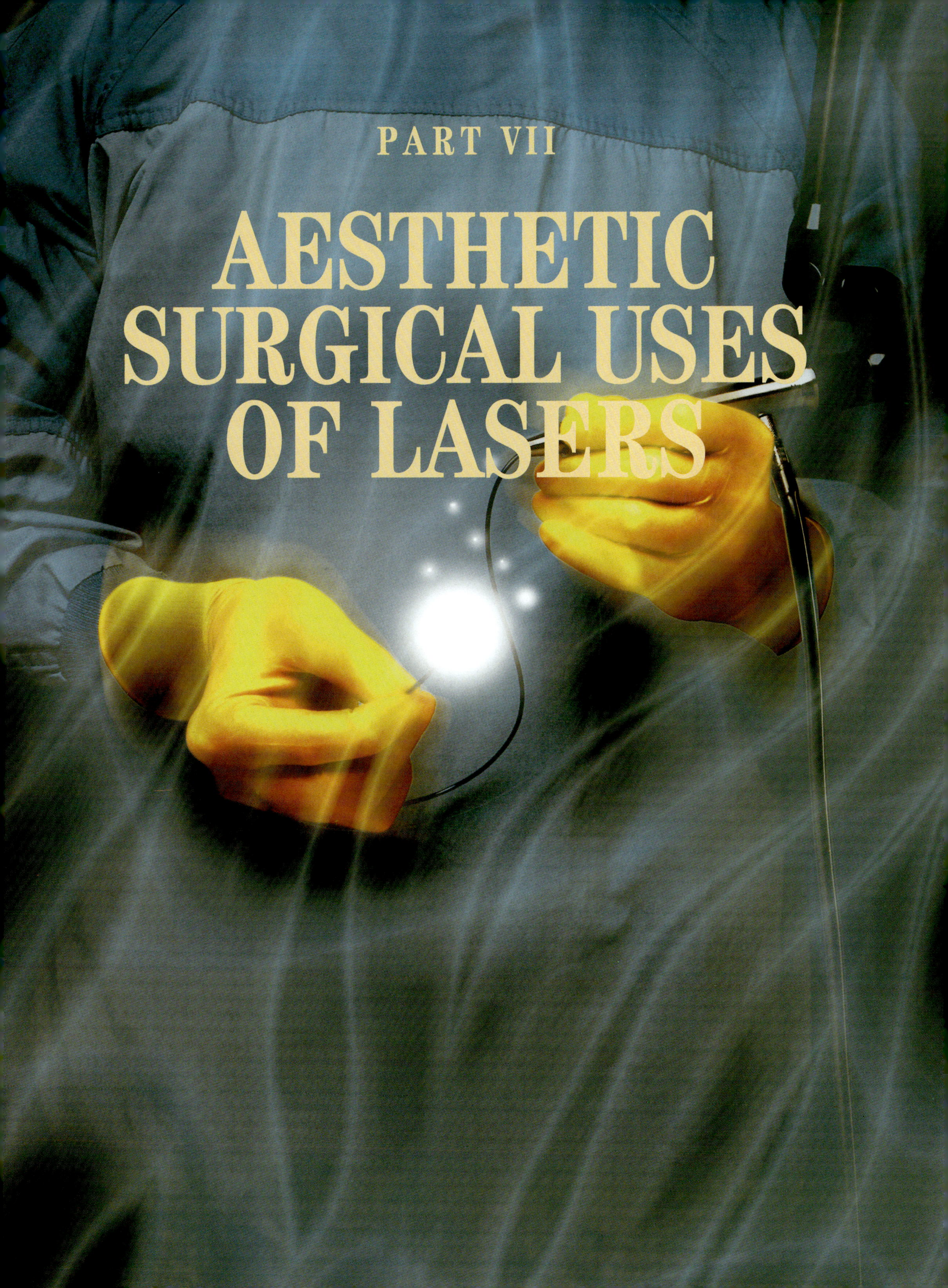

PART VII
AESTHETIC
SURGICAL USES
OF LASERS

CHAPTER 35

Lasers in Aesthetic Facial Surgery: An Overview

GREGORY S. KELLER AND VICTOR G. LACOMBE

Lasers have achieved almost universal acceptance in the field of facial plastic surgery. However, their usefulness is debated in the field of "cutting" aesthetic surgery. Originally, one of the issues debated involved whether the additional costs of using a laser were justified by advantages to the surgeon and patient. Although cost is always a significant issue, now many surgeons have already purchased carbon dioxide (CO_2) lasers for resurfacing, which means the lasers are also available for cutting at little additional cost.

Advantages of using a laser to cut tissue are the lack of bleeding, diminished swelling, and improved surgical field. Disadvantages include the cumbersome nature of the instrument itself, additional safety needs that include wearing eye protection and evacuating smoke (although this is not different from electrosurgery), and additional cost if the laser has not already been purchased.

SPECIFIC USES

Physicians most commonly use lasers for aesthetic and reconstructive blepharoplasty (also known as an "eye lift"), which is discussed more extensively in Chapters 37 and 38. The laser provides a bloodless field for precision surgery, and swelling and postoperative recovery time appear to be diminished.[1–3]

Lasers are also used to resurface the underside of neck lift flaps. William Cook has previously reported this use,[4] and Chapter 39 exclusively covers this topic. Our own histologic evaluations have shown that extremely low doses of laser light seem to cause an inflammatory reaction that may cause neck flap shrinkage and/or enhanced adherence to underlying tissues. There is no effect on the dermal collagen in terms of thermal injury or shrinkage because a layer of subdermal fat covers the skin from below. Long-term follow-up data are currently unavailable.

Proponents of the use of lasers for endoscopic fore-headplasty cite diminished ecchymosis and swelling as advantages. The laser primarily cuts the small expressive muscles, resulting in diminished bleeding and subsequent ecchymosis.[5–7] The procerus and depressor muscles are located away from the supratrochlear nerves and are the most amenable targets. The orbicularis oris muscle, lateral to the supraorbital nerve, is also distanced from the main sensory nerve bundles and is easily incised with the laser, although the surgeon must be careful not to penetrate the skin. The corrugator muscle is more difficult to incise with the laser, and one must use caution around the larger vessels and supratrochlear nerve branches.

Other surgeons use the laser to sever the branch of the frontal nerve that goes to the corrugator muscle. The orbicularis oris lateral to the supraorbital nerve is severed at the level of and slightly superior to the brow. The nerve is anterior to the muscle. As it is severed, the corrugator relaxes. Whether this denervation technique is as effective

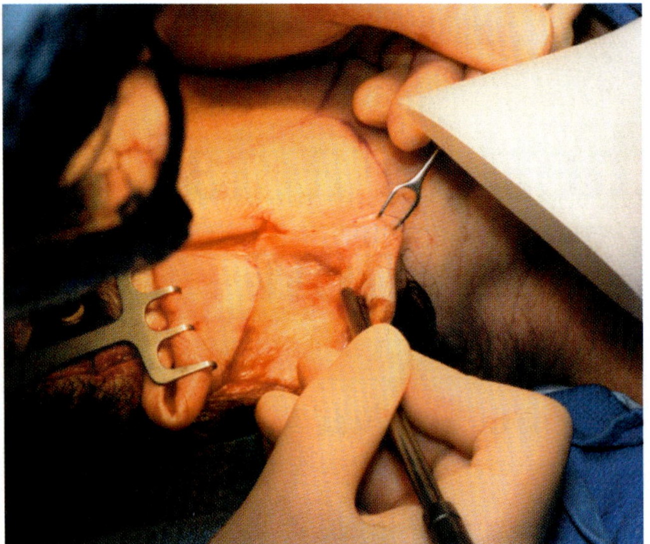

Figure 35–1. A Sharplan XJ150 CO_2 laser in use for elevating a postauricular flap.

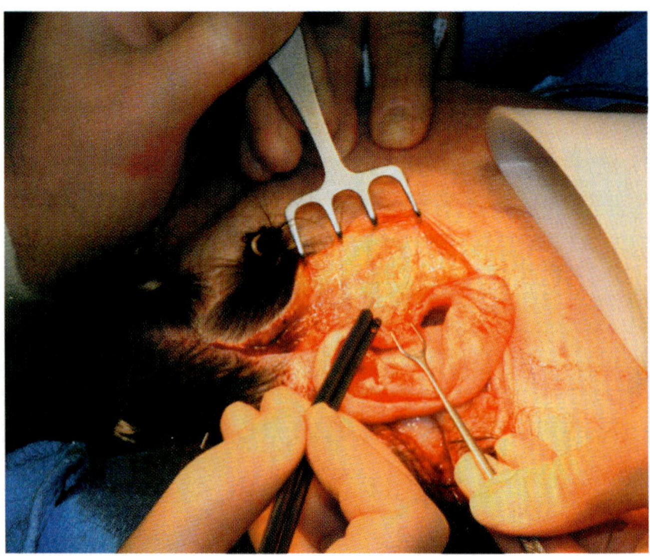

Figure 35–2. Bloodless elevation of the preauricular region during rhytidectomy.

or long-lasting as myotomy is as yet unknown. It is the senior author's (GSK) opinion that myotomy is the only technique that is effective in the long term.

The laser is able to "find" areolar planes in face-lift surgery to easily allow quick and bloodless anatomic dissection (Fig. 35–1 and 35–2). The platysma, sub-mandibular aponeurotic system (SMAS), and orbicularis oris muscle may be severed bloodlessly with the laser

as well. The laser may also be used in a variety of face-lift planes (Fig. 35–3), provided that areolar tissue is present. Distorted tissue planes can be one of the primary obstacles to laser-assisted face-lift surgery. Reported results of laser use for face-lift surgery suggest that the recovery period is less severe than with "cold knife" surgery and that swelling and ecchymosis appear to be diminished.[8,9]

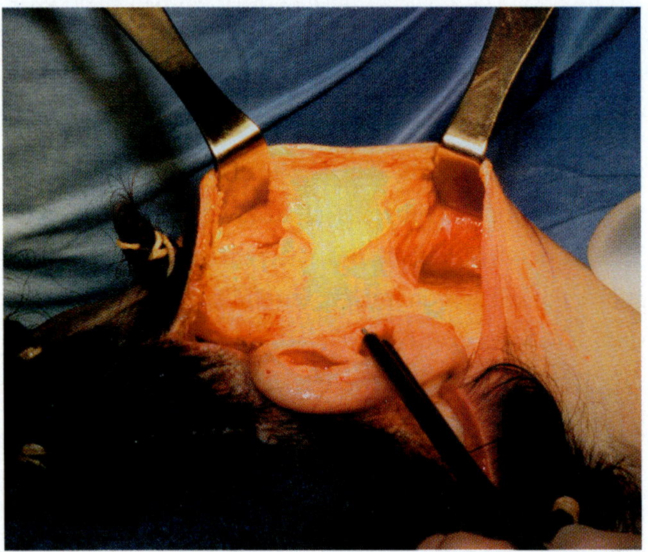

Figure 35–3. The CO_2 laser can be used safely both in superficial planes, such as the temporal region on the left, and in deeper planes, such as the suprafibromuscular level on the right.

CONCLUSIONS

Whether laser use in aesthetic facial plastic surgery contributes to a better outcome is a matter of debate. The laser is already the surgical tool of choice for many physicians, but whether the additional cost and presence of the large laser equipment in the operating room justify the diminished bleeding and reduced postoperative ecchymosis and swelling remains a contested issue. The most common procedure currently performed with the laser is blepharoplasty, and many surgeons have reported substantial benefits. For other procedures, it is the individual surgeon's responsibility to determine whether the benefits inherent to laser surgery are worthwhile. Further practical experience on a widespread scale and documentation in the literature will ultimately define the laser's utility in aesthetic surgery.

REFERENCES

1. Baker SS, Pham RT. Lateral canthal tendon suspension using the carbon dioxide laser: A modified technique. *Dermatol Surg.* 1995;21:1071–1073.
2. Baker SS. Carbon dioxide laser ptosis surgery combined with blepharoplasty. *Dermatol Surg.* 1995;21:1065–1070.
3. Trelles MA, Baker SS, Ting J, Toregard BM. Carbon dioxide laser transconjunctival lower lid blepharoplasty complications. *Ann Plast Surg.* 1996;37:465–468.
4. Cook WR Jr. Laser neck and jowl liposculpture including platysma laser resurfacing, dermal laser resurfacing, and vaporization of subcutaneous fat. *Dermatol Surg.* 1997;23:1143–1148.
5. Griffin JE Jr, Frey BS, Max DP, Epker BN. Laser-assisted endoscopic forehead lift. *J Oral Maxillofac Surg.* 1998;56:1040–1048.
6. Choo PH, Carter SR, Seiff SR. Carbon dioxide laser-assisted endoscopic forehead lift. *Plast Reconstr Surg.* 1999;103:294–298.
7. Rosenberg GJ. The subperiosteal endoscopic laser forehead (SELF) lift. *Plast Reconstr Surg.* 1998;102:493–501.
8. Hutcherson R, Keller GS. Endoscopic techniques in facial rejuvenation surgery. *Facial Plast Surg.* 1996;12:303–310.
9. Ramirez OM, Pozner JN. Subperiosteal minimally invasive laser endoscopic rhytidectomy: the SMILE facelift. *Aesthetic Plast Surg.* 1996;20:463–470.

CHAPTER 36

Laser Rhytidectomy

WILLIAM H. BEESON

The aim of rhytidectomy is to (1) provide a smooth contour and tighten jowls, (2) elevate sagging cheeks, (3) elevate the downward lines of facial expression to a "more youthful" posterosuperior orientation, (4) reduce the problems of buccal labial folds, and (5) reduce redundancy and bulkiness in the submental and cervical regions.

It is paramount to obtain a natural, unoperated look. Patients want incisions to be hidden in natural creases and natural hairlines to be maintained as much as possible. They also want to avoid obvious lines of demarcation between surgically rejuvenated areas and areas that have not been altered surgically. For these reasons, rhytidectomy procedures must address age-related changes in the cervical, malar, and lateral temporal areas.

TRADITIONAL VERSUS LASER FACE-LIFT SURGERY

Traditional face-lift surgery is associated with several significant complications and adverse effects, such as prolonged convalescence, discomfort, postoperative edema, and the possibility of hematoma. It is interesting to note that multiple surveys have shown hematoma to be the most frequent adverse sequela. Although postoperative hematomas reportedly occur in 4 to 7% of patients, it is widely believed that hematomas not requiring surgical

drainage occur much more frequently and may be encountered in up to 15% of face-lift procedures. Therefore, hematoma is a major concern with face-lift surgery.

In addition to desiring a natural, rested appearance after rhytidectomy, patients want to return to normal work and social activities quickly. Moreover, they want this fast recovery to be accompanied by a minimal amount of discomfort. For these reasons, the carbon dioxide (CO_2) laser has become an important part of the facial surgeon's armamentarium.

Traditionally, the CO_2 laser has been the workhorse of laser facial surgery. Major advantages of the CO_2 laser have included decreased pain, reduced swelling and bruising, a bloodless surgical field, and additional hemostasis. Advent of the high-energy, pulsed CO_2 laser has added two new elements to this list: char-free surgery and accelerated wound healing.

High-energy CO_2 lasers are gain-switching lasers. The various waveforms of these lasers are produced by gain switching the lasing medium, or gas mixture, of the laser. In gain-switching mode, the laser power supply generates a very high pulse of current that "pumps" the gas mixture, producing a burst of optical power typically two times in excess of its normal capacity.

Numerous surgeons have advocated use of the CO_2 laser in facial surgery. Dr. G.S. Keller has worked with both potassium-titanyl-phosphate (KTP) and CO_2 lasers (personal communication, 1996). Both Drs. Capriotti and

Morrow have advocated use of the CO_2 laser for rhytidectomy (personal communications, 1996). Until recently, the problems associated with laser face lifts were both technical and pathophysiologic.

Technical problems included the large, cumbersome handpiece, which made flap elevation very difficult. In addition, there were the inherent laser safety issues that complicated the surgical procedure. Pathophysiologically, healing of the CO_2 laser incision has been shown by Mittelman and Apfelberg[1] to be inferior to that of the cold knife incision. For the reasons previously stated, new technical advances of the high-energy CO_2 laser have rectified these problems. Some authors now believe that wound healing associated with high-energy CO_2 lasers is comparable with that of traditional scalpel incisions and may even be accelerated. Pogrel and colleagues[2] have shown accelerated wound healing with high-energy CO_2 lasers as compared with traditional scalpel incisions. Yu and colleagues[3] have shown that the expression of growth factors in CO_2 laser incisions and scalpel incisions is essentially the same. Allen[4] has confirmed elevated levels of tissue growth factors TB-1 and TB-2 in association with high-energy CO_2 laser treatment.

The fiber-optic delivery system is a technical advancement that enables surgeons to maintain tactile sensation while using the CO_2 laser and greatly facilitates flap elevation. In addition, the fiber-optic delivery system allows maintenance of the Gaussian waveform of the laser energy so that the precise energy level selected is delivered at the tip of the fiber. This is not true with traditional waveguides and is a significant technologic improvement.

Previous studies have shown the benefits of electrosurgical dissection. Reduced blood loss, bloodless dissection of tissue planes affording better anatomic visualization, sealing of lymphatic channels, and more rapid hemostasis have been noted. In addition, with the absence of sharp instruments in the surgical field, there is a reduction in the chance of intraoperative transmission of blood-borne diseases, such as acquired immune deficiency syndrome.[5] Another study has also shown that electrical dissection results in no histologic evidence of fibrosis, inflammation, or necrosis in the early postoperative period. In addition, no deleterious effects on tissue flaps were seen with elevation by either lasers or electrocautery, as compared with sharp tissue dissection of cutaneous flaps.[6]

LASER-TISSUE INTERACTIONS

To fully appreciate what can be achieved with a high-energy CO_2 laser, one must have a thorough understanding of laser-tissue interactions. Tissue injury results when the CO_2 laser light is absorbed by the water in facial tissues. This releases heat that irreversibly ablates tissue proteins and creates three zones of tissue damage: (1) carbonized eschar, (2) a surrounding zone of coagulative necrosis, and (3) a sheath of edema that surrounds the ablated site. The volume of tissue ablated varies directly with the power and intensity of the laser. Of significance, the collagen in the zone of coagulative necrosis becomes somewhat mummified, which can result in delayed dermal healing for a number of months. This is why healing after CO_2 laser surgery has not been as efficacious compared with healing after the cold knife technique.

If one could reduce the zone of coagulative necrosis, there would be more rapid healing and less scarring. The high-energy CO_2 laser, which achieves very high energy levels in a very short period of time, produces individual pulses that never exceed 600 microseconds (less than the thermal relaxation time of tissue). The result is little or no collateral tissue damage (i.e., coagulative necrosis) and more efficacious wound healing. The high-energy, short-pulsed, laser energy is absorbed by the water in facial tissues, resulting in almost immediate tissue vaporization and dispersal of heat as steam in the laser plume and not as collateral thermal trauma to tissues.

COMPARATIVE STUDIES

Beeson and Keller[7] evaluated face-lift patients and compared incisional wound healing for the high-energy CO_2 laser versus traditional cold-steel techniques. Patients (28 women and 2 men) averaged the same age in each category (range, 40 to 71 years). The contralateral methodology involved performing a laser face lift on one side of the patient's face and a conventional cold-steel undermining technique on the opposite side. This approach was used in 10 patients, who were then compared with 10 patients who underwent bilateral face lift using the laser technique and 10 patients who underwent a conventional cold-steel face lift.

A high-energy, direct-current CO_2 laser was used in all laser patients. All surgeries were performed by the same surgeon while the patients were under intravenous sedation, and pressure dressings were removed on the first postoperative day. No drains were employed. Complications, length of procedure, degree of patient discomfort, and time to total resolution of bruising were monitored in each patient. The patient, physician, and nurse observers, as well as the operative surgeon, monitored each patient on a daily basis until all edema and ecchymosis were classified as resolved by all monitors.

Results

No complications were noted in the 30 patients observed; no hematomas, infections, flap necrosis, alopecia, or paresthesias occurred.

Technically, laser surgery required more operative time compared with the traditional cold-steel technique ($\sim$23% longer). With experience, the disparity between the operative times of the two techniques decreased markedly. However, laser rhytidectomy is still more time-consuming than traditional cold-steel undermining.

The point of maximal bruising and ecchymosis occurred between the third and fifth postoperative days with the laser and between the fourth and seventh postoperative days with the cold-steel technique. There was a significant difference in terms of total resolution of swelling and ecchymosis. In the contralaterally treated group, bruising resolved in 10.8 days on the laser side versus 21.8 days on the cold-steel side, a difference of approximately 50%. In laser face-lift patients, bruising

resolved in 7.6 days, whereas in the cold steel patients, bruising resolved in 23.1 days. Because there can be crossover edema and ecchymosis due to submental undermining, it is not surprising to note a greater percentage variation between the two technique-specific groups.

Patient satisfaction could not be evaluated objectively because there were no controls. Laser patients did experience significantly less discomfort and required less postoperative pain medication than did their counterparts.

Conclusions

The study concluded that laser rhytidectomy required a slight increase in surgical time. However, as the surgeon became more experienced with the technique, operative time significantly decreased. There was a marked reduction in swelling and bruising with laser face lift, as compared with traditional cold-steel technique. There appeared to be no aesthetic difference in the quality of incisions between the two techniques. Laser face-lift patients appear to have decreased pain and required less pain medication. However, this was a subjective result with no clinical controls. Overall, CO_2 laser face-lift surgery was well accepted by patients and appeared to provide a quicker return to work and normal social activities.

LASER PROTOCOL
PATIENT SELECTION AND PREPARATION

The ideal rhytidectomy candidate is a thin, fair-skinned, middle-aged person in good health with minimal subcutaneous adipose tissue and moderate skin laxity in the jowl and cervicomental regions. Individuals with prominent zygomatic eminences may obtain even further enhancement through accentuation of their strong, attractive underlying osseous framework.

Conversely, overweight individuals with thick, hyperpigmented skin may experience less than optimal results. Individuals who have large, ptotic submandibular glands and those with a hyoid bone in an extremely inferior position obtain a more obtuse cervicomental angle that makes them more susceptible to a "double chin" or "turkey neck" deformity. Although improvement in the cervical area is possible for these individuals, their anatomic variation dictates less than optimal results.

Anesthesia

Laser surgery is usually performed under conscious sedation (monitored anesthesia care). A tumescent technique is used for regional anesthesia and hydrodissection, as advocated by Klein.[8] Advantages of this technique include a prolonged anesthetic effect (~18 hours after surgery), which markedly decreases the amount of postoperative analgesics needed. Klein has shown that peak plasma levels of lidocaine occur 12 to 18 hours following infiltration. Clinical local anesthesia is maintained for up to 18 hours after injection. Excellent vasoconstriction is obtained, and hydrodissection via the infiltration technique facilitates flap elevation in the superficial, subdermal plane.

The anesthetic solution contains 0.1% lidocaine with epinephrine 1:100,000 and is prepared by adding 1000 mg of lidocaine (100 mL 1% lidocaine), 1 mg of epinephrine (1 mL of 1:100,000), and 12.5 mEq sodium bicarbonate (1 mEq/mL) to 1000 mL normal saline (0.9% NaCl). The intravenous infusion bag containing this solution is then placed in a pneumatic blood delivery pouch, and the pressure is elevated to facilitate filling of a rapid, multidose 3-mL syringe. A 6-in, 18-gauge infusion needle is used for infiltration of the anesthetic solution.

Safety

Proper laser safety precautions are taken. Moist towels are placed around the treatment site and over the patient's eyes. Metal protective eye shields for the patient may also be used, and all personnel should wear laser masks and protective eye shields. The orifice of the smoke evacuator tube is held within 2 cm of the source to remove the laser

plume, and the used smoke evacuator tubing is treated as biohazardous waste.

TECHNIQUE

We use a direct-current, high-energy CO_2 laser with a fiber-optic delivery system (Sharplan XJ-150/Fiberlase Fiber Optic Delivery System; Sharplan Lasers, Inc., Allendale, NJ) to elevate tissues in the subdermal plane.

Incisions

Incisions are outlined preoperatively with a skin scribe, and hair is braided and taped prior to the patient being moved into surgery (Fig. 36–1). Incisions are placed in periauricular creases (Fig. 36–2), and a retrotragal incision is used in women. The incision is then carried into the postauricular sulcus to approximately the low external auditory canal. At this point, the incision is carried horizontally into the hairline and then to the postoccipital region for approximately 4 to 5 cm. A gentle curving (lazy-S) configuration is used. This posterior extension

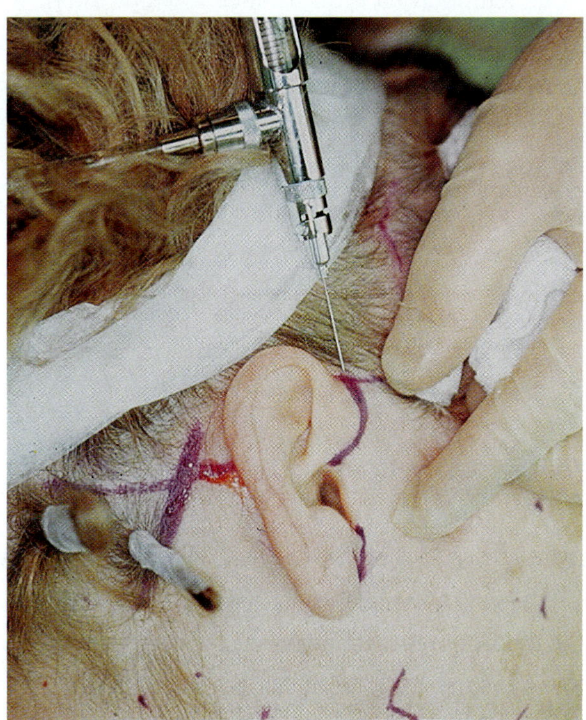

Figure 36–1. A tumescent infiltration technique is used to administer regional anesthesia and perform hydrodissection. Note that incisions have already been outlined with a skin scribe and hair has been braided and taped.

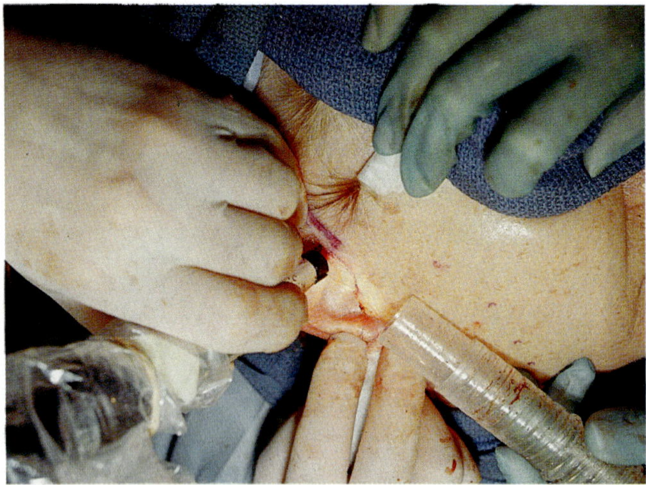

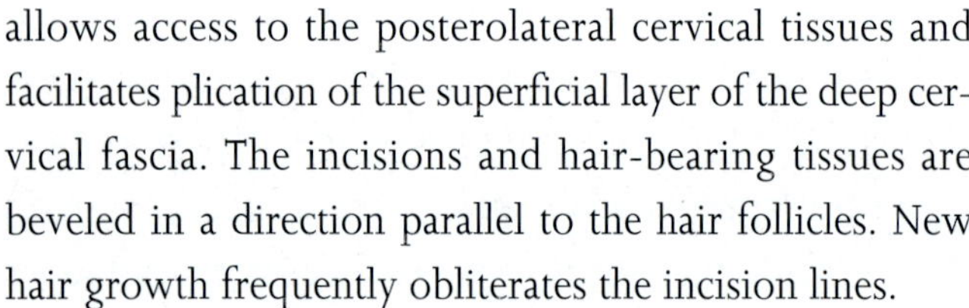

Figure 36–2. The high-energy CO_2 laser with a 125-mm handpiece is used to make the skin incision. The smoke evacuator is kept within 2 cm of the dissection site.

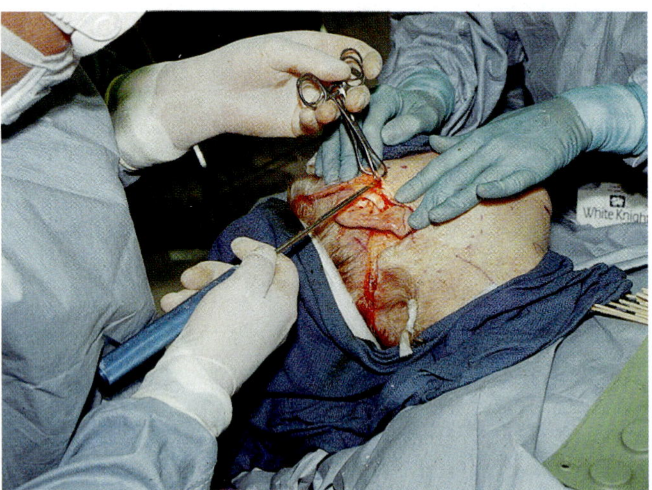

Figure 36–3. A dissection cannula is used to tunnel the subdermal plane in both the pre- and postauricular areas.

allows access to the posterolateral cervical tissues and facilitates plication of the superficial layer of the deep cervical fascia. The incisions and hair-bearing tissues are beveled in a direction parallel to the hair follicles. New hair growth frequently obliterates the incision lines.

The temporal incision parallels a gentle curve with the hairline approximately 1 cm into the hair-bearing area, where follicle density is sufficient to hide the scar. The primary advantage of this hair-sparing incision is that it preserves the important temporoperiauricular hair tuft. An incision placed more posteriorly may displace the hairline posterosuperiorly with flap redraping, producing an unnatural appearance. A secondary lift, or "tuck up" procedure, further increases this distortion.

Undermining

Undermining is performed in the subdermal plane in the periauricular and posterior cervical areas and in the subgaleal plane in the pretemporal region. Blunt undermining is used in the transition zone between the subgaleal and subdermal regions in the area where the frontal branch of the facial nerve courses on a plane tangent to a line drawn 5 cm below the tragus to 0.1 to 0.5 cm from the lateral portion of the eyebrow. Subdermal tunnels are created with a dissecting cannula (Fig. 36–3). The tissue

is placed under tension with retractors, and the CO_2 laser with the Fiberlase handpiece is used for dissection in a subdermal plane (Figs. 36–4, 36–5, and 36–6). The laser easily dissects intervening connective tissue between the undermined tunnels. Tactile perception should essentially reveal a minimal amount of tissue drag. As one moves more superficially into a dermal plane, there is more resistance. Although this procedure results in meticulous hemostasis, vessels over 2 mm in size (often noted in the postauricular-occipital area) require bipolar cautery for more appropriate hemostasis.

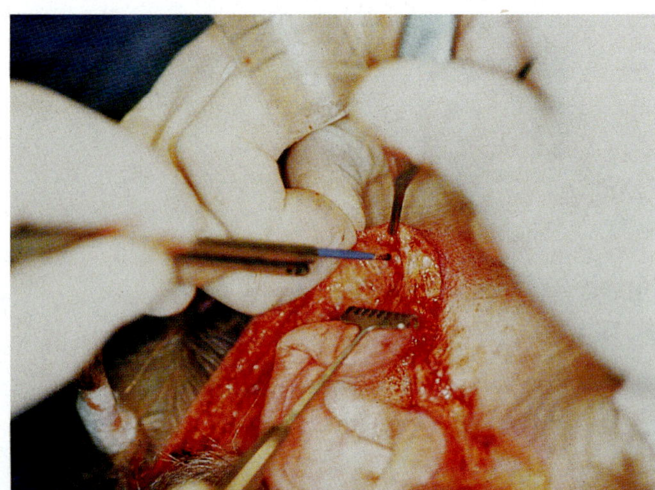

Figure 36–4. The skin flap is elevated in a subdermal plane using the CO_2 laser. The fiber-optic handpiece allows for tactile sensation and facilitates flap elevation.

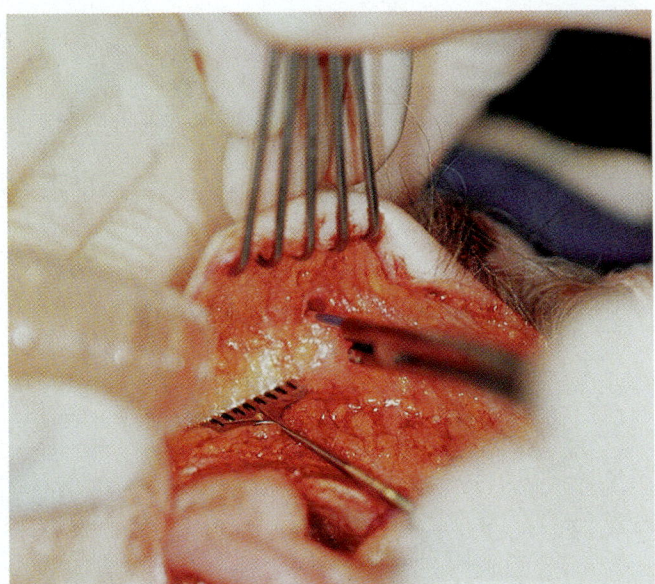

Figure 36–5. A rake retractor provides tension on the flap.

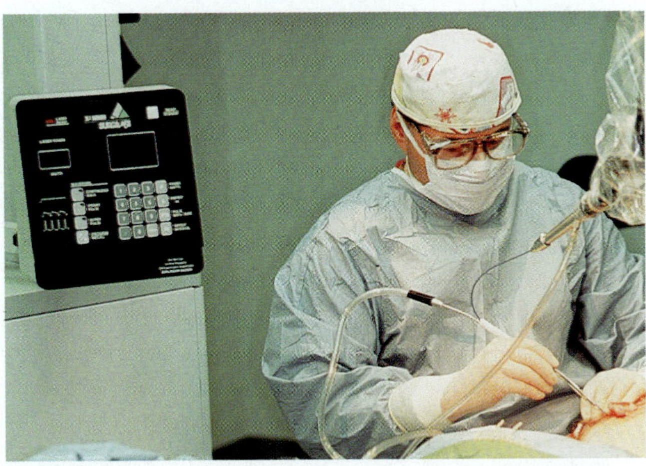

Figure 36–6. Dissection with the CO_2 laser provides a bloodless surgical field and facilitates anatomic dissection. The fiber-optic handpiece allows the articulating arm to be out of the surgical field and facilitates use of the CO_2 laser for the surgical dissection.

An open liposuction technique is then used to remove excess adipose tissue (Fig. 36–7). Facial liposuction facilitates dissection and allows better contouring. A liposuction cannula is used to remove adipose tissue and achieve contouring in the pre- and postauricular areas prior to using plication sutures. Liposuction allows better contouring along the angle of the mandible and helps to eliminate or markedly reduce the "puckered" appearance seen immediately after rhytidectomy when a plication technique is employed.

Plication of the Superficial Musculoaponeurotic System

Superficial musculoaponeurotic system (SMAS) tissue is plicated with 2-0 Ethibond suture (Fig. 36–8). The first plication stitch runs from the angle of the mandible to the

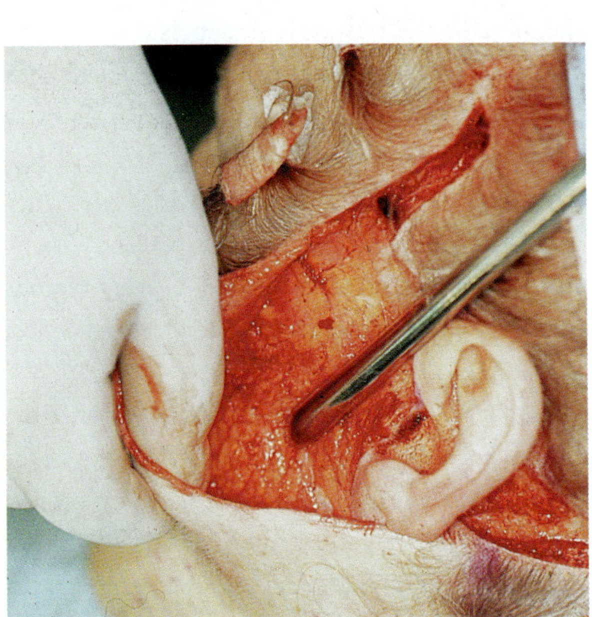

Figure 36–7. An open liposuction technique is used to remove adipose tissue in the pre- and postauricular areas.

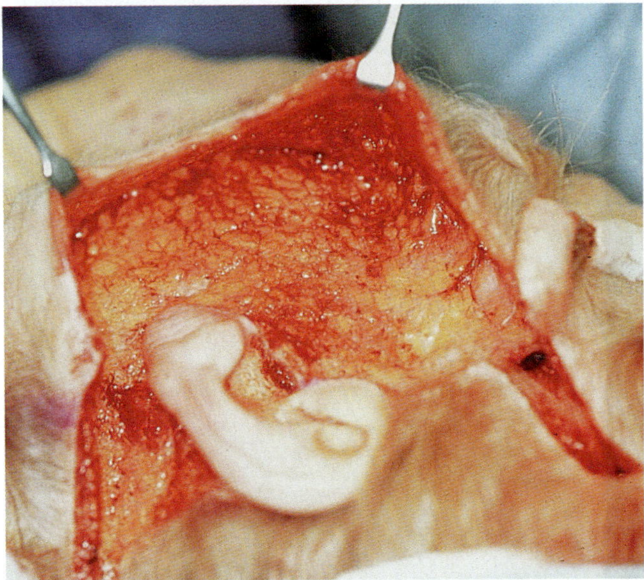

Figure 36–8. Plication of SMAS is performed using 2-0 Ethibond suture. The first plication suture supports tissue from the angle of mandible to the tragus.

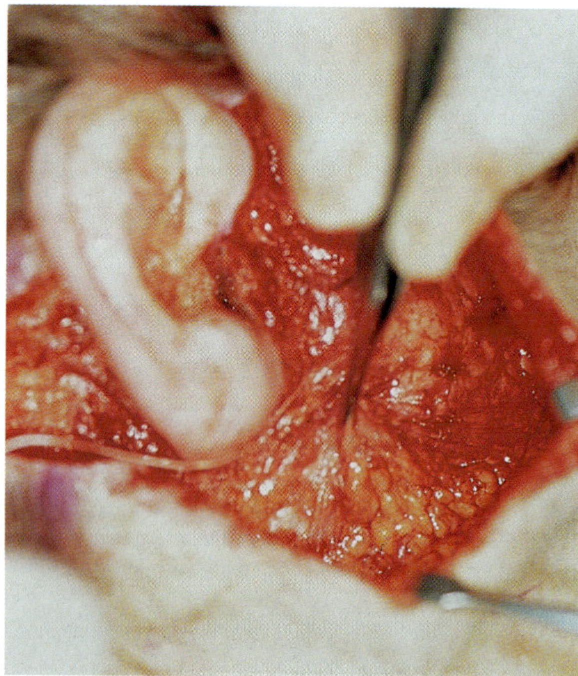

Figure 36–9. Additional SMAS plication sutures are used to advance tissue in a posterosuperior direction in the preauricular area.

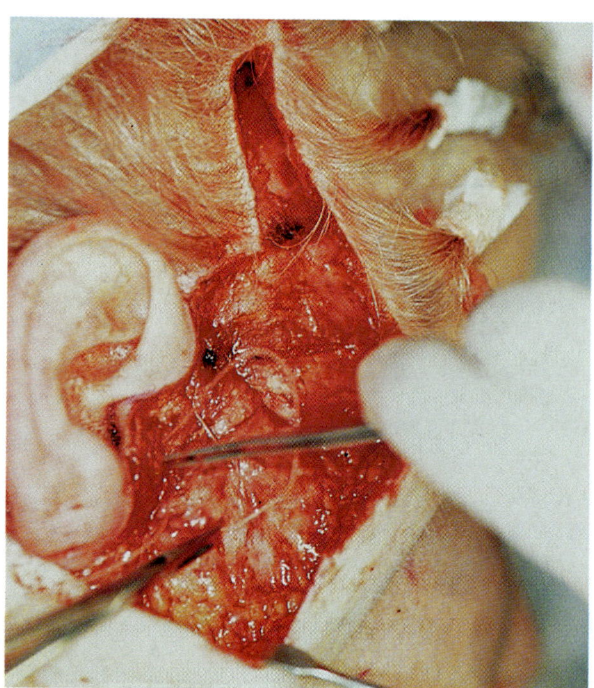

Figure 36–10. The superficial layer of the deep cervical fascia is plicated with 2-0 Ethabon suture in the postauricular-occipital area.

inferior margin of the tragus. This provides elevation in the posterosuperior direction and is the key positioning suture. Additional plicating sutures are placed in the preauricular and postauricular areas along selected vectors to provide the desired aesthetic result (Figs. 36–9 and 36–10). Great care

is taken to ensure that the plication sutures are inverted to lessen foreign-body reaction and extrusion.

Tailoring the Skin Flap

The skin flap is draped in a posterosuperior direction. The skin in the inferior lobular area can be advanced to the apex of the postauricular incision. To avoid a step-off, the postauricular hairline is advanced antero-superiorly (Fig. 36–11). Regional tailoring is then accomplished along the posterior auricular tissue to rotate in a clockwise manner toward the auricle (Fig. 36–12). Redundant tissue is excised. Stainless steel autostaples are used in the hair-bearing regions to position the skin flap and to provide for wound closure (Fig. 36–13).

The anterior flap is draped in a posterosuperior direction and lined with the vector running from the tragus to Darwin's tubercle (Fig. 36–14). The flap is tailored with anchoring staples placed at the junction of the frontotemporal auricular margin. The frontotemporal tissue is then advanced superiorly, with great care taken to avoid excess tension on the flap (Figs. 36–15A and B).

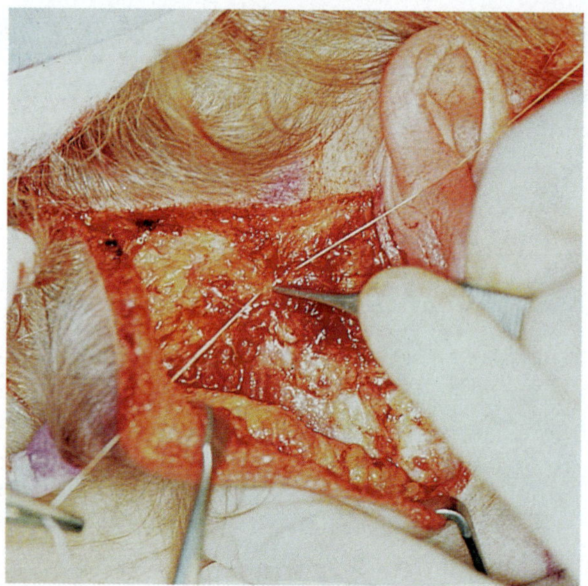

Figure 36–11. The postauricular hairline is lined to prevent a "step-off" deformity.

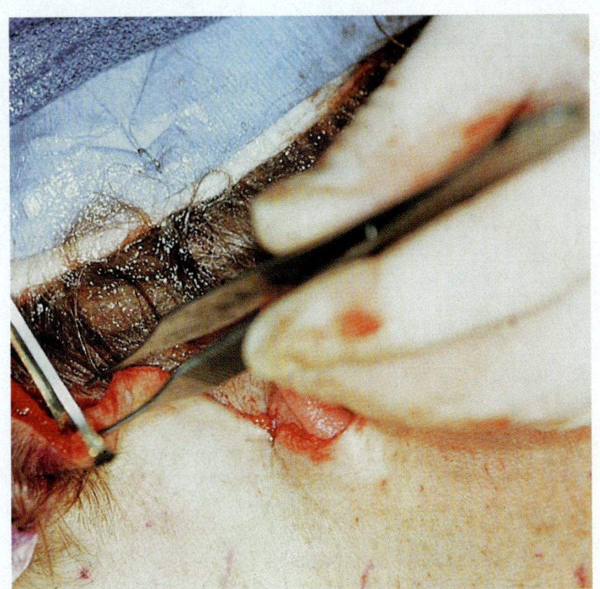

Figure 36–12. The skin flap is rotated in the posterior occipital area in a clockwise fashion, and redundant tissue is excised.

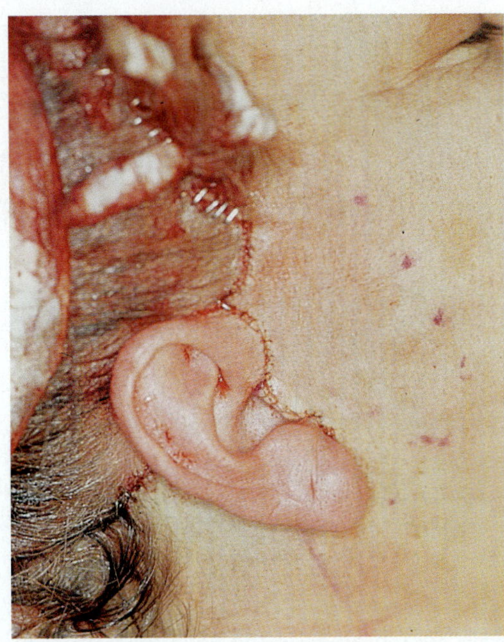

Figure 36–13. Autostaples are used to close the wound in hair-bearing tissues.

Redundant tissue is excised, and skin staples are used in the hair-bearing tissues (Fig. 36–15C).

A multiclosure technique with 4-0 clear Prolene suture supports deep dermal structures in both the pre-and postauricular areas, whereas 6-0 mild chromic suture is used to oppose cutaneous margins in the preauricular area (Fig. 36–16). Finally, 5-0 plain catgut suture is used to close the postauricular incision.

Submental Lipectomy

Submental lipectomy is the final phase of the rhytidectomy procedure, which is performed last to maintain the soft tissue attachments in the area along the cheek lift, thus providing additional traction but facilitating dissection by maintaining support in the submental region. In addition, it prevents asymmetric tension and distortion of cutaneous tissues. By undermining the submental region after tension has been placed bilaterally on the malar and postauricular areas, the surgeon is able to eliminate a tethered and potentially asymmetric appearance by allowing for equilibration of vector forces from undermining of the submental area with lateral extension into the previously dissected malar and lateral cervical regions. It also allows the surgeon to evacuate any blood that has accumulated in the posterior auricular and malar areas secondary to the previous dissection. The face-lift dressing is then placed immediately after the submental

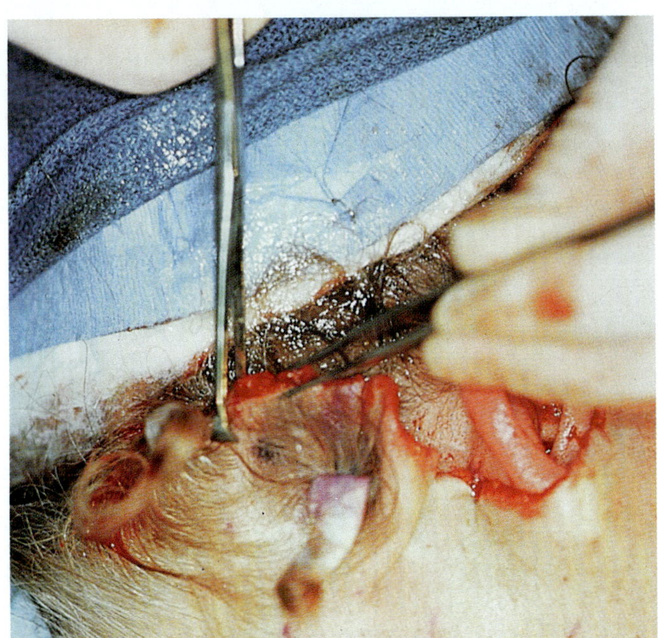

Figure 36–14. The skin flap in the pretragal area is positioned in a posterosuperior vector line that runs from the tragus to Darwin's tubercle. Positioning the flap in this direction results in a posterosuperior elevation.

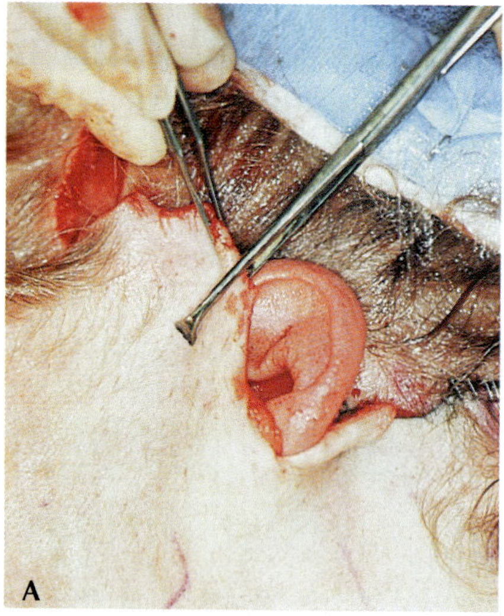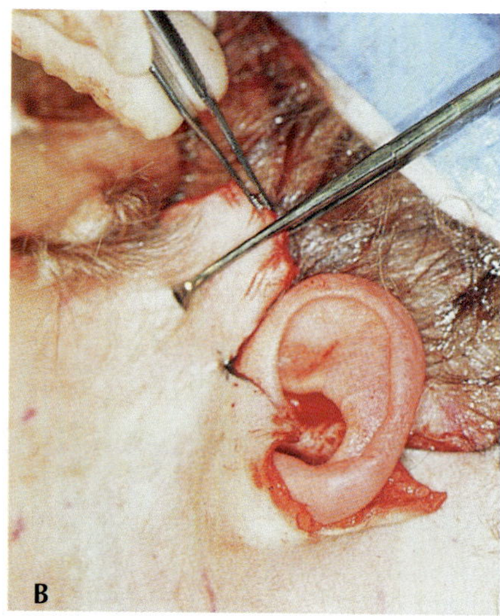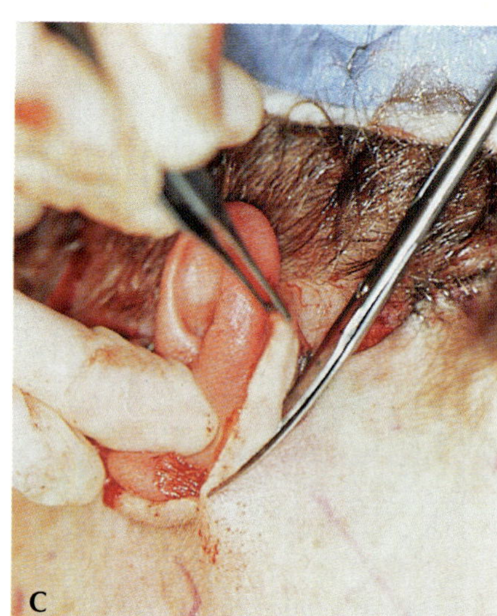

Figure 36–15. (A, B) The skin flap is contoured, and (C) redundant tissue is excised.

lipectomy, which obviates the need for drains and minimizes postoperative bruising.

A small stab incision is made in the submental crease (Fig. 36–17). Sharp undermining is performed using scissors in a subdermal plane to provide a more uniform plane of dissection and to maximize the amount of adipose tissue that can be removed with liposuction. The liposuction cannula is used with the orifice remaining away from the dermis at all times so as to avoid injury to the dermal vascular plexus. Liposuction is performed down to the level of the hyoid bone and the anterior margins of the sternocleidomastoid muscle bilaterally.

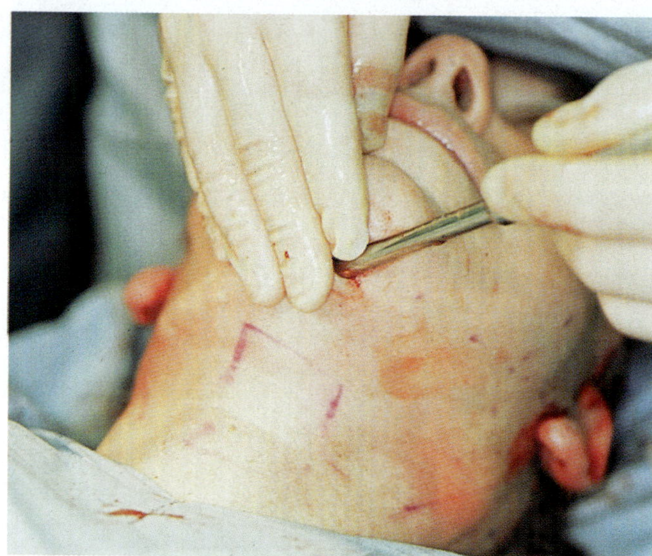

Figure 36–16. A multilayer closure with 4-0 clear Prolene suture to oppose deep dermal structures and interrupted and interlocking 6-0 mild chromic suture to oppose cutaneous margins are used in the preauricular area.

Figure 36–17. A stab incision is performed in the submental area, and liposuction is performed. Great care is taken to prevent the orifice of the cannula from injuring the subdermal plexis. Liposuction is continued to the level of the hyoid bone inferiorly and to the anterior border of the sternocleidomastoid muscle bilaterally.

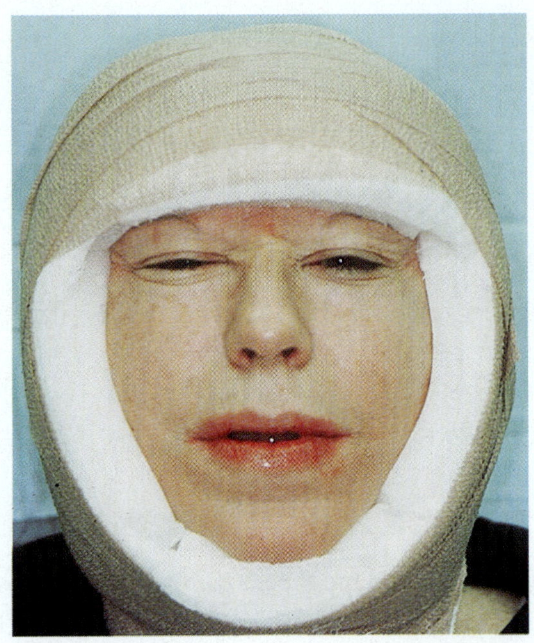

Figure 36–18. A pressure dressing consisting of Reston Foam, Kerlix, and Coban is used as a postoperative dressing. It is removed the morning following surgery. No drains are employed.

POSTOPERATIVE CARE

The hair is washed, and a pressure dressing in the periauricular areas consisting of telfa, followed by Reston Foam, Kerlix, and Coban, is applied (Fig. 36–18). No drains are employed. The dressing is removed the following morning, and the patient is instructed to use ice compresses over the areas of dissection for the next 48 hours.

The stainless-steel autostaples are removed after 7 days, and most patients are able to return to normal social and work activities within 7 to 10 days. Hydrogen peroxide and bacitracin ointment are applied three to four times per day to the cutaneous incisions. Patients are instructed to shower frequently to minimize crusting in hair-bearing tissues.

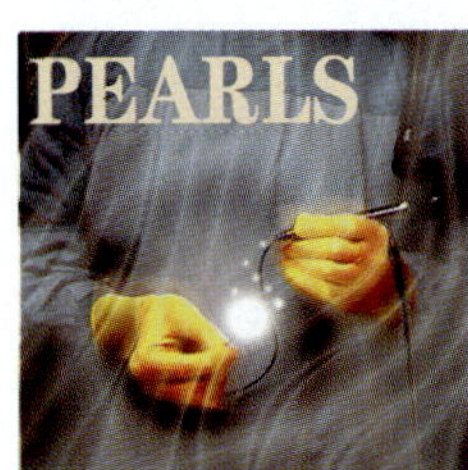

- Hematoma is the most frequent adverse sequela of traditional face-lift surgery. Although the incidence of postoperative hematoma is quite low, hematomas that don't require surgical drainage probably occur much more frequently.

- The CO_2 laser has always had several advantages over traditional cold-steel techniques (e.g., decreased pain, reduced swelling and bruising, a bloodless surgical field, and additional hemostasis). The high-energy, pulsed CO_2 laser now allows for char-free surgery and accelerated wound healing.

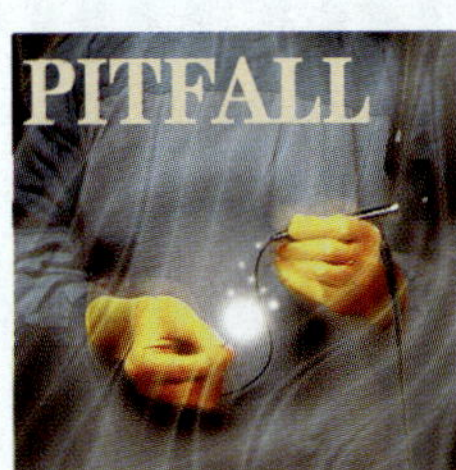

- Laser surgery requires more operative time compared with the traditional cold-steel technique, but as the operator gains experience, operative time with the laser decreases markedly. Despite this decrease, laser rhytidectomy is still more time-consuming than traditional cold-steel undermining.

REFERENCES

1. Mittelman H, Apfelberg D. *Ann Plast Surg.* 1990;2.
2. Pogrel MA, Pham HD, Gutenhoner M, Stem R. Profile of hyaluronidase activity distinguishes carbon dioxide laser from scalpel wound healing. *Ann Surg.* 1993;217:196–200.
3. Yu W, Naim JO, Lanzafame RJ. Expression of growth factors in early wound healing in rat skin. *Lasers Surg Med.* 1994;15:281–289.
4. Allen J. Histologic analysis of wounds following high-energy CO_2 laser resurfacing. Paper presented at: Annual Meeting of the American Academy of Facial Plastic and Reconstructive Surgery; Washington, DC: September, 1997.
5. Gellman CL, et al. The effect of lasers, electrocautery, and sharp dissection on cutaneous flaps. *Plast Reconstr Surg.* 1994;94:829–833.
6. Bateman SN, Noorily AD, McGuff HS. Sharp dissection, electrosurgery, and argon-enhanced electrosurgery in porcine skin flaps. *Otolaryngol Head Neck Surg.* 1966;114:435–442.
7. Beeson WH, Keller G. Laser facelift—comparison of cold steel technique. Paper presented at: American Academy of Cosmetic Surgery Annual Scientific Meeting; February, 1995; Los Angeles, CA.
8. Klein JA. Tumescent technique for regional anesthesia permits lidocaine doses of 35 mg per kilogram for liposuction. *J Dermatol Surg Oncol.* 1994;16:248–263.

CHAPTER 37

Laser Blepharoplasty with the Sharplan XJ150

MAURICE M. KHOSH AND WAYNE F. LARRABEE

Use of the carbon dioxide (CO_2) laser as a cutting tool has been advocated since the introduction of medical lasers in 1964.[1] Cutting is accomplished by heating the tissue to the point of vaporization. At the same time, however, thermal energy from the laser may be conducted to adjacent tissues, where coagulative necrosis occurs. Currently, delivery modes in CO_2 are broadly categorized as continuous wave (CW) or pulsed. The CW mode offers better hemostatic control but greater collateral thermal damage. Pulsed and ultrashort-pulsed modes cause less thermal conduction and, therefore, less adjacent tissue necrosis.

In the human epithelium and mucosa, the CW CO_2 laser at 6 W causes irreversible thermal damage 200 to 250 μm outside the margin of the incision. In the subepidermal collagen, laser incisions exhibit less marginal necrosis, and thermal damage extends to only 60 μm beyond the incision.[2] Thermal coagulative necrosis beyond wound edges offers both advantages and disadvantages. Thermal energy seals small blood vessels (<0.5 mm), lymphatic vessels, and small sensory nerves, which is associated with decreased bleeding and reduced postoperative edema and pain in laser blepharoplasty. These same local tissue effects, however, delay wound healing.

LASER VERSUS SCALPEL

The CO_2 laser offers several advantages versus scalpel technique for blepharoplasty. There is less bleeding and, therefore, enhanced intraoperative visualization. Postoperatively, there is less edema and ecchymosis, which leads to faster patient recovery.[3–7] Some investigators claim reduced postoperative pain.[5] Long-term results from laser blepharoplasty do not seem to differ from those of the more traditional methods. Reported advantages of reduced operative time and diminished postoperative pain have been disputed by Mittelman and Apfelberg.[8]

The greatest disadvantage of using lasers for blepharoplasty is the added cost. Staff needs to be trained in laser safety techniques, and additional staff may be necessary for handling the new equipment. The surgeon must meticulously adhere to laser safety protocols because of the risk of accidental burns. In upper blepharoplasty surgery, thermal insult from the laser delays dermal healing. Sutures should remain in place 1 or 2 days longer than those for scalpel incisions. Box 37–1 lists the advantages and disadvantages of laser blepharoplasty.

CLINICAL EXPERIENCE

We use the Sharplan XJ150 laser (Allendale, NJ) to perform incisions and skin resurfacing in the SurgiPulse mode, which delivers couplets of large energy peaks in very short pulse durations (less than the thermal relaxation time for skin). SurgiPulse allows vaporization of tissue with reduced thermal conduction and, therefore,

Box 37–1. Advantages and Disadvantages of Laser Blepharoplasty

Advantages
 Less bleeding
 Less operative time
 Less ecchymosis
 Earlier patient recovery
 Less swelling
Disadvantages
 Expense
 Extra personnel
 Training
 Delayed wound healing
 Safety hazards

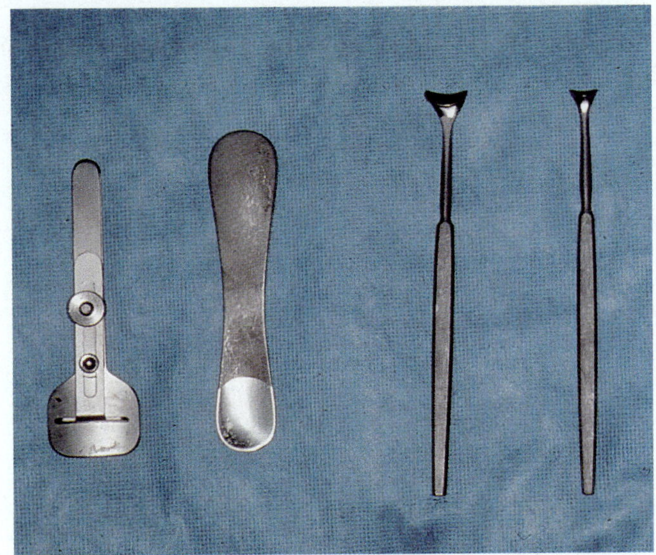

Figure 37–1. Laser blepharoplasty instruments (left to right): small Desmarres retractor, large Desmarres retractor, Jaeger bone plate, David-Baker clamp.

minimizes surrounding tissue damage. Carbon dioxide laser resurfacing of the skin is achieved using the FeatherTouch optical scanner.

TREATMENT PROTOCOL

Preoperative patient evaluation, medical and ophthalmologic history, and physical examination are performed as for other laser procedures. The amount of excess skin and protruding fat is estimated for each eye. For lower lid blepharoplasty candidates, lower lid laxity is assessed with a distraction or snap test. The incision sites, expected discomforts, and risks of surgery are explained to the patient during the preoperative consultation. Routine laser safety precautions, including laser masks, protective goggles for the staff and eye shields for the patient, and a smoke evacuator, are used. Typical laser blepharoplasty instruments are shown in Figure 37–1.

In our practice, blepharoplasty is commonly performed with other cosmetic procedures under general anesthesia. As an isolated procedure, blepharoplasty can be performed under general anesthesia or local anesthesia with sedation. When local anesthesia is chosen, topical anesthesia of the conjunctiva is accomplished by placing two drops of 4% tetracaine in each eye. Local anesthesia

using 1% lidocaine with 1:100,000 epinephrine is employed in all patients.

Upper Blepharoplasty

Skin markings identifying the supratarsal fold are drawn while the patient is in the supine position. If the supratarsal fold is ill-defined, measurements from the contralateral eyelid are used. The superior extent of the incision is determined by pinching the skin between the supratarsal fold and its proposed upper limit until the lid everts slightly. To minimize the risk of suboptimal scarring, extension of incisions medially past the punctum and laterally past the bony orbital rim should be avoided. Once the skin markings have been drawn satisfactorily, each upper lid is infiltrated in a subcutaneous plane with a few milliliters of local anesthetic. Ten minutes are allowed for hemostasis to take effect.

We use the David-Baker clamp (Byron Medical, Tucson, AZ) for corneal protection and skin retraction (Fig. 37–2). To avoid skin damage at the site of the clamp jaw, overtightening of the clamp should be avoided. The laser is set at 6 W in continuous mode with a focused beam diameter of 0.2 mm. The skin is incised steadily at a rate of 1 to 1.5 cm/s (Fig. 37–3). If advanced too

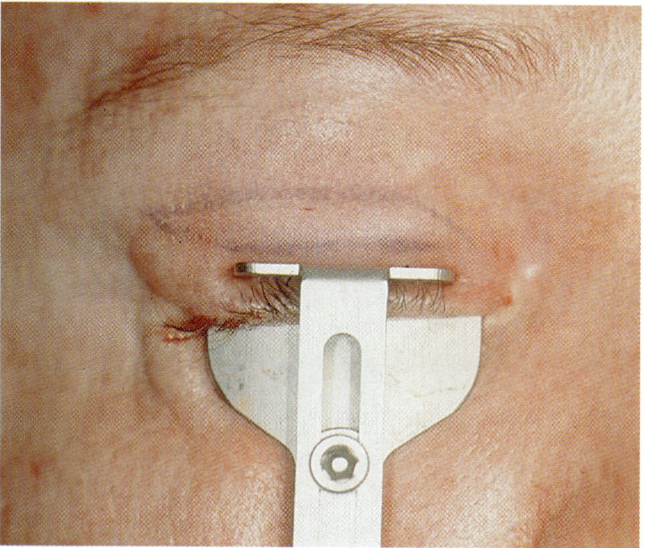

Figure 37–2. David-Baker clamp in place for upper blepharoplasty.

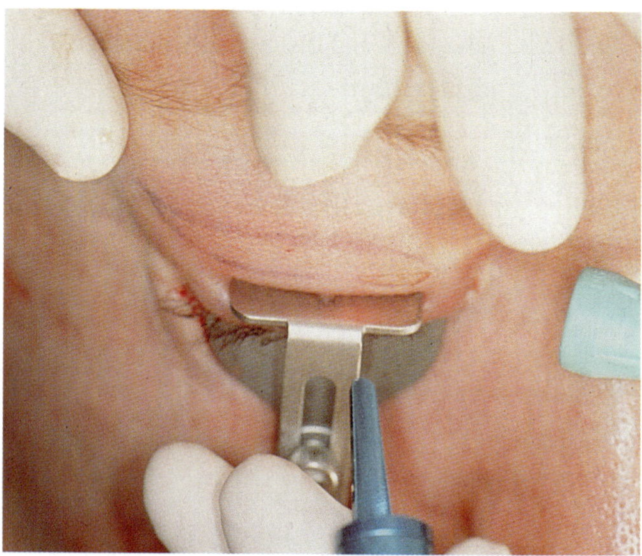

Figure 37–3. Upper eyelid skin incision with laser.

rapidly, the laser fails to cut the skin completely. If advanced too slowly, the levator aponeurosis and conjunctiva can be injured. To remove the skin, the lateral corner of the incision is grasped, and the skin is undercut and separated from the underlying muscle. A Jaeger bone plate (Byron Medical, Tucson, AZ) is used as a "backstop" when undercutting the skin. Cotton-tipped applicators soaked in saline provide countertraction if necessary.

Next, a 5-mm width of orbicularis muscle extending the length of the incision is removed to expose the sep-

tum and the underlying fat compartments. The orbital septum is incised along its entire length. Because of the flattening effect of the David-Baker clamp, identification of the medial fat pad can be somewhat difficult. Once the fat pads have been identified, each is grasped with a pair of fine pickups and gently retracted. (Excess force while retracting the fat pads can cause vessel injury and lead to bleeding.) Excess fat is cut with the laser while the Jaeger bone plate is in place (Fig. 37–4). The laser seals small blood vessels while in defocused mode. Larger vessels are cauterized with a bipolar cautery. The contralateral upper lid is treated in a similar manner. Then, the wound is closed with a subcuticular running 6-0 polypropylene suture.

Lower Blepharoplasty

We almost exclusively use the transconjunctival approach for lower lid blepharoplasty. Excess lower lid skin is treated with laser resurfacing or pinch excision. The transconjunctival approach to the lower lid offers several advantages over the transcutaneous method. It is less likely to alter the shape of the lower lid or cause scleral show because it avoids violation of the orbital septum and the orbicularis muscle. It avoids skin incisions and is faster. The transconjunctival approach is safer in sec-

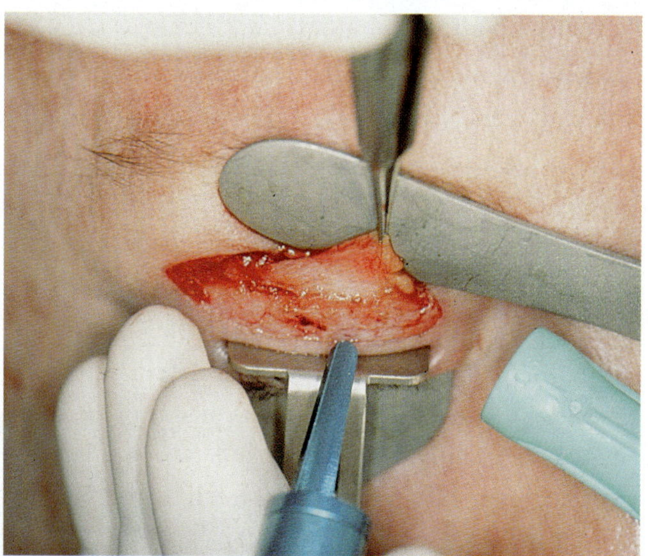

Figure 37–4. Excision of upper lid fat with laser.

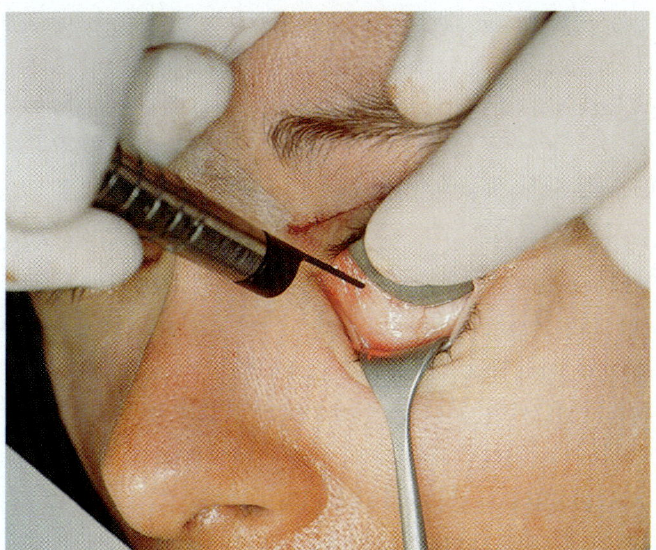

Figure 37–5. Scleral shield and DeMaris retractor in place during the conjunctival incision for lower blepharoplasty.

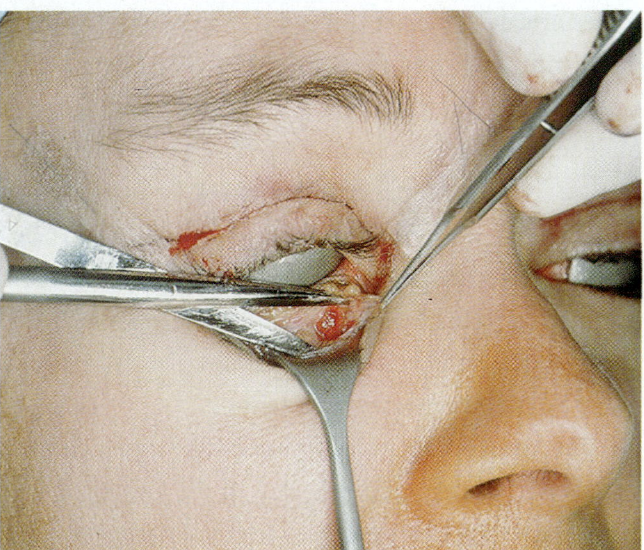

Figure 37–6. Identification of the inferior oblique muscle prior to fat excision.

ondary blepharoplasty procedures. During transconjunctival lower lid blepharoplasty, it is important to identify the inferior oblique muscle to avoid inadvertent injury.

The lower lid conjunctiva is injected with 1 to 1.5 mL of local anesthesia. The scleral shield is placed and the lower lid retracted with a Desmarres retractor or two dull double hooks. The conjunctiva is incised with continuous motion of the laser. The assistant adjusts the retractor as the laser advances the incision. This incision is typically about 5 mm inferior to the inferior lid margin

or about 2 mm inferior to the lower edge of the tarsus (Fig. 37–5). The assistant gently retracts and everts the upper eyelid to move the upper eyelashes away from the laser beam.

A second pass of the laser is usually required to cut the capsulopalpebral fibers and the lower lid retractors. Next, the inferior oblique muscle is identified with fine instruments (Fig. 37–6). The fat pockets are each separately opened with the laser. The medial fat pad has a distinguishing pale-yellow color. The lower lid fat pads are treated sequentially. The edge of each fat pad is grasped with fine pickups and gently retracted anterosuperiorly. While exerting gentle pressure on the globe, excess fat is excised with the laser until the remaining fat is flush with the orbital rim. The Desmarres retractor is used as a backstop during laser trimming of the fat pads (Fig. 37–7). Lateral and medial fat pads should be assessed carefully because underresection is not uncommon. The lateral fat pads in particular tend to be obscured by the lateral orbital rim.

Large angular vessels are always present in the medial fat pad and need to be carefully avoided or adequately cauterized to avoid troublesome bleeding. Once the fat pads have been trimmed, the retractor is removed and the lower lid reexamined. The lateral and medial fat pads

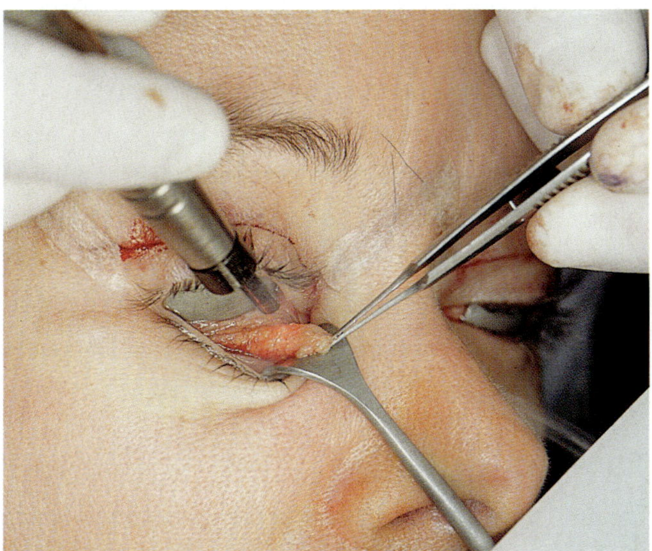

Figure 37–7. Excision of lower eyelid fat.

sometimes need further trimming. In assessing adequacy of fat trimming, one should not confuse underresected fat with the skin bulge that can be caused by the inferior oblique muscle. Additionally, swelling or bulge inferior or lateral to the orbital rim should not be attributed to the orbital fat. Hemostasis is meticulously checked. Conjunctival edges are not sutured unless a large gap exists. If necessary, conjunctival edges can be approximated with buried 6-0 fast-absorbing catgut sutures. The contralateral lower lid is treated in a similar fashion.

The transconjunctival blepharoplasty approach does not allow treatment of excess skin in the lower lid. This area must be treated separately by laser resurfacing or pinch excision. Preoperative assessment of lower lid tone dictates the need for a lid-tightening procedure. When lid tightening is indicated, we perform modified lateral tarsal strip and canthoplasty as described by Anderson and Gordon.[9]

Lower Lid Resurfacing

Skin resurfacing of the lower lid with the CO_2 laser quite effectively removes fine wrinkles and crepiness in the lower lid. We use the Sharplan XJ150 laser with the FeatherTouch optical scanner set at 36 W with a 4-mm spot size. Patients with a history of isotretinoin (e.g., Accutane) use within 2 years and patients with Fitzpatrick skin type IV or higher are advised against laser resurfacing. Prophylactic antiviral therapy is employed in all patients undergoing laser resurfacing. The inferior limit of resurfacing is symmetrically marked on the skin prior to the start of the procedure. An infraorbital nerve block with 1 to 2 mL of local anesthesia is used in addition to any sedation or general anesthesia.

Using the wooden end of a moist cotton-tipped applicator, the lower eyelashes are retracted superiorly while skin resurfacing is started a distance of 2 mm from the lid margin. Working in a cephalad-to-caudad direction, resurfacing is carried to the previously marked margins. A single laser pass with minimal-to-no overlap of laser spots is used. The assistant retracts the cheek and lateral orbital area during the procedure. At the end of the

procedure, the skin is wiped clean with moist gauze. Flexzan (3M Medical-Surgical Division, St. Paul, MN) wound dressing is applied to the resurfaced area.

Pinch Skin Excision

Pinch excision of redundant lower lid can effectively address dermatochalasia of the lower lid skin. The lower lid skin is injected with 1 to 2 mL of local anesthetic mixed with hyaluronidase. After 5 minutes, the skin is pinched with Bishop Harmon (1:10) pickups in a medial-to-lateral direction. The upper end of the pinch is kept close to the lid margin, similar to a subciliary approach for blepharoplasty. The lower extent of the pinch excision is dictated by the extent of skin excess. The skin to be excised is demarcated and then excised with scissors in a lateral-to-medial direction. The remaining edges of excised skin should now lay in close proximity. The skin is closed with a running subcuticular 6-0 polypropylene suture.

POSTOPERATIVE CARE

Cold saline-soaked gauze or gel pads are used continuously for 24 hours after surgery. The patient is asked to keep the head of the bed elevated and to avoid coughing, straining, and lifting for 7 days. Any visual disturbance or severe orbital pain should be reported immediately. Bacitracin ophthalmic ointment is applied to skin incisions four times daily until the sutures are removed. The Flexzan dressing is removed on postoperative day 4. Thereafter, Catrix ointment (Donell Der Medex, New York, NY) or bacitracin ophthalmic ointment is applied to the resurfaced area until reepithelialization is complete. In the pre- and postoperative periods, avoidance of both smoking and nonsteroidal antiinflammatory medication use is stressed. Figures 37–8 and 37–9 show some patients before and after laser blepharoplasty.

COMPLICATIONS

The most dreaded complication in blepharoplasty is blindness. DeMere and colleagues, in a survey of 16,000 oph-

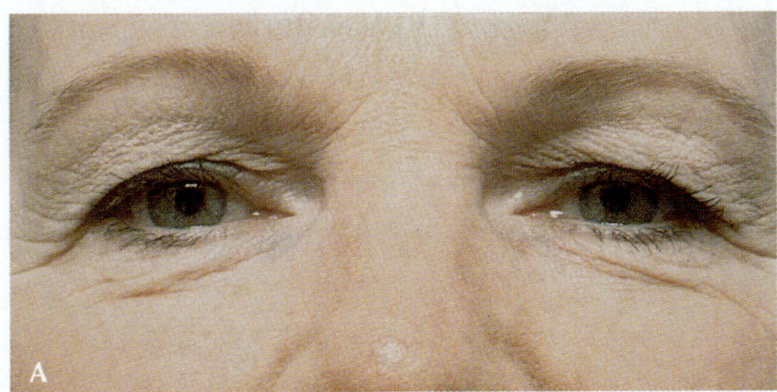

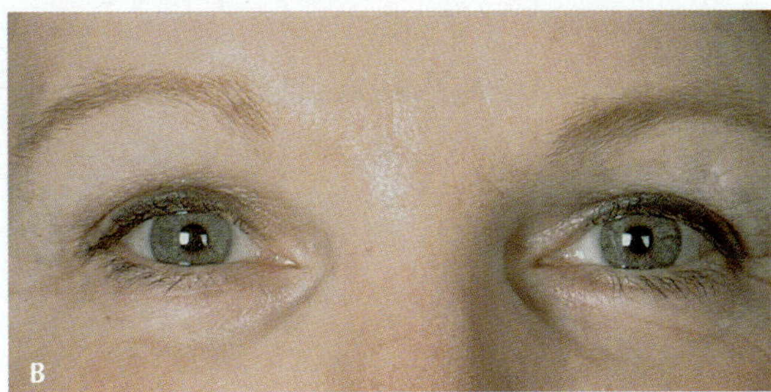

Figure 37–8. (A) Preoperative photograph. (B) Appearance 4 months after bilateral upper and lower blepharoplasty and full-face CO_2 laser resurfacing.

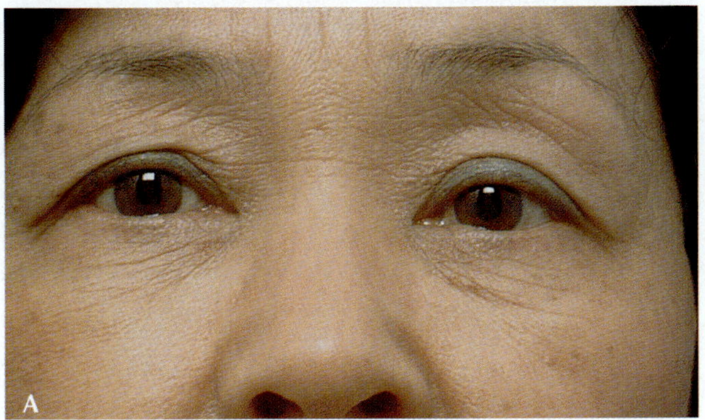

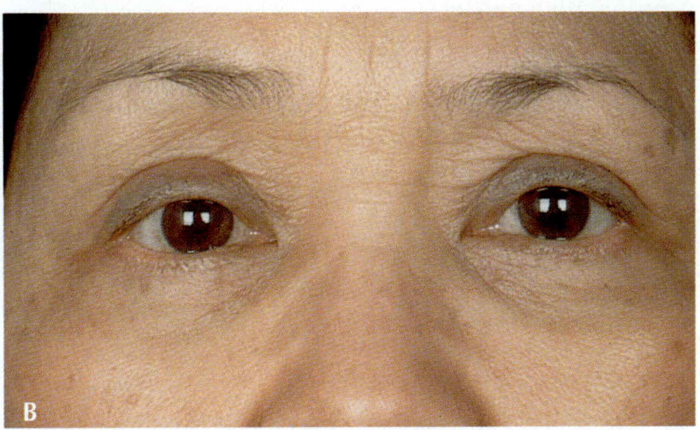

Figure 37–9. (A) Preoperative photograph. (B) Appearance 6 months after bilateral upper and lower blepharoplasty and periorbital CO_2 laser resurfacing.

thalmologists, found that 0.04% of 98,514 eyelid operations resulted in blindness.[10] Callahan studied 68 cases of blindness and found all to be associated with intraoperative or postoperative hemorrhage.[11] Optic nerve damage from spasm of the central retinal artery and/or posterior ciliary artery secondary to unipolar cautery use has also been theorized as another cause of blindness.[12] The effects of the laser on the risk of blindness or orbital hematoma have not been studied, so it remains speculative whether laser blepharoplasty reduces such risks.

Thermal damage to the dermis can lead to delayed wound healing and wound dehiscence in upper lid incisions. It is advisable to leave sutures in the skin for an extra 1 or 2 days to allow for adequate wound healing. Lid ptosis is a possible complication that may be specifically related to use of the laser. Excessive depth of penetration by the laser while incising the skin or orbital septum can result in levator aponeurosis injury. If recognized during the procedure, the aponeurosis should be repaired promptly. Singed eyelashes and chemosis are some of the other risks in laser blepharoplasty. Upper eyelid asymmetry is one of the frequent complications of blepharoplasty and is not affected by use of the laser. Secondary procedures may be necessary to achieve lid symmetry.

One of the more common complications of lower eyelid blepharoplasty is related to eyelid retraction caused by anterior lamellar shortening. Consequences can vary in severity from mild scleral show to ectropion.[13–17] The transconjunctival approach reduces the risk of lower lid retraction by maintaining the anterior lamella intact. Skin resurfacing or pinch excision of the lower lid can be complicated by lower lid retraction. The risk of this complication can be minimized by careful assessment of lower lid tone prior to surgery.

CONCLUSIONS

The CO_2 laser is an effective tool in blepharoplasty. Laser sealing of small vessels makes the operative procedure faster and less bloody. In the immediate postoperative period, there is reduced edema, less ecchymosis, and a more rapid recovery for the patient. Use of the laser necessitates an understanding of the laser-tissue interactions, an educated operating room staff, and strict adherence to laser safety standards. Appropriate use of the laser in cosmetic blepharoplasty reduces morbidity in the early postoperative period.

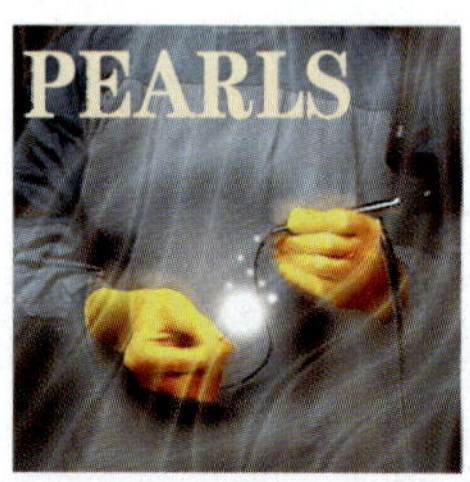

- The transconjunctival approach for lower lid blepharoplasty offers several advantages over the transcutaneous method because it is less likely to alter the shape of the lower lid or cause scleral show, avoids skin incisions, and is faster.
- The surgical assistant assumes a hands-on role in laser blepharoplasty by adjusting the retractor as the laser advances the incision and keeping the eyelashes away from the laser beam.
- It is important to correctly identify and assess the fat pads because underresection, especially of the lateral and medial fat pads, is not uncommon. The lateral fat pads in particular tend to be obscured by the lateral orbital rim. Fat pads may also be confused with muscular structures and other swelling or bulges that most definitely should not be resected.

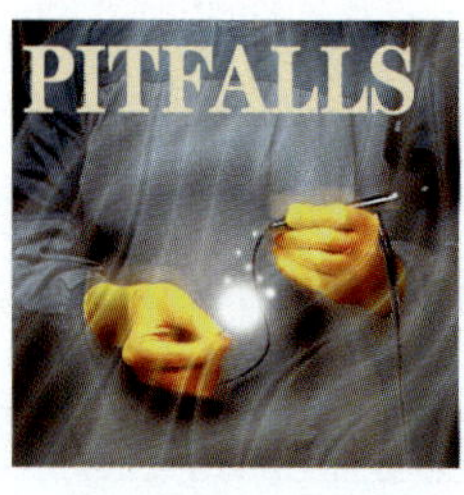

- Although the transconjunctival blepharoplasty approach works well for removing excess fat from the lower lid, the procedure does not allow treatment of excess skin in the lower lid. This area must be treated separately by laser resurfacing or pinch excision. A modified lateral tarsal strip and canthoplasty is recommended.

- The risk of blindness after blepharoplasty is minimal but nonetheless associated with intraoperative or postoperative hemorrhage and optic nerve damage from local artery spasm. It remains speculative whether laser blepharoplasty reduces the risk of blindness.

REFERENCES

1. Patel CKN. Continuous-wave laser action of vibrational-rotational transitions of CO_2. *Phys Rev.* 1964;136A:1187–1193.
2. Ben-Bassat M, Ben Bessat M, Kaplan I. A study of the ultrastructural features of the cut margin of skin and mucous membrane specimens excised by carbon dioxide laser. *J Surg Res.* 1976;21:77–84.
3. Glassberg E, Babapour R, Lask G. Current trends in laser blepharoplasty. *Dermatol Surg.* 1995;21:1060–1063.
4. Baker SS, Muenzler WS, Small RG, Leonard JE. Carbon dioxide laser blepharoplasty. *Ophthalmology.* 1984;91:238–244.
5. David LM. The laser approach to blepharoplasty. *Dermatol Surg Oncol.* 1988;14:741–746.
6. Morrow DM, Morrow LB. CO_2 laser blepharoplasty—a comparison with cold-steel surgery. *Dermatol Surg Oncol.* 1992;18:307–313.
7. David LM, Sanders G. CO_2 laser blepharoplasty: a comparison to cold steel and electrocautery. *J Dermatol Surg Oncol.* 1987;13:110–114.
8. Mittelman H, Apfelberg DB. Carbon dioxide laser blepharoplasty—advantages and disadvantages. *Ann Plast Surg.* 1990;24:1–6.
9. Anderson RL, Gordon DD. The tarsal strip procedure. *Arch Ophthalmol.* 1979;97:2193–2196.
10. DeMere M, Wood T, Austin W. Eye complications with blepharoplasty or other eyelid surgery. *Plast Reconstr Surg.* 1974;53:634–636.
11. Callahan M. Prevention of blindness after blepharoplasty. *Ophthalmology* 1983;90:1047–1051.
12. Castanares S. Complications of blepharoplasty. *Clin Plast Surg.* 1978;5:139–165.
13. Baylis HI, Sutcliff RT. Conjunctival approach to lower eyelid blepharoplasty. *Adv Ophthalmol Plast Reconstr Surg.* 1983;2:43–54.
14. Edgerton MT. Causes and prevention of lower eyelid ectropion following blepharoplasty. *Plast Reconstr Surg.* 1972;43:367–373.
15. Levine MR, Boynton J, Tenzel RR, Miller GR. Complications of blepharoplasty. *Ophthalmol Surg.* 1975;6:53–57.
16. McCord CD. Techniques in blepharoplasty. *Ophthalmol Surg.* 1979;10;40–55.
17. Wiggs EO. Blepharoplasty complications. *Trans Am Acad Ophthalmol Otolaryngol.* 1976;81:603–606.

CHAPTER 38

Coherent UltraPulse Carbon Dioxide Laser Blepharoplasty

DAVID B. APFELBERG

Lasers have assumed a permanent role in facial cosmetic surgery. In addition to skin resurfacing for rhytids and photoaging, the laser may be used as a "light knife" or scalpel for hemostatic incision. Blepharoplasty (also known as an "eye lift") with the carbon dioxide (CO_2) laser demonstrates a marked diminution in postoperative edema, ecchymosis, and pain versus conventional scalpel/cautery techniques. Lower blepharoplasty using the transconjunctival approach combined with laser resurfacing to tighten the skin and eliminate fine rhytids also eliminates lower eyelid scars.

CARBON DIOXIDE LASER VERSUS CONVENTIONAL SURGERY

Several authors have investigated and compared wound healing with the CO_2 laser versus conventional surgery. Hambley and associates, in animal and microscopic studies, have shown that there is more damage to the skin from the standard CO_2 laser incision when compared with scalpel incisions on the basis of clinical evaluation, histopathology of reepithelialization, and measurement of tensile strength.[1] Norris and Mullarky compared incisions made by the scalpel and the CO_2 laser in pig skin and found no difference at 30 days, although the initial reepithelialization and tensile strength were diminished in the CO_2 laser incision in the first 2 weeks.[2] Mittelman, Keating, and Smoller studied facial skin incised by scalpel, cautery, CO_2 laser, 532-nm potassium titanyl phosphate: yttrium-aluminum-garnet (KTP:YAG) laser, and standard 1064-nm YAG laser.[3] They concluded that the acute stage of healing demonstrated greater tissue injury from lasers and cautery. Although the lasers were more hemostatic than the scalpel (with the YAG laser performing slightly better than the CO_2 laser), the lasers caused epithelial and dermal injury to varying degrees, the CO_2 laser being slightly better than the YAG lasers (532 and 1064 nm). All studies were done with conventional continuous wave (CW) or superpulsed lasers, and not the currently available short-pulse, high-energy lasers.

Precursors for the development of CO_2 laser blepharoplasty came from development of the laser for surgery of the eye and adnexa. Beckman and associates in 1980 described numerous uses of the laser to treat ocular (e.g., glaucoma, scleral lesions) and adnexal lesions, including lid tumors and hemangiomas.[4] Wesley and Bond also described use of the CO_2 laser for lymphangiomas, hemangiomas, and anticoagulated patients.[5] Korn and Glotzbach have repaired medial ectropion by CO_2 laser resection of conjunctiva/tarsus-inferior muscle.[6]

Initial claims of the benefit of the CO_2 laser for blepharoplasty were made by Baker and colleagues in 1984 when they reported results in 40 patients monitored for about 16 months.[7] They concluded that the CO_2 laser improved intraoperative hemorrhage and postoperative ecchymosis and edema. Baker updated his experience in 1992 and described the use of the David-Baker clamp for protection of the eye and retraction of tissue.[8]

David and Sanders, in contralateral comparison studies, reported better results on the CO_2 laser side than on the regular scalpel/cautery side.[9] David further described CO_2 laser techniques, including the transconjunctival lower blepharoplasty approach,[10,11] as did Trelles and colleagues[12] and Spadoni and Cain[13] (nurses working in Dr. David's practice). Morrow and Morrow compared laser blepharoplasty with conventional blepharoplasty in a contralateral study of 10 patients and concluded that the laser reduced operating time, bleeding, bruising, swelling, and postoperative pain and resulted in a shorter recovery time.[14] Mittleman and Apfelberg, in a contralateral study in 1990, were not able to demonstrate significant differences between laser and regular blepharoplasty.[15] However, the study was not done totally with the laser and so was not consistent with previous studies. Beeson, Kabaker, and Keller noted that the superpulsed CO_2 laser required less operative time and was associated with less bruising and swelling compared with contralateral scalpel/cautery surgery, especially when the surgeon was experienced in use of the laser.[16] In 1992, Morrow and Morrow reported a series of 110 lower face lifts using the CO_2 laser as the only cutting instrument.[17] These authors felt that laser use resulted in less postoperative bruising, swelling, pain, and discomfort. In a contralateral study with the YAG laser using sapphire tips, Apfelberg demonstrated less bruising and swelling on the laser blepharoplasty side when compared with the conventional surgery side.[18] Apfelberg has reported his results with CO_2 laser blepharoplasty and face lift plus resurfacing in large series of patients.[19–22]

CLINICAL EXPERIENCE

The Coherent UltraPulse Model 5000 CO_2 laser (Coherent, Palo Alto, CA) used in the series discussed in this chapter represents a significant advance over previous CW CO_2 laser technology because the laser almost achieves a "cold incision." The laser tube is supercharged with high doses of radiofrequency energy for a very short time (pulse duration), which results in a buildup of laser power within the tube that may be delivered to tissue in short durations (known as "ultrapulses"). Each pulse delivers higher power than is normally possible with a CW or superpulsed laser. The UltraPulse achieves high power over one millionth of a second (1 microsecond). The pulses may be repeated at a certain rate (pulse per second = hertz). For example, an average power of 5 W would have a repetition rate of 25 Hz, pulse width (or time on) of 314 microseconds, time off of 39,686 microseconds, and an energy-per-pulse of 250 mJ.

Clinically, at 3 to 5 W of power, 15 to 25 mJ of continuous power, and a 0.2-mm spot size, excellent hemostatic cutting may be achieved. Defocusing accomplishes coagulation, and eyelid skin and fat can be excised easily and almost bloodlessly (0 to 0.5 mL for all four lids). Skin, muscle, and fat may all be resected with the laser without the need for cross-clamping or crushing these structures. These tissues are easily incised because ultrapulses result in vaporization or incision without char or thermal injury to tissue. Because the thermal relaxation time of skin is established to be around 695 to 700 microseconds, the short pulse does not allow accumulation of heat. Also, the delay (time off) between pulses permits the minimal level of heat that has accumulated in surrounding areas to dissipate before the next burst of laser energy is delivered. The result is extremely precise vaporization or cutting, which means there is no need to cut back wound edges prior to closure, and there is minimal risk of scarring or prolonged healing time.

TECHNIQUE

Ophthalmic anesthetic solution and ophthalmic antibiotic ointment are applied before protective eye shields are inserted. The laser is set at 4 W of continuous power with a 0.2-mm focused handpiece pointed at focal length

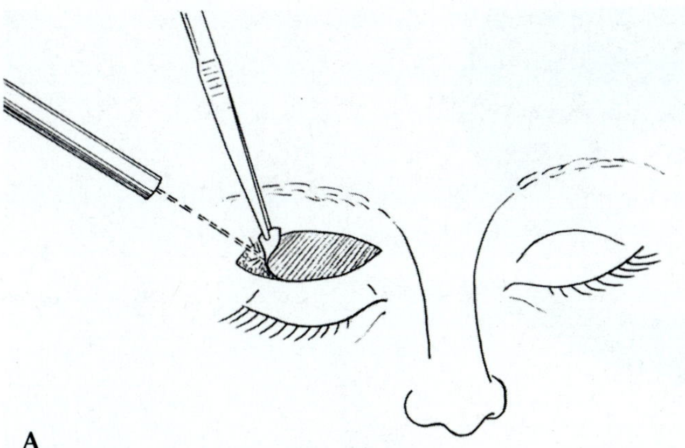

A

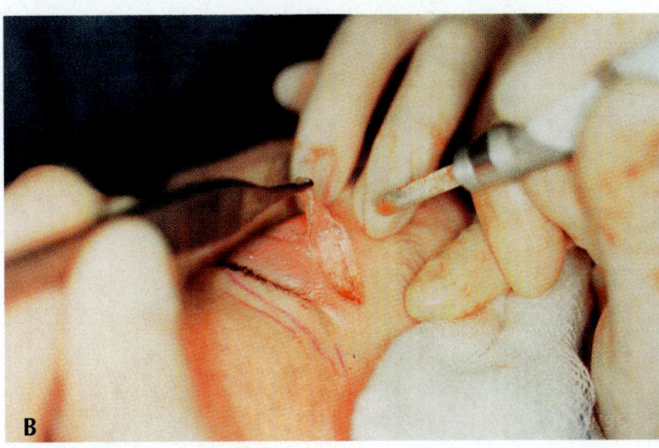

B

Figure 38–1. Skin and muscle are resected by tangentially focused laser utilizing a cotton-tipped applicator (A) or a moist tongue blade (B) as a backstop.

and directed toward tissue that is placed under traction for easier separation. Skin and muscle are first circumscribed and then resected (Fig. 38–1). Moistened applicators or tongue blades or specially designed dull-finish metalshields are placed as a "backstop" behind tissue that is elevated for removal by the laser so that the beam will not strike tissue beyond the area to be removed (Fig. 38–2); alignment may be checked by directing the laser toward a moist tongue blade. Other safety factors that must be observed include smoke evacuation and moist gauze draping of adjacent skin.

The orbital septum is opened with the laser, and fat is resected over a backstop (Fig. 38–3). The eye shields are removed immediately after the procedure is completed to prevent corneal edema.

Transconjunctival blepharoplasty may be accomplished safely and bloodlessly as well. The laser is used to incise the conjunctiva (Fig. 38–4). Fat is delivered and resected by the laser against a backstop (Fig. 38–5). The laser has no electrical potential, so fat may be draped directly across a small metal retractor and removed without fear of electric shock transmission or burns of the skin.

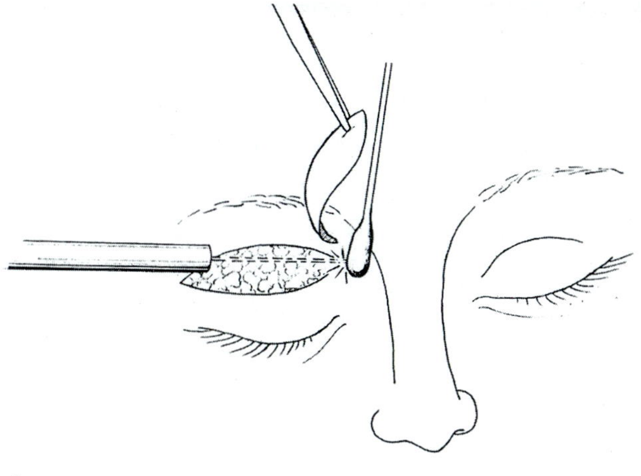

A

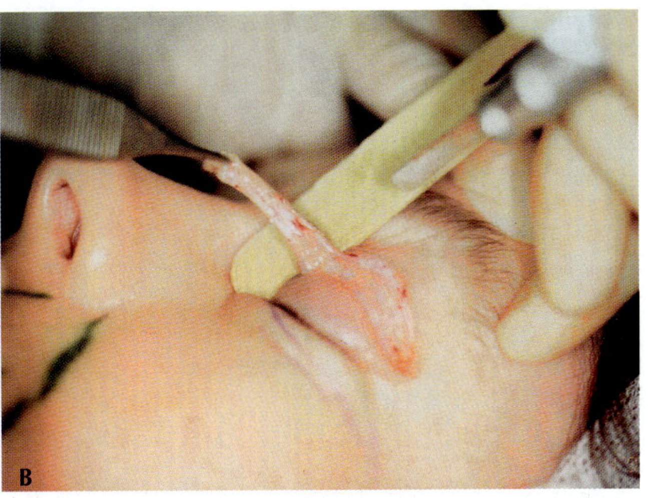

B

Figure 38–2. The 0.2-mm spot-size focused beam is used to incise skin and muscle (A, B).

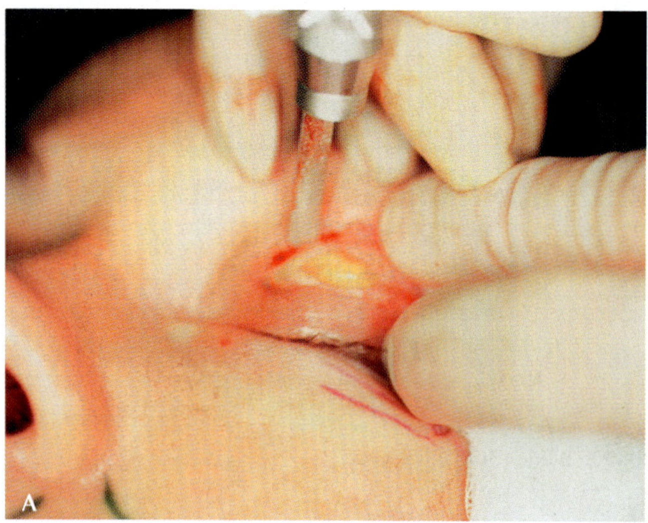

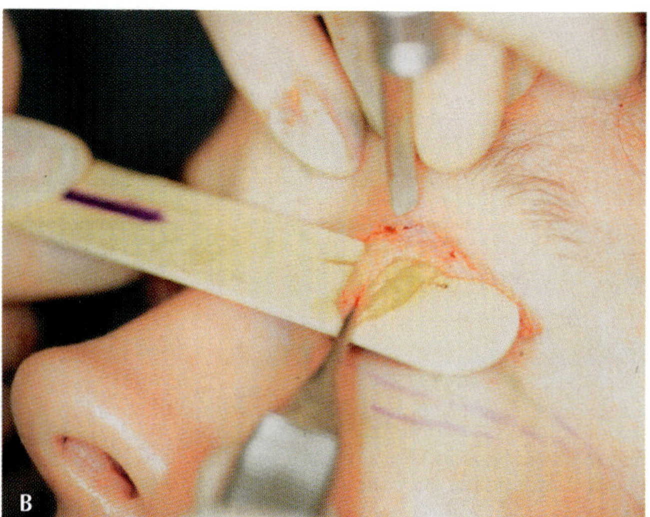

Figure 38–3. The orbital septum is opened with the laser (A), and fat is resected over a backstop (B).

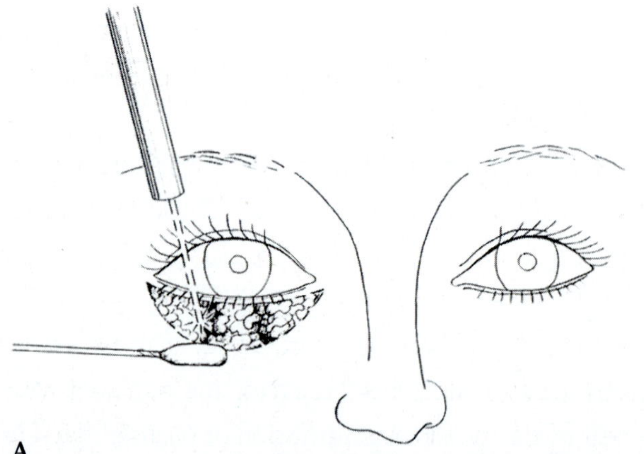

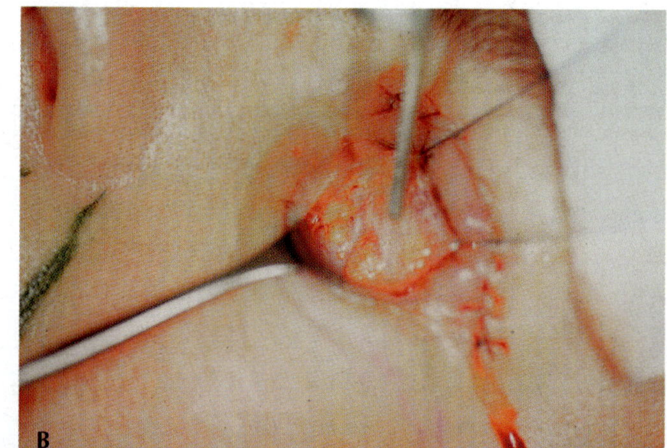

Figure 38–4. A transconjunctival incision is made with the laser (A, B).

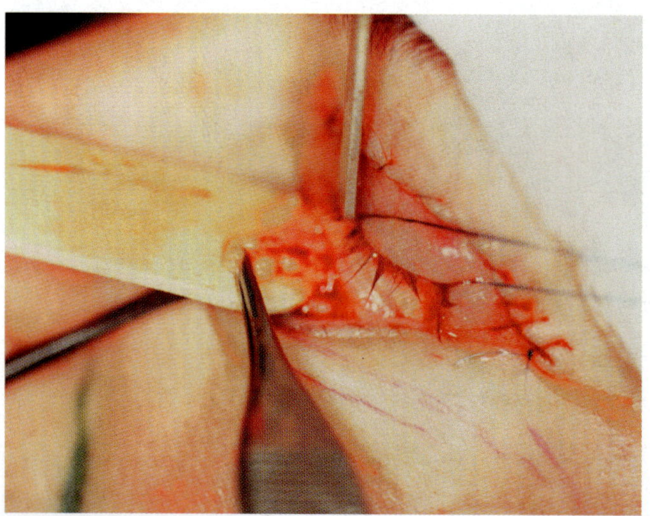

Figure 38–5. Fat is resected with the laser over a backstop.

RESULTS

Between 1991 and 1999, we treated 81 blepharoplasty patients and 21 meloplasty/blepharoplasty patients using the UltraPulse CO_2 laser (Table 38–1). Of the 102 patients, 11 were male and 91 were female, with an average age of 51.3 years (blepharoplasty).

Use of the laser did not significantly affect the duration of the procedure, and there were no laser-related complications. The results of this series were very encouraging. Occasionally, patients reported no use of any analgesic agent (5%). Approximately one third of blepharoplasty patients recorded very minor blood loss (<5 mL) for all four lids, whereas blood loss for the

Table 38–1. Carbon Dioxide Laser Cosmetic Surgery

Procedure	No. of Patients	Gender	Averge Age (y)	EBL (mL)	Final Healing (d)
Blepharoplasty	81	7 M, 74 F	48.5	7.7	11.6
Meloplasty/ blepharoplasty	21	4 M, 17 F	62.2	60.0	12.6

whole blepharoplasty group averaged just 7.7 mL. Postoperative swelling, ecchymosis, pain, and discomfort were markedly reduced in all patients (Fig. 38–6). Some patients examined 1 day postoperatively exhibited very little bruising and swelling, and some were completely free of residual ecchymosis and swelling after 1 week. The average time for bruising and swelling to disappear totally was 8.9 days (range, 4 to 17 days) in blepharoplasty

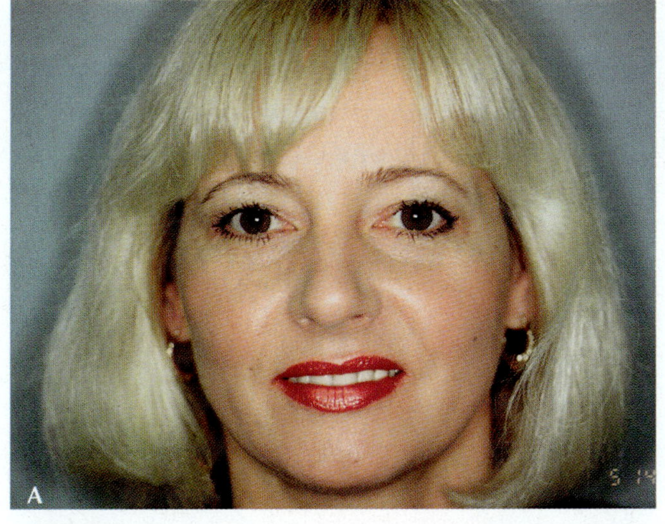
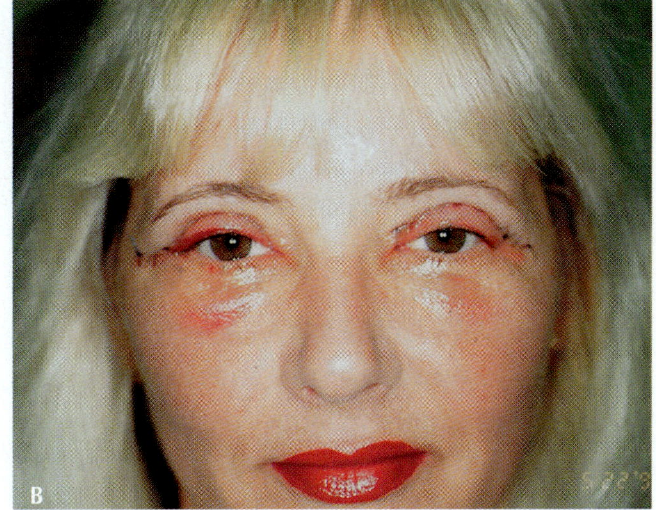
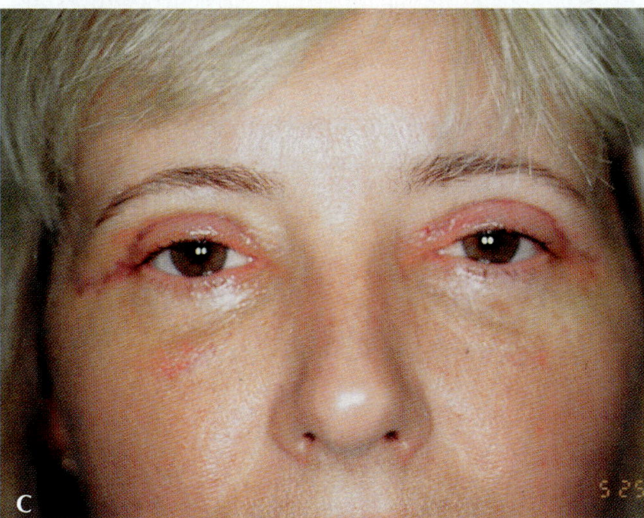
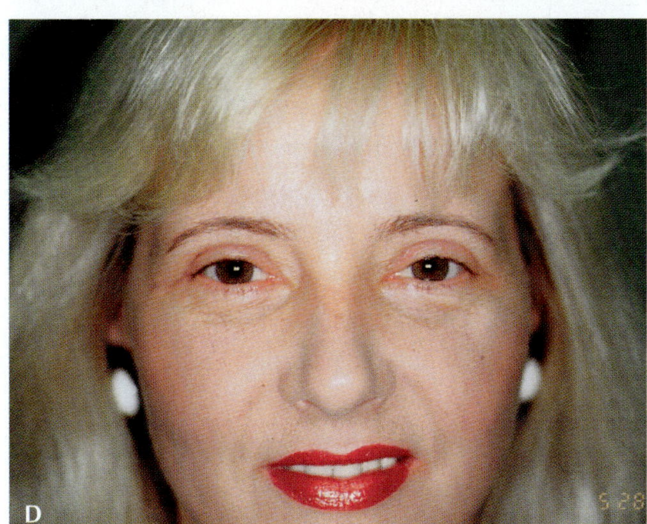

Figure 38–6. (A) A 46-year-old woman with moderate upper blepharochalasia and fullness of the lower lids. (B) Appearance 3 days following upper blepharoplasty and transconjunctival lower blepharoplasty. (C) Appearance 6 days following surgery, showing markedly decreased bruising and swelling. (D) All bruising and swelling are completely gone 9 days postoperatively.

patients. Three of four patients who underwent laser blepharoplasty in one eye and standard blepharoplasty in the contralateral eye demonstrated resolution of bruising and swelling 3 to 5 days earlier on the laser side. Many patients were able to resume normal work activities and social interactions in 7 to 10 days, as opposed to 14 to 17 days for patients who have conventional procedures.

CONCLUSIONS

Use of the laser has facilitated facial cosmetic procedures and enhanced results in the immediate postoperative period. Operative time does not change, and the excellent hemostasis benefits the surgeon because visibility is enhanced and vital structures can be dissected relatively bloodlessly. Consequently, patients experience less ecchymosis and edema in the postoperative period. Contralateral studies have demonstrated that the recovery period is shortened by one third (i.e., from an average of 14 to 17 days with the standard scalpel to 7 to 11 days with the laser),[18] which means that patients can return to work or social activities sooner. Many patients experience little or no pain following the laser procedure. By 3 weeks after the procedure, no difference can be detected between the scalpel- and laser-treated sides.

Further advantages include a positive marketing or practice enhancement factor because many patients are interested in lasers or are already familiar with the perceived benefits. Although mere interest or familiarity alone certainly would not adequately justify an expensive laser purchase, preferences must be considered.

There are also disadvantages associated with laser use. Lasers, accessories, and maintenance can cost from $65,000 to $125,000. Logistically, one must consider storage for a relatively large and bulky piece of equipment and support materials such as fibers, tips, and peripheral devices. Lasers may require special electrical power requirements and plumbing for water cooling. Like any other high-tech equipment, lasers may be subject to "down time" or malfunction; fortunately, this is a relatively rare occurrence. When in use, lasers produce noise and heat in the operating room environment.

Misdirected firing may burn adjacent tissue. Eye safety for the patient and all personnel in the room must be observed, as well as other safety measures (e.g., smoke evacuation, access warning signs). Special training for the physician and the nursing staff is also required. Most surgeons find laser surgery slightly more cumbersome and awkward than regular surgery, although this factor diminishes with experience.

Because patients are charged more for laser surgery, and the surgeon may find the laser's size and noise make its use slightly more awkward than standard surgery, the laser is not recommended for every facial cosmetic procedure. Patients who need to return to work or social activity as soon as possible should be offered the laser, as should patients who are attracted to procedures specifically because of laser availability. Any patient with a coagulation disorder, who claims "easy bruising," or who has inadvertently taken aspirin or antiinflammatory agents prior to surgery is a good candidate for laser use because of the excellent hemostasis achieved with the laser. Currently, 75% of all blepharoplasties and 50% of all face lifts are performed with the laser.

The laser provides intraoperative and early postoperative advantages but no difference from standard techniques late postoperatively. It is just one more tool in the surgeon's armamentarium, and most procedures also include scissors, scalpel, and cautery. Surgical judgment in patient selection, appropriate tissue resection and tension of closure, and adequate hemostasis must still be exercised, keeping in mind that skin healing and scars are not affected by the laser.

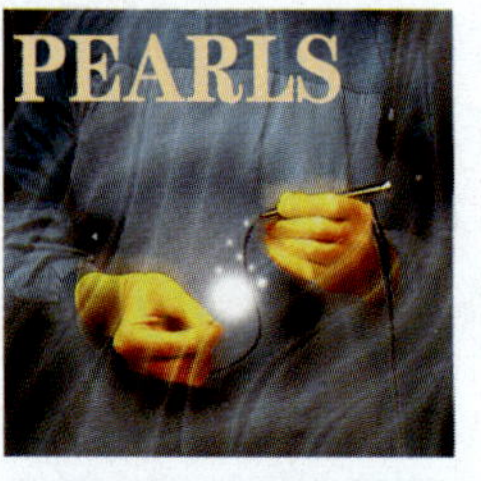

- Carbon dioxide laser blepharoplasty evolved from development of the laser for surgery of the eye and adnexa (e.g., glaucoma, scleral lesions, lid tumors, hemangiomas, lymphangiomas, and medial ectropion).
- The UltraPulse CO_2 laser represents a significant advance in laser technology because the laser almost

achieves a "cold incision" by having a shorter pulse than the relaxation time of the skin, which means that heat does not accumulate to cause thermal damage.

- The laser has no electrical potential, so fat may be draped directly across a small metal retractor and removed without fear of electric shock transmission or burns of the skin.

- Eyelid skin and fat can be excised easily and almost bloodlessly with the UltraPulse CO_2 laser, thereby enhancing the surgeon's visual field.

- Many patients are interested in lasers or are already familiar with the perceived benefits, which may increase the acceptability of laser procedures. However, scalpel surgery still retains a place in the surgeon's practice.

- The laser is not recommended for every facial cosmetic procedure, but may be ideal when the patient needs to return to work or social activity very quickly. Any patient who has a coagulation disorder, is easily bruised, or has inadvertently taken aspirin or antiinflammatory agents prior to surgery is a good candidate for laser surgery.

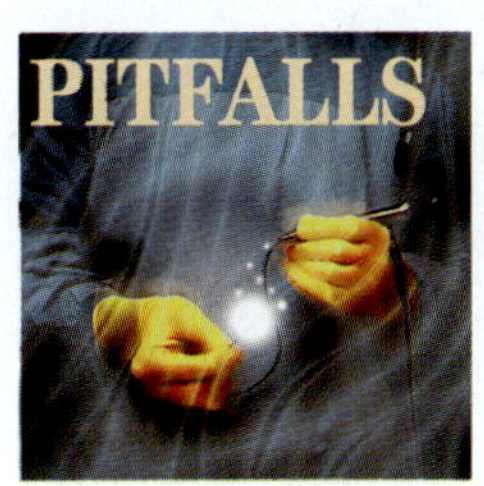

- The laser, its accessories, and maintenance are very expensive and present storage problems. Like any other high-tech equipment, lasers may occasionally experience down time or malfunction.

- Misdirected firing of the laser may burn adjacent tissue. Use of the laser necessitates implementation of several safety measures. The physician and the nursing staff must be properly trained to institute these safety procedures and use the laser effectively and responsibly. Most surgeons find laser surgery slightly more cumbersome and awkward than standard surgery, although this factor diminishes with experience.

REFERENCES

1. Hambley R, Hebda P, Abell E, et al. Wound healing of skin incisions produced by ultrasonically vibrating knife, scalpel, electrosurgery and carbon dioxide laser. *J Dermatol Surg Oncol.* 1988;14:1213–1271.

2. Norris CW, Mullarky MB. Experimental skin incisions made with the carbon dioxide laser. *Laryngoscope.* 1982;92:416–419.

3. Mittelman H, Keating W, Smoller BR. Evaluation of acute human tissue injury using various lasers in facial surgery. In Facial Plastic surgery Clinics of North America, pp 173–179.

4. Beckman H, Fuller TA, Boyman R, et al. Carbon dioxide laser surgery of the eye and adnexa. *Ophthalmology.* 1980;87:999–1000.

5. Wesley RE, Bond JB. Carbon dioxide laser in ophthalmic plastic and orbital surgery. *Ophthalmic Surg.* 1985;18:631–633.

6. Korn EL, Glotzbach RK. Carbon dioxide laser repair of medial ectropion. *Ophthalmic Surg.* 1988;19:653–657.

7. Baker SS, Muenzler WS, Small RG, Leonard JE. Carbon dioxide laser blepharoplasty. *Ophthalmology.* 1984;91:238–243.

8. Baker SS. Carbon dioxide laser upper lid blepharoplasty. *Am J Cosmet Surg.* 1992;9:141–145.

9. David LM, Sanders G. Carbon dioxide laser blepharoplasty: a comparison to cold steel and electro-cautery. *J Dermatol Surg Oncol.* 1987;13:110–114.

10. David LM. The laser approach to blepharoplasty. *J Dermatol Surg Oncol.* 1988;1:741–746.

11. David LM, Abergel RP. Carbon dioxide laser blepharoplasty: conjunctival temperature during surgery. *J Dermatol Surg Oncol.* 1989;15:421–423.

12. Trelles MA, Sanchez J, Sala P, Elspas S. Surgical removal of lower eyelid fat using the carbon dioxide laser. *Am J Cosmet Surg.* 1992;9:149–152.

13. Spadoni D, Cain CL. Laser blepharoplasty. The transconjunctival method. *AORN J.* 1988;47:1184–1194.

14. Morrow DM, Morrow LB. Carbon dioxide laser blepharoplasty. *J Dermatol Surg Oncol.* 1992;18:307–313.

15. Mittelman HM, Apfelberg DB. Carbon dioxide laser blepharoplasty: advantages and disadvantages. *Ann Plast Surg.* 1990;24:1–6.

16. Beeson WM, Kabaker S, Keller GS. Carbon dioxide laser blepharoplasty, a comparison to an electro surgery. *Int J Aesthetic Restorative Surg.* 1994;2:33–36.

17. Morrow DM, Morrow LB. Carbon dioxide laser assisted lower facelift: a preliminary report. *Am J Cosmet Surg.* 1992;9:159–168.

18. Apfelberg DB. YAG laser meloplasty and blepharoplasty. *Aesthetic Plast Surg.* 1995;19:231–235.

19. Apfelberg DB. Ultrapulse carbon dioxide laser resurfacing and facial cosmetic surgery. *Can J Plast Surg.* 1995;3:1–4.

20. Apfelberg DB. The ultrapulse carbon dioxide laser with computer pattern generator automatic scanner for facial cosmetic surgery and resurfacing. *Ann Plast Surg.* 1996;36:522–529.

21. Apfelberg DB. A critical appraisal of high-energy pulsed carbon dioxide laser resurfacing for acne scars. *Ann Plast Surg.* 1997;38:95–101.

22. Apfelberg DB. Ultrapulse carbon dioxide laser with CPG scanner for full-face resurfacing for rhytids, photoaging, and acne scars. *Plast Reconstr Surg.* 1997;99:1817–1825.

CHAPTER 39

Weekend Laser Neck Lift

GREGORY S. KELLER AND VICTOR G. LACOMBE

Treatment of the aging neck but not the aging face is controversial. Many patients are more disturbed by aging of the neck than facial aging and often seek a more limited procedure than a face lift for treatment of their neck ptosis.

Although most surgeons agree that younger patients can benefit from modification of the underlying neck structure with liposuction to remove genetic fat deposits or from platysmaplasty to tighten ptotic neck structures, there is disagreement about whether neck lift alone is sufficient for older patients. Younger patients have more elastic skin and can expect contraction over the cavity produced by the removal of the neck fat. Older patients have skin that is less elastic and contractile and have trouble eliminating the space between the skin and platysma muscle produced by liposuction and platysmaplasty. Consequently, some surgeons feel that such skin (also known as a "wattle") needs to be excised in older patients, and many feel that a full face lift is required for older patients who have significant sagging. These surgeons argue that only by operating on the neck does one lose the upward pull on the platysma muscle generated by the submandibular aponeurotic system (SMAS) portion of the cheek lift. In addition, a face lift can rotate upward and excise redundant skin, which cannot be accomplished with liposuction and a neck lift alone.

Nonetheless, there are published techniques for segmental neck lifts that do not involve face lifts.[1-4] These techniques can be divided into posterior platysmaplasty techniques, anterior platysmaplasty techniques, and combined techniques.

TECHNIQUE

Posterior approach techniques allow skin to be drawn back and resected from the postauricular hairline incision. With backward rotation of the flap, the anterior cavity that is produced by liposuction or anterior platysmaplasty can be effaced by directing the skin backward against the platysma muscle. Anterior neck lifting usually involves liposuction and a pulling together of the platysma muscles in the midline. The resulting space formed anteriorly between the skin and the tightened platysma muscle is not effaced and can form a seroma.

To obtain contraction of the redundant skin, Dr. W.R. Cook Jr. has adopted the novel tactic of lasing the skin from the platysma side of the flap. His theory is that laser treatment of the underside of the flap produces sufficient additional contraction of neck skin so that patients of any age may undergo a "weekend laser neck lift" without the need for a face lift or a postauricular incision. He uses the Coherent UltraPulse 5000 laser (Coherent, Palo Alto, CA) in a defocused mode to treat the midportion of the neck through a 2.5-cm midline incision, using a low power setting of 7 W. The theoretical problem with this procedure is the potential for damage to the subdermal plexus and necrosis of the overlying skin. However, Dr. Cook estimates that he treats only 20% of the surface area because he uses a crisscrossing pattern.

PERSONAL EXPERIENCE

We have used a Surgilase XJ150 laser with a flexible waveguide and pulses of 35 mJ/cm^2 to perform a procedure similar to Dr. Cook's. This laser's chief advantage is that the waveguide can be inserted into a small incision to lase the entire undersurface of the flap, not just the central portion. In 20 patients to date, we have encountered no delayed healing or necrosis.

The actual procedure involves liposuction of the neck and jowls employing the tumescent technique. This is followed by anterior platysmaplasty with "corset" suturing to the level of the hyoid, as well as excisional release of the platysma in the midline at the level of the hyoid. Finally, the undersurface of the flap and platysma is lased prior to closure of the incision. An elastic neck support is worn day and night for 4 days postoperatively.

We make an anterior submental incision with cold steel 2 to 2.5 cm below the submental crease. Using a Klein injection needle (Bernesco), the neck and jowls are injected with Klein tumescent solution. Then, using size 8 to 12 Klein needle cannulas at low suction pressures, the neck and jowls are suctioned aggressively.

Excess platysma muscle is clamped in the midline and excised. The platysma muscle is imbricated together in the midline with interrupted horizontal mattress sutures to the level of the hyoid. A triangle of platysma muscle is then removed below the suture line.

The Surgilase XJ150 laser set to 35 mJ/cm^2 with a flexible fiberoptic waveguide lases the undersurface of the flap in a checkerboard pattern. This energy level minimally affects the underlying tissue; there is no peeling or other evidence of dermal damage. The platysma muscle underlying the flap is also lased in a similar checkerboard fashion, although higher energy levels may be used.

Box 39–1 describes some of the subjective conclusions based on the brief history of our technique. It is our impression that use of the laser for liposculpture of the neck and platysmaplasty produces some skin contraction and extends the usefulness of this procedure to an older population. The ideal patient is still younger with excess submental fat and good skin elasticity. The procedure gives a "good" result to the less demanding patient who simply wants to reduce the neck wattle, but it is less useful for thin patients with inelastic skin (Figs. 39–1 and 39–2).

Box 39–1. Conclusions about the Surgilase XJ150 Laser Neck Lift

1. There is some tightening and contraction of neck skin.
2. There have been no seromas in our patients.
3. The posterior-approach neck lift with platysmal incision and rotation produces more dramatic results with the same healing period but does not require the wearing of a neckband for 4 days.
4. Patients with submental fat accumulations were happy with the results of the procedure. Older, thin patients with skin elasticity problems were not as happy with their improvement. Edema associated with this procedure lasts up to 8 to 9 months, so the poorer results in this patient group frequently are not seen immediately.
5. Platysmal bands with an anterior corset procedure are not eliminated indefinitely; they usually recur about 18 to 24 months after the procedure.
6. The laser produces little, if any, thermal injury to the flap. The mechanism of skin tightening is still being investigated, although mild contraction can be visualized.
7. Patients with very high expectations are generally not satisfied with the level of jowl improvement.

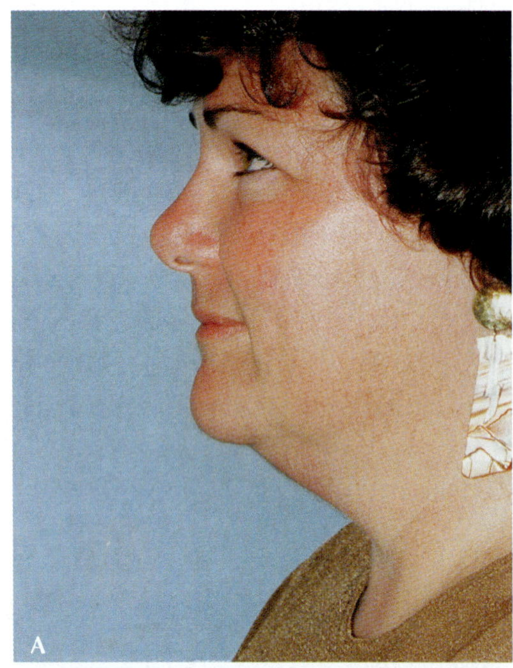
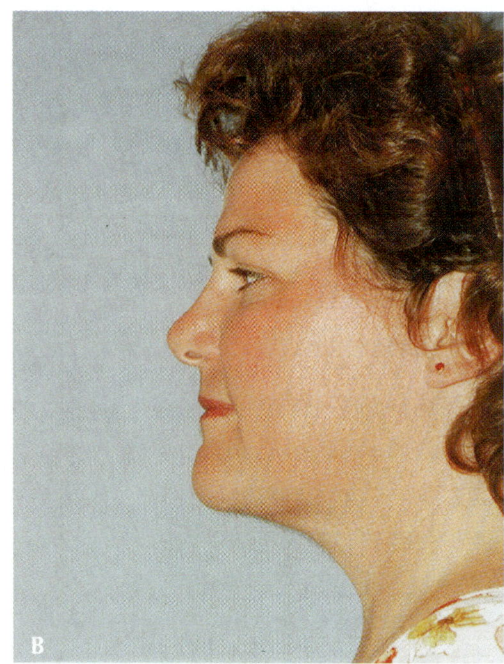
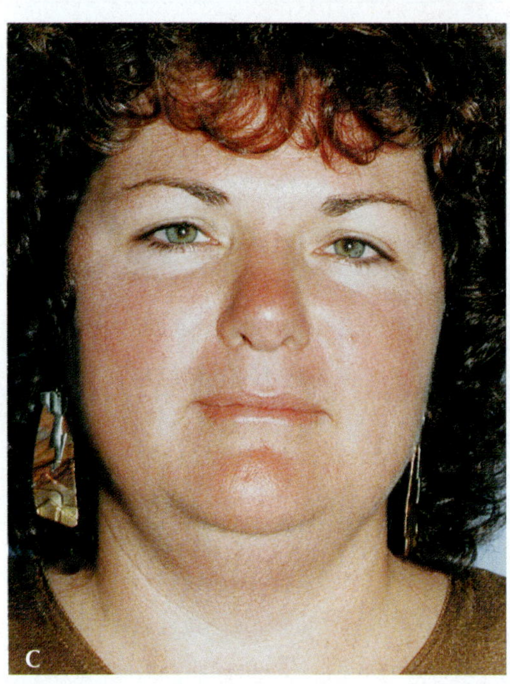
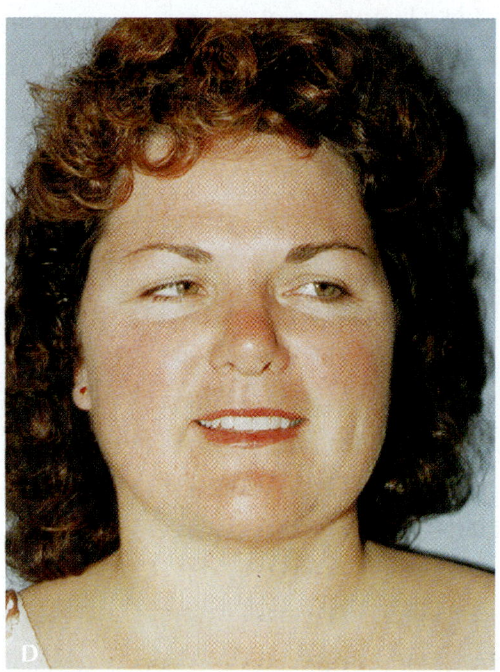

Figure 39–1. Preoperative (A, C, E, G) and postoperative (B, D, F, H) views of a young woman with excessive submental fat. Left, frontal, right, and three-quarters views. Note improvement in jawline definition.

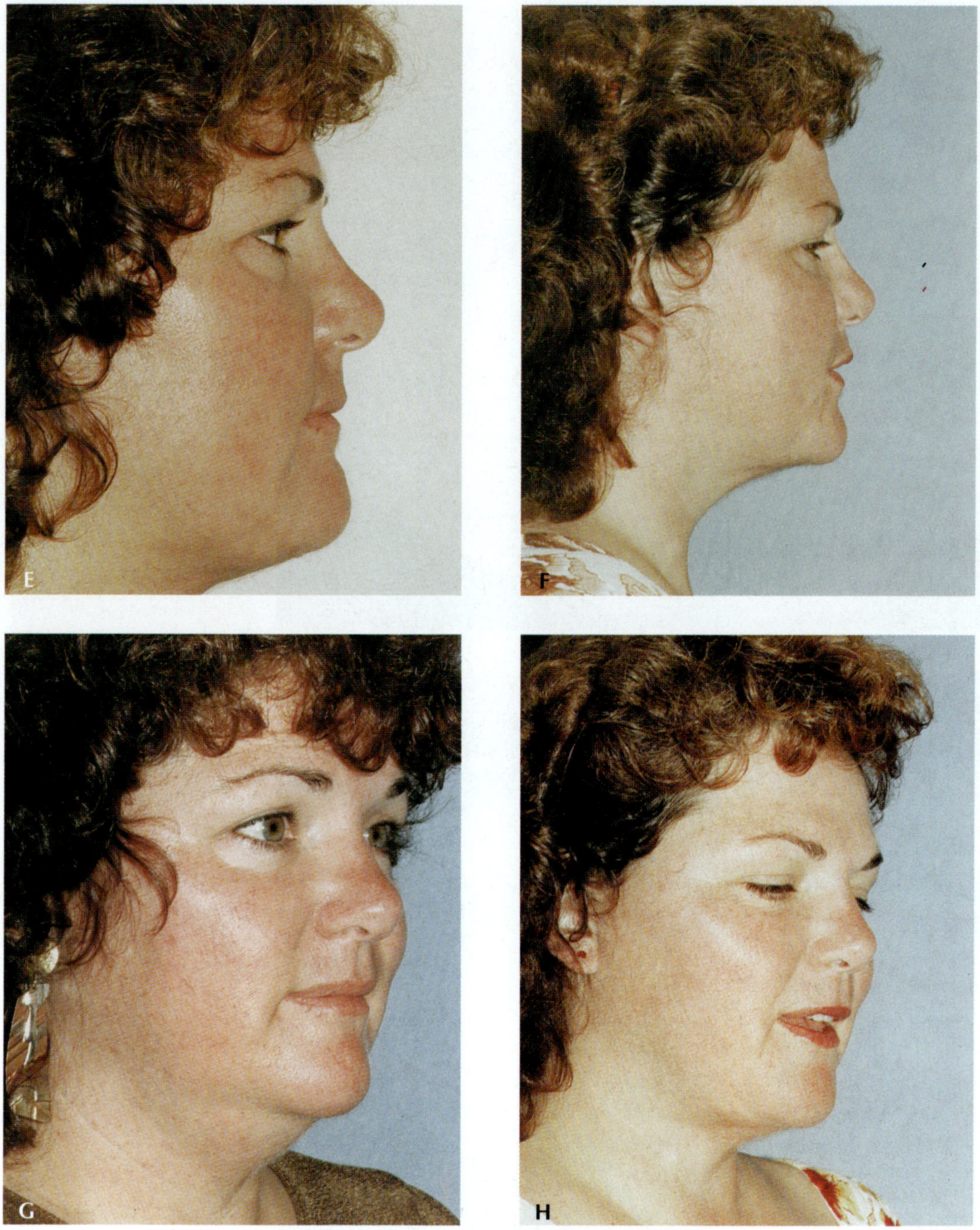

Figure 39–1. *(continued)*

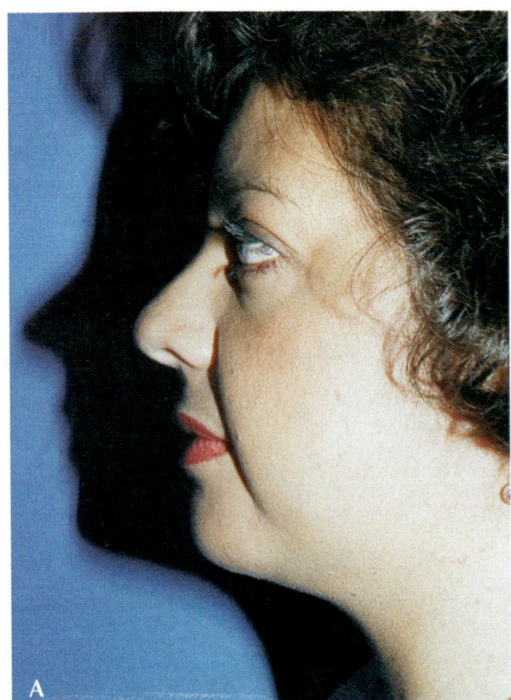
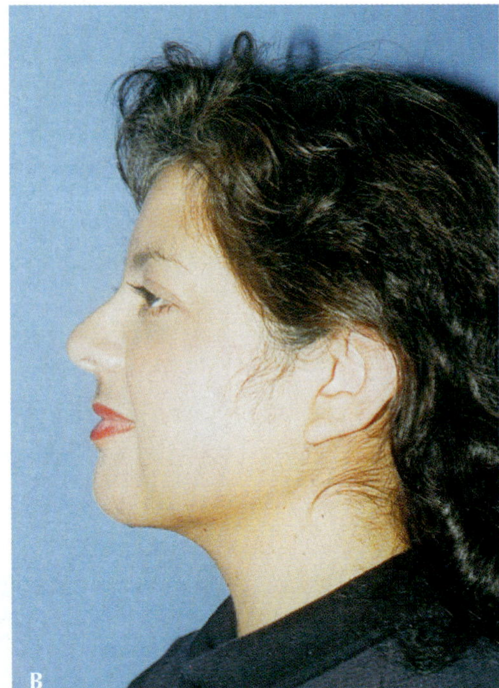
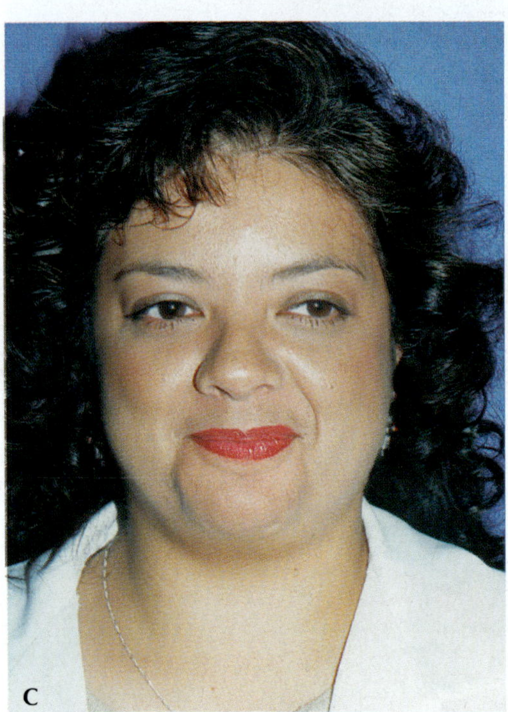
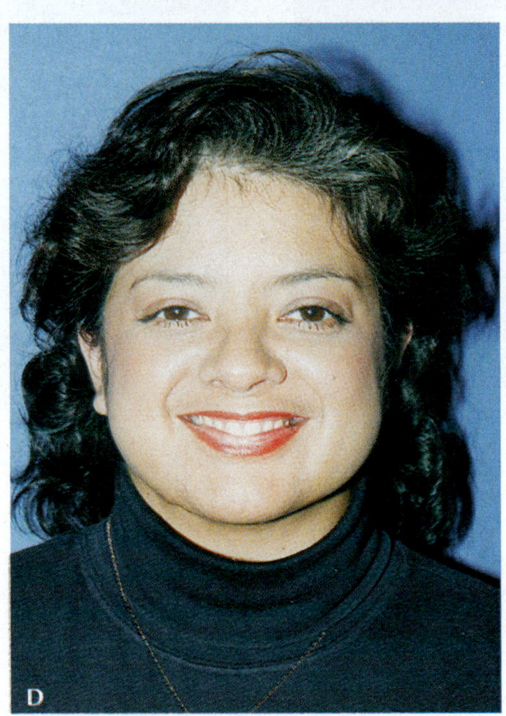

Figure 39–2. Preoperative (A, C, E, G) and postoperative (B, D, F, H) views of a young woman with excessive submental fat. Left, frontal, right, and three-quarters views. Younger patients have good skin elasticity and are able to redrape effectively after aggressive liposuction.

Figure 39–2. *(continued)*

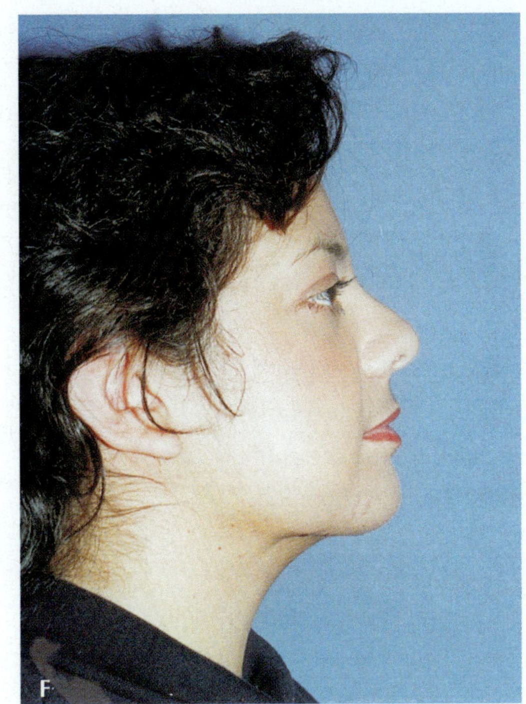

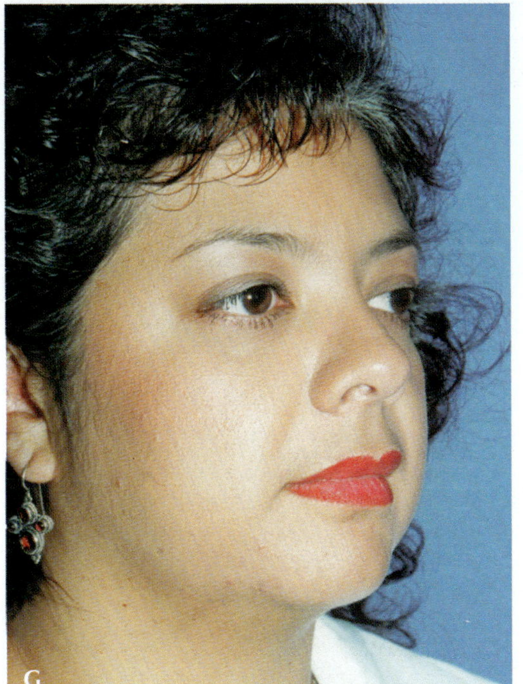

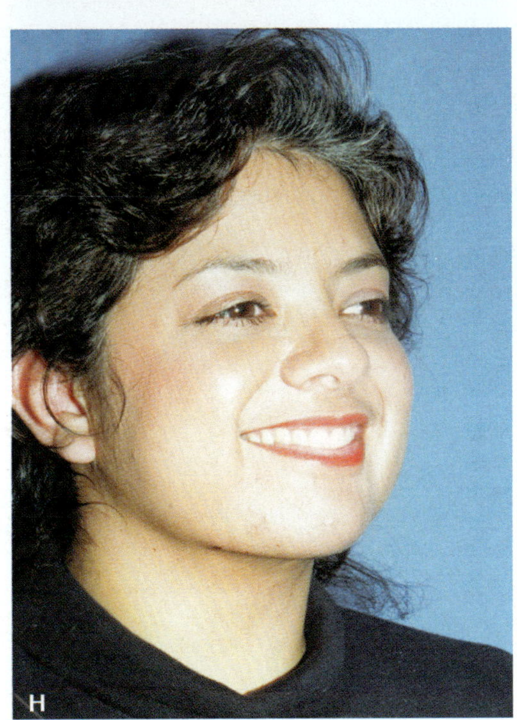

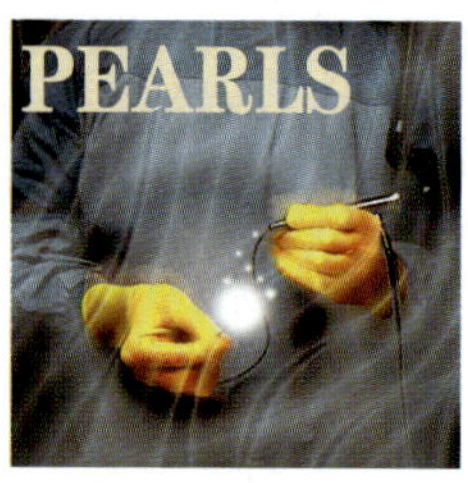

- The novel tactic of lasing the skin from the platysma side of the flap has successfully produced sufficient additional contraction of neck skin so that patients of any age may undergo a "weekend laser neck lift" without the need for a face lift or a postauricular incision.

- The chief benefit of using the Surgilase XJ150 laser with a flexible waveguide is that the waveguide can be inserted into a small incision to lase the entire undersurface of the flap, not just the central portion.

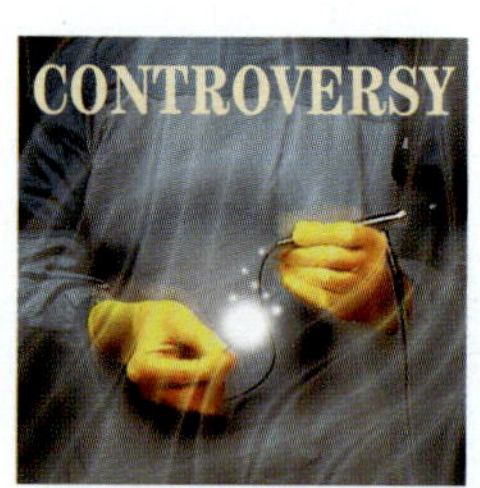

- Although younger patients definitely benefit from a neck lift without a concomitant face lift, there is disagreement about whether a neck lift alone is sufficient for older patients; some surgeons feel that such skin needs to be excised, whereas others feel that a full face lift is required for older patients.

REFERENCES

1. Cook WR Jr. Laser neck and jowl liposculpture including platysmal laser resurfacing, dermal laser resurfacing and vaporization of subcutaneous fat. *Dermatol Surg.* 1997;23: 1143–1148.
2. Ramirez OM. Cervicoplasty: nonexcisional anterior approach. *Plast Reconstr Surg.* 1997;99:1576–1585.
3. Coleman WP. Liposuction. In: Coleman W, Hanke C, Alt T, eds. *Cosmetic Surgery of the Skin.* Philadelphia: BC Decker Inc.; 1991:213–238.
4. Pitman G. Face and neck. In: Pitman G, ed. *Liposuction in Aesthetic Surgery.* St. Louis: Quality Medical Publishing Inc.; 1993: 111–167.

CHAPTER 40

Skin Resurfacing Using Bipolar Cautery

VICTOR G. LACOMBE, W. GREGORY CHERNOFF, AND GREGORY S. KELLER

There is a great deal of interest surrounding skin resurfacing modalities and their potential for rhytid reduction. From chemical peels, to dermabrasion, to lasers, physicians have taken technologies and applied them to cosmetic surgery. A recent innovation in electrosurgery is now being applied to skin resurfacing. The Refinity Coblation system, as it is being called by the parent company (McGhan, Santa Barbara, CA), employs bipolar electrical current in an ionic fluid medium to allow for cold ablation of tissue (Fig. 40–1). The application of the electrical current and the formation of a plasma layer are unique to this new use of a familiar surgical tool. Initially applied to arthroscopic procedures with good success, a skin resurfacing unit was subsequently developed using the same technology. Multiple gold electrodes act as end-plates for the electrical current, which makes an arc and returns to the probe. The current passes through saline or lactated Ringer's solution and creates charged ionic particles. A voltage gradient develops between the plasma and the soft tissue when applied to the skin and enough energy is generated to cause dissociation of molecular bonds within the tissue. This leads to cell lysis and ablation of the tissue. The effects are limited to the area in contact with the plasma layer. This method of ablation is similar to that achieved with the excimer lasers used for corneal sculpting and refractive surgery.

HISTORY OF ELECTROSURGERY

In 1891, d'Arsonval was the first to use a high frequency electrosurgical device.[1] William Bovie later developed the first adaptable generator for both cutting and coagulating currents.[2] The basic theory behind electrosurgery is that as current passes through tissue it meets resistance, which generates heat. Depending on the frequency, application, voltage, and amperage of the current, the effect on tissue varies. A continuous wave creates cutting whereas an intermittent current allows for coagulation. Electrodessication, electrofulguration, electrocoagulation, and electrolysis are all variations on the theory.[3]

THEORY

With the Refinity system and Coblation, the electrical current remains in the fluid medium, and charged particles from the saline plasma transmit energy to the superficial layer of the skin to cause ablation. Temperatures at the skin level reach only 60 to 100°C. This is much lower than that seen with many resurfacing lasers that may generate up to 600°C at the tissue level. It is high enough to allow for hemostasis and heating of collagen to induce contraction. The spread of the thermal energy is low because only tissue in contact with the plasma layer receives energy and low temperatures are dissipated

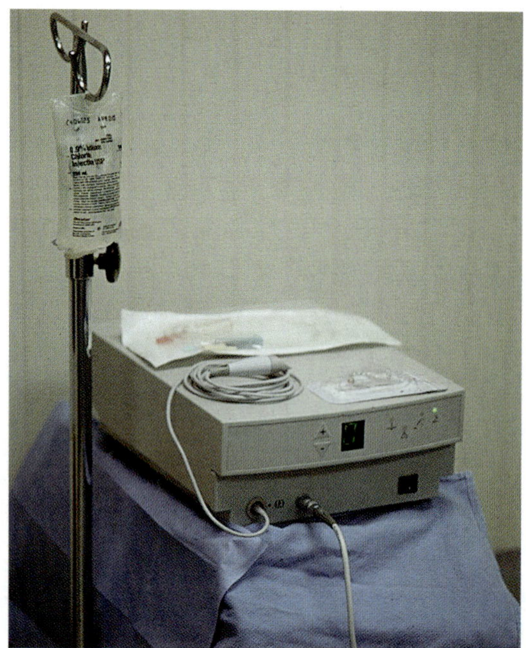

Figure 40–1. The Refinity system with all the necessary components. Saline, tubing handpiece, sterile tip, and footpedal cable all attach to the main unit. Small size makes for an easily portable unit.

rapidly in surrounding tissues. As a result ablation with little residual thermal injury is expected.[4]

STUDY DESIGN

Although this technology has much physics and theory behind it, clinical usage for cosmetic surgery is in its early stages. Preliminary studies were performed in Canada and a multicenter phase II trial is underway in the United States. The device has already been approved for general dermatologic use. There are, however, no studied parameters of ideal power settings or numbers of passes necessary to achieve good results for rhytids. Furthermore, there have been no studies of the histologic effects of the system.

In our study, we set out to achieve two goals. The first was to determine what the actual histologic effects of the system were on facial skin and the second, how treated areas would respond.

HISTOLOGIC EFFECTS

Our methods included the treatment of preauricular skin of patients prior to undergoing rhytidectomy

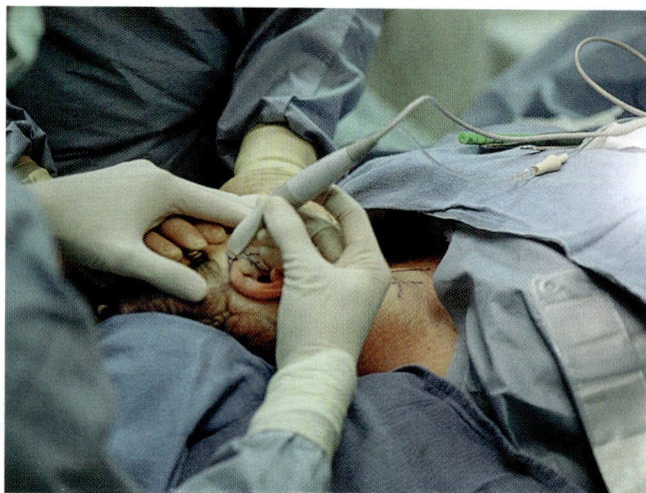

Figure 40–2. Clinical use intraoperatively prior to facelift procedure. Sterile draping and gowns are necessary for resurfacing purposes only.

(Fig. 40–2). The test area was treated with 1 to 6 passes at various power settings. Once the treatment was completed the skin was harvested, fixed in formalin, and sent for evaluation by an independent pathologist. Patients each gave informed consent; had they not, the harvested skin would have been discarded during the procedure.

RESULTS

Full thickness epidermal ablation was seen with either one or two passes. The initial ablation reached an average of 80 μ with an additional 20 μ of thermal injury. Up to six additional passes saw little to no increase in depth of ablation and up to 60 μ of thermal injury. A total of 64 samples from eight patients have been examined. Further samples are still being collected to help determine the optimal parameters in a statistically significant manner.

CLINICAL EFFECTS

Ten volunteers who desired resurfacing of periocular rhytids were also treated with the Refinity system. All patients were instructed on postresurfacing wound care, given oral antiviral and antibiotic prescriptions, and followed closely postoperatively. Patients signed consent forms similar to those used with laser resurfacing. Only periocular areas were treated and all patients received only local anesthetic infiltration.

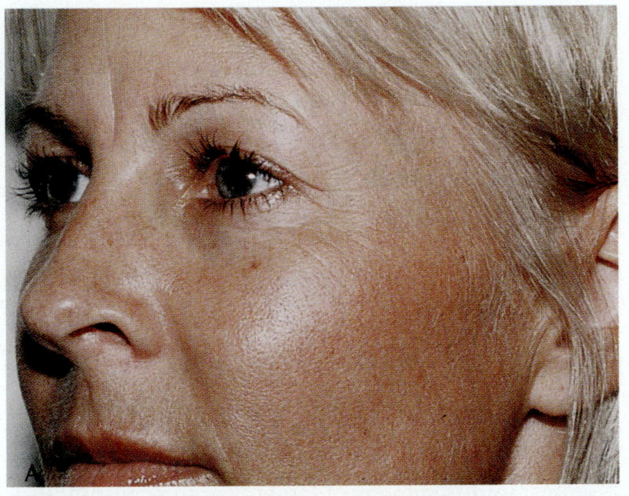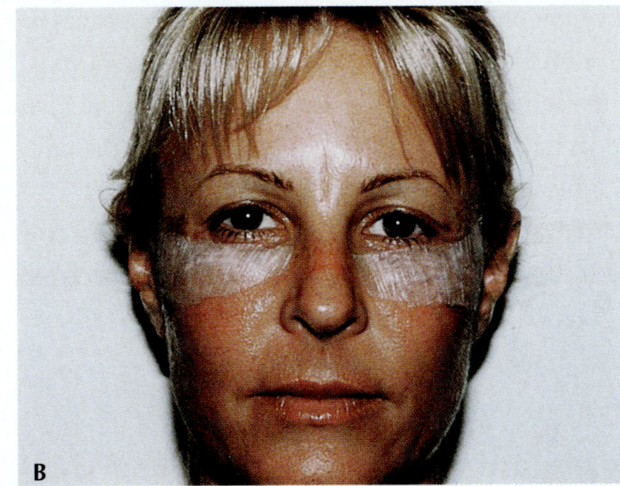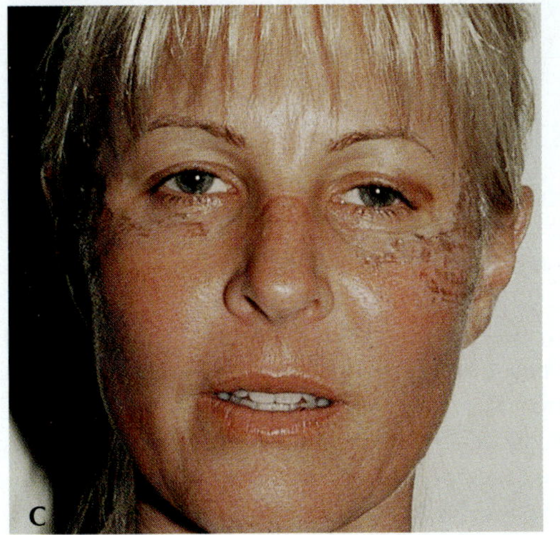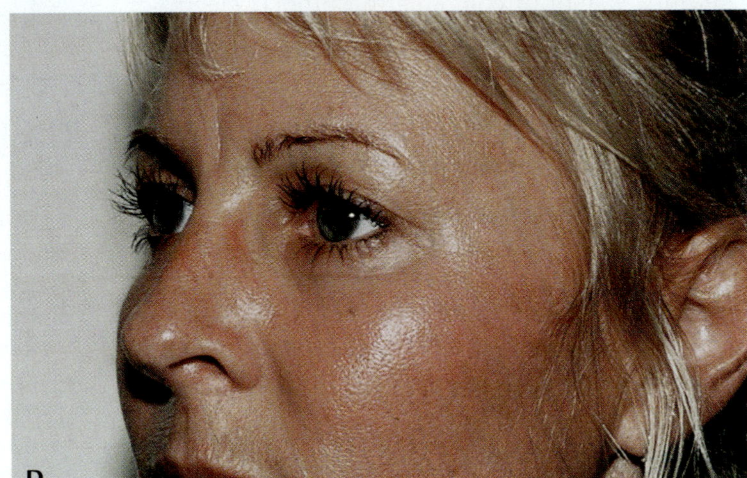

Figure 40–3. A 35-year old patient. (A) Preoperative view, prior to resurfacing. (B) 2 days, (C) 4 days, and (D) 4 months postoperatively.

Clinical Results

The power setting used was 4, which is 125 W, and two passes were performed over the area. Clinically the wound that was created was very similar to those seen with laser resurfacing. Semiocclusive dressing was used and reepithelialization was seen to occur by an average of 7 days, with a range of 5 to 10 days. Posttreatment erythema was mild and lasted an average of 3 to 4 weeks. Of note, when the healing was complete, there was a noticeable improvement in fine lines and crepey skin of the lower eyelid. There was also improvement in the area of the crow's feet. However, deep rhytids in this area were not completely obliterated with the two passes of the Refinity (Fig. 40–3).

THEORETICAL ADVANTAGES

In the field of skin resurfacing, the Refinity system appears to offer several advantages. It provides a controlled depth of ablation, low surface skin temperatures, and minimal thermal injury. The histologic findings are that this system provides deeper ablation than several passes of the erbium laser and causes less thermal injury than even a single pass with the carbon dioxide (CO_2) laser. The time to reepithelialization was comparable to that of laser wounds and erythema was intermediate to that of erbium and CO_2 lasers. Long-term resolution of rhytids has yet to be determined, but in the short term, results are promising and patients were very satisfied with their results.

CONCLUSIONS

In addition to its clinical effects, the Visage system is small, quiet, portable, and safe. No eye protection is required and there is no need for smoke evacuation. The potential for its widespread use is great because the unit costs a fraction of conventional lasers on the market.

Disadvantages of the system include the need for saline to be dripped onto the field, which can become annoying, and the fact that deeper ablation, if necessary or desired, may not be possible.

CONCLUSIONS

The Refinity system of cold ablation bipolar electrocautery for skin resurfacing appears to have adapted a familiar surgical tool to a new application. Certainly the extensive science and research of laser medicine and laser resurfacing contributed to the development of this device. The goals of precise tissue ablation with minimal thermal necrosis and thermal injury have been well thought out. Although the Refinity system is a relative newcomer in the field of skin resurfacing, it appears to have good potential in that realm. Further clinical tests remain to be performed before its place in the spectrum of resurfacing and rejuvenating modalities is determined.

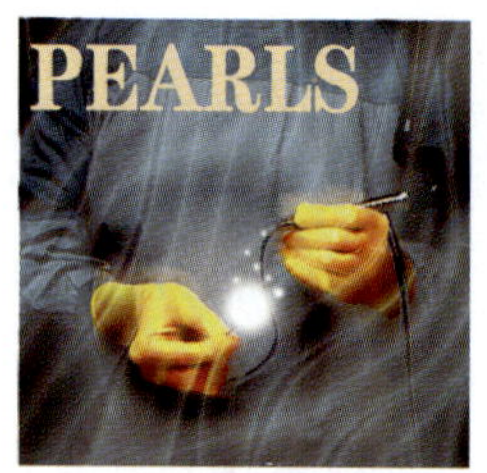

- It is important during treatment that the handpiece and electrodes remain perpendicular to the treatment area.
- The tip becomes coated with ablated tissue fragments and must be wiped with a moist gauze from time to time. Wiping the skin also removes debris and allows for more effective tissue interaction with the handpiece.
- The original handpiece came with a smaller tip size, but newer 1-cm tips are currently available. This allows for rapid treatment of larger areas because with each pass, a large area is being treated.

REFERENCES

1. d'Arsonval A. Action physiologique des courants alternatifs. *Soc Biol.* 1891;43:283–286.
2. Goldwyn RM. Bovie: The man and the machine. *Ann Plast Surg.* 1979;2:135–153.
3. Olhoffer IH, Leffell DJ. What's new in electrosurgery? Coblation: a new method for facial resurfacing. *Aesthetic Dermatology and Cosmetic Surgery* 1999;1:31–33.
4. Eggers PE, Thalipyal HV, Grekin RA. Coblation: a newly described method of soft tissue surgery. *Res Outcomes Cosmet Reconstr Surg.* 1998;1:1–3.

CHAPTER 41

Skin Rejuvenation for Sun Damage, Aging, and Rosacea Using Intense Pulsed Light

PATRICK H. BITTER, SR. AND GEOFFERY PAUL NASE

Current trends in aesthetic treatment of facial skin call for an effective adjunct to laser skin resurfacing. Younger, more active patients in great numbers seek treatment, which offers a return to a more youthful appearance through restoration of even color and smoothness, relief from pigmentary sun damage, fine lines, and wrinkles, and, often, the redness and flushing associated with rosacea. In addition, this patient group requires treatments that are short and pain-free, and allow immediate return to all activities.

Following more than 20 years of treatment of vascular lesions using the flashlamp-excited pulsed dye laser, a new laser-like intense pulsed light (IPL) device was developed that treats these conditions with success and answers the essential lifestyle criteria when used in a carefully administered program. This new IPL nonablative skin rejuvenation technique, marketed as PhotoFacial™, now has a clinical history of more than 3,000 treatments with excellent patient acceptance.

USE OF INTENSE PULSED LIGHT

IPL differs from laser light in that, rather than monochromatic single wavelength, IPL emits a noncoherent, broad spectrum light. The Multilight or Epilight device (ESC/Sharplan, Needham, MA, USA) used in the PhotoFacial procedure emits with each pulse a spectrum extending from 500 nm to 1,200 nm. To customize the light energy delivery for a given procedure, the operator employs a cutoff filter, or light guide, of designated wavelength, below which the spectrum is selectively eliminated (Fig. 41–1).

The IPL system, as used in the PhotoFacial procedure, conforms to the principle of selective photothermolysis.[1]

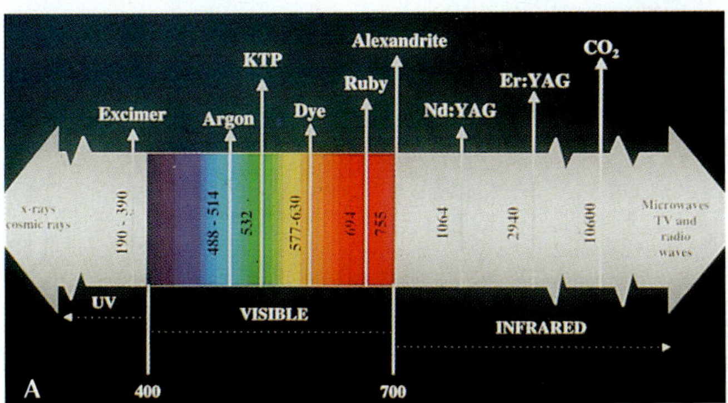

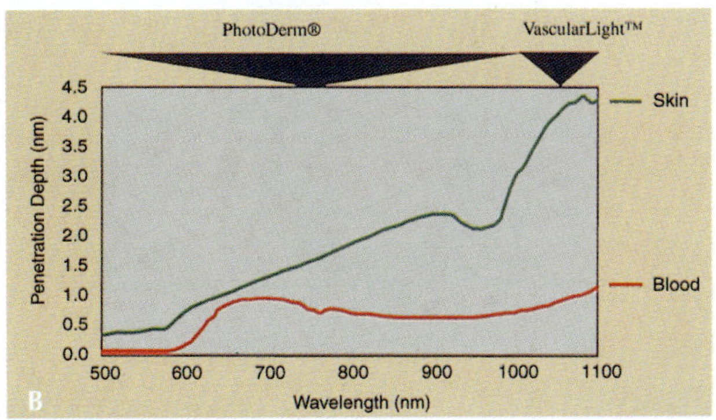

Figure 41–1. (A) The electromagnetic spectrum. (B) Penetration depth for various wavelengths used for treatment of facial abnormalities.

For dilated vessels, as seen in patients with sun damage and rosacea, the light energy with high absorption by hemoglobin and oxyhemaglobin reaches the dermal capillary bed and selectively destroys the abnormal vessels.[2] For pigmentary abnormalities, as seen in patients with aging and sun damage, the IPL energy is selectively absorbed by melanin, which destroys the abnormally pigmented cells, resulting in a more even complexion.

The operator controls all aspects of the light pulse, including cutoff wavelength (nm), energy level (Joules/cm^2), pulse duration (milliseconds), pulse pattern (single, double, or triple), and delay time between pulses (milliseconds). This allows for precise control of light energy, which in this procedure is utilized for customization for skin type, procedure progress, and other variables.

All controls are computer driven, and the system houses a patient database that automatically records the parameters of the treatment and treatment history for each patient.

FACIAL TELANGIECTASIAS

The IPL system was developed with a fundamental application of treatment of benign vascular lesions, such as facial telangiectasias. In initial studies,[3] not only did IPL perform this successfully and without the unsightly purpura associated with the pulsed dye laser, it had the added benefit of reducing the redness associated with these conditions. It was soon recognized that this technology could be effective in relieving the redness and flushing of the face and chest associated with rosacea (Fig. 41–2).

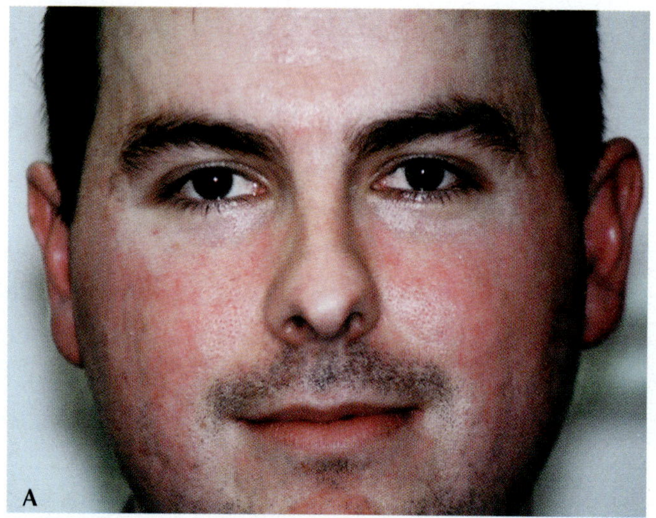
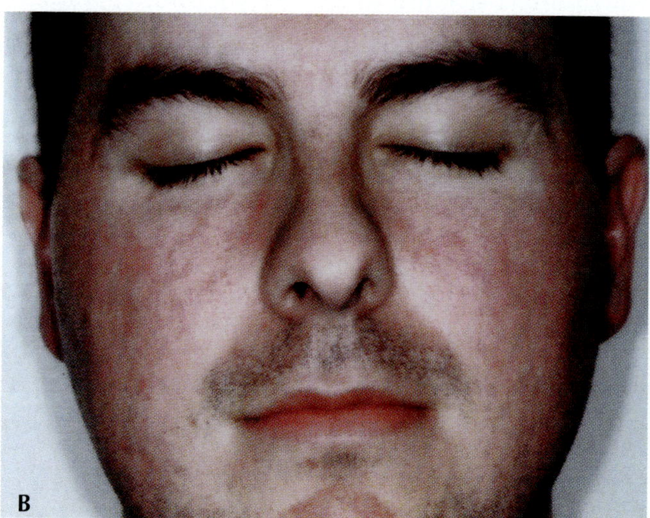
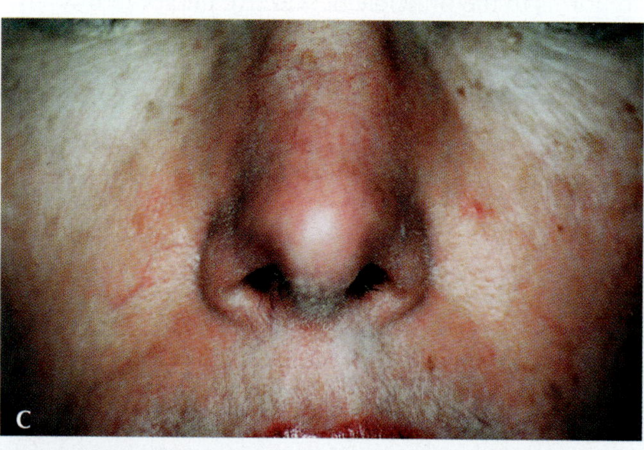
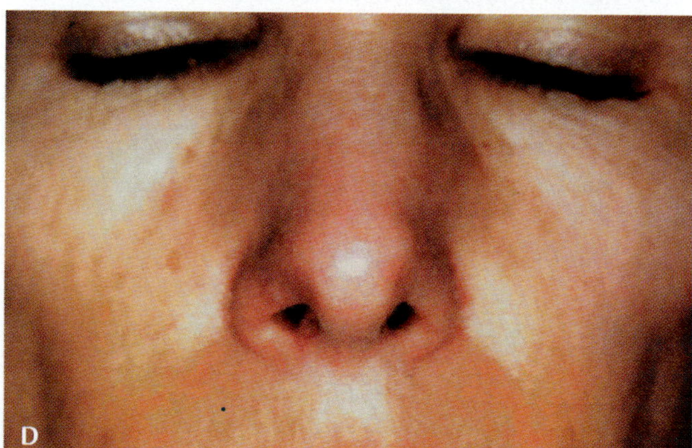
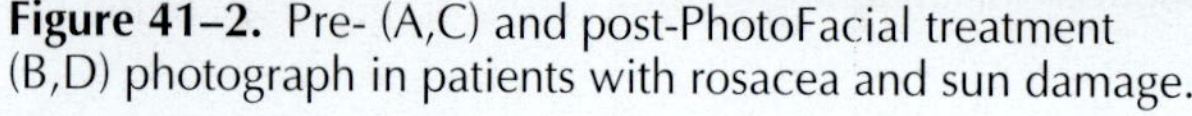

Figure 41–2. Pre- (A,C) and post-PhotoFacial treatment (B,D) photograph in patients with rosacea and sun damage.

ROSACEA

As reported by the Rosacea Society, rosacea sufferers number more than 13 million in the United States alone. This is a chronic skin disorder affecting the face, characterized by redness and telangiectasias, and is punctuated by episodes of inflammation with papules, pustules, and swelling.

The underlying causes of rosacea have not been elucidated yet. It is most likely multifactorial (e.g., abnormality of facial blood vessels, nerves, connective tissue, locally released vasoactive factors, and complex interactions between each system). There are four basic stages through which rosacea sufferers may progress: pre-rosacea, mild, moderate, and severe forms. Pre-rosacea refers to the stage where a person flushes or blushes to a stimulus, but returns immediately to normal when the stimulus is removed. The progression of pre-rosacea to bouts of flushing and blushing that do not dissipate for hours or days is now considered to be directly related to microvascular dysfunction or damage. In support of this, Neuman and Frithz[4] recently reported that biopsies of vascular lesions from rosacea patients demonstrated moderate to severe damage to endothelial and smooth muscle cells. In addition, these same biopsies showed evidence of abnormal fusion of capillaries and angiogenesis. Taken together, rosacea-related alterations in endothelial cells, vascular smooth muscle, formation of new inflammatory shunt vessels, and angiogenesis could explain why the rosacea-related red face, flushing, and blushing worsens over time. In effect, it is plausible that alterations in microvascular structure and function allow for more intense bouts of blood flow and inflammation, resulting in even more microvascular damage—a vicious and progressive cycle.

Therefore, therapy should be centered around the removal of damaged and dysfunctional microvessels such that new thicker walled microvessels with normal plump endothelial cells are laid down. Previous treatment of the acute inflammatory episodes have consisted of avoidance of heat, cold, sunlight, alcohol, and stress. Physicians have used tetracyclines, dapsone, erythromycin, chloramphenicol, metronidazole, clonidine, and Accutane with limited success. Topical treatments with antibiotics, sulfa preparations, and topical steroids have also been used. Indeed, steroid use ultimately compounds the problem by causing more reddening, flaring, and atrophy. None of these treatments remove the abnormal vessels. Electrocautery treats only those larger visible vessels, and not without pain, bleeding, and frustration of both practitioner and patient.

Yellow light lasers have been used for telangiectatic vessels on the face and legs. The copper bromide laser was found to be poorly suited for diffuse erythema and very large vessels such as the vessels of the nasal alae. This correlated with vessel size: Smaller telangiectasias responded well, but the small vessels (<100 microns) responsible for facial blushing, and the larger vessels (>300 microns) responsible for the vessels of the nasal alae, did not respond. Yellow light has limited penetration due to its interaction with pigment found in the superficial vascular plexus; thus it cannot destroy some of the deeper, larger vessels.

More advanced use of lasers, particularly the dye lasers first introduced in the mid-1980s, held more hope.[5,6] In addition to thermal damage produced by the absorption of the 577 to 585 nm wavelength, the photoacoustic "shock wave" damage resulting from rapid absorption of the energy by the oxyhemoglobin molecule also promotes purpura. This unsightly purpura was enough for some patients to seclude themselves for 2 weeks or refuse further treatment (Fig. 41–3).

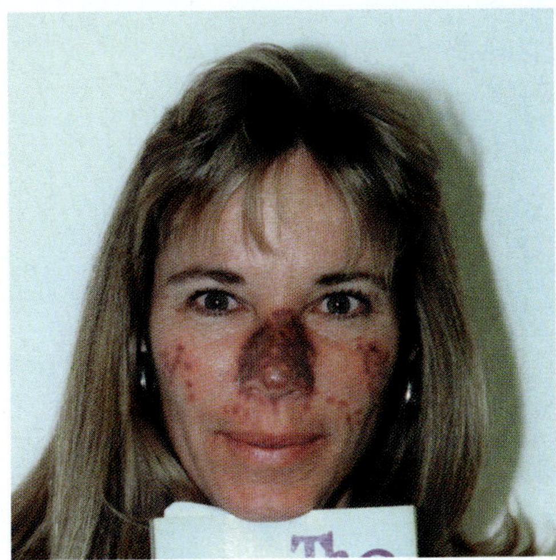

Figure 41–3. Patient with purpura, typical after flash pump dye laser treatment.

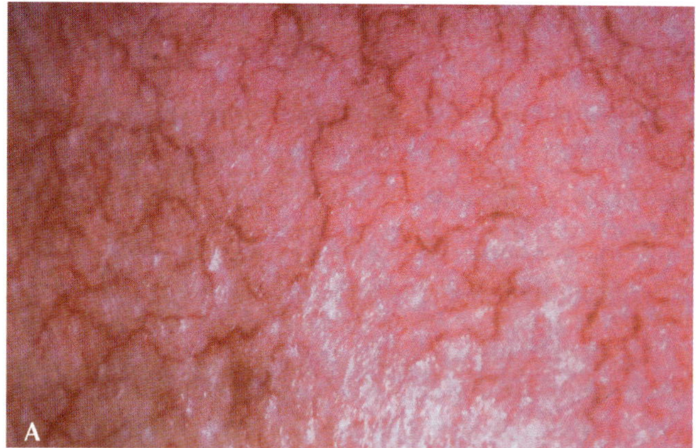

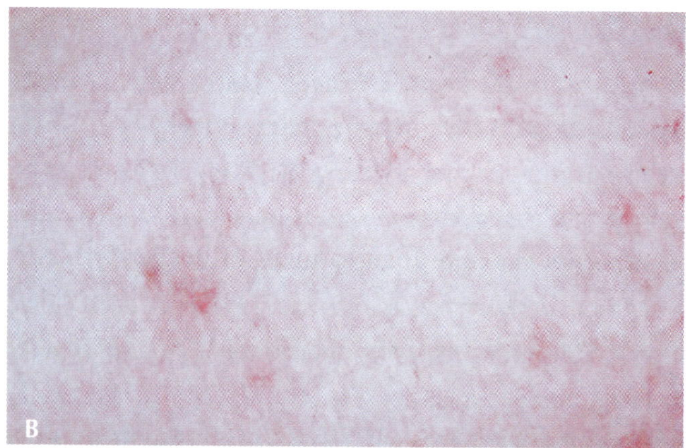

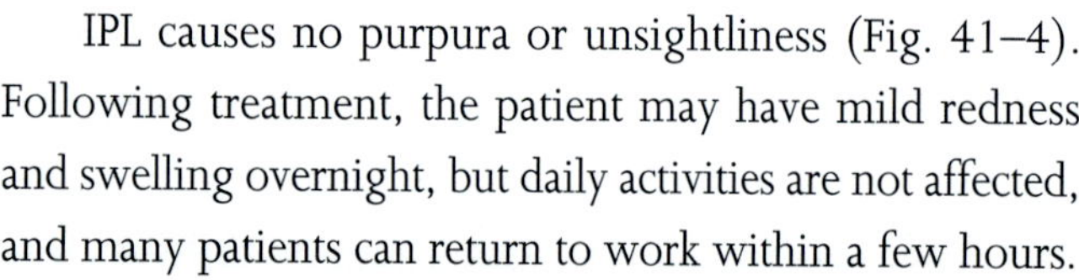

Figure 41–4. Closeup of moderate to severe rosacea after four to six treatments.

IPL causes no purpura or unsightliness (Fig. 41–4). Following treatment, the patient may have mild redness and swelling overnight, but daily activities are not affected, and many patients can return to work within a few hours.

ABNORMAL PIGMENTATION

Further development of IPL has demonstrated that treatment of the entire face, rather than spots of outbreak, provides dividends in the treatment of abnormal pigmentation due to sun damage, aging, and menopause.

This technique has also been used for dark circles under the eyes. The basis for improvement is the selective absorption of pulsed light energy by high concentrations of pigment within the abnormal cells. This leads to cell death, with sloughing of the pigmented population of cells over the course of 2 to 4 days. Because normal cells are left unaffected, this improvement occurs without blistering, destruction of epithelium, or excessive redness. The pigmented areas may demonstrate some slight, temporary erythema around the edges as well as darkening as they are pushed to the surface (Fig. 41–5).

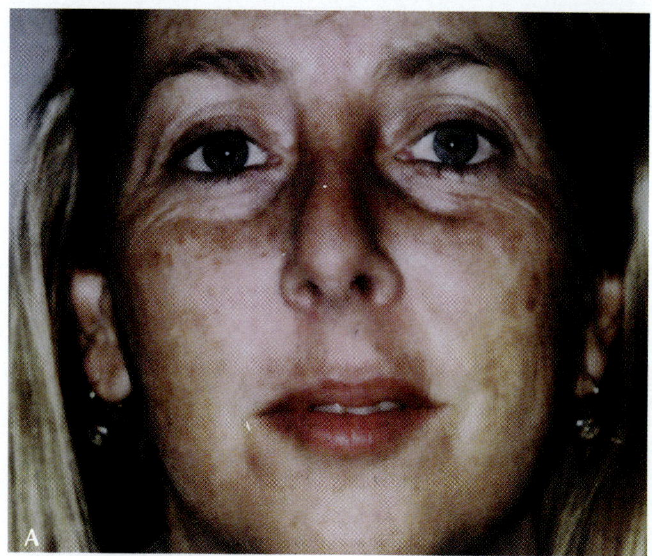

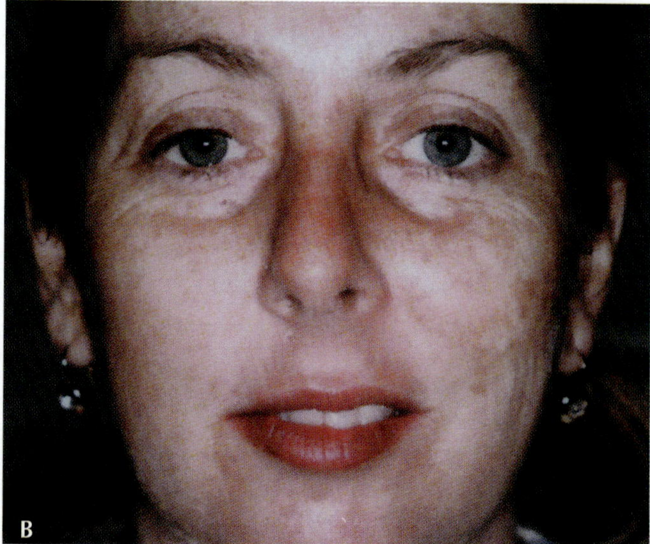

Figure 41–5. Pre- (A) and post-treatment (B) photographs of patient with sun damage.

SKIN TEXTURE ABNORMALITIES AND OTHER USES

IPL has demonstrated an improvement in fine lines and wrinkles, as well as reduction in pore size, possibly due to new collagen deposition in the dermis. This technique is not effective for treatment of deeper wrinkles and sagging skin treated with laser resurfacing and traditional surgical techniques. IPL has also been used effectively to treat psoriasis of the face, to reduce erythema following laser skin resurfacing, and to treat acne scarring.

THE PHOTOFACIAL TECHNIQUE

The PhotoFacial technique consists of a series of IPL treatments, usually five treatments scheduled over 4 months. A full patient history and three high-quality facial photographs are taken. The IPL is performed on the full face after administration of topical analgesia. The parameters are set as follows:

1. Fitzpatrick skin type is entered.
2. Selected cutoff filter/light guide is installed. This is typically 550, 570, or 590 nm.
3. Energy level is entered. This variable depends on the skin type, treatment progress, and other factors. It may be as low as 30 J/cm^2 to as high as 56 J/cm^2. This is a key area for advanced training and patient experience. Excessive energy can burn the epidermis.
4. Pulse duration is entered, typically 2.0 to 3.5 msec.
5. Pulse pattern and pulse delay are entered. Higher energy levels are typically delivered in double and triple pulses, allowing an interval for thermal relaxation of the vascular structures.
6. The treatment is accomplished using chilled gel to couple the rectangular light guide surface to the skin. A single pass is performed over the whole face with minimal overlap.

PHOTOFACIAL PATIENT SATISFACTION

Fifty-seven patients with rosacea were chosen randomly and evaluated to determine the overall success with the PhotoFacial protocol. Patient satisfaction was high, as evidenced by improved scores for erythema, flushing, eradication of telangiectatic vessels, uneven pigmentation, and skin texture. The reduction of fine lines and acne rosacea flares were not as dramatic (Fig. 41–6).

ADVERSE REACTIONS, CAUTIONS, AND EVALUATION OF RESULTS

The PhotoFacial technique has been remarkably free of adverse reactions. Practitioners are cautioned, however, that pitfalls in treatment do exist.

The most difficult patients to treat are those with Fitzpatrick skin type I who have a long history of sun exposure. In these patients, connective tissue is so fragile that IPL parameters selected for optimal relief of redness may damage the skin, with a higher incidence of purpura, swelling, and blistering. In such cases, suboptimal parameters must be used early in treatment until the connective tissue supporting the dermal vasculature is strengthened and the target tissue is reduced in size. The standard five-treatment program is usually extended in this patient group.

Judging the results of this technique in rosacea patients can be difficult. Patients have different triggers for precipitating rosacea outbreaks and facial flushing. Among these triggers are alcohol, spicy foods, stress, heat, cold, and exercise. A patient may enter the physician's office under the effect of one or more of these influences, clearly exhibiting symptoms. By the time treatment is complete, the patient has undergone a period of soothing relaxation in the physician's office that resolves the flushing episode. This effect can give the physician a false sense of accomplishment.

Improvement in skin condition continues for 30 to 45 days following the fifth or final treatment. Final evaluation should not be made until that time. Sun-damaged pigment such as solar lentigos respond to the IPL

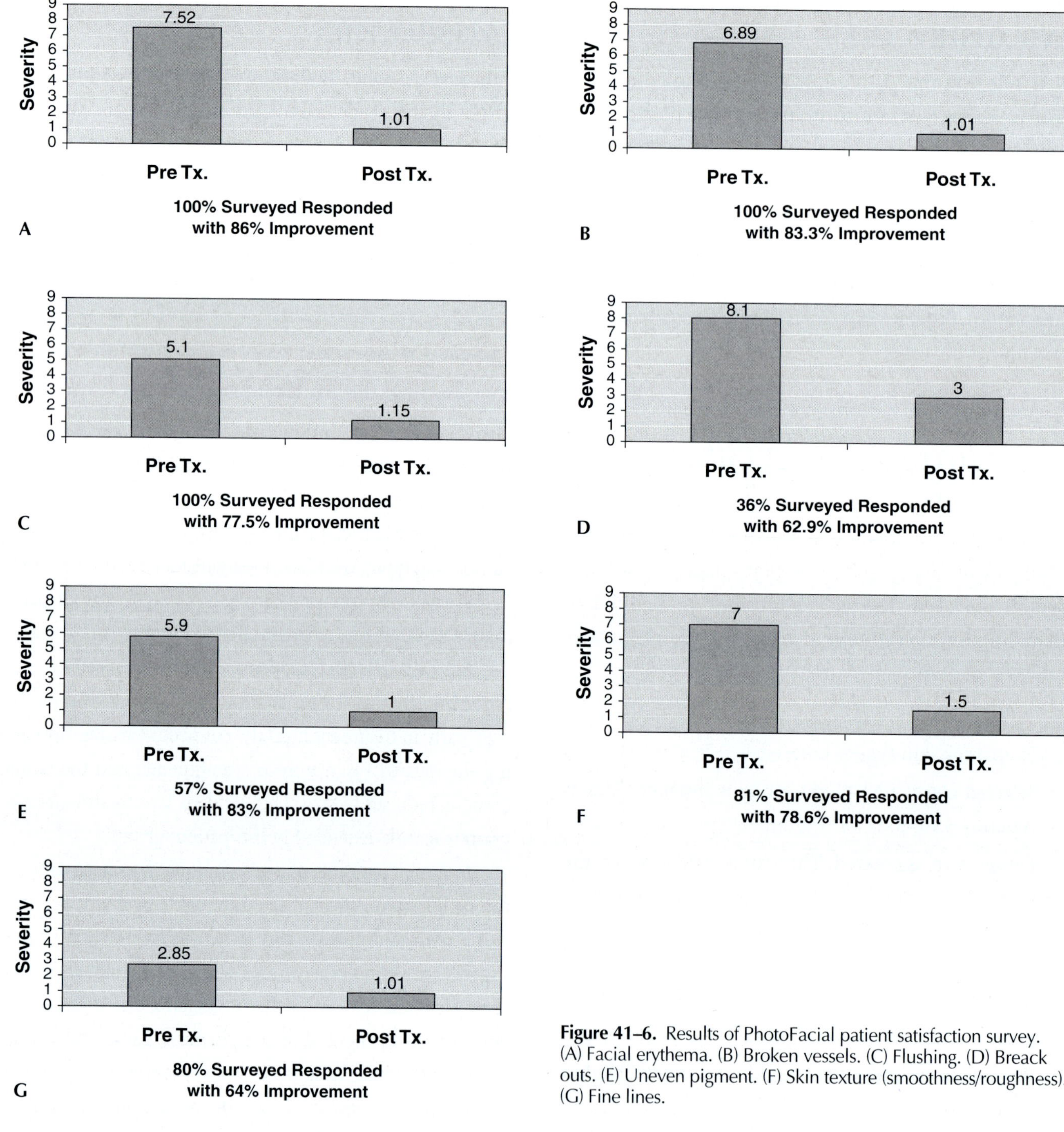

Figure 41–6. Results of PhotoFacial patient satisfaction survey. (A) Facial erythema. (B) Broken vessels. (C) Flushing. (D) Break outs. (E) Uneven pigment. (F) Skin texture (smoothness/roughness). (G) Fine lines.

treatment by becoming pyknotic, shriveling, and sloughing off in 2 to 4 days.

RELATED STUDIES

Recent research indicates that long pulsed intense light can improve superficial rhytides in a nonablative manner. Goldberg[7] studied patients with class I periorbital rhytides receiving one to three treatment sessions similar to the PhotoFacial technique. Of 20 subjects, 10 showed significant improvement, 7 showed mild improvement, and 3 showed no improvement.

Zelickson et al.[8] demonstrated that both the pulsed dye laser and IPL can induce clinical and histologic improvement in actinically damaged skin.

CONCLUSIONS

Working within the constraints of the lifestyles of active, working patients requiring brief, relatively pain-free facial treatments with no down time, the IPL nonablative skin rejuvenation technique PhotoFacial provides superior cosmetic results. Specifically, the treatment offers relief from the redness and flushing symptoms of rosacea, improved smoothness and texture of facial skin, reduction of the pigmentary signs of photoaging, restoration of even color, and reduction of fine lines and wrinkles.

REFERENCES

1. Anderson RR, Parrish JA. Selective photothermolysis: Precise microsurgery by selective absorption of pulsed radiation. *Science* 1983;220:524.

2. Goldman MP, Fitzpatrick RE. Treatment of cutaneous vascular lesions. In: Goldman MP, Fitzpatrick RE, eds. *Cutaneous Laser Surgery: The Art and Science of Selective Photothermolysis.* St. Louis: Mosby; 1994:19–105.

3. Goldman M. Treatment of benign vascular lesions with the PhotoDerm VL High Intensity Pulsed Light Source. *Adv Dermatol.* 1997;13:503–521.

4. Neuman, Frithz. Capillaropathy and capillaroneogenesis in the pathogenesis of rosacea. *Int J Dermatol.* 1998;34(4): 263–266.

5. Polla LL, Tan OT, Garden JM, Parrish JA. Tunable pulsed dye laser for the treatment of benign cutaneous vascular ectasia. *Dermatologica* 1987;174:11–17.

6. Jacques SL. The role of Skin Optics in Diagnostic and therapeutic uses of laser. In: Steiner R, Kaufman R, Lanthaler M, Braun-falco O, eds. *Lasers in Dermatology.* Berlin: Springer Verlag; 1992:8–19.

7. Goldberg. American Society of Lasers in Surgery and Medicine, 1999.

8. Zelickson et al. American Society of Lasers in Surgery and Medicine, 1999.

Index

Page numbers in *italics* indicate figures.
Page numbers followed by "t" indicate tables.